BONE MARROW
PATHOLOGY

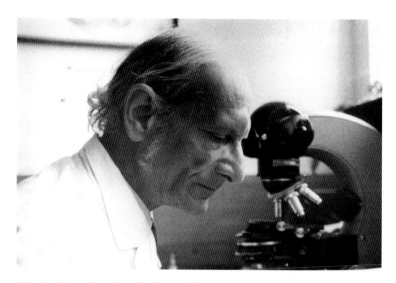

This book is dedicated to the late Professor David A. G. Galton

BONE MARROW PATHOLOGY

BARBARA J. BAIN

MBBS, FRACP, FRCPath
Professor of Diagnostic Haematology,
St Mary's Hospital Campus of Imperial College Faculty of Medicine,
Imperial College, London
and Honorary Consultant Haematologist,
St Mary's Hospital, London

DAVID M. CLARK

MD, MRCP (UK), FRCPath
Consultant Histopathologist,
Path Links, North Lincolnshire and Goole Hospitals NHS Foundation Trust,
Honorary Consultant Histopathologist,
Nottingham University Hospitals NHS Trust, Nottingham
and Special Lecturer in Pathology,
University of Nottingham

BRIDGET S. WILKINS

DM, PhD, FRCPath
Consultant in Haematopathology,
Guy's and St Thomas' Hospitals NHS Foundation Trust, London,
Honorary Senior Lecturer in Haematopathology,
King's College, London

FOURTH EDITION

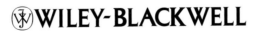

WILEY-BLACKWELL

A John Wiley & Sons, Ltd., Publication

This edition first published 2010, © 1992, 1996, 2001, 2010 by Barbara J. Bain, David M. Clark, Bridget S. Wilkins

Blackwell Publishing was acquired by John Wiley & Sons in February 2007. Blackwell's publishing program has been merged with Wiley's global Scientific, Technical and Medical business to form Wiley-Blackwell.

Registered office: John Wiley & Sons Ltd, The Atrium, Southern Gate, Chichester, West Sussex, PO19 8SQ, UK

Editorial offices: 9600 Garsington Road, Oxford, OX4 2DQ, UK
The Atrium, Southern Gate, Chichester, West Sussex, PO19 8SQ, UK
111 River Street, Hoboken, NJ 07030-5774, USA

For details of our global editorial offices, for customer services and for information about how to apply for permission to reuse the copyright material in this book please see our website at www.wiley.com/wiley-blackwell

The right of the author to be identified as the author of this work has been asserted in accordance with the Copyright, Designs and Patents Act 1988.

Library of Congress Cataloging-in-Publication Data

Bain, Barbara J.
    Bone marrow pathology / Barbara J. Bain, David M. Clark, Bridget S. Wilkins. – 4th ed.
        p. ; cm.
    Rev. ed. of: Bone marrow pathology / Barbara J. Bain . . . [et al.]. 3rd ed. 2001.
    Includes bibliographical references and index.
    ISBN 978-1-4051-6825-0
    1. Bone marrow – Histopathology. I. Clark, David M., MD. II. Wilkins, Bridget, 1959–
III. Bone marrow pathology. IV. Title.
    [DNLM: 1. Bone Marrow Diseases – pathology. 2. Bone Marrow – pathology. WH 380 B162b 2010]
    RC645.7.B35 2010
    616.4′107–dc22
                                                                2009034632

A catalogue record for this book is available from the British Library.

Set in 9 on 11.5 pt Meridien by SNP Best-set Typesetter Ltd., Hong Kong
Printed and bound in Singapore by Fabulous Printers Pte Ltd

1 2010

CONTENTS

PREFACE TO THE
FOURTH EDITION

In this book we have set out to provide a practical guide to bone marrow diagnosis, based on an integrated assessment of peripheral blood and bone marrow aspirate films, trephine biopsy sections and supplementary investigations. We believe that a trephine biopsy specimen should not be examined and interpreted in isolation. We have therefore discussed the clinical context of bone marrow diagnosis and have given equal weight to cytological and histological features. Since bone marrow diagnosis is no longer based on morphological features alone we have also discussed in detail the role of immunophenotypic, cytogenetic and molecular genetic analysis.

We have dealt very fully with haematological disorders for which bone marrow examination is commonly performed. However, we have also sought to be comprehensive, including information on uncommon and rare disorders so that the book will serve as a useful reference source. When possible, we have illustrated rare as well as common conditions and have cited the relevant scientific literature extensively. In this edition magnifications are given as the microscope objective used for photography rather than as the magnification on the printed page.

To facilitate use of the book in diagnostic laboratories we have extended the 'Problems and pitfalls' sections and have added new diagnostic algorithms and summary boxes, which we believe will be of value. We hope that haematologists and histopathologists will continue to find *Bone Marrow Pathology* a useful aid in their day-to-day practice and that trainees in these disciplines will find it indispensable.

BJB, DMC, BSW

ACKNOWLEDGEMENTS

We should like to thank our many friends and colleagues in North America, Europe, Africa, Asia and Australia who have provided illustrations or have permitted us to photograph microscopic slides from their personal collections. They are individually acknowledged in the legends of specific figures. In addition we should like to thank our technical and medical colleagues in St Mary's Hospital, Hammersmith Hospital, Nottingham University Hospital, Path Links and St Thomas' Hospital for the direct and indirect help they have given us in the preparation of this edition. We are also grateful for the comments and feedback given to us by readers of the previous editions and individuals attending the postgraduate courses on which we teach.

Our special thanks go to Dr Irvin Lampert, for his invaluable contributions as co-author of the first three editions of this book, and for the friendship and wisdom he has generously shared with us for more than 20 years.

This book is dedicated to the late Professor David Galton (1922–2006) who taught us and countless other haematologists and histopathologists a great deal over many years. Those who had the opportunity to work with him admired him for his exceptional diagnostic skills, his humility and his mindfulness of patients as individuals. He is much missed.

BJB, DMC, BSW

ABBREVIATIONS

aCML	atypical chronic myeloid leukaemia	CML	chronic myeloid leukaemia
AIDS	acquired immune deficiency syndrome	CMML	chronic myelomonocytic leukaemia
AILD	angioimmunoblastic lymphadenopathy with dysproteinaemia	CMV	cytomegalovirus
		CNS	central nervous system
		CT	computerized tomography
		del	deletion
ALCL	anaplastic large cell lymphoma	DIC	disseminated intravascular coagulation
ALIP	abnormal localization of immature precursors	DLBCL	diffuse large B-cell lymphoma
ALL	acute lymphoblastic leukaemia	DNA	deoxyribonucleic acid
ALPS	autoimmune lymphoproliferative syndrome	EBER	Epstein–Barr early RNA
		EBNA	Epstein–Barr nuclear antigen
AML	acute myeloid leukaemia	EBV	Epstein–Barr virus
ANAE	alpha-naphthyl acetate esterase	EDTA	ethylene diamine tetra-acetic acid
APAAP	alkaline phosphatase–anti-alkaline phosphatase	EGIL	European Group for the Immunological Classification of Leukaemia
ATLL	adult T-cell leukaemia/lymphoma		
ATRA	all-*trans*-retinoic acid	EMA	epithelial membrane antigen
BFU	burst-forming unit	ER	oestrogen receptor
BL	Burkitt lymphoma	ET	essential thrombocythaemia
BM	bone marrow	FAB	French–American–British (co-operative group)
BSAP	B-cell-specific activator protein		
c	cytoplasmic	FBC	full blood count
CAE	chloroacetate esterase	FISH	fluorescence *in situ* hybridization
CD	cluster of differentiation		
CDA	congenital dyserythropoietic anaemia	G-CSF	granulocyte colony-stimulating factor
CEA	carcino-embryonic antigen	GM-CSF	granulocyte–macrophage colony-stimulating factor
CEL	chronic eosinophilic leukaemia		
CFU	colony-forming unit	GMS	Grocott's methenamine silver (stain)
CGH	comparative genomic hybridization		
		GPI	glycosyl phosphatidylinositol
CGL	chronic granulocytic leukaemia	GVHD	graft-versus-host disease
CHAD	cold haemagglutinin disease	Hb	haemoglobin concentration
CK	cytokeratin	H&E	haematoxylin and eosin (stain)
CLL	chronic lymphocytic leukaemia		

HEMPAS	hereditary erythroid multinuclearity with positive acidified serum lysis test	NK	natural killer
		NLPHL	nodular lymphocyte-predominant Hodgkin lymphoma
HER2	human epidermal growth factor receptor 2		
		NOS	not otherwise specified
HHV	human herpesvirus	NSE	non-specific esterase
HIV	human immunodeficiency virus	PAS	periodic acid–Schiff (stain)
		PB	peripheral blood
HL	Hodgkin lymphoma	PBS	phosphate-buffered saline
HLA	human leucocyte antigen	PcAb	polyclonal antibody
HTLV-I	human T-cell lymphotropic virus I	PCR	polymerase chain reaction
		PEL	primary effusion lymphoma
i	isochromosome	PET	positron emission tomography
idic	isodicentric chromosome	Ph	Philadelphia (chromosome)
Ig	immunoglobulin	PLL	prolymphocytic leukaemia
IGH	immunoglobulin heavy chain (gene locus)	PMF	primary myelofibrosis
		PNET	primitive neuroectodermal tumour/s
IHC	immunohistochemistry		
IL	interleukin	PNH	paroxysmal nocturnal haemoglobinuria
inv	inversion		
IPSID	immunoproliferative small intestinal disease	POEMS	polyneuropathy, organomegaly, endocrinopathy, M protein, skin changes (syndrome)
IPSS	International Prognostic Scoring System		
		PSA	prostate-specific antigen
ISH	*in situ* hybridization	PSAP	prostate-specific acid phosphatase
ITD	internal tandem duplication		
JMML	juvenile myelomonocytic leukaemia	PV	polycythaemia vera
		RA	refractory anaemia
KIR	killer inhibitory receptor	RAEB	refractory anaemia with excess of blasts
LDH	lactate dehydrogenase		
LGL	large granular lymphocyte/s	RAEB-T	refractory anaemia with excess of blasts in transformation
LMP	latent membrane protein		
MALT	mucosa-associated lymphoid tissue	RARS	refractory anaemia with ring sideroblasts
McAb	monoclonal antibody	RARS-T	refractory anaemia with ring sideroblasts and thrombocytosis
MDS	myelodysplastic syndrome/s		
M : E	myeloid : erythroid	RCC	refractory cytopenia of childhood
MGG	May–Grünwald–Giemsa (stain)		
MGUS	monoclonal gammopathy of undetermined significance	RCMD	refractory cytopenia with multilineage dysplasia
MPAL	mixed phenotype acute leukaemia	RCUD	refractory cytopenia with unilineage dysplasia
MPN	myeloproliferative neoplasm/s	REAL	Revised European American Lymphoma (classification)
MPO	myeloperoxidase		
MRD	minimal residual disease	RN	refractory neutropenia
mRNA	messenger ribonucleic acid	RNA	ribonucleic acid
MSB	Martius scarlet blue (stain)	RQ-PCR	real time quantitative polymerase chain reaction
NEC	non-erythroid cell/s		
NHL	non-Hodgkin lymphoma	RT	refractory thrombocytopenia

RT-PCR	reverse transcriptase polymerase chain reaction	SNP	single nucleotide polymorphism
SB	Southern blot	t	translocation
SBB	Sudan black B	TAR	thrombocytopenia-absent radii (syndrome)
SD	standard deviation		
SLL	small lymphocytic lymphoma	TBS	Tris-buffered saline
		TCR	T-cell receptor
SLVL	splenic lymphoma with villous lymphocytes	*TCR*	T-cell receptor (gene locus)
		TdT	terminal deoxynucleotidyl transferase
SM-AHNMCD	systemic mastocytosis with associated clonal, haematological non-mast cell lineage disease (WHO classification)	TNF	tumour necrosis factor
		TPO	thrombopoietin
		TRAP	tartrate-resistant acid phosphatase
SmIg	surface membrane immunoglobulin	TTF1	thyroid transcriptase factor 1
		WBC	white blood cell count
SMZL	splenic marginal zone lymphoma	WHO	World Health Organization
		ZN	Ziehl–Neelsen (stain)

ONE

THE NORMAL BONE MARROW

The distribution of haemopoietic marrow

During extra-uterine life haemopoiesis is normally confined to the bone marrow, which occupies interstices within bone. An understanding of normal bone structure is necessary for interpreting bone marrow specimens. Bones are composed of cortex and medulla. The cortex is a strong layer of compact bone; the medulla is a honeycomb of cancellous bone, the interstices of which form the medullary cavity and contain the bone marrow. Bone marrow is either red marrow, containing haemopoietic cells, or yellow marrow, which is largely adipose tissue. The distribution of haemopoietic marrow is dependent on age. In the neonate virtually the entire bone marrow cavity is fully occupied by proliferating haemopoietic cells; haemopoiesis occurs even in the phalanges. As the child ages, haemopoietic marrow contracts centripetally, being replaced by fatty marrow. By early adult life haemopoietic marrow is largely confined to the skull, vertebrae, ribs, clavicles, sternum, pelvis and the proximal half of the humeri and femora; however, there is considerable variation between individuals as to the distribution of haemopoietic marrow [1]. In response to demand, the volume of the marrow cavity occupied by haemopoietic tissue expands.

The organization of the bone marrow

Bone

The cortex and the medulla differ functionally as well as histologically. Bone may be classified in two ways. Classification may be made on the basis of the macroscopic appearance into: (i) compact or dense bone with only small interstices that are not visible macroscopically; and (ii) cancellous (or trabecular) bone with large, readily visible interstices. Bone may also be classified histologically on the basis of whether there are well-organized osteons in which a central Haversian canal is surrounded by concentric lamellae composed of parallel bundles of fibrils (lamellar bone) (Fig. 1.1) or, alternatively, whether the fibrils of the bone are in disorderly bundles (woven or spongy bone) (Fig. 1.2).

The cortex is a solid layer of compact bone that gives the bone its strength. It is composed largely of lamellar bone but also contains some woven bone. The lamellar bone of the cortex consists of either well-organized Haversian systems or angular fragments of lamellar bone, which occupy the spaces between the Haversian systems; in long bones there are also inner and outer circumferential lamellae. Extending inwards from the cortex is an anastomosing network of trabeculae, which partition the medullary space (Fig. 1.3). The medullary bone is trabecular or cancellous bone; it contains lamellae but the structure is less highly organized than that of the cortex. Most of the cortical bone is covered on the external surface by periosteum, which has an outer fibrous layer and an inner osteogenic layer. At articular surfaces, and more extensively in younger patients, bone fuses with cartilage rather than being covered by periosteum. The bony trabeculae and the inner surface of the cortex are lined by endosteal cells; most of these are flattened endosteal cells that can be histologically inapparent but there are some actively osteogenic cells (osteoblasts) and occasional osteoclasts, both more numerous in children. Osteocytes are found within lacunae in bony trabeculae and in

Bone Marrow Pathology. By Barbara Bain, David Clark and Bridget Wilkins. © 2010, Blackwell Publishing.

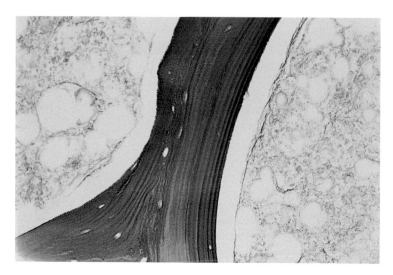

Fig. 1.1 Bone marrow (BM) trephine biopsy section showing normal bone structure; the trabeculae are composed of lamellar bone. Paraffin-embedded, reticulin stain ×20.

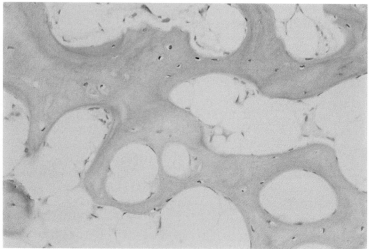

Fig. 1.2 BM trephine biopsy section showing woven bone (pale pink; without lamellae) in a hypocellular but otherwise unremarkable bone marrow. Paraffin-embedded, haematoxylin and eosin (H&E) ×20.

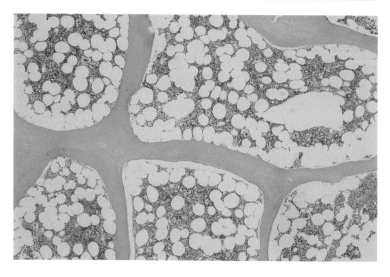

Fig. 1.3 BM trephine biopsy section showing normal bone structure; there are anastomosing bony trabeculae. Paraffin-embedded, H&E ×5.

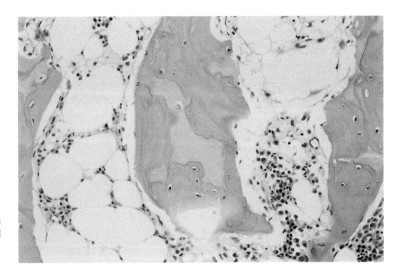

Fig. 1.4 BM trephine biopsy section from a child showing endochondrial ossification in an island of cartilage. Paraffin-embedded, H&E ×20.

cortical bone. Although osteoblasts and osteoclasts share the surface of the bone trabeculae, they originate from different stem cells. Osteoblasts, and therefore osteocytes, are of mesenchymal origin, being derived from the same stem cell as chondrocytes and probably also stromal fibroblasts. Osteoclasts, however, are derived from a haemopoietic stem cell, being formed by fusion of cells of the monocyte lineage.

The cells that give rise to bone-forming cells are designated osteoprogenitor cells; they are flattened, spindle-shaped cells that are capable of developing into either osteoblasts or chondrocytes, depending on micro-environmental factors. Osteoblasts synthesize glycosaminoglycans of the bone matrix and also the collagenous fibres that are embedded in the matrix, thus forming osteoid or non-calcified bone; subsequently mineralization occurs. Bone undergoes constant remodelling. In adult life, remodelling of the bone takes place particularly in the subcortical regions. Osteoblasts add a new layer of bone to trabeculae (apposition) while osteoclasts resorb other areas of the bone; up to 25% of the trabecular surface may be covered by osteoid. The osteoclasts, which are resorbing bone, lie in shallow hollows, known as Howship's lacunae, created by the process of resorption, while osteoblasts are seen in rows on the surface of trabecular bone or on the surface of a layer of osteoid. As new bone is laid down, osteoblasts become enclosed in bone and are converted into osteocytes. The bone that replaces

osteoid is woven bone; this, in turn, is remodelled to form lamellar bone. The difference between the two can be easily appreciated by microscopy using polarized light. The organized structure of lamellar bone, with bundles of parallel fibrils running in different directions in successive lamellae, gives rise to alternating light and dark layers when viewed under polarized light. This structure is also easily seen in Giemsa- and reticulin-stained sections.

Trephine biopsy specimens from children may contain cartilage as well as bone, and endochondrial bone formation may be observed (Figs 1.4 and 1.5). Transition from resting cartilage to proliferating and hypertrophic cartilage can be observed, followed by a zone of calcifying cartilage, invading vessels and bone. Mature cartilage can also be seen in trephine biopsy specimens from adults (Fig. 1.6).

Other connective tissue elements

Haemopoietic cells of the bone marrow are embedded in a connective tissue stroma, which occupies the intertrabecular spaces of the medulla. The stroma is composed of fat cells and a meshwork of blood vessels, branching fibroblasts, macrophages, a few myelinated and non-myelinated nerve fibres and a small amount of reticulin. Stromal cells include cells that have been designated reticulum or reticular cells. This term probably includes two cell types of different origin. Phagocytic reticulum cells are macrophages and originate from a haemopoietic progenitor. Non-phagocytic reticulum or

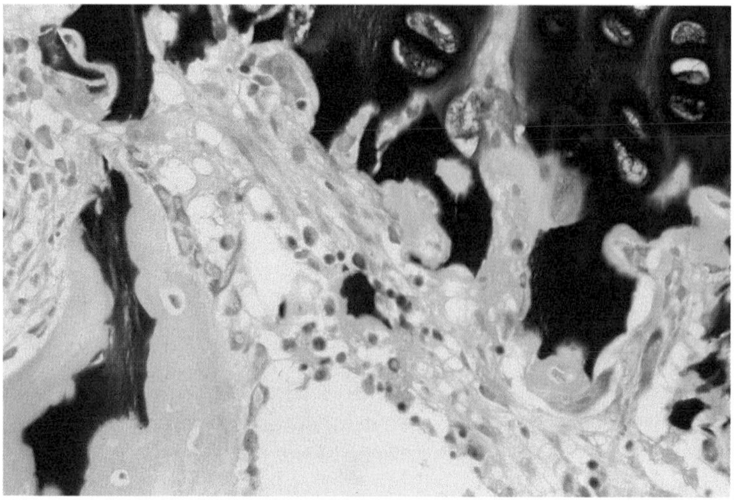

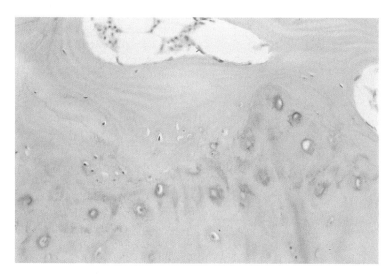

Fig. 1.5 BM trephine biopsy section from a child showing endochondrial ossification; a bony spicule with a core of cartilage is lined by osteoblasts. Paraffin-embedded, Giemsa stain ×40.

Fig. 1.6 BM trephine biopsy section from an adult showing cartilage adjacent to the cortex. By contrast with childhood appearances, a well-defined layer of cortical bone separates this cartilage from the bone marrow. Cartilage cells are dispersed singly or in small groups and are not aligned into columns, as they are in childhood. Paraffin-embedded, H&E ×20.

reticular cells are closely related to fibroblasts, adventitial cells of sinusoids (see below) and probably also osteoblasts and chondrocytes. They differ from phagocytic reticulum cells in that the majority are positive for alkaline phosphatase. There is a close interaction between haemopoietic cells and their micro-environment, with each modifying the other.

The blood supply of the marrow is derived in part from a central nutrient artery, which enters long bones at mid-shaft and bifurcates into two longitudinal central arteries [2]. Similar arteries penetrate flat and cuboidal bones. There is a supplementary blood supply from cortical capillaries, which pen-etrate the bone from the periosteum. Branches of the central artery give rise to arterioles and capillaries, which radiate towards the endosteum and mainly enter the bone, subsequently turning back to re-enter the marrow and open into a network of thin-walled sinusoids [2]. Only a minority of capillaries enter the sinusoids directly without first supplying bone. The sinusoids drain into a central venous sinusoid, which accompanies the nutrient artery. Sinusoids are large, thin-walled vessels through which newly formed haemopoietic cells enter the circulation. They are often collapsed in paraffin-embedded histological sections and are therefore not readily seen. In the presence of

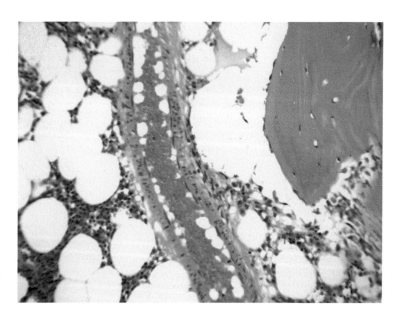

Fig. 1.7 BM trephine biopsy section showing a longitudinal section of an arteriole. Paraffin-embedded, H&E ×20.

marrow sclerosis, these vessels are often held open and are then very obvious. The walls of sinusoids consist of endothelial cells, forming a complete cover with overlapping junctions, and an incomplete basement membrane. The outer surface is clothed by adventitial cells – large, broad cells that branch into the perivascular space and therefore provide scaffolding for the haemopoietic cells, macrophages and mast cells. Adventitial cells are thought to be derived from fibroblasts; they are associated with a network of delicate extracellular fibres, which can be demonstrated with a reticulin stain. Reticulin fibres are concentrated close to the periosteum as well as around blood vessels. It is likely that both adventitial cells and fibroblasts can synthesize reticulin [3], which is a form of collagen. Arterioles are easily recognized both in longitudinal section (Fig. 1.7) and in cross-section. Capillaries may also be visible. Collapsed sinusoids and capillaries are better visualized with the use of an immunohistochemical stain for an endothelial cell-associated antigen.

The marrow fat content varies inversely with the quantity of haemopoietic tissue. Fat content also increases as bone is lost with increasing age. Marrow fat is physiologically different from subcutaneous fat. The fat of yellow marrow is the last fat in the body to be lost in starvation. When haemopoietic tissue is lost very rapidly it is replaced by interstitial mucin (gelatinous transformation). Subsequently this mucin is replaced by fat cells.

Haemopoietic and other cells

Haemopoietic cells lie in cords or wedges between the sinusoids. In man, normal haemopoiesis, with the exception of some thrombopoiesis at extramedullary sites, is confined to the interstitium. In pathological conditions haemopoiesis can occur within sinusoids. Mature haemopoietic cells enter the circulation by passing transcellularly, through sinusoidal endothelial cells [2]. The detailed disposition of haemopoietic cells will be discussed below.

Bone marrow also contains lymphoid cells, small numbers of plasma cells and mast cells (see below).

Examination of the bone marrow

Bone marrow was first obtained from living patients for diagnostic purposes during the first decade of the twentieth century, but it was not until the introduction of sternal aspiration in the late 1920s that this became an important diagnostic procedure. Specimens of bone marrow for cytological and histological examination may be obtained by aspiration biopsy, by core biopsy using a trephine needle or an electric drill, by open biopsy and at autopsy. The two most important techniques, which are complementary, are aspiration biopsy and trephine biopsy.

Bone marrow aspiration causes only mild discomfort to the patient. A trephine biopsy causes moderate discomfort and, in an apprehensive patient, sedation can be useful. Intravenous midazolam, 2–10 mg, is a commonly employed agent. Guidelines for safe sedation practice must be followed [4]. In children, aspiration and trephine biopsies are often performed under general anaesthesia.

All bone marrow aspirates and needle biopsies require informed consent. Local policies should be followed as to whether written consent is required, but this is becoming customary.

Bone marrow aspiration

Aspiration biopsy is most commonly carried out on the sternum or the ilium. Aspiration from the medial surface of the tibia can yield useful diagnostic specimens up to the age of 18 months, but is mainly used in neonates in whom other sites are less suitable. Aspiration from ribs and from the spinous processes of vertebrae is also possible but is now little practised. Sternal aspiration should be carried out from the first part of the body of the sternum, at the level of the second intercostal space. Aspiration from any lower in the sternum increases the risks of the procedure. Aspiration from the ilium can be from either the anterior or the posterior iliac crest. Aspiration from the anterior iliac crest is best carried out by a lateral approach, a few centimetres below and posterior to the anterior superior iliac spine. Approach through the crest of the ilium with the needle in the direction of the main axis of the bone is also possible but is more difficult because of the hardness of the bone. Aspirates from the posterior iliac crest are usually taken from the posterior superior iliac spine. When aspiration is carried out at the same time as a trephine biopsy it is easiest to perform the two procedures from adjacent sites. This necessitates the use of the ilium. If a trephine biopsy is not being carried out there is a choice between the sternum and the iliac crest. Either is suitable in adults and older children, although great care must be exercised in carrying out sternal aspirations. In a study of 100 patients in whom both techniques were applied, sternal aspiration was found to be technically easier and to produce a suitable diagnostic specimen more frequently, although on average the procedure was more painful, both with regard to bone penetration and to the actual aspiration [5]. Sternal aspiration is also more dangerous (see below), and is unsuitable for use in young children. Posterior iliac crest aspiration is suitable for children, infants and many neonates. Tibial aspiration is suitable for very small babies but has no advantages over iliac crest aspiration in older infants.

Bone marrow specimens yielded by aspiration are suitable for the following: preparation of wedge-spread films and films of crushed marrow fragments; study of cell markers (by flow cytometry or on films or cytospin preparations); cytogenetic study; ultrastructural examination; culture for microorganisms; culture to study haemopoietic precursors; and the preparation of histological sections of fragments. Cytogenetic analysis is most often indicated in suspected haematological neoplasms but it also permits rapid diagnosis of suspected congenital karyotypic abnormalities such as trisomy 18; diagnosis is possible within a day, in comparison with the 3 days needed if peripheral blood lymphocytes are used.

Bone marrow aspiration may fail completely, this being referred to as a 'dry tap'. Although this can happen when bone marrow histology is normal, a dry tap usually indicates significant disease, most often metastatic cancer, chronic myeloid leukaemia, primary myelofibrosis or hairy cell leukaemia [6], with associated fibrosis. On other occasions only blood is obtained (a 'blood tap'); this is often also the result of bone marrow disease causing fibrosis.

Trephine biopsy of bone marrow

Trephine or needle biopsy is most easily carried out on the iliac crest, either posteriorly or anteriorly, as described above. The posterior approach appears now to be more generally preferred. If a trephine biopsy and a bone marrow aspiration are both to be carried out, they can be performed through the same skin incision but with two areas of periosteum being infiltrated with local anaesthetic and with the needle being angled in different directions. A single-needle technique in which aspiration is followed by core biopsy should not be used as the quality of the core biopsy may be inadequate [7]. Core biopsy specimens, obtained with a trephine needle, are suitable for histological sections, touch preparations (imprints) and electron microscopy. A touch preparation is particularly important when it is not possible to obtain an aspirate since it allows cytological details to be studied [8]. In addition, touch preparations may show more neoplastic cells than are detected in an aspirate; they may also demonstrate bone marrow infiltration when it is not detected in an aspirate, for example in hairy cell leukaemia, multiple myeloma or lymphoma [9]. Touch preparations may be made either by touching the core of bone on a slide or rolling the core gently between two slides. Biopsy specimens can be used for cytogenetic study but aspirates are much more suitable. Frozen sections of trephine biopsy specimens are possible but they are not usually very satisfactory because of technical problems, including difficulty in cutting sections, poor adhesion of sections to glass slides during staining procedures and poor preservation of morphological detail. They are rarely used now that immunohistochemistry can be readily applied to fixed tissues. Histological sections may be prepared from fixed biopsy specimens which have either been decalcified and paraffin-embedded or have been embedded in resin without prior decalcification.

Processing of trephine biopsy specimens

The two principal methods of preparation of fixed trephine biopsy specimens have advantages and disadvantages. Problems are created because of the difficulty of cutting tissue composed of hard bone and soft, easily torn bone marrow. Alternative approaches are to decalcify the specimen or to embed it in a substance that makes the bone marrow almost as hard as the bone. Decalcification can be achieved with weak organic acids, e.g. formic acid and acetic acid, or by chelation, e.g. with ethylene diamine tetra-acetic acid (EDTA). Decalcification and paraffin-embedding lead to considerable shrinkage and some loss of cellular detail. Because sections are thicker than those from resin-embedded specimens, cellular detail is harder to appreciate. Some cytochemical activity is lost; for example, chloroacetate esterase activity is lost when acid decalcification is used. Immunological techniques are more readily applicable to paraffin-embedded than to resin-embedded specimens. Resin-embedding techniques are more expensive and, for laboratories that are processing only small numbers of trephine biopsy specimens, are technically more difficult. There is no shrinkage, preservation of cellular detail is excellent and the thinness of the sections means that fine cytological detail can be readily appreciated. Some enzyme activities, for example chloroacetate esterase, are retained. Immunological techniques can be applied, but excessive background staining is often a problem. Although excellent results are achieved with resin-embedded specimens it is now also possible to get very good results for both histology and immuno-histochemistry with paraffin-embedding and this is the technique used in the authors' laboratories. Resins with differing qualities are available for embedding. Methyl methacrylate requires lengthy processing and is therefore not very suitable for routine diagnostic laboratories. Glycol methacrylate is more satisfactory; however, when cellularity is low, sections tend to tear and, in this circumstance, a small amount of decalcification may be useful. Methods which we have found satisfactory are given in the Appendix.

Relative advantages of aspiration and core biopsy

Bone marrow aspiration and trephine biopsy each have advantages and limitations. The two procedures should therefore be regarded as complementary. Bone marrow aspirates are unequalled for demonstration of fine cytological detail. They permit a wider range of cytochemical stains and immunological markers than is possible with histological sections and are also ideal for cytogenetic and molecular genetic studies. Aspiration is particularly useful, and may well be performed alone, when investigating patients with suspected iron deficiency anaemia, anaemia of chronic disease, megaloblastic anaemia and acute leukaemia. Trephine biopsy is essential for diagnosis when a 'dry tap' or 'blood tap' occurs as a consequence of the marrow being fibrotic or very densely cellular. Only a biopsy allows a complete assessment of marrow architecture and of the pattern of distribution of any abnormal infiltrate. This technique is particularly useful in investigating suspected aplastic or hypoplastic anaemia, lymphoma, metastatic carcinoma, myeloproliferative neoplasms and diseases of the bones. We have also found trephine biopsy generally much more useful than bone marrow aspiration when investigating patients with the advanced stages of human immunodeficiency virus (HIV) infection in whom hypocellular, non-diagnostic aspirates are common. It should not be forgotten, however, that trephine biopsy undoubtedly causes more pain to the patient than does aspiration.

Complications of bone marrow aspiration and trephine biopsy

Complications of bone marrow aspiration and trephine biopsy are rare.

Sternal aspiration is more hazardous than iliac crest aspiration and trephine biopsy. Although deaths are very rare, at least 21 have been reported and we are aware of four further fatalities, not reported in the scientific literature; deaths have been consequent mainly on laceration of vessels or laceration of the heart with pericardial tamponade. The risk may be greater when bones are abnormally soft, as in multiple myeloma [10]. Sternal aspiration may also be complicated by pneumothorax or pneumopericardium and sternomanubrial separation has been observed in one patient.

Although haemorrhage is rare following iliac crest aspiration and uncommon following trephine biopsy it is, nevertheless, the most frequently observed serious complication, sometimes requiring blood transfusion and occasionally leading to, or contributing to, death [11]. Haemorrhage may be either intra-abdominal [12], retroperitoneal [11] or into the buttock and thigh [11], in the latter two circumstances with the risk of nerve compression [11,13,14]. Risk factors are heparin or warfarin therapy, coagulation factor deficiencies, von Willebrand's disease, disseminated intravascular coagulation, thrombocytopenia, functional platelet defects (either disease related – myeloid neoplasms or resulting from the presence of a paraprotein – or the result of aspirin or other antiplatelet agents) and a diagnosis of a myeloproliferative neoplasm. Haemorrhage is also occasionally a problem when a biopsy is carried out on bone with an abnormal vasculature, for example in Paget's disease. Severe retroperitoneal haemorrhage has also been observed in patients with osteoporosis. Correction of any coagulation defect is advisable, when possible. Prolonged firm pressure is advised in patients with thrombocytopenia or functional platelet defects and, when clinically appropriate, pre-procedure platelet transfusion should be considered.

Damage to the lateral cutaneous nerve of the thigh occurs rarely and is suggestive of poor technique. In patients with osteosclerosis, needles may break. Infection is a rare complication. Other rare complications include avulsion fracture at the biopsy site [15], pneumoretroperitoneum [16], implantation of malignant cells in the track of the biopsy needle in plasmacytoma and non-Hodgkin lymphoma [17,18], prolonged leak of serous fluid in a patient with nephrotic syndrome [19] and later development of exostosis [20].

Other techniques

It is occasionally necessary to obtain a bone marrow specimen by open biopsy under a general anaesthetic. This is usually only required when a specific lesion has been demonstrated at a relatively inaccessible site, by radiology, magnetic resonance imaging or bone scanning.

At autopsy, specimens of bone marrow for histological examination are most readily obtained from the sternum and the vertebral bodies, although any bone containing red marrow can be used. Unless the autopsy is performed soon after death, the cytological detail is often poor.

Cellularity

Bone marrow cellularity can be assessed most accurately in histological sections (Fig. 1.8) although assessment can also be made from aspirated bone marrow fragments in wedge-spread films (Fig. 1.9). Specimens that are suitable for histological assessment of cellularity are: aspirated fragments; needle or open biopsy specimens; and autopsy specimens. The cellularity of the bone marrow in health depends on the age of the subject and the site from which the marrow specimen was obtained. It is also influenced by technical factors, since decalcification and paraffin-embedding lead to some shrinkage of tissue in comparison with resin-embedded specimens; estimates of cellularity based on the former

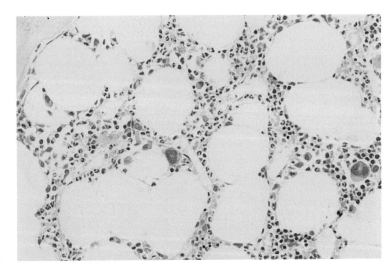

Fig. 1.8 Section of normal BM: normal distribution of all three haemopoietic lineages; note the megakaryocyte adjacent to a sinusoid. Resin-embedded, H&E ×20

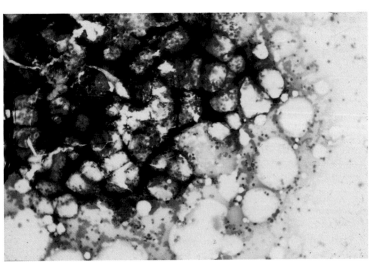

Fig. 1.9 Aspirate of normal BM: fragment showing normal cellularity. May–Grünwald–Giemsa (MGG) ×40.

are approximately 5% lower than estimates based on the latter [21].

The cellularity of histological sections can be assessed most accurately by computerized image analysis or, alternatively, by point-counting using an eyepiece with a graticule; the process is known as histomorphometry. Results of the two procedures show a fairly close correlation [21,22]. Cellularity can also be assessed subjectively. Such estimates are less reproducible and may lead to some under-estimation of cellularity but show a reasonable correlation with histomorphometric methods; in one study the mean cellularity was 78% by histomorphometry (point-counting) and 65% by visual estimation, with the correlation between the two methods being 0.78 [21]. Bone marrow cellularity is expressed as the percentage of a section that is occupied by haemopoietic tissue. However, the denominator may vary. The cellularity of sections of fragments is expressed in terms of haemopoietic tissue as a percentage of the total of haemopoietic and adipose tissue. In the case of a trephine biopsy, however, the cellularity may be expressed either as a percentage of the entire biopsy (including bone) [23] or as a percentage of the marrow cavity [21,24]. There are advantages in the latter approach, in which the area occupied by bone is excluded from the calculation, since the

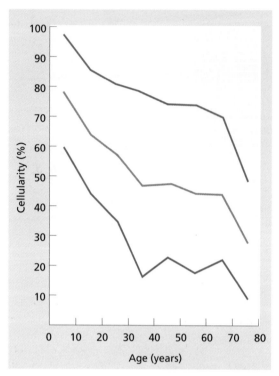

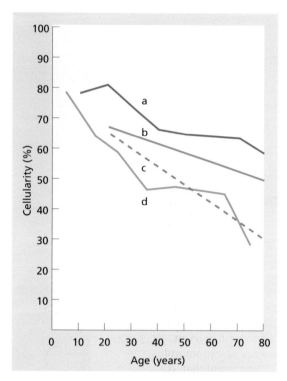

Fig. 1.10 Mean and 95% range of cellularity at various ages of anterior iliac crest bone marrow which has been decalcified and paraffin-embedded. Cellularity is expressed as a percentage of the bone marrow cavity. (Calculated from Hartsock *et al.* [24].)

Fig. 1.11 Mean value of bone marrow cellularity at various ages expressed as a percentage of bone marrow cavity: (a) iliac crest, autopsy, not decalcified (recalculated from Frisch *et al.* [23]); (b) iliac crest, autopsy, not decalcified [26]; (c) sternum, biopsy, not decalcified [27]; and (d) ilium, autopsy, decalcified [24].

percentages obtained are then directly comparable with measurements made on histological sections of aspirated fragments or estimates made from fragments in bone marrow films.

The bone marrow of neonates is extremely cellular, negligible fat cells being present. Cellularity decreases fairly steadily with age, with an accelerated rate of decline above the age of 70 years [23–27] (Figs 1.10 and 1.11). The decreasing percentage of the marrow cavity occupied by haemopoietic tissue is a consequence both of a true decline in the amount of haemopoietic tissue and of a loss of bone substance with age requiring adipose tissue to expand to fill the larger marrow cavity. In subjects with osteoporosis this effect can be so great that even young persons who are haematologically normal may have as little as 20% of their marrow cavity occupied by haemopoietic cells [25]. In haematologically normal subjects without

bone disease, typical reported rates of decline in average marrow cellularity (expressed as a percentage of haemopoietic cells plus adipose cells) are: from 64% in the second decade to 29% in the eighth decade in the iliac crest [24]; from 85% at age 20 years to 40% at age 60, also in the iliac crest [25]; and from 66% at age 20 to 30% at age 80 in the sternum [27].

Bone marrow cellularity also depends on the site of biopsy. Study of the two tissues by the same techniques has shown that the cellularity of lumbar vertebrae is, on average, about 10% more than the cellularity of the iliac crest [6]. Vertebrae are also more cellular than the sternum. Because of the considerable dependence of the assessment of cellularity on methods of processing and counting, it is much more difficult to make generalizations when different tissues have not been assessed by

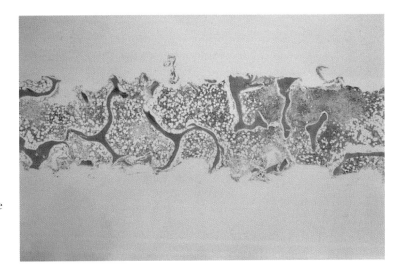

Fig. 1.12 A section of a trephine biopsy specimen of adequate size from a patient with Hodgkin lymphoma showing only a small area of infiltration at one end of the specimen, illustrating how a small biopsy may miss focal lesions. Paraffin-embedded, H&E ×2.5. (By courtesy of Dr K. Maclennan.)

the same techniques. Bennike *et al.* [5], in comparing the two sites in 100 subjects, considered the sternum to be on average somewhat more cellular than the iliac crest. However, comparison of the results of histomorphometric studies by different groups found that, comparing a single study of the sternum with four studies of the iliac crest, the sternum was generally *less* cellular [23–27]. It should be noted that the lowest estimates of iliac crest cellularity are from a study using decalcified, paraffin-embedded bone marrow specimens [24] while the highest estimates are from a study using non-decalcified, resin-embedded specimens [23]. Some studies have been conducted on biopsy specimens [27] and others on specimens obtained at autopsy [23,24,26]. Because of such technical considerations it is difficult to make any generalizations about normal bone marrow cellularity. However, it is possible to say that, except in extreme old age, cellularity of less than 20% is likely to be abnormal, as is cellularity of more than 80% in those above 20 years of age.

In making a subjective assessment of the cellularity of films prepared from aspirates, the cellularity of fragments is of more importance than the cellularity of trails, although occasionally the presence of quite cellular trails – despite hypocellular fragments – suggests that the marrow cellularity is adequate. An average fragment cellularity between 25% and 75% is usually taken to indicate normality, except at the extremes of age.

Because of the variability of cellularity from one intertrabecular space to the next, it is not possible to assess marrow cellularity if few fragments are aspirated or if a biopsy core is of inadequate size. In particular, a small biopsy sample containing only a small amount of subcortical marrow does not allow assessment of cellularity since this area is often of low cellularity, particularly in the elderly. A biopsy specimen containing at least five or six intertrabecular spaces is desirable, not only for an adequate assessment of cellularity but also to give a reasonable probability of detecting focal bone marrow lesions (Fig. 1.12). This requires a core of 20–30 mm in length.

Haemopoietic cells

A multipotent stem cell gives rise to all types of myeloid cell: erythrocytes and their precursors; granulocytes and their precursors; macrophages, monocytes and their precursors; mast cells; and megakaryocytes and their precursors (Fig. 1.13). It should be mentioned that the term 'myeloid' can be used with two rather different meanings. It is used to indicate all cells derived from the common myeloid stem cell and also to indicate only the granulocytic and monocytic lineages, as in the expression 'myeloid:erythroid ratio'. It is usually evident from the context which sense is intended but it is important to avoid ambiguity in using this

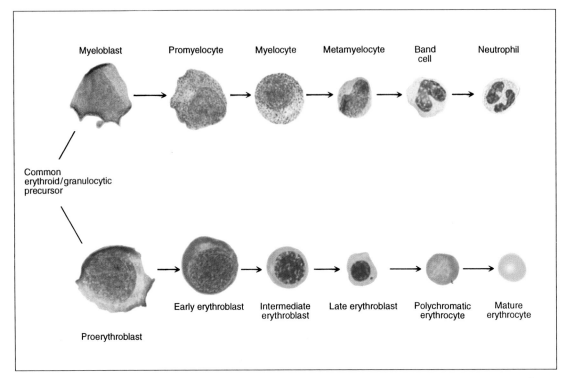

Fig. 1.13 A semi-diagrammatic representation of granulopoiesis and erythropoiesis. Cell division occurs up to the myelocyte and intermediate erythroblast stages.

term. The common myeloid stem cell and stem cells committed to the specific myeloid lineages cannot be identified morphologically but it is likely that they are cells of similar size and appearance to a lymphocyte. The various myeloid lineages differ both morphologically and in their disposition in the bone marrow. The normal bone marrow contains, in addition to myeloid cells, smaller numbers of lymphoid cells (including plasma cells) and the stromal cells, which have been discussed above.

Erythropoiesis

Cytology

Precursors of erythrocytes are designated erythroblasts. The term normoblast can also be used but has a narrower meaning; 'erythroblast' includes all recognizable erythroid precursors whereas 'normoblast' is applicable only when erythropoiesis is normoblastic. There are at least five generations of

erythroblasts between the morphologically unrecognizable erythroid stem cell and the erythrocyte. Erythroblasts develop in close proximity to a macrophage, the cytoplasmic processes of which extend between and around individual erythroblasts. Several generations of erythroblasts are associated with one macrophage, the whole cluster of cells being known as an erythroblastic island [28]. Intact erythroblastic islands are sometimes seen in bone marrow films (Fig. 1.14). Erythroblasts are conventionally divided, on morphological grounds, into four categories – proerythroblasts and early, intermediate and late erythroblasts. An alternative terminology is: proerythroblast, basophilic erythroblast, early polychromatophilic erythroblast and late polychromatophilic erythroblast. The term orthochromatic erythroblast is best avoided since the most mature erythroblasts are only orthochromatic (that is acidophilic, with the same staining characteristics as mature red cells) when erythropoiesis is abnormal.

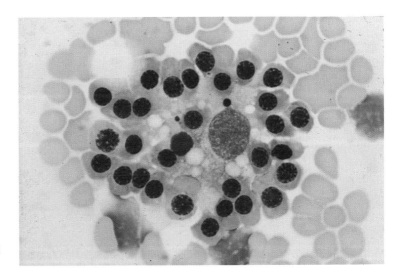

Fig. 1.14 BM aspirate: an erythroid island. MGG ×100.

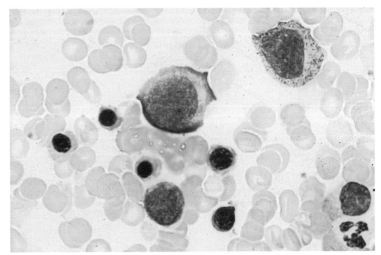

Fig. 1.15 Aspirate of normal BM: a proerythroblast, intermediate erythroblast, four late erythroblasts, a myelocyte, large and small lymphocytes and a neutrophil. MGG ×100.

Proerythroblasts (Fig. 1.15) are large round cells with a diameter of 12–20 μm and a large round nucleus. The cytoplasm is deeply basophilic with a pale perinuclear zone, attributable to the Golgi apparatus, sometimes being apparent. The nucleus has a finely granular or stippled appearance and contains several nucleoli.

Early erythroblasts (Fig. 1.16) are smaller than proerythroblasts and more numerous. The nucleocytoplasmic ratio is somewhat lower. They have strongly basophilic cytoplasm and a granular or stippled chromatin pattern without visible nucleoli. A perinuclear halo, which is less strongly basophilic than the rest of the cytoplasm, may be apparent.

Intermediate erythroblasts (Figs 1.15 and 1.16) are smaller again, with a lower nucleocytoplasmic ratio than that of the early erythroblast, less basophilic cytoplasm and moderate clumping of the chromatin. They are more numerous than early erythroblasts.

Late erythroblasts (Figs 1.15 and 1.16) are smaller and more numerous than intermediate erythroblasts. They are only slightly larger than mature red cells. Their nucleocytoplasmic ratio is lower than that of the intermediate erythroblast and the chromatin is more clumped. The cytoplasm is only weakly basophilic and in addition has a pink tinge due to the increased amount of haemoglobin.

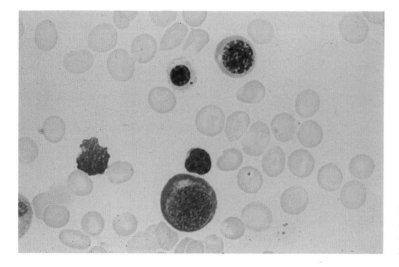

Fig. 1.16 Aspirate of normal BM: early, intermediate and late erythroblasts and a lymphocyte. MGG ×100.

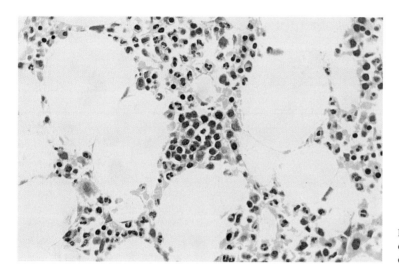

Fig. 1.17 Section of normal BM: an erythroid island (centre). Resin-embedded, H&E ×40.

Because of the resultant pinky-blue colour the cell is described as polychromatophilic.

Late erythroblasts extrude their nuclei to form polychromatophilic erythrocytes, which are slightly larger than mature erythrocytes. These cells can be identified by a specific stain as reticulocytes; when haemopoiesis is normal they spend about 2 days of their 3-day life span in the bone marrow.

Small numbers of normal erythroblasts show atypical morphological features such as irregular nuclei, binuclearity and cytoplasmic bridging between adjacent erythroblasts [29].

Histology

Erythroblastic islands (Figs 1.17 and 1.18) are recognizable as distinctive clusters of cells in which one or more concentric circles of erythroblasts closely surround a macrophage. The erythroblasts that are closer to the macrophage are less mature than the peripheral ones. The central macrophage sends out extensive slender processes, which envelop each erythroblast. The macrophage phagocytoses defective erythroblasts and extruded nuclei; nuclear and cellular debris may therefore be recognized in the cytoplasm and a Perls' stain (see page

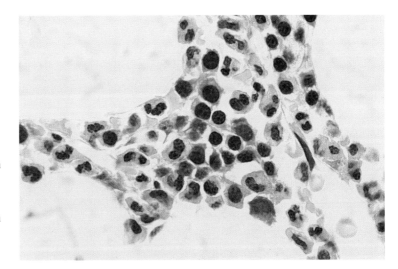

Fig. 1.18 Section of normal BM: an erythroid island containing intermediate and late erythroblasts and a haemosiderin-laden macrophage; a Golgi zone is seen in some of the intermediate erythroblasts. Resin-embedded, H&E ×100.

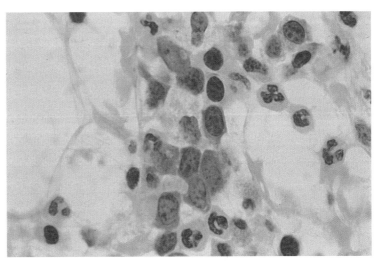

Fig. 1.19 Section of normal BM: an erythroid island containing early and intermediate erythroblasts. Resin-embedded, Giemsa ×100.

57) may demonstrate the presence of haemosiderin. Erythropoiesis occurs relatively close to marrow sinusoids although it is probable that, as in the rat [30], only a minority of erythroblastic islands actually abut on sinusoids.

Early erythroblasts (Fig. 1.19) are large cells; they have relatively little cytoplasm and large nuclei with dispersed chromatin and multiple small, irregular or linear nucleoli often abutting on the nuclear membrane. The nuclei are rounder than those of myeloblasts but, in contrast to the nuclei of early erythroid cells in bone marrow aspirates of healthy subjects, in histological sections some appear ovoid or slightly irregular. More mature erythroid cells have condensed nuclear chromatin and cytoplasm that is less basophilic. The chromatin in the erythroblast nuclei is evenly distributed and, as chromatin condensation occurs, an even, regular pattern is retained.

There are four features that are useful in distinguishing erythroid precursors in the marrow from other cells: (i) in normal bone marrow they occur in distinctive erythroblastic islands containing several generations of cells of varying size and maturity; (ii) erythroblasts adhere tightly to one another; (iii) their nuclei are round; and (iv) in late erythroblasts the chromatin is condensed in a regular manner whereas nuclei of small lym-

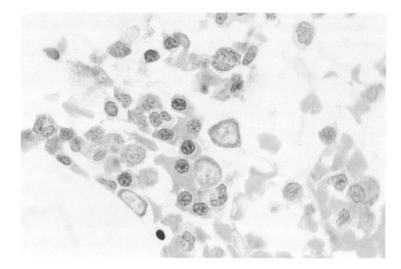

Fig. 1.20 Section of normal BM: erythroid island containing three early, one intermediate and numerous late erythroblasts; note the cytoplasmic basophilia of early erythroblasts. Resin-embedded, Giemsa ×100.

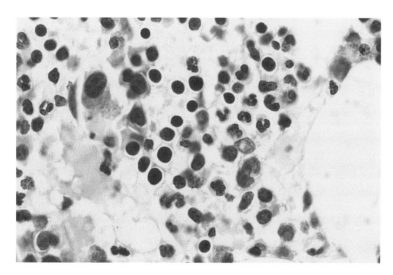

Fig. 1.21 Section of normal BM: erythroid island showing intermediate and late erythroblasts with haloes surrounding the nuclei. Paraffin-embedded, H&E ×100.

phocytes show coarse clumping. With a Giemsa stain (Fig. 1.20), the intense cytoplasmic basophilia with a small, negatively staining Golgi zone adjacent to the nucleus is also distinctive. In paraffin-embedded specimens (Fig. 1.21), artefactual shrinking of cytoplasm of later erythroblasts can be useful in distinguishing them from lymphocytes. Shrinkage artefact is absent in resin-embedded sections, in which the identification of erythroid cells is aided by their syncytial appearance (Fig. 1.22).

When the bone marrow is regenerating rapidly, erythroid islands may be composed of cells all of which are at the same stage of maturation. This results in some islands consisting only of immature elements. A similar pattern is sometimes seen when erythropoiesis is abnormal, for example in myelodysplasia, in which the intramedullary death of erythroblasts is a major mechanism.

The identification of abnormal erythroblasts can be more difficult than the identification of their normal equivalents, for example, if well-organized erythroblastic islands are not present or if they contain only immature cells. When there is any difficulty in recognizing erythroid precursors their identity can be confirmed by cytochemical or immunocytochemical staining (see page 71).

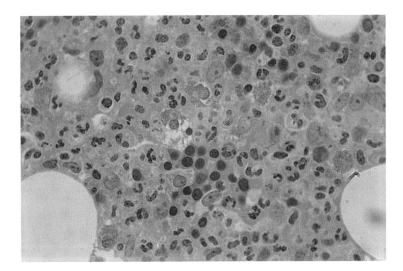

Fig. 1.22 Syncytial appearance of erythroblasts in an erythroid island in sections from a trephine biopsy specimen. Resin-embedded, H&E ×60.

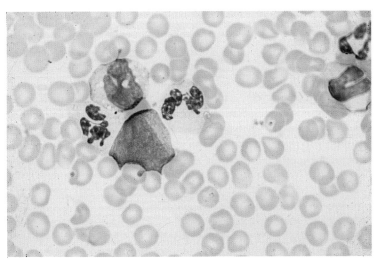

Fig. 1.23 Aspirate of normal BM: a myeloblast, three neutrophils and two monocytes; the myeloblast has a high nucleocytoplasmic ratio, a diffuse chromatin pattern and a nucleolus. MGG ×100.

Granulopoiesis

Cytology

There are at least four generations of cells between the morphologically unrecognizable committed granulocyte–monocyte precursor and the mature granulocyte, but cell division does not necessarily occur at the same point as maturation from one stage to another. The first recognizable granulopoietic cell is the myeloblast (Figs 1.23 and 1.24). It is similar in size to the proerythroblast, about 12–20 μm. It is more irregular in shape than a proerythroblast and its cytoplasm is moderately rather than strongly basophilic. The chromatin pattern is diffuse and there are several nucleoli. Myeloblasts are generally defined as being cells that lack granules but, in the context of the abnormal myelopoiesis of acute myeloid leukaemia and the myelodysplastic syndromes, primitive cells with granules may also be accepted as myeloblasts. Myeloblasts are capable of cell division and mature to promyelocytes.

Promyelocytes (Fig. 1.24) have a nucleolated, slightly indented nucleus, a Golgi zone and primary or azurophilic granules, which are reddish-purple with a Romanowsky stain. Promyelocytes are larger than myeloblasts, usually 15–25 μm, and their cytoplasm is often more strongly basophilic.

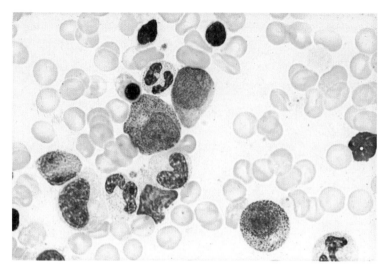

Fig. 1.24 Aspirate of normal BM: a myeloblast and a promyelocyte (centre), a myelocyte (lower right), a metamyelocyte, band forms, a neutrophil and a late erythroblast; the promyelocyte is larger than the myeloblast and is showing some chromatin condensation but with persisting nucleoli, well-developed cytoplasmic granulation and a Golgi zone. MGG ×100.

By light microscopy, promyelocytes of the three granulocytic lineages cannot easily be distinguished, but by ultrastructural examination the distinction can be made. Promyelocytes are capable of cell division and mature to myelocytes.

Myelocytes (Fig. 1.24) are smaller than promyelocytes and are quite variable in size – from 10 to 20 μm. Their nuclei show partial chromatin condensation and lack nucleoli. Their cytoplasm is less basophilic than that of promyelocytes and specific neutrophilic, eosinophilic and basophilic granules can now be discerned, staining lilac, orange-red and purple, respectively. Eosinophil myelocytes may also contain some granules that take up basic dyes and stain purple; these differ ultrastructurally from the granules of the basophil lineage and are best designated pro-eosinophilic granules. There are probably normally at least two generations of myelocytes so that at least some cells of this category are capable of cell division. Late myelocytes mature to metamyelocytes, which are 10–12 μm in diameter and have a markedly indented or U-shaped nucleus (Fig. 1.24). The metamyelocyte is not capable of cell division but matures to a band form with a ribbon-shaped nucleus. The band cell, in turn, matures to a polymorphonuclear granulocyte with a segmented nucleus and specific neutrophilic, eosinophilic or basophilic granules. The bone marrow is a major reservoir for mature neutrophils.

Histology

Myeloblasts (Fig. 1.25) are the earliest granulocyte precursors identifiable histologically; they are present in small numbers and are most frequently found adjacent to the bone marrow trabecular surfaces or to arterioles. They are fairly large cells with round to oval nuclei and one to five relatively small nucleoli. There is no chromatin clumping. They have relatively little cytoplasm. They are readily distinguished from lymphoid cells by the absence of chromatin clumping and the presence of nucleoli. Myeloblasts are far outnumbered in normal marrows by the promyelocytes (Figs 1.25 and 1.26) and myelocytes (Fig. 1.26), which are recognized by their granularity. Primary and neutrophilic granules may be seen as faintly eosinophilic granules in good quality haematoxylin and eosin (H&E)-stained sections, but they are best seen with a Giemsa stain. Granules of cells of eosinophil lineage are large, refractile and more strongly eosinophilic. They are therefore easily recognized on both H&E and Giemsa stains. Basophil granules are water-soluble and, since trephine biopsy specimens are fixed in aqueous fixatives, basophils are not recognizable in histological sections. As maturation occurs, granulocytic precursors are found progressively more deeply in the haemopoietic cords but away from the sinusoids. When they reach the metamyelocyte stage, they appear to move towards the sinusoids and, at the polymorphonuclear

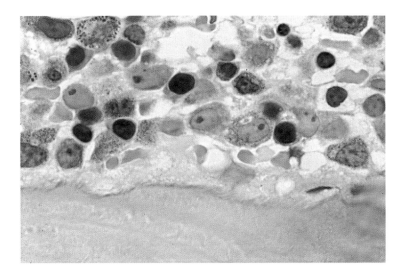

Fig. 1.25 Section of normal BM: myeloblasts and promyelocytes adjacent to a bony trabecula. Resin-embedded, H&E ×100.

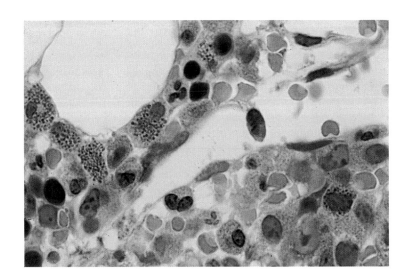

Fig. 1.26 Section of normal BM: promyelocytes, myelocytes and maturing neutrophils and eosinophils adjacent to a sinusoid. Resin-embedded, H&E ×100.

granulocyte stage, cross the wall to enter the circulation.

In undecalcified resin-embedded sections, and in sections from specimens decalcified using EDTA, the chloroacetate esterase stain is a reliable marker of neutrophil haemopoiesis from the promyelocyte stage onwards. Overnight incubation of acid-decalcified sections in a buffer at pH 6.8 partly restores chloroacetate esterase activity. Alternatively, the identity of cells of the granulocytic lineage can be confirmed by immunocytochemistry.

Monocytopoiesis

Cytology

Monocytes are derived from a morphologically unrecognizable common granulocytic–monocytic precursor. The earliest morphologically recognizable precursor is a monoblast, a cell which is larger than a myeloblast with abundant cytoplasm showing a variable degree of basophilia and with a large, round nucleus. Monoblasts are capable of division and mature into promonocytes, which are

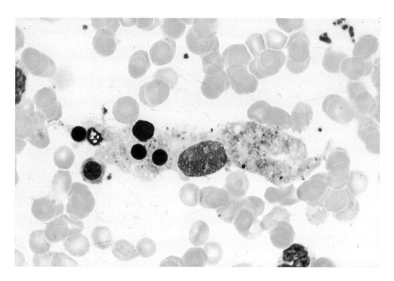

Fig. 1.27 Aspirate of normal BM: a macrophage containing granular and refractile debris and several normoblast nuclei. MGG ×100.

similar in size to promyelocytes; they have nucleoli, some degree of nuclear lobulation and azurophilic cytoplasmic granules. Promonocytes mature into monocytes, which migrate rapidly into the peripheral blood. Monocytes are 12–20 μm in diameter. They have a lobulated nucleus and abundant cytoplasm, which is weakly basophilic. The cytoplasm may contain small numbers of fine azurophilic granules and often has a ground-glass appearance, in contrast to the clear cytoplasm of a lymphocyte.

Monocytes mature into macrophages (Fig. 1.27) in the bone marrow as well as in other tissues. These are large cells, 20–30 μm in diameter, of irregular shape, with a low nucleocytoplasmic ratio and voluminous weakly basophilic cytoplasm. When relatively immature, they may have an oval nucleus with a fairly diffuse chromatin pattern. When mature, the nucleus is smaller and more condensed and the cytoplasm may contain lipid droplets, recognizable degenerating cells and amorphous debris; an iron stain commonly shows the presence of haemosiderin. Bone marrow macrophages may develop into various storage cells, which will be discussed in later chapters.

Both monocytes and their precursors are quite infrequent among marrow cells partly because monocytes, in contrast to mature neutrophils, are released rapidly into the peripheral blood rather than being stored in the bone marrow. Macrophages (histiocytes), however, are readily apparent.

Histology

Monocytes are recognized in histological sections of the marrow as cells that are larger than neutrophils with lobulated nuclei; monocyte precursors are not usually recognizable. In haematologically normal subjects, only small numbers of randomly distributed monocytes are present.

Macrophages (Fig. 1.28) are identified as irregularly scattered, relatively large cells with a small nucleus and abundant cytoplasm. In thin sections, only the cytoplasm may be visible, the nucleus being out of the plane of the section. Phagocytosed debris may be prominent in the cytoplasm. Some are associated with erythroblasts (forming erythroblastic islands), plasma cells or lymphoid nodules. Immunohistochemistry of trephine biopsy sections highlights a prominent network of dendritic macrophages dispersed through the stroma (Fig. 1.29).

Megakaryopoiesis and thrombopoiesis

Cytology

Megakaryocytes arise from haemopoietic stem cells via a common megakaryocyte–erythroid progenitor cell that gives rise to erythroid precursors and megakaryoblasts. The latter are small, proliferative cells with diploid nuclei, not generally recognizable in normal bone marrow. In normal marrow, the earliest morphologically recognizable cell in the megakaryocyte lineage is the megakaryocyte itself although, when haemopoiesis is abnormal, mega-

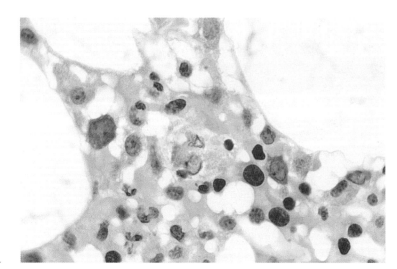

Fig. 1.28 Section of normal BM: a macrophage containing cellular debris. Resin-embedded, H&E ×100.

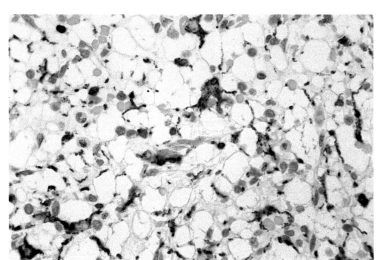

Fig. 1.29 Section of trephine biopsy specimen showing a network of dendritic macrophages. Paraffin-embedded, immunoperoxidase with CD68 monoclonal antibody ×50.

karyoblasts of similar size and morphology to myeloblasts can sometimes be recognized. Megakaryocytes undergo endoreduplication as they mature, resulting in large cells (30–160 μm) with a marked degree of heterogeneity in both nuclear DNA content (ploidy) and nuclear size. Endoreduplication is encountered only rarely in any other mammalian cell. It is promoted by upregulation of cyclin D3 and is believed to contribute to the high productive capacity of megakaryocytes for platelet components [31]. Megakaryocytes can be classified by their ploidy level. In normal marrow they range from 4 N (tetraploid) to 32 N with the dominant ploidy category being 16 N.

Megakaryocytes can also be classified on the basis of their nuclear and, more particularly, their cytoplasmic characteristics into three stages of maturation [32]. Group I megakaryocytes (Fig. 1.30) have strongly basophilic cytoplasm and a very high nucleocytoplasmic ratio. Group II megakaryocytes have a lower nucleocytoplasmic ratio and cytoplasm that is less basophilic; the cytoplasm contains some azurophilic granules. Group III megakaryocytes (Fig. 1.31) have plentiful weakly basophilic cytoplasm containing abundant azurophilic granules; the cytoplasm at the cell margins is agranular. Group III megakaryocytes are mature cells, capable of producing platelets and no longer synthesizing

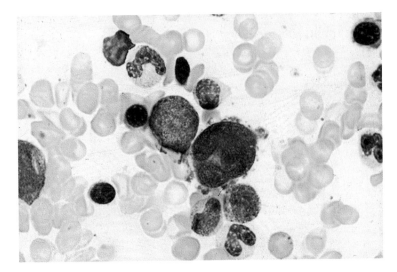

Fig. 1.30 Aspirate of normal BM: an immature megakaryocyte with a polyploid nucleus showing little chromatin condensation: the cytoplasm is scanty and basophilic. MGG ×100.

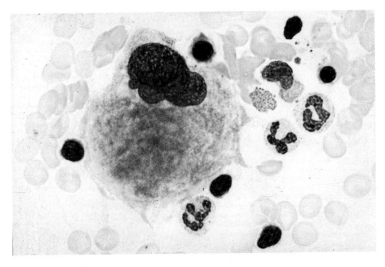

Fig. 1.31 Aspirate of normal BM: a mature megakaryocyte with a lobulated nucleus and voluminous granular cytoplasm. MGG ×100.

DNA. There is some correlation between the three stages of maturation and ploidy level. All stages of maturation include megakaryocytes that are 8 N, 16 N and 32 N, but 4 N megakaryocytes are confined to group I and 32 N megakaryocytes are more numerous in group III. The nuclei of the great majority of normal polyploid megakaryocytes form irregular lobes joined by strands of chromatin. A minority have either a non-lobated nucleus or more than one nucleus. Platelet production involves aggregation of components within the cell cytoplasm, segregation within a demarcation membrane system and organization into proplatelets. The latter are then shed directly into bone marrow sinusoids in a highly coordinated process of cytoplasmic fragmentation. The final stage in megakaryocyte maturation is an apparently bare nucleus (actually with a thin cytoplasmic rim), the great bulk of the cytoplasm having been shed into sinusoids as platelets (Fig. 1.32).

Megakaryocyte proliferation and platelet production are primarily regulated by interactions between thrombopoietin (TPO) and its cell surface receptor, MPL [33]. An increased demand for platelets, for example due to peripheral destruction, leads to an increase in ploidy level and cell size, apparent in a bone marrow film as an increased volume of cytoplasm and a large, usually well-

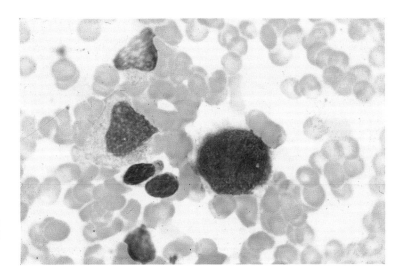

Fig. 1.32 Aspirate of normal BM: a late megakaryocyte which has shed most of its cytoplasm as platelets. MGG ×100.

lobated nucleus. It should be noted that whether or not megakaryocytes appear to be producing platelets shows little correlation with the number of platelets being produced. In patients with thrombocytosis, particularly with essential thrombocythaemia, there are often many 'budding' megakaryocytes but in autoimmune thrombocytopenia, in which platelet production is also greatly increased, 'budding' megakaryocytes are quite uncommon.

It is necessary to assess megakaryocyte numbers as well as morphology. In films of an aspirate this can only be a subjective assessment – that megakaryocytes are decreased, normal or increased. A more accurate assessment can be made from histological sections of aspirated fragments or from sections of trephine biopsy specimens. Somewhat fewer megakaryocytes are seen in sections of aspirated fragments than in trephine biopsies, possibly because these large cells are not as readily aspirated as smaller marrow cells.

Megakaryocytes may 'engulf' other haemopoietic cells (lymphocytes, erythrocytes, erythroblasts and granulocytes and their precursors), a process known as emperipolesis (Fig. 1.33). This process differs from phagocytosis in that the engulfed cells have entered dilated cavities in the demarcation membrane system rather than being in phagocytic vacuoles; on examination of bone marrow films the cells within the megakaryocyte are observed to be intact and morphologically normal.

Identification of megakaryocytes is aided by cytochemistry and immunocytochemistry (see pages 63 and 71).

Histology
Megakaryocytes are by far the largest of normal bone marrow cells, their size being related to their ploidy. They have plentiful cytoplasm and usually a lobulated nucleus. The chromatin pattern is finely granular and evenly dispersed. With a Giemsa stain, demarcation of platelets within the cytoplasm is apparent.

Megakaryocytes are most frequently found associated with sinusoids, at some distance from bony trabeculae (Figs 1.8, 1.34 and 1.35). They are found in a paratrabecular position only when haemopoiesis is abnormal. Serial sections show that, in normal marrow, all megakaryocytes abut on sinusoids [34]. Megakaryocytes lie directly outside the sinusoid and discharge platelets by protruding cytoplasmic processes through endothelial cells; such processes break up into platelets. 'Bare nuclei' which have shed almost all their cytoplasm in this manner can be recognized in histological sections (Fig. 1.36) as well as in bone marrow films. Intact megakaryocytes and bare nuclei can also enter the circulation and are seen within vessels in histological sections of lung, spleen, liver and other organs. Multiple mitotic figures are sometimes observed in megakaryocytes (Fig. 1.37). Emperipolesis is readily observed in histological sections (Fig. 1.38).

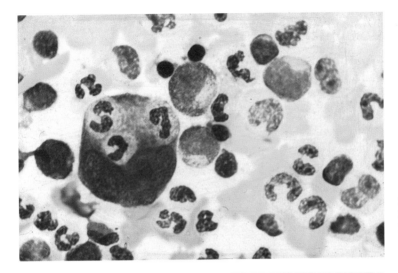

Fig. 1.33 Aspirate of non-infiltrated BM from a patient with Hodgkin lymphoma: a mature megakaryocyte exhibiting emperipolesis. MGG ×100.

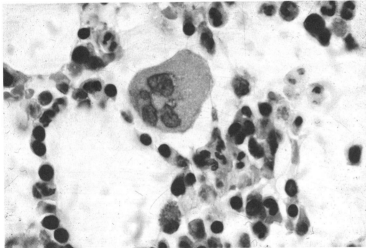

Fig. 1.34 Section of normal BM showing cells of all haemopoietic lineages including a normal megakaryocyte with finely granular cytoplasm. Paraffin-embedded, Giemsa ×100.

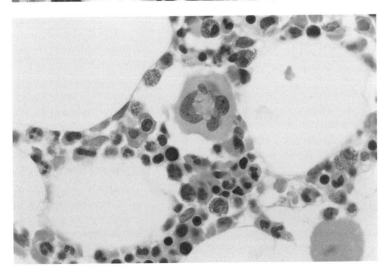

Fig. 1.35 Section of normal BM showing a normal megakaryocyte and other normal haemopoietic cells. Paraffin-embedded, H&E ×100.

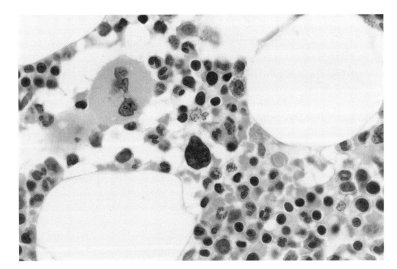

Fig. 1.36 Section of normal BM showing a normal mature megakaryocyte and a 'bare' megakaryocyte nucleus. Paraffin-embedded, H&E ×100.

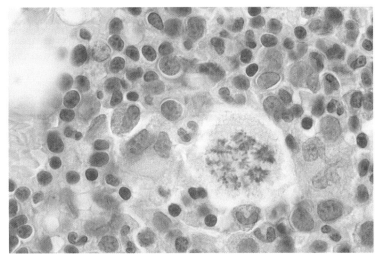

Fig. 1.37 Section of a trephine biopsy specimen from a patient with polycythaemia vera showing two megakaryocytes, one of which shows multiple mitotic figures; note shrinkage haloes around the intermediate and late erythroblasts. Paraffin-embedded, H&E ×100.

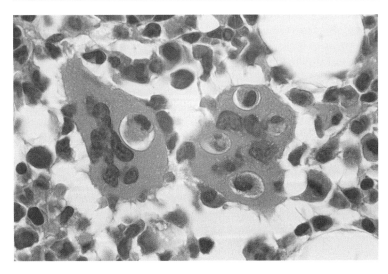

Fig. 1.38 Section of a trephine biopsy specimen from a patient with AIDS: two megakaryocytes show prominent emperipolesis; in normal marrow emperipolesis is less striking. Paraffin-embedded, H&E ×100.

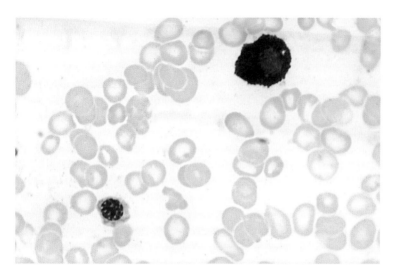

Fig. 1.39 Aspirate of normal BM: a mast cell and a normoblast; the mast cell has a round nucleus and cytoplasm packed with deeply basophilic granules. MGG ×100.

In assessing the morphology of megakaryocytes, it is important to remember that the megakaryocyte is a very large cell and only a cross-section of it is being examined. It is therefore not possible to determine the size or degree of nuclear lobulation of single megakaryocytes. However, by examining a large number of cells it is possible to form a judgement as to the average size of the megakaryocytes, the size distribution, the average degree of lobulation, and whether there are abnormal features such as micromegakaryocytes or an increased number of non-lobulated megakaryocytes (see pages 211 and 212).

When haemopoiesis is normal, megakaryocytes do not form clusters of more than two or three cells. Larger clusters of megakaryocytes are seen in regenerating marrow, following chemotherapy and bone marrow transplantation, and also in various pathological states; this feature is diagnostically useful.

Megakaryocytes can be quantified by counting their number per unit area, or a subjective impression can be formed as to whether they are present in decreased, normal or increased numbers. Depending on the processing and staining techniques employed, estimates of mean megakaryocyte number in normal marrow vary from 7 to 15 per mm^2 [35]. If an immunocytochemical technique is used, estimates are considerably higher, with the mean normal value being 25 per mm^2; this

is probably because more small megakaryocytes and megakaryocyte precursors are recognized [35].

Mast cells

Cytology
Mast cells (Fig. 1.39) are derived from the multipotent myeloid stem cell. In bone marrow films they appear as oval or elongated cells varying in size from 5 to 25 μm. The nucleus is central, relatively small and either round or oval. The cytoplasm is packed with granules that stain deep purple with Romanowsky stains. Mast cells can be distinguished from basophils by the different nuclear characteristics (non-lobulated nucleus with less chromatin clumping) and by the fact that the granules do not obscure the nucleus.

Histology
Mast cells are rare in normal marrow. They are difficult to recognize in H&E-stained histological sections because the granules do not stain distinctively. They are readily recognizable in a Giemsa stain (Fig. 1.40) in which the granules stain metachromatically; their vivid purple colour make them conspicuous. Mast cell granules also give positive reactions for chloroacetate esterase, are periodic

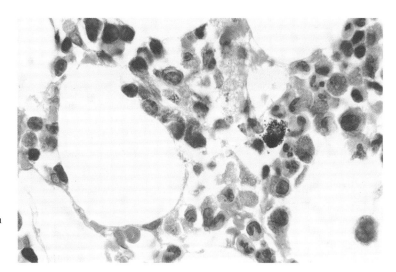

Fig. 1.40 Section of a trephine biopsy specimen from a patient with renal failure: a mast cell and maturing granulocytes. Resin-embedded, Giemsa ×100.

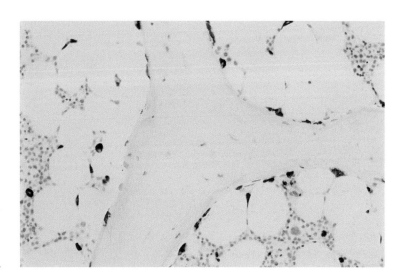

Fig. 1.41 Section of a trephine biopsy specimen showing a reactive increase in interstitial and paratrabecular mast cells. Paraffin-embedded, immunoperoxidase, mast cell tryptase (McAb AA1) ×20.

acid–Schiff (PAS) positive and stain metachromatically with toluidine blue. They show tartrate-resistant acid phosphatase activity in EDTA- but not acid-decalcified specimens. Mast cells are distributed irregularly in the medullary cavity but are most numerous near the endosteum, in the periosteum, in association with the adventitia of small blood vessels and at the periphery of lymphoid nodules or aggregates [36]. They appear as elliptical or elongated cells with an average diameter of 12 μm. Their cytoplasmic projections stretch out between haemopoietic cells. Their distribution and cytological features can be demonstrated by immunohistochemistry (Figs 1.41 and 1.42).

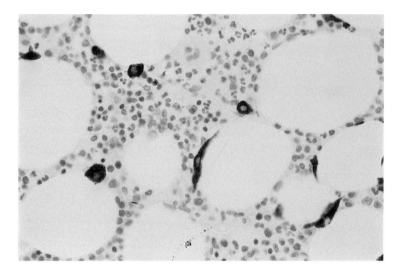

Fig. 1.42 Sections of a trephine biopsy specimen showing a reactive mast cell increase; note that some mast cells are round and some are spindle-shaped. Paraffin-embedded, immunoperoxidase, mast cell tryptase (McAb AA1) ×40.

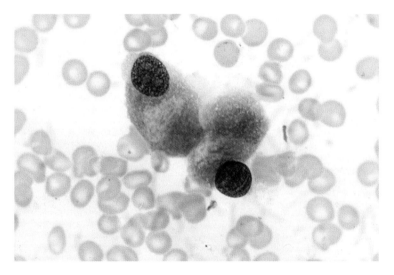

Fig. 1.43 Aspirate of normal BM: two osteoblasts; note the eccentric nucleus and basophilic cytoplasm. These cells can be distinguished from plasma cells by their larger size and the position of the Golgi zone, which is not immediately adjacent to the nucleus. MGG ×100.

Osteoblasts and osteoclasts

Osteoblasts and osteoclasts differ in their origin but have complementary functions. Osteoblasts have a common origin with other mesenchymal cells and are responsible for bone deposition. Osteoclasts are formed by fusion of cells of monocyte lineage and are responsible for dissolution of bone.

Cytology
Osteoblasts (Fig. 1.43) are mononuclear cells with a diameter of 20–50 μm. They have an eccentric nucleus, moderately basophilic cytoplasm and a Golgi zone that is not in apposition to the nuclear membrane. The nucleus shows some chromatin condensation and may contain a small nucleolus. Osteoblasts can be distinguished from plasma cells, to which they bear a superficial resemblance, by the lesser degree of chromatin condensation and the separation of the Golgi zone from the nucleus. Osteoblasts are uncommon in bone marrow aspirates of healthy adults but, when present, often appear in small clumps. They are much more numerous in the bone marrow of children and adolescents.

Osteoclasts (Fig. 1.44) are multinucleated giant cells with a diameter of 30–100 μm or more. Their nuclei tend to be clearly separate, uniform in

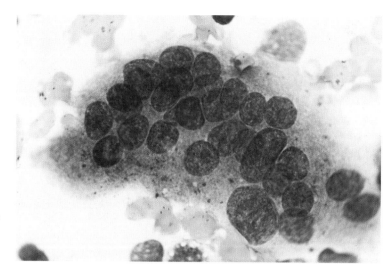

Fig. 1.44 Aspirate of normal BM: an osteoclast; note the highly granular cytoplasm and the multiple nuclei which are uniform in size and have indistinct, medium-sized, single nucleoli. MGG ×100.

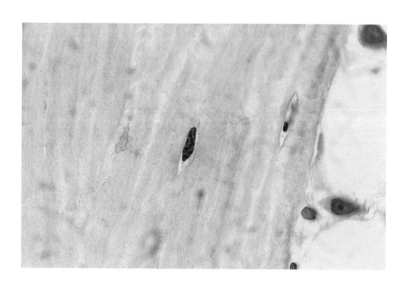

Fig. 1.45 Section of normal BM: a bone spicule containing an osteocyte; note the myeloblasts in the adjacent marrow. Resin-embedded, H&E ×100.

appearance and slightly oval with a single lilac-staining nucleolus. The voluminous cytoplasm contains numerous azurophilic granules, which are coarser than those of megakaryocytes. Osteoclasts are not commonly seen in marrow aspirates of healthy adults but are much more often seen in aspirates from children.

Histology

Osteocytes, osteoblasts and osteoclasts in histological sections are identified by their position and their morphological features. Osteocytes (Fig. 1.45) lie within bone lacunae. Osteoblasts (Figs 1.46 and 1.47) appear in rows along a bone spicule or a layer of osteoid and their eccentric nuclei and prominent Golgi zones are apparent. A decline in number per unit area of bone occurs during the second and third decades [37]. Osteoclasts (Fig. 1.48) are likely to be found on the other side of a spicule from osteoblasts or some distance away. They are identified as multinucleated cells lying in hollows known as Howship's lacunae. A decline in numbers occurs during the first and second decades [37]. They show tartrate-resistant acid phosphatase activity in EDTA- but not acid-decalcified specimens.

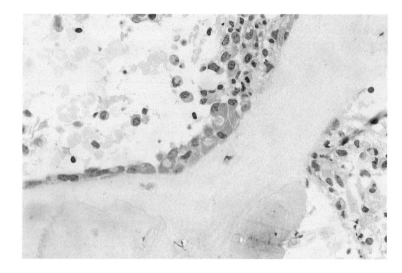

Fig. 1.46 Section of BM from a patient with Fanconi anaemia: the trabecula is lined by osteoblasts; note the distinct Golgi zones which do not abut on the nuclear membrane. Resin-embedded, H&E ×40.

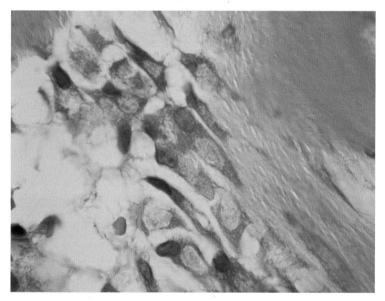

Fig. 1.47 Trephine biopsy sections showing normal osteoblasts in the bone marrow of a child. Golgi zones are very clearly shown; the nuclei are oval and some contain a small nucleolus. Paraffin-embedded, H&E ×100.

Fat cells

Fat cells are almost always recognizable in bone marrow specimens, exceptions being found in very young infants and when the bone marrow is markedly hypercellular.

Cytology

Stromal fat cells are present mainly in aspirated fragments. Since the fat dissolves during processing the cytoplasm appears completely empty. In iso-lated fat cells (Fig. 1.49), an oval nucleus, either peripheral or central, is present within apparently empty cytoplasm.

Histology

In sections of bone marrow, the fat cells appear in clusters, separated by haemopoietic tissue. They are often particularly prominent adjacent to trabeculae. Fat cells appear as empty spaces with an oval nucleus at one edge of the cell.

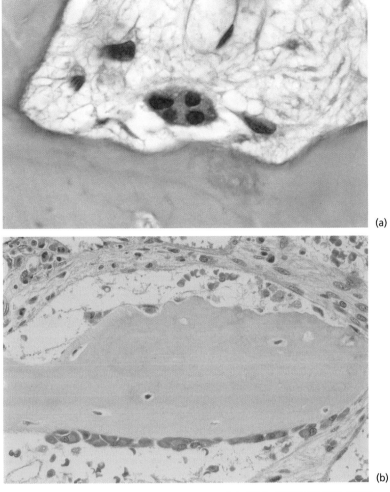

(a)

(b)

Fig. 1.48 (a) Section of BM from a patient with renal osteodystrophy: an osteoclast with four nuclei. Paraffin-embedded, H&E ×100. (b) Section of BM showing a bone spicule; one side is lined with osteoblasts while the other shows Howship's lacunae, two of which contain osteoclasts. Paraffin-embedded, H&E ×40.

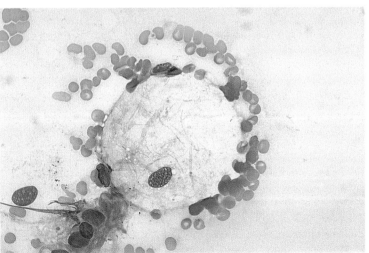

Fig. 1.49 BM aspirate showing a fat cell. MGG ×50.

Lymphopoiesis

Lymphocytes

Both B and T lymphocytes share a common origin with myeloid cells, all of these lineages being derived from a pluripotent stem cell. The bone marrow contains mature cells and precursor cells of both T- and B-lymphoid lineages. T cells are more numerous among mature cells whereas among precursor cells those of B lineage are more frequent.

Cytology

Bone marrow lymphocytes are small cells with a high nucleocytoplasmic ratio and scanty, weakly basophilic cytoplasm. The nuclei show some chromatin condensation but the chromatin often appears more diffuse than that of peripheral blood lymphocytes. Lymphocytes are not very numerous in the marrow in the first few days of life but otherwise during infancy they constitute a third to a half of bone marrow nucleated cells [38]. Numbers decline during childhood and in adults they do not generally comprise more than 15–25% of nucleated cells, unless the marrow aspirate has been considerably diluted with peripheral blood. If there is no haemodilution they usually account for approximately 10% of nucleated cells. The majority of lymphocytes in normal bone marrow are CD8-positive T lymphocytes.

The bone marrow of healthy children may show significant numbers of immature cells with a cytological resemblance to leukaemic lymphoblasts, referred to as haematogones (see pages 310–311); these are B-lymphocyte precursors.

Histology

Normal marrow contains scattered interstitial lymphocytes and, sometimes, small lymphoid nodules or follicles. Estimates of lymphocyte numbers based on histological sections are considerably lower than those based on aspirates. In one study approximately 10% of bone marrow cells were lymphocytes, with the ratio of T to B cells being 6:1 [39]. In another investigation of a small number of subjects, not all of whom were strictly normal, the T:B cell ratio was 4–5:1 [40]. In a third study, median numbers were of the order of 2%, representing approximately equal numbers of B and T

cells; the range of B cells, identified by CD20 reactivity, was 0% to 5.97%, while the range of T cells, identified by CD45R0 reactivity, was 0% to 6.7% [41]. In contrast to the peripheral blood, CD8-positive T lymphocytes are more numerous in the marrow than CD4-positive cells. Lymphocytes appear to concentrate around arterioles near the centre of the haemopoietic cords. Lymphoid follicles of normal marrow have small blood vessels at their centre and may contain a few macrophages, peripheral mast cells or plasma cells. Lymphoid follicles are discussed further on page 132.

Plasma cells

Cytology

Plasma cells (Fig. 1.50) are infrequent in normal bone marrow in which they rarely constitute more than 1% of nucleated cells. In healthy children they are even less frequent [42]. They are distinctive cells with a diameter of 15–20 μm and an eccentric nucleus, moderately basophilic cytoplasm and a prominent paranuclear Golgi zone. The cytoplasm may contain occasional vacuoles and sometimes stains pink with a May–Grünwald–Giemsa (MGG) stain, consequent on the presence of carbohydrate. The nuclear chromatin shows prominent coarse clumps, although the clock-face chromatin pattern that is often discernible in histological sections is usually less apparent in films. Occasional normal plasma cells have two or more nuclei. Plasma cells may occur in small clumps and may be detected within aspirated marrow fragments and around capillaries.

Histology

Normal marrow contains scattered interstitial plasma cells but plasma cells may also be associated with macrophages and are preferentially located around capillaries (Fig. 1.51). Typical mature plasma cells in histological sections are readily identified by their eccentric nuclei and prominent Golgi zones. The chromatin is coarsely clumped and often distributed at the periphery of the nucleus with clear spaces between the chromatin clumps, giving the appearance of a cartwheel or clock-face. In Giemsa-stained sections the cytoplasm, with the exception of the Golgi zone, is deeply basophilic.

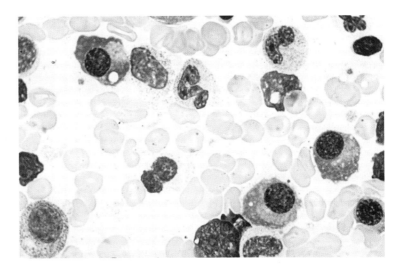

Fig. 1.50 Aspirate of BM from a patient with an inflammatory condition: three plasma cells; note the basophilic cytoplasm, eccentric nucleus and Golgi zone adjacent to the nucleus. MGG ×100.

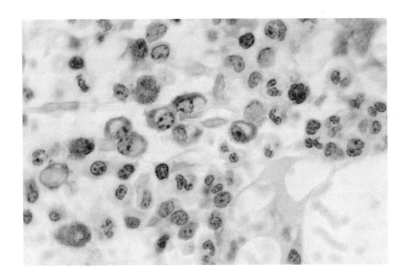

Fig. 1.51 Section of BM from patient with Hodgkin lymphoma (without marrow infiltration): pericapillary plasma cells, neutrophils, eosinophils and erythroblasts. Resin-embedded, Giemsa ×100.

The cellular composition of bone marrow

Cytology

The cellular composition of aspirated bone marrow is determined by the volume of the aspirate since the larger the volume aspirated the more sinusoidal blood is sucked into the aspirate. Dilution of marrow with blood leads to a higher percentage of lymphocytes and mature granulocytes and a lower percentage of granulocyte and erythroid precur-

sors. Dresch *et al.* [43] found, for example, that as the volume of aspirate from the sternum increased from 0.5 to 4.5 ml, the total concentration of nucleated cells fell to about one sixth; the percentage of granulocyte precursors (myeloblasts to metamyelocytes) declined from approximately 55% to approximately 30%, while the percentage of mature neutrophils showed a more than twofold rise. Ideally, a cell count should be performed on films prepared from the first one or two drops of aspirated marrow. If large volumes are required for further tests a second syringe can be applied to the needle after the syringe containing the first few drops has been removed. The differential count is then representative of the cellular composition of the bone marrow.

Determining the cellular composition of marrow requires that large numbers of cells be counted so that a reasonable degree of precision is achieved. This is particularly important when the cell of interest is one that is normally infrequent, such as the myeloblast or the plasma cell. A 500 cell count provides a reasonable compromise between what is desirable and what is practicable. The cell count should be performed in the trails behind fragments so that the cells counted represent cells that have come from fragments rather than contaminating peripheral blood cells. Alternatively, the cell count can be performed on squashed bone marrow fragments. Because some cells, for example plasma cells and lymphocytes, are distributed unevenly through the marrow it is important to count the trails behind several fragments or several squashed fragments. Because cells of different lineages may not be released from the fragments into the trails to the same extent there may not be good correlation between differential counts on wedge-spread films and squash preparations. It is likely that counts on the latter are more valid. However, counts are usually performed on wedge-spread films and hence published reference ranges are based on such counts.

It is customary and useful to determine the myeloid:erythroid (M:E) ratio of aspirated marrow since consideration of this value, together with an assessment of the overall cellularity, allows an assessment of whether erythropoiesis and granulopoiesis are reduced, normal or increased. It is simplest to include in the myeloid component all granulocytes and their precursors and any monocytes and their precursors. However, some haematologists exclude mature neutrophils and others include neutrophils but exclude eosinophils, basophils and monocytes. These inclusions and exclusions will make a slight difference to what is regarded as a normal M:E ratio but their effects are heavily outweighed by differences caused by different aspiration volumes. The larger the volume of the aspirate the higher the M:E ratio, particularly if mature neutrophils are included in the count.

The bone marrow at birth has major erythroid and myeloid components with few lymphocytes and very few plasma cells [38,42,44,45] (Fig. 1.52). The percentage of erythroid cells declines steeply in the first weeks [44,45]. The percentage of lymphocytes increases during the first month and remains at a high level until 18 months of age [38]. In children above the age of 2 years, the proportions of different cell types do not differ greatly from those in normal adult bone marrow. However, children may have increased numbers of immature lymphoid cells (see pages 310–311). Typical values determined for the cellular composition of normal marrow at various ages are shown in Tables 1.1 and 1.2 [29,38,44–50]. Bain [29] found a significantly higher proportion of granulocytes in the bone marrow of women than of men. This was not observed in a smaller cohort studied by den Ottolander [51].

The bone marrow of healthy volunteers shows a low proportion of cells with features that could be regarded as dysplastic, such as erythroid cells showing cytoplasmic bridging or megakaryocytes with non-lobulated nuclei [52]. Fernández-Ferrero and Ramos, studying haematologically normal surgical patients, found the frequency of these minor dysplastic features to increase with age [53].

Histology

It is possible to perform differential counts and estimate an M:E ratio from resin-embedded bone marrow biopsy sections [54,55] although this is rarely necessary in practice. Such counts have the potential to be more accurate than those obtained from aspirates since there is no dilution with sinusoidal blood. It is also possible that larger cells or cells adjacent to trabeculae might be less likely to be aspirated. However, an element of inaccuracy is introduced by the fact that larger cells appear at more levels of the biopsy and so are more likely to be counted in any given section. Lack of dilution by blood means that the estimated M:E ratio is likely to be lower than that determined from an aspirate. This is borne out by the results of a study of 13 healthy subjects which found a mean M:E ratio of 1.52 with a range of 1.36–1.61 [54].

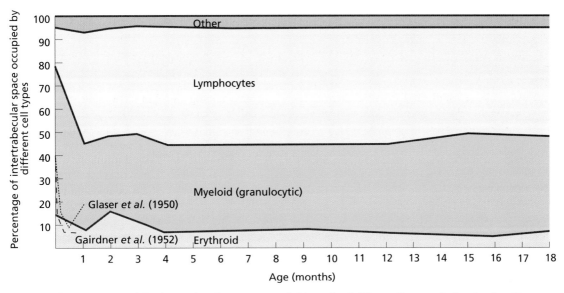

Fig. 1.52 The percentage of the intertrabecular space occupied by cells of different lineages during the first 18 months of life, derived from Rosse *et al.* [38]; the higher initial erythroid percentage and sharp fall in erythroblast number observed by Glaser *et al.* [44] and Gairdner *et al.* [45] are shown as dotted lines.

Interpretation of bone marrow aspirates and trephine biopsies

Examination of a bone marrow aspirate in isolation permits cytomorphological features to be ascertained but does not permit full interpretation of the findings. The haematologist must also know the age and sex of the patient, the full blood count and relevant clinical details, and must have examined a peripheral blood film. Similarly, examination of trephine biopsy sections in isolation permits detection of histomorphological abnormalities but not a full assessment of a case. The pathologist should beware of the risks of either over-interpreting biopsy findings or failing to offer an adequate interpretation because of lack of consideration of clinical and haematological features and aspirate findings. It is desirable that trephine biopsy specimens are either reported by a haematopathologist able also to interpret bone marrow aspirates or that the histopathologist and haematologist examine aspirate films and biopsy sections together. It should be appreciated that a trephine biopsy is just one part of a jigsaw puzzle and it may not always be possible to make a definitive diagnosis. Sometimes it is

desirable to seek a second opinion. When this is so, it is essential that the haematopathologist is sent full clinical and haematological information. Films of the peripheral blood and the bone marrow aspirate should accompany trephine biopsy specimens being sent for a second opinion, with all material being carefully labelled and dated.

Examination of bone marrow aspirate films

A minimum of three or four films should always be stained and examined. These should include a Perls′-stained film for all initial diagnostic aspirates. If there is a likelihood of infiltration of the marrow and the first films do not show any abnormality, it is important to stain and examine a larger number.

Bone marrow films should first be examined under low power (×10 objective) in order to assess cellularity and megakaryocyte numbers and to scan the entire film for any abnormal infiltrate. The film should then be examined with a ×40 or ×50 objective, which will allow appreciation of most morphological features. At this stage, all cell populations should be specifically and systematically examined from the point of view of both numbers and morphology – the erythroid lineage, granulocytic

Table 1.1 Mean values (observed range) for bone marrow cells in healthy infants and children.

	Birth [38] (n = 57)	0–24 hours [45] (n = 19)	8–10 days [44] (n = 23)	3 months [45] (n = 12)
M:E ratio	4.4	1.2	1.35	2.4
Myeloblasts (%)	0.3*	1.0 (0.5–2)	1.0 (0–3)	1.5 (0–4)
Promyelocytes (%)	0.8	1.5 (0.5–5)	2.0 (0.5–7)	2.0 (1.5–5)
Myelocytes (%)	4	4.0 (1–9)	4.0 (1–11)	5.0 (0.5–16)
Metamyelocytes (%)	19	14.0 (4.5–25)	18.0 (7–35)	11.0 (3–33)
Bands (%)	29 ⎫	22.0 (10–40)	20.0 (11–45)	15.0 (2–24)
Neutrophils (%)	7 ⎭			
Eosinophil series (%)	2.7	3.5 (1–8)†	3.0 (0–6)†	2.5 (0–6)†
Basophil series (%)	0.12	– (0–1.5)†	– (0–1)†	– (0–0.5)
Monocytes(%)	0.9	– (0–2.5)†	1.0 (0–3)	0.5 (0–1)
Erythroid (%)	14.5	39.5 (23.5–70)†	7.5 (0–20.5)†	16.0 (3.5–33.5)†
Lymphocytes (%)	15	12.0 (4–22)	37.0 (20–62)	47.0 (31–81)
Plasma cells (%)	0	0	0	0

E, erythroid; M, myeloid.
*'Unknown blasts'.
†Approximate (sum of ranges for different categories).

Table 1.2 Mean values (95% ranges) for bone marrow cells in sternal or iliac crest aspirates of healthy adult Caucasians.

	20–29 years [47] Males and females (n = 28), sternum	20–30 years [48] Males (n = 52), sternum	20–30 years [48] Females (n = 40), sternum
Volume aspirated (ml)	≤0.5	0.2	0.2
M:E ratio	3.34	–	–
Myeloblasts (%)	1.21 (0.75–1.67)	1.32 (0.2–2.5)	1.2 (0.1–2.3)
Promyelocytes (%)	2.49 (0.99–3.99)	1.35 (0–2.9)	1.65 (0.5–2.8)
Myelocytes (%)	17.36 (11.54–23.18)	15.0 (7.5–22.5)	16.6 (11.4–21.8)
Metamyelocytes (%)	16.92 (11.4–22.44)	15.7 (9.2–22)	15.8 (11.0–20.6)
Band cells (%)	8.70 (3.58–13.82)	10.5 (3–17.9)	8.3 (4–12.4)
Neutrophils (%)	13.42 (4.32–22.52)	20.9 (9.9–31.8)	21.7 (11.3–32)
Eosinophils (%)	2.93 (0.28–5.69)*	2.8 (0.1–5.6)*	3 (0–7.2)*
Basophils (%)	0.28 (0–0.69)*	0.14 (0–0.38)	0.16 (0–0.46)
Monocytes (%)	1.04 (0.36–1.72)	2.3 (0.5–4)	1.61 (0.2–3)
Erythroblasts (%)	19.26 (9.12–29.4)†	12.9 (4.1–21.7)	11.5 (5.1–17.9)
Lymphocytes (%)	14.60 (6.66–22.54)	16.8 (7.2–26.3)	18.1 (10.5–25.7)
Plasma cells (%)	0.46 (0–0.96)	0.39 (0–1.1)	0.42 (0–0.9)

E, erythroid; M, myeloid.
*Including eosinophil and basophil myelocytes and metamyelocytes.
†Approximate (sum of ranges for different categories of erythroblast).
‡Promyelocytes were categorized either with myeloblasts or with myelocytes.
§Neutrophils plus precursors : erythroblasts.
‖Including basophil precursors and mast cells.
¶Neutrophil plus eosinophil myelocytes: mean and range: 8.9 (2.14–15.3); band cells included in neutrophil category; macrophages: mean and range: 0.4 (0–1.3).

Table 1.1 (continued)

3 months [38] (n = 24)	1 year [38] (n = 12)	18 months [38] (n = 19)	2–6 years [46] (n = 12)	2–9 years [47] (n = 13)
4.9	4.8	5	5.8 (2–13)	5.3
0.6*	0.5*	0.4*	1.0	1.3 (0.7–1.8)
0.8	0.7	0.6	0.5	2.8 (0.8–4.8)
2	2	2.5	17	26.7 (18–35)†
12	11	12	20	22.0 (15.7–29)
15	14	14	11	4.5 (0.9–8)
3.5	6	6	10	8.3 (2.6–14)
2.5	2	3	6	1.2 (0–2.5)
0.1	0.1	0.1	–	0
0.7	1.5	2	0.4	0
12	8	8	13	12.5 (9.5–22.3)†
44	49	46	21	18.2 (8.5–28)
0	0.03	0.06	–	0.13 (0.05–0.41)

Table 1.2 (continued)

17–45 years [49] Males (n = 42) and females (n = 8), sternum	Age not stated [50] Males (n = 12), sternum	21–56 years [29] Males (n = 30) and females (n = 20), iliac crest	Age not stated [51] Males (n = 53) and females (n = 14), site not stated
3	–	0.1–0.2	–
6.9	2.3 (1.1–3.5)§	2.4 (1.4–3.6)	2.2 (0.8–3.6)
1.3 (0–3)	0.9 (0.1–1.7)	1.4 (0–3)	0.4 (0–1.3)
–‡	3.3 (1.9–4.7)	7.8 (3.2–12.4)	13.7 (8–19.4)
8.9 (3–15)	12.7 (8.5–16.9)	7.6 (1.9–13.3)¶	
8.8 (4–15)	15.9 (7.1–24.7)	4.1 (2.3–5.9)	
23.9 (12.5–33.5)	12.4 (9.4–15.4)	–	35.5 (22.2–48.8)
18.5 (9–31.5)	7.4 (3.8–11)	34.2 (23.4–45)¶	
1.9 (0–5.5)	3.1 (1.1–5.2)*	2.2 (0.3–4.2)	1.7 (0.2–3.3)
0.2 (0–1)	<0.1 (0–0.2)‖	0.1 (0–0.4)	0.2 (0–0.6)
2.4 (0–6)	0.3 (0–0.6)	1.3 (0–2.6)	2.5 (0.5–4.6)
9.5 (2.5–17.5)	25.6 (15–36.2)	25.9 (13.6–38.2)	23.6 (14.7–32.6)
16.2 (7.5–26.5)	16.2 (8.6–23.8)	13.1 (6–20)	16.1 (6.0–26.2)
0.3 (0–1.5)	1.3 (0–3.5)	0.6 (0–1.2)	1.9 (0–3.8)

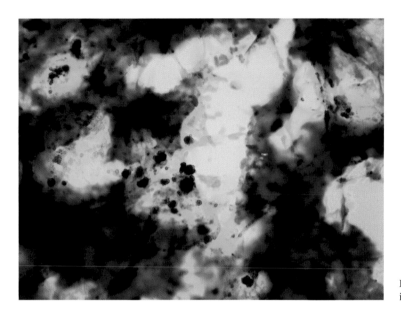

Fig. 1.53 BM aspirate showing increased haemosiderin. MGG ×50.

lineages including eosinophils and basophils, megakaryocytes, lymphocytes and plasma cells. Consideration should be given to whether there is an increased number of mast cells, macrophages, osteoblasts or osteoclasts and whether any non-haemopoietic cells are present. Fragments should be examined not only to assess cellularity but also to determine if any cells have been preferentially retained in the fragments, e.g. mast cells or myeloma cells. Increased storage iron can also sometimes be detected in fragments stained by MGG, haemosiderin having a greenish tinge (Fig. 1.53). Only when a thorough assessment of several films has been carried out with a ×40 or ×50 objective should the film be examined under high power (×100) with oil immersion in order to assess fine cytological detail. A differential count of cells in the trails behind several fragments is best carried out under high power but only after assessment of whether there is any increase of minority populations, for example blast cells or plasma cells, confined to one film or to the cell trail behind one fragment. It can be useful to have an oil immersion ×50 or ×60 objective as well as a ×100 as it is then easy to switch between lenses for an overall and more detailed view of the same area. Perls-stained films should similarly be examined under low power to assess storage iron, with a ×40 or ×50

objective to detect abnormally prominent siderotic granulation and with a ×100 objective to assess whether siderotic granulation is reduced, normal or increased.

Films of squashed bone marrow fragments should similarly be examined in a systematic manner.

Reporting a bone marrow aspirate

The report of a bone marrow aspirate should commence with the clinical details given to the haematologist and a record of the full blood count and peripheral blood film appearances at the time of bone marrow aspiration. There should then be a statement as to the site of aspiration, the texture of the bone and the ease of aspiration. The aspirate report should include an assessment of overall cellularity, an M:E ratio and a description of each lineage. Storage iron in fragments and siderotic granules in cells should be described. If a trephine biopsy was performed this should be stated and, if a trephine biopsy would normally have been expected but was not performed or was unsuccessful, this should also be included in the report. Any supplementary tests for which samples were taken, for example immunophenotyping, cytogenetic analysis or molecular genetic analysis, should be listed so that the clinician is aware that other results are to be expected. Finally, a brief summary of significant findings should be made and an interpretation offered, bearing in mind that this might be the only part of the report read by some clinicians. Reports should distinguish between factual statements and opinions. The description of the aspirate should be purely factual whereas it is useful for the final summary to include an explanation of the significance of the findings and, when relevant, suggestions for further tests. The level of certainty of any opinion should be expressed by careful use of terms such as 'diagnostic of', 'suggestive of' or 'consistent with'. If an attempted aspirate fails or there is a 'dry tap' a report should be issued stating this. The report should be signed or computer-authorized by the haematologist or haematopathologist responsible for it.

Examination of trephine biopsy sections

The interpretation of trephine biopsy sections is often viewed as one of the more difficult areas of surgical pathology. This is probably because the organized structure of haemopoietic tissue is not as readily apparent as that of many other tissues. However, as the preceding part of this chapter illustrates, the bone marrow is actually highly organized, with the various elements maturing in different micro-anatomical sites. Failure to recognize this and failure to identify individual categories of cell may lead to a lack of systematic analysis, with diagnoses being made only by a process of pattern recognition. Conversely, the haematologist, although experienced in cytology, may be unfamiliar with the interpretation of tissue sections, in which architectural features are often of prime importance.

A systematic approach, which is essential for accurate diagnosis, requires a working knowledge of the normal micro-anatomy and the pathological changes that may occur, coupled with a methodical examination of the various component parts. Initially, the whole section should be examined at low power, preferably using a ×4 objective. This allows a general impression of the biopsy specimen to be gained, including overall cellularity and megakaryocyte number and distribution. Abnormalities of the bone are often apparent at this magnification. It should also be noted if the biopsy specimen is too small, or is composed largely of cortical bone

and subcortical marrow, or shows crush artefact or other artefactual distortion of the architecture. Focal lesions, such as granulomas or infiltrates of metastatic tumour or lymphoma, are often better appreciated on low power examination. Following this, the bone, haemopoietic elements and marrow stromal elements should be studied using medium power (×10 or ×20 objective) and a high power dry objective (×40 or ×60); examination under oil immersion (×100 objective) is not necessary as a routine but is often useful to study fine cytological detail. The bone should be examined for trabecular thickness, number of osteoblasts and osteoclasts, and presence and number of Howship's lacunae; undecalcified resin-embedded sections should be assessed for the quantity of osteoid (see Chapter 11). With a little experience, visual estimations of the marrow cellularity, of the relative amounts of granulocytic and erythroid elements, and of any deviations from normal can easily be made. The next step is to examine the various haemopoietic elements for the following features:

1 *Erythroid series*: the proportion of erythroid cells and relative proportions of cells at different stages of maturation; presence, appearance and location of erythroblastic islands; morphology of erythroblasts including any evidence of dyserythropoiesis.

2 *Granulocytic series*: the proportion of granulocytic cells (eosinophil and neutrophil lineages); morphology and relative proportions of immature and mature granulocytic precursors; position of immature precursors (promyelocytes and myeloblasts); morphology of granulocytic cells.

3 *Megakaryocytes*: number of megakaryocytes; megakaryocyte morphology (cell size and nuclear features) and localization; presence or absence of megakaryocyte clusters.

4 *Lymphoid cells*: number, localization and morphology of lymphocytes; presence, position and morphology of lymphoid aggregates; number, localization and morphology of plasma cells.

5 *Macrophages and mast cells*: number of macrophages; presence of haemophagocytosis; intracellular microorganisms (usually fungi or protozoa); evidence of lysosomal storage disorders such as Gaucher's disease; granulomas; mast cell numbers, morphology and localization.

It is easy to neglect the stromal elements, yet these are disturbed in a variety of conditions.

Important changes that should be noted include: oedema; gelatinous change; necrosis; fibrosis; ectasia of sinusoids; vasculitis; amyloid deposition; and bone abnormalities.

A stain for reticulin should be examined in every case. In some laboratories an iron stain is examined in all cases but this is not the policy in the authors' laboratories. Choice of further histochemical or immunohistochemical stains is dependent on clinical features and histological findings.

Obviously, in many cases, as when there is heavy infiltration by leukaemic cells or metastatic carcinoma, the above scheme is modified.

Reporting trephine biopsy sections

The trephine biopsy report [56] should include a statement as to the length of the biopsy specimen and its integrity. The report of the microscopic appearance should describe the cellularity and any abnormalities in bone, stroma or haemopoietic tissue. The reticulin stain and, if performed, the iron stain should be described. In sections from a resin-embedded specimen, iron stores should be graded; with a decalcified biopsy specimen an assessment should be made as to whether stainable iron is absent, present or increased but further grading should not be attempted (see pages 57–60). Any other histochemical or immunohistochemical stains should be described. In describing the results of immunohistochemistry, antibodies with a CD designation should be identified by the appropriate CD number.

Following a description of biopsy histology, a conclusion should be given in which all relevant findings are summarized and interpreted (as for the bone marrow aspirate, bearing in mind that many clinical staff will read only the summary). The level of certainty of any opinion should be expressed by careful use of terms such as 'diagnostic of', 'suggestive of' or 'consistent with'. If the report is provisional, either because further investigations are pending or because a second opinion is being sought, this should be stated clearly in the concluding summary. The report must be signed or computer-authorized by the responsible pathologist or haematologist.

Guidelines, integrated reporting and audit

Guidelines for best practice in performing, processing and reporting bone marrow aspirates and tre-

phine biopsies have been published [57,58]. If sedation is employed, guidelines for safe practice should be followed [4].

Optimal practice dictates that, for haematological neoplasms, an integrated final report should be assembled. This should include the results of all tests performed on a bone marrow aspirate and trephine biopsy specimen, interpreted in the context of full clinical and haematological information. When appropriate, results of peripheral blood analyses (e.g. clonality studies, immunophenotyping, molecular analysis, human T-cell lymphotropic virus I (HTLV-I) serology) should also be included. For the National Health Service in England and Wales, this advice is included in a guideline from the National Institute for Clinical Excellence, *Improving Outcomes Guidance for Haematological Cancers* [59]. Ideally, information technology systems should facilitate the development of integrated reports.

Periodic audit of clinical and laboratory procedures is advised and national schemes to document morbidity and mortality are recommended.

Artefacts

Various artefacts in bone marrow aspirates and trephine biopsy specimens need to be recognized so that they are not misinterpreted as evidence of disease. Artefacts are of three main types: (i) introduced by the biopsy process or by processing in the laboratory; (ii) consequent on extraneous material or tissue being included in the biopsy; and (iii) resulting from previous tissue damage at the biopsy site. The latter group are not, strictly speaking, artefacts since what is observed are real changes in the tissues. Nevertheless, they are potentially misleading in the same way as artefacts and will therefore be considered here.

Cytology

If bone marrow is anticoagulated in EDTA and if delay then occurs in making films, storage artefacts can develop and can simulate dyserythropoiesis [60]. Such features may include nuclear lobulation and fragmentation and cytoplasmic vacuolation. Processing artefacts can be induced in bone marrow aspirates by inadequate drying of the film, poor fixation or prolonged storage of the film prior to

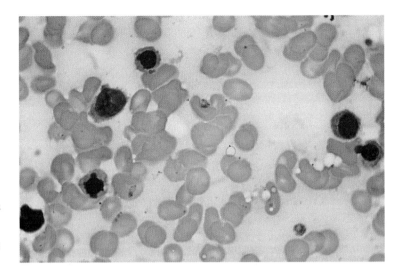

Fig. 1.54 BM aspirate showing the effect of fixing and staining the film before adequate drying has occurred; the erythroblast nuclear content appears to have leaked into the cytoplasm. MGG ×100.

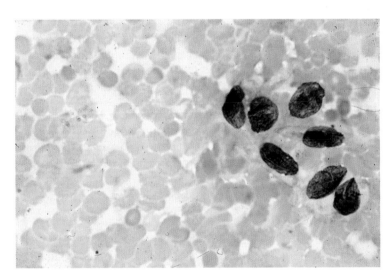

Fig. 1.55 Vena cava scraping showing endothelial cells; similar cells are occasionally observed in BM aspirates. MGG ×100. (By courtesy of Dr Marjorie Walker, London.)

fixation and staining. If slides are fixed before they have dried adequately there is an appearance suggesting that nuclear contents are leaking into the cytoplasm and cellular outline is indistinct (Fig. 1.54). Water uptake into methanol used in fixation causes refractile 'inclusions' in red cells and poor definition of cellular details. Delayed fixation and staining of archival bone marrow slides usually leads to a strong blue or turquoise tint to the film; this can be avoided by fixing slides prior to storage although this limits their subsequent uses.

If an aspirate is partly clotted, small bone marrow clots may be mistaken for bone marrow particles, leading to a mistaken attempt to assess cellularity or the presence or absence of storage iron in the clot. The presence of fibrin strands and the lack of any organized structure of the apparent particle is a clue to its true nature. In patients with essential thrombocythaemia, solid clumps of large numbers of platelets can also be mistaken for bone marrow fragments.

Extraneous non-haemopoietic cells that may appear in bone marrow aspirates include endothelial cells (Fig. 1.55) and epithelial cells (Fig. 1.56). Endothelial cells may appear in masses and be pleomorphic. It is important that they are not confused with tumour cells. They have weakly basophilic cytoplasm and oval nuclei, which appear grooved.

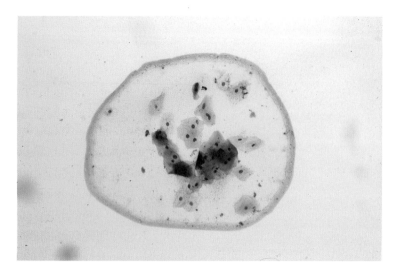

Fig. 1.56 BM aspirate, epithelial cells. MGG ×10.

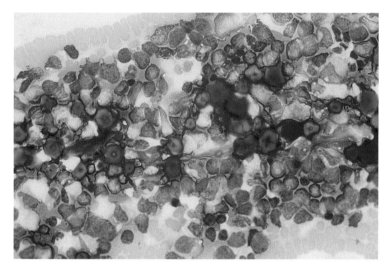

Fig. 1.57 Crystals of glove powder in a BM aspirate. MGG ×40.

Epithelial cells, both nucleated and anuclear, are more readily recognized by their voluminous, opaque, powder-blue cytoplasm. Extraneous material that may appear in bone marrow aspirate films includes crystals of glove powder. These are blue with an MGG stain (Fig. 1.57) and red with a PAS stain.

Abnormalities in bone marrow aspirates may result from a previous biopsy performed at the same site a short time before. Increased numbers of macrophages, including foamy macrophages, can be found. The scars of previous biopsies are usually apparent and repeat biopsies should be carried out from the other side of the pelvis or a centimetre or so away from any recent biopsy on the same side. It should also be noted that, if the pelvis has previously been irradiated, biopsies will show bone marrow hypoplasia or aplasia which is not indicative of the appearance of the bone marrow at other sites. Biopsy of previously irradiated bone marrow should therefore generally be avoided.

If imprints are made from trephine biopsy specimens containing cartilage, for example in children, there may be deposition of purple granular material in the imprint [61].

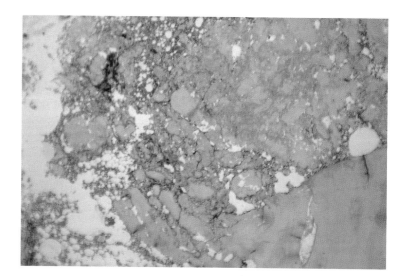

Fig. 1.58 BM trephine biopsy section, crushed bone. Paraffin-embedded, H&E ×20.

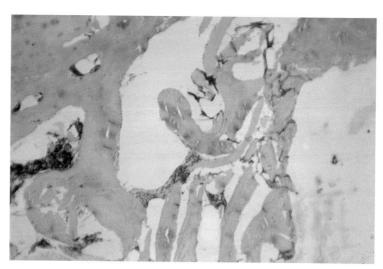

Fig. 1.59 BM trephine biopsy section showing apparently empty intertrabecular spaces consequent on squeezing of the biopsy specimen. Paraffin-embedded, H&E ×10.

Histology

A trephine biopsy specimen that is too short or a biopsy that is performed at the wrong angle may mean that the specimen includes only subcortical bone, which is often markedly hypocellular. This can create a mistaken impression of aplastic anaemia. Performing a biopsy and processing the specimen can induce crumbling of bone to amorphous material (Fig. 1.58), or bone marrow tissue may be absent from the intertrabecular spaces (Fig. 1.59). The latter artefact may be related to the use of blunt needles since it does not appear to be a problem with disposable needles. Torsion artefact

(Fig. 1.60) is common. The elongated nuclei that are produced by twisting should not be confused with the nuclei of fibroblasts. Usually, twisted bone marrow is not interpretable but sometimes it is possible to recognize neoplastic cells, e.g. myeloma cells or carcinoma cells, despite the artefact.

Artefacts can be introduced during fixation. If formol-saline is used as a fixative, it is necessary to allow at least 18 hours for fixation. If more rapid fixation is required then a protein precipitant formulation should be used. Poor fixation leads to glassy nuclei in which detailed structure cannot be recognized (Fig. 1.61). Poor fixation is aggravated

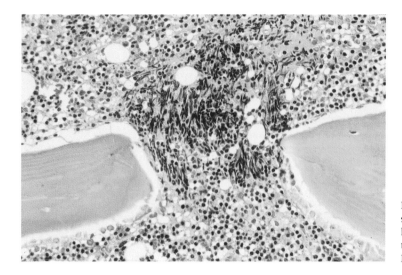

Fig. 1.60 BM trephine biopsy section from a patient with chronic lymphocytic leukaemia showing torsion artefact. Paraffin-embedded, H&E ×20.

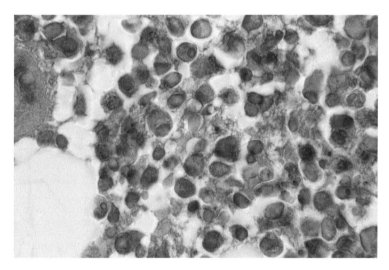

Fig. 1.61 BM trephine biopsy section showing nuclei which appear glassy and homogeneous as a consequence of fixation artefact. Paraffin-embedded, H&E ×100.

by the use of strong decalcifying agents. Often it is impossible to give any reliable interpretation of a poorly fixed marrow. Another fixation-related problem is deposition of formalin pigment. Formalin pigment is blackish-brown and should be distinguished from haemosiderin, which is golden brown (Fig. 1.62). If biopsy specimens are fixed in mercury-based fixatives, such as B5, inadequate washing may lead to cells being obscured by a precipitate [62]; however, it should be noted that in many counties mercury-based fixatives are prohibited on environmental and safety grounds.

Both excessive and inadequate decalcification can lead to artefactual changes. Excessive decalci-

fication leads to loss of cellular detail (particularly nuclear detail) and poor uptake of haematoxylin. Inadequate decalcification leads to the presence of a central core of undecalcified bone in the centre of bony spicules. This makes it difficult to produce high quality thin sections and the sections tend to tear.

Artefacts induced during processing are most often a problem in paraffin-embedded tissue. Some degree of shrinkage artefact is usual. This is most apparent with erythroblasts for which the halo that surrounds the nucleus can be an aid to identification. Shrinkage artefact also leads to megakaryocytes appearing within large empty spaces (Fig.

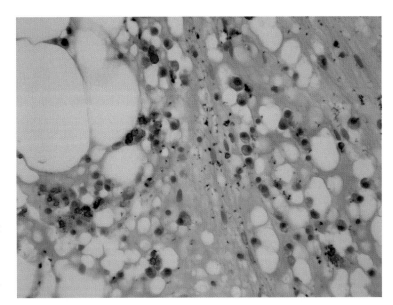

Fig. 1.62 BM section from a patient with multiple myeloma showing both increased haemosiderin (golden brown) and formalin pigment (black). Paraffin-embedded, H&E ×50.

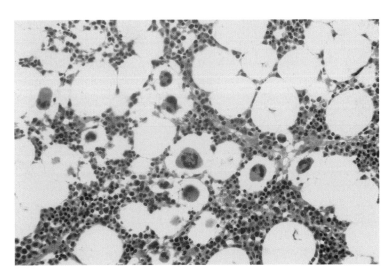

Fig. 1.63 BM trephine biopsy section showing megakaryocytes surrounded by an empty space as a consequence of shrinkage artefact. Paraffin-embedded, H&E ×40.

1.63). The use of a blunt knife can lead to tearing of sections or to the sections appearing banded (Fig. 1.64). Bony trabeculae may be lost during processing leaving gaps in the section (Fig. 1.65).

Artefactual inclusion of extraneous tissue in the biopsy specimen is not uncommon. Trephine biopsy samples, particularly from children, may include cartilage (Fig. 1.66). Pieces of skin (Fig. 1.67), adipose tissue, striated muscle (Fig. 1.68), hair follicles (Fig. 1.69) and sweat glands (Figs 1.69 and 1.70) can be introduced into the biopsy specimen during the biopsy process. Occasionally syn-

ovium (Fig. 1.71), or even a gouty tophus (Fig. 1.72), is included in the specimen. Other extraneous material can be transferred from the blade used in cutting sections and can be embedded with the bone marrow biopsy specimen (Fig. 1.73). Tissue from other biopsy specimens can contaminate the water bath in which sections are floated prior to mounting on glass slides. Such tissue may adhere to the trephine biopsy specimen or to the glass slide adjacent to the section, and may thus appear to represent part of the trephine biopsy specimen. Sometimes the abnormal tissue that is

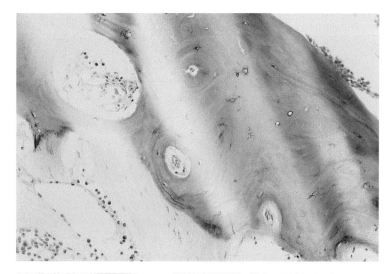

Fig. 1.64 BM trephine biopsy specimen showing an artefact caused by using a blunt knife. Paraffin-embedded, H&E ×40.

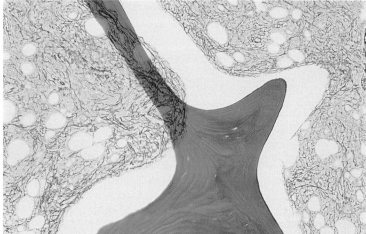

Fig. 1.65 BM trephine biopsy specimen showing displacement of bony trabeculae; if trabeculae are completely displaced confusion with dilated sinusoids can occur. Paraffin-embedded, reticulin stain ×10.

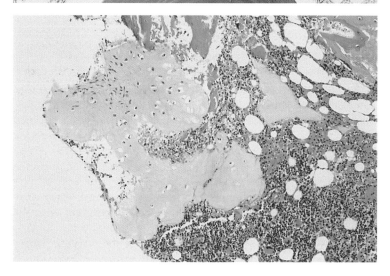

Fig. 1.66 An inclusion of paediatric cartilage in a trephine biopsy specimen. Paraffin-embedded, H&E ×20.

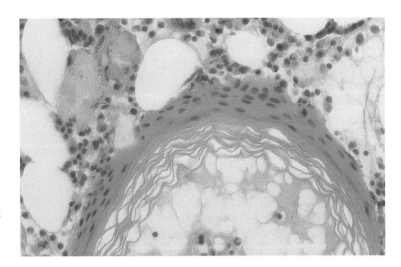

Fig. 1.67 BM trephine biopsy showing a piece of epidermis which has been driven into the biopsy specimen. Paraffin-embedded, H&E ×50.

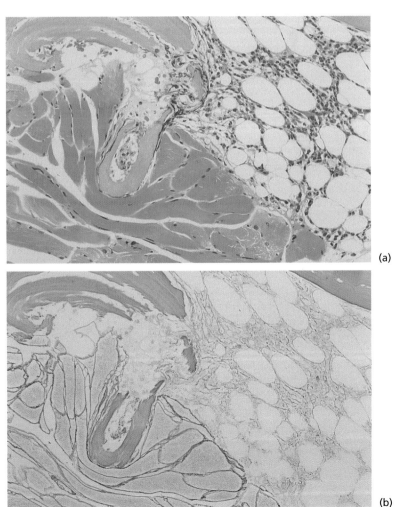

(a)

(b)

Fig. 1.68 Trephine biopsy showing striated muscle which has been driven into the biopsy specimen.
(a) Paraffin-embedded, H&E ×40.
(b) Paraffin-embedded, reticulin stain ×40.

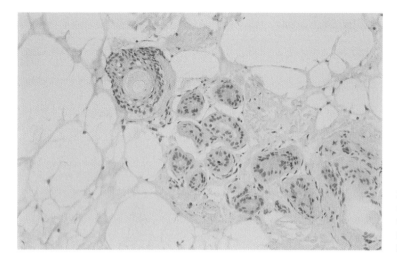

Fig. 1.69 A hair follicle and ducts of a sweat gland which have been driven into a trephine biopsy specimen. Paraffin-embedded, H&E ×10.

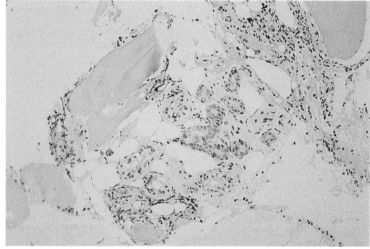

(a)

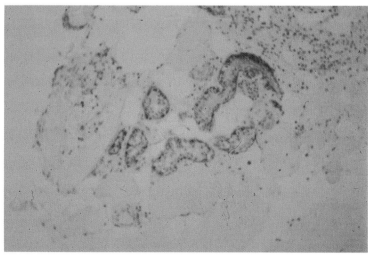

(b)

Fig. 1.70 BM trephine biopsy showing sweat glands which have been driven into the biopsy. (a) Paraffin-embedded, Giemsa ×10. (b) Immunohistochemistry with an antibody to smooth muscle actin demonstrating the myoepithelial cells of the sweat gland. Paraffin-embedded, immunoperoxidase ×10.

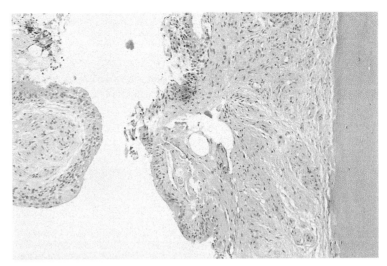

Fig. 1.71 Section of BM trephine biopsy specimen showing synovium on the periosteal surface of cortical bone. Paraffin-embedded, H&E ×10.

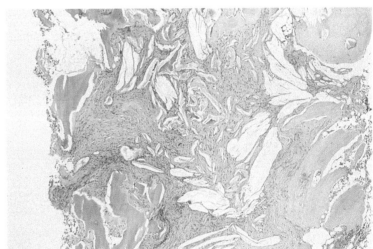

Fig. 1.72 Section of trephine biopsy specimen showing a gouty tophus which has been driven into the bone marrow; the empty spaces represent areas where uric acid has been removed during processing. Paraffin-embedded, H&E ×10.

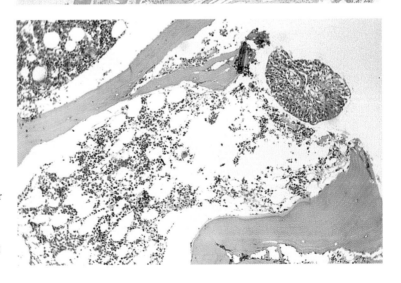

Fig. 1.73 BM trephine biopsy specimen showing dysplastic bladder epithelium which has been embedded with the biopsy as a result of contamination during processing. Paraffin-embedded, H&E ×10.

inadvertently included is dysplastic or neoplastic. Examination of reticulin stains can be helpful if there is doubt as to whether or not abnormal tissue is an intrinsic part of the biopsy specimen. If foreign tissue has been transferred with a knife, it will not be present if repeat sections are cut. However, sometimes extraneous tissue that was floating in a solvent solution is actually included in the block and will therefore also be present in repeat sections. Histopathology laboratories need good practices for dealing with small friable biopsy specimens to avoid this problem and both haematologists and histopathologists must be aware of this potential problem. In a last resort the unexplained tissue can

be dug out of the block and human leucocyte antigen (HLA) typed against the trephine biopsy specimen or any other candidate specimen to establish its true origin.

Artefacts can be induced by a previous aspiration or trephine biopsy at the same site. A bone marrow aspiration performed immediately before a trephine biopsy usually causes haemorrhage, disruption of the tissue and loss of haemopoietic cells. Occasionally the actual track of the aspiration needle is apparent (Fig. 1.74). This artefact can be avoided if the aspiration and trephine biopsy needles are introduced several millimetres apart and angled somewhat differently. This can be done

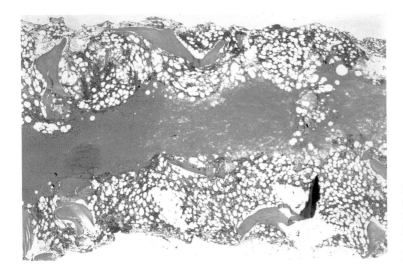

Fig. 1.74 BM trephine biopsy specimen showing a needle track from a bone marrow aspiration performed immediately before the trephine biopsy. Paraffin-embedded, H&E ×4.

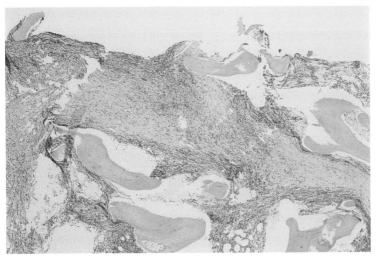

Fig. 1.75 BM trephine biopsy specimen showing a linear scar resulting from damage by a previous biopsy at the same site. Paraffin-embedded, H&E ×5.

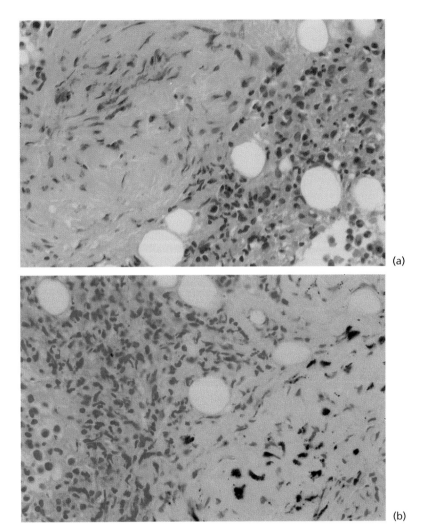

(a)

(b)

Fig. 1.76 Section of BM trephine biopsy specimen from an intravenous drug abuser with Hodgkin lymphoma showing a bone marrow scar; there is deposition of haemosiderin in the scar. (a) Paraffin-embedded, H&E ×40. (b) Paraffin-embedded, Perls' stain ×40.

even if they are inserted through the same skin incision. A biopsy performed some time previously may lead to the pathological specimen showing fat necrosis, with focal collections of foamy macrophages, or granulation tissue. A biopsy performed inadvertently at the site of a healing fracture produces a similar histological picture. There is initially granulation tissue, increased reticulin deposition and new bone formation; this can be confused with myelofibrosis [63]. Subsequently, granulation tissue is usually replaced by adipose tissue in which islands of haemopoietic cells develop. A trephine

biopsy (Fig 1.75) or other localized bone marrow damage (Fig 1.76) can result in a biopsy specimen showing a scar which, in the case of a previous trephine biopsy, may be linear. Scars should not be confused with fibrosis resulting from other pathological processes.

References

1 Hashimoto M (1962) Pathology of bone marrow. *Acta Haematol (Basel)*, **27**, 193–216.

2 de Bruyn PPH (1981) Structural substrates of bone marrow function. *Semin Hematol*, **18**, 179–193.

3 Wickramasinghe SN (1975) *Human Bone Marrow*. Blackwell Scientific Publications, Oxford.

4 Barlow D, Bell GD, Chalmers AH, Charlton JE, Halligan A, Hayward R et al. (2001) *Implementing and Ensuring Safe Sedation Practice for Healthcare Procedures in Adults*. Report of an Intercollegiate Working Party chaired by the Royal College of Anaesthetists.

5 Bennike T, Gormsen H and Moller B (1956) Comparative studies of bone marrow punctures of the sternum, the iliac crest, and the spinous process. *Acta Med Scand*, **155**, 377–396.

6 Humphries J (1990) Dry tap bone marrow aspiration: clinical significance. *Am J Hematol*, **35**, 247–250.

7 Islam A (2007) Bone marrow aspiration before bone marrow core biopsy using the same bone marrow biopsy needle: a good or bad practice? *J Clin Pathol*, **60**, 212–215.

8 James LP, Stass SA and Schumacher HR (1980) Value of imprint preparations of bone marrow biopsies in hematologic diagnosis. *Cancer*, **46**, 173–177.

9 Aboul-Nasr R, Estey EH, Kantarjian HM, Freireich EJ, Andreeff M, Johnson BJ and Albitar M (1999) Comparison of touch imprints with aspirate smears for evaluating bone marrow specimens. *Am J Clin Pathol*, **111**, 753–758.

10 Marti J, Antón E and Valent C (2004) Complications of bone marrow biopsy. *Br J Haematol*, **124**, 557–558.

11 Bain BJ (2003) Bone marrow biopsy morbidity and mortality. *Br J Haematol*, **121**, 949–951.

12 Gupta S, Meyers ML, Trambert J and Billett HH (1992) Massive intra-abdominal bleeding complicating bone marrow aspiration and biopsy in multiple myeloma. *Postgrad Med J*, **68**, 770.

13 Salem P, Wolverson MK, Reimers HJ and Kudva GC (2003) Complications of bone marrow biopsy. *Br J Haematol*, **121**, 821.

14 Le Dieu R, Luckit J and Sundarasun M (2003) Complications of trephine biopsy. *Br J Haematol*, **121**, 822.

15 Stellon A, Davies A and Williams R (1985) Avulsion of the anterior superior iliac spine complicating bone biopsy. *Postgrad Med J*, **61**, 625–626.

16 Williams NP and Ford GA (1986) Pneumoretroperitoneum following iliac crest trephine. *Br J Radiol*, **59**, 935–937.

17 Kansara G, Hussain M and Dimauro J (1989) A case of plasmacytoma in muscle as a complication of needle track seeding after percutaneous bone marrow biopsy. *Am J Clin Pathol*, **91**, 604–606.

18 Fowler N, Asatiani E and Cheson B (2008) Needle track seeding after bone marrow biopsy in non-Hodgkin lymphoma. *Leuk Lymphoma*, **49**, 156–158.

19 Bain BJ (2004) Bone marrow biopsy morbidity – report of 2003. *Clin Lab Haematol*, **26**, 315–318.

20 Murphy WA (1977) Exostosis after iliac bone marrow biopsy. *Am J Roentgenol*, **129**, 1114–1115.

21 Kerndrup G, Pallesen G, Melsen F and Mosekilde L (1980) Histomorphometric determination of bone marrow cellularity in iliac crest biopsies. *Scand J Haematol*, **24**, 110–114.

22 Al-Adhadh AN and Cavill I (1983) Assessment of cellularity in bone marrow fragments. *J Clin Pathol*, **36**, 176–179.

23 Frisch B, Lewis SM, Burkhardt R and Bartl R (1985) *Biopsy Pathology of Bone and Marrow*. Chapman & Hall, London.

24 Hartsock RJ, Smith EB and Petty CS (1965) Normal variations with ageing of the amount of hematopoietic tissue in bone marrow from the anterior iliac crest; a study made from 177 cases of sudden death examined by necropsy. *Am J Clin Pathol*, **43**, 326–331.

25 Meunier P, Aaron J, Edouard C and Vignon G (1971) Osteoporosis and the replacement of cell populations of the marrow by adipose tissue. *Clin Orthopaed*, **80**, 147–154.

26 Courpron P, Meunier P, Edouard C, Bernard J, Bringuier J-P and Vignon G (1973) Données histologiques quantitatives sur le vieillissement osseux humain. *Rev Rhum*, **40**, 469–482.

27 Bryon PA, Gentilhomme O and Fiere D (1979) Étude histologique quantitative du volume et de l'hétérogénéité des adipocytes dans les insuffisance myéloïdes globales. *Pathol Biol*, **27**, 209–213.

28 Bessis M (1958) L'Îlot érythroblastique, unité fonctionelle de la moelle osseuse. *Rev Hematol*, **13**, 8–11.

29 Bain BJ (1996) The bone marrow aspirate in healthy subjects. *Br J Haematol*, **94**, 206–209.

30 Mohandas N and Prenant M (1978) Three-dimensional model of bone marrow. *Blood*, **51**, 633–643.

31 Ravid K, Lu J, Zimmet JM and Jones MR (2002) Roads to polyploidy; the megakaryocyte example. *J Cell Physiol*. **190**, 7–20.

32 Queisser U, Queisser W and Spiertz B (1971) Polyploidization of megakaryocytes in normal humans and patients with idiopathic thrombocytopenia and with pernicious anaemia. *Br J Haematol*, **20**, 489–501.

33 Deutch VR and Tomer A (2006) Megakaryocyte development and platelet production. *Br J Haematol*, **134**, 453–466.

34 Tavassoli M and Aoki M (1989) Localization of megakaryocytes in the bone marrow. *Blood Cells*, **15**, 3–14.

35 Thiele J and Fischer R (1991) Megakaryocytopoiesis in human disorders: diagnostic features of bone marrow biopsies. An overview. *Virchows Archiv (A)*, **418**, 87–97.

36 Johnstone JM (1954) The appearance and significance of tissue mast cells in the human bone marrow. *J Clin Pathol*, **7**, 275–280.

37 Frisch B and Bartl R (1999) *Biopsy Interpretation of Bone and Bone Marrow: Histology and immunohistology in paraffin and plastic*, 2nd edn. Arnold, London.

38 Rosse C, Kraemer MJ, Dillon TL, McFarland R and Smith NJ (1977) Bone marrow cell populations of normal infants: the predominance of lymphocytes. *J Lab Clin Med*, **89**, 1225–1240.

39 Thaler J, Greil R, Dietze O and Huber H (1989) Immunohistology for quantification of normal bone marrow lymphocyte subsets. *Br J Haematol*, **73**, 576–577.

40 Horny H-P, Wehrmann M, Griesser H, Tiemann M, Bultmann B and Kaiserling E (1993) Investigation of bone marrow lymphocyte subsets in normal, reactive, and neoplastic states using paraffin-embedded biopsy specimens. *Am J Clin Pathol*, **99**, 142–149.

41 O'Donnell LR. Alder SL, Balis AJ, Perkins SL and Kjeldsberg CR (1995) Immunohistochemical reference ranges for B lymphocytes in bone marrow biopsy paraffin sections. *Am J Clin Pathol*, **104**, 517–523.

42 Steiner ML and Pearson HA (1966) Bone plasmacytic values in children. *J Pediatr*, **68**, 562–568.

43 Dresch C, Faille A, Poieriero O and Kadouche J (1974) The cellular composition of normal human bone marrow according to the volume of the sample. *J Clin Pathol*, **27**, 106–108.

44 Glaser K, Limarzi L and Poncher HG (1950) Cellular composition of the bone marrow in normal infants and children. *Pediatrics*, **6**, 789–824.

45 Gairdner D, Marks J and Roscoe JD (1952) Blood formation in infancy. Part I. The normal bone marrow. *Arch Dis Child*, **27**, 128–133.

46 Diwany M (1940) Sternal marrow puncture in children. *Arch Dis Child*, **15**, 159–170.

47 Jacobsen KM (1941) Untersuchungen über das Knochenmarkspunktat bei normalen Individuen verschiedener Altersklassen. *Acta Med Scand*, **106**, 417–446.

48 Segerdahl E (1935) Über sternalpunktionen. *Acta Med Scand*, **64** (Suppl.), 1–105.

49 Vaughan SL and Brockmyr F (1947) Normal bone marrow as obtained by sternal puncture. *Blood*, **1** (Special issue), 54–59.

50 Wintrobe MM, Lee RG, Boggs DR, Bithell TC, Athens JW and Foerster J (1974) *Clinical Hematology*, 7th edn. Lea & Febiger, Philadelphia.

51 den Ottolander GJ (1996) The bone marrow aspirate in healthy subjects. *Br J Haematol*, **95**, 574–575.

52 Bain BJ (1996) The bone marrow aspirate of healthy subjects. *Br J Haematol*, **94**, 206–209.

53 Fernández-Ferrero S and Ramos F (2001) Dyshaemopoietic bone marrow features in healthy subjects are related to age. *Leuk Res*, **25**, 187–189.

54 Dancy JT, Deubelbeiss KA, Harker LA and Finch CA (1976) Neutrophil kinetics in man. *J Clin Invest*, **58**, 705–715.

55 Wilkins BS and O'Brien CJ (1988) Techniques for obtaining differential cell counts from bone marrow trephine biopsy specimens. *J Clin Pathol*, **41**, 558–561.

56 Bain BJ. Bone marrow. In: Domizio P and Lowe D (eds) *Reporting Histopathology Sections*. Chapman & Hall, London, 1997.

57 Bain BJ (2001) Bone marrow aspiration. *J Clin Pathol*, **54**, 657–663.

58 Bain BJ (2001) Bone marrow trephine biopsy. *J Clin Pathol*, **54**, 737–742.

59 http://www.nice.org.uk/nicemedia/pdf/NICE_HAEMATOLOGICAL_CSG.pdf (accessed 21/1/2009).

60 Wang LJ and Glasser L (2001) Spurious dyserythropoiesis. *Am J Clin Pathol*, **117**, 57–59.

61 Anand M, Kumar R, Paniker N and Karak A (2003) Cartilage in bone marrow biopsy and purple granular deposits in the biopsy touch. *J Clin Pathol*, **56**, 883.

62 Foucar K (2001) *Bone Marrow Pathology*, 2nd edn. ASCP Press, Chicago.

63 Salgado C, Feliu E, Blade J, Rozman M, Aguilar JL and Rozman C (1992) A second bone marrow biopsy as a cause of a false diagnosis of myelofibrosis. *Br J Haematol*, **80**, 407–409.

TWO

SPECIAL TECHNIQUES APPLICABLE TO BONE MARROW DIAGNOSIS

Peripheral blood samples, bone marrow aspirates and trephine biopsy specimens are suitable for many diagnostic investigations in addition to routine microscopy of Romanowsky-stained blood and bone marrow films and haematoxylin and eosin (H&E)-stained histological sections. Some of these techniques, for example Perls' stain to demonstrate haemosiderin in a bone marrow aspirate, are so often useful that they are performed routinely, whereas other techniques are applied selectively. This chapter will deal predominantly with special techniques that are applicable to bone marrow aspirates and trephine biopsy sections but reference will be made to the peripheral blood where this is the more appropriate tissue for study.

Bone marrow aspirate films are stained routinely with a Romanowsky stain such as a May–Grünwald–Giemsa (MGG) or Wright–Giemsa stain. Other diagnostic procedures that may be of use in individual cases include cytochemistry, immunophenotyping (by immunocytochemistry or, more usually, flow cytometry), cytogenetic and molecular genetic analysis, ultrastructural examination, culture for microorganisms and culture for assessment of haemopoietic progenitor cells.

In most countries, histological sections cut from bone marrow trephine biopsy specimens are stained routinely with H&E. Most laboratories also use silver stains routinely to demonstrate reticulin and some employ, in addition, a Giemsa stain, a Perls' stain or both. We recommend the routine use of H&E, Giemsa and reticulin stains. Giemsa staining permits the easy identification of mast cells, facilitates recognition of plasma cells and helps in

making a distinction between early erythroid cells and myeloblasts. If a Giemsa stain is not performed routinely then it is important that it is used whenever necessary for these indications. Other techniques that may be applied to trephine biopsy sections include a wider range of cytochemical stains, immunohistochemistry, cytogenetic and molecular genetic analysis (particularly *in situ* hybridization) and ultrastructural examination.

Cytochemical and histochemical stains

Cytochemical stains on bone marrow aspirates

Perls' stain for iron

A Perls' or Prussian blue stain (Figs 2.1 and 2.2) demonstrates haemosiderin in bone marrow macrophages and within erythroblasts. Consequently it allows assessment of both the amount of iron in reticulo-endothelial stores and the availability of iron to developing erythroblasts.

Assessment of storage iron requires that an adequate number of fragments are obtained. A minimum of seven fragments in one or more bone marrow films need to be examined in order to state with reasonably reliability that bone marrow iron is absent [1]. A bone marrow film or squash preparation will contain both intracellular and extracellular iron, the latter being derived from crushed macrophages. It is usual to base assessment of iron stores mainly on intracellular iron since iron stains are prone to artefactual deposits and it can be difficult to distinguish between extracellular iron and artefact. Iron stores may be assessed as normal, decreased or increased or may be graded as 1+ to 6+ as shown in Table 2.1 [2,3], grades of 1+ to 3+

Bone Marrow Pathology. By Barbara Bain, David Clark and Bridget Wilkins. © 2010, Blackwell Publishing.

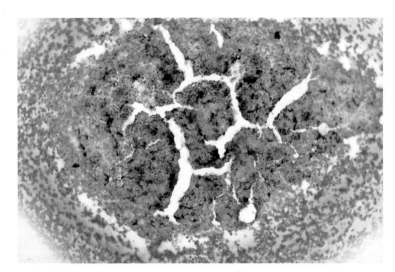

Fig. 2.1 Aspirate of normal bone marrow (BM): bluish-black iron in macrophages in a fragment. Perls' stain ×40.

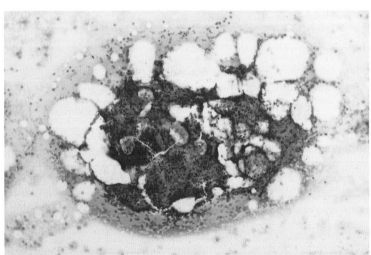

Fig. 2.2 Aspirate of normal BM: a fragment with no stainable iron. Perls' stain ×40.

Table 2.1 Grading of bone marrow storage iron [2,3].

0	No stainable iron
1+	Small iron particles just visible in reticulum cells using an oil objective
2+	Small, sparse iron particles in reticulum cells, visible at lower power
3+	Numerous small particles in reticulum cells
4+	Larger particles with a tendency to aggregate into clumps
5+	Dense, large clumps
6+	Very large clumps and extracellular iron

being considered normal. Alternatively, iron stores may be graded as 1+ to 4+ [4,5]. In routine practice, grading as absent, scanty, reduced, normal or increased is also a practical approach.

Examination of a Perls' stain of a bone marrow film allows adequate assessment of erythroblast iron as long as a thinly spread area of the film is examined with optimal illumination. A proportion of normal erythroblasts have a few (one to five) fine iron-containing granules randomly distributed in the cytoplasm (Fig. 2.3). Such erythroblasts are designated sideroblasts. In haematologically normal subjects with adequate iron stores, 20–50% of bone marrow erythroblasts are sideroblasts [6–8].

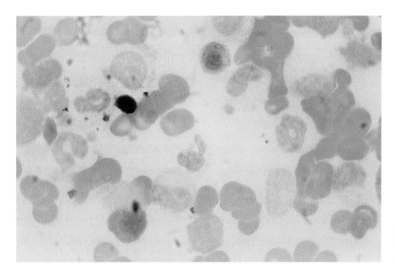

Fig. 2.3 BM aspirate from a healthy volunteer showing a normal sideroblast. Perls' stain ×100.

Examination of an iron stain allows detection not only of an increased or decreased proportion of sideroblasts but also of abnormal sideroblasts. The latter include those in which siderotic granules are merely increased in size and number and those in which granules are also distributed abnormally within the cytoplasm, being sited in a ring around the nucleus rather than randomly (ring sideroblasts).

In certain pathological conditions, plasma cells contain haemosiderin inclusions, which are irregular in shape and relatively large. With an MGG stain they are greenish black (Fig. 2.4a). Their nature is confirmed by a Perls' stain (Fig. 2.4b). Haemosiderin inclusions in plasma cells are observed mainly in iron overload (for example in haemochromatosis and transfusional siderosis) and in chronic alcoholism [9].

Problems and pitfalls Since iron is distributed irregularly within bone marrow macrophages it is necessary to assess a minimum of seven fragments before concluding that storage iron is absent or reduced. If necessary, a Perls' stain can be performed on more than one bone marrow film. Stain deposit on the slide must be distinguished from haemosiderin. Careful examination will show that it is not related to cells and is often in another plane of focus. It will also be present beyond the area of the film of bone marrow.

Other cytochemical stains

Cytochemical stains are employed mainly in the investigation of acute leukaemia and the myelodysplastic syndromes (MDS); such stains are used less with the increasing use of immunophenotyping but still have a role. In acute leukaemia there may be numerous blast cells in the peripheral blood and it is then useful to perform cytochemical stains on blood and bone marrow in parallel. Cytochemical investigation of suspected MDS should be performed on bone marrow films since there are usually only small numbers of immature cells in the peripheral blood.

The techniques recommended for diagnosis and classification of acute leukaemia are either myeloperoxidase or Sudan black B staining, to identify cells showing granulocytic differentiation, plus a non-specific esterase or combined esterase stain, to identify cells showing monocytic differentiation. Enzyme cytochemistry for either α-naphthyl butyrate esterase or α-naphthyl acetate esterase is suitable as a 'nonspecific' esterase staining method for the identification of monocytic differentiation. In a combined esterase stain either of these methods is combined with demonstration of naphthol AS-D chloroacetate esterase (chloroacetate esterase), the latter to show granulocytic differentiation. The application of these stains will be discussed in Chapter 4.

Other cytochemical stains that are occasionally used include toluidine blue to demonstrate the

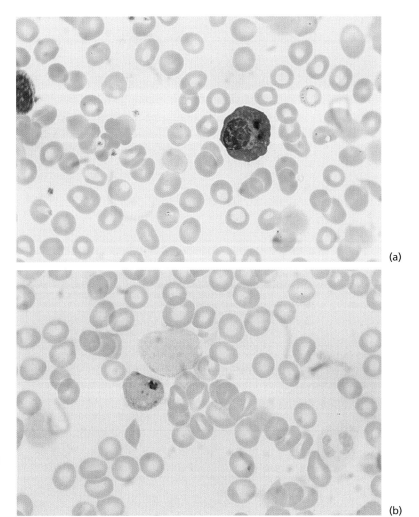

(a)

(b)

Fig. 2.4 BM aspirate from a patient with chronic alcoholism showing haemosiderin in plasma cells: (a) May–Grünwald–Giemsa (MGG) ×100; (b) Perls' stain ×100.

metachromatic granules in basophils and mast cells and staining of cells of mast cell lineage for ε-aminocaproate. When immunophenotyping is available, periodic acid–Schiff (PAS) and acid phosphatase stains are redundant in the investigation of acute leukaemias, although differences can be observed between different types of acute lymphoblastic and acute myeloid leukaemia [10,11]. Either a Sudan black B or a myeloperoxidase stain should also be used in cases of suspected MDS to facilitate the detection of Auer rods.

Cytochemistry now has little place in the investigation of lymphoproliferative disorders. However,

the demonstration of tartrate-resistant acid phosphatase activity is still of value in the diagnosis of hairy cell leukaemia, particularly when a large panel of appropriate immunophenotyping reagents is not available.

Histochemical stains on trephine biopsy sections

Perls' stain for haemosiderin
Because of the irregular distribution of iron within bone marrow macrophages a biopsy may show the presence of iron when none has been detected in

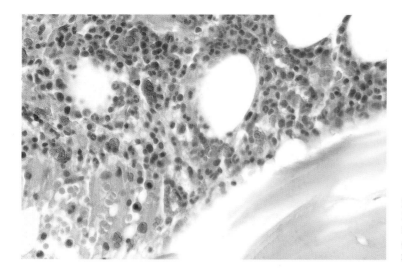

Fig. 2.5 Section of BM showing haemosiderin within macrophages in an HIV-positive patient with iron overload. Paraffin-embedded, H&E ×40.

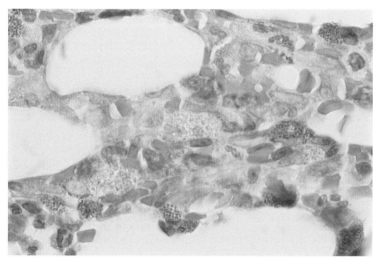

Fig. 2.6 Section of BM trephine biopsy specimen showing haemosiderin in stromal macrophages demonstrated by Giemsa staining. A distinctive yellow-green colour is obtained that is easily visible against background haemopoietic cell staining. Paraffin-embedded, Giemsa ×100.

an aspirate. Haemosiderin can often be detected, particularly when it is increased, as golden brown refractile pigment in unstained or H&E-stained sections (Fig. 2.5). In a Giemsa-stained section it is greenish-blue (Fig. 2.6). An iron stain (Fig. 2.7) can be successfully carried out using either resin-embedded or paraffin-embedded biopsy specimens. However, resin-embedded specimens give more reliable results. Decalcification of a paraffin-embedded specimen, by acid decalcification, leads to some leaching out of iron [12]. Resin-embedded samples are also superior for the detection of ring sideroblasts or other abnormal sideroblasts. These can sometimes also be detected in paraffin-embedded

bone marrow fragments but not in decalcified trephine biopsy sections. However, no technique for processing and staining a biopsy specimen allows assessment of whether siderotic granules are normal or decreased; this requires an iron stain of an aspirate. Haemosiderin deposits in plasma cells may, however, be sufficiently large that they can be detected on sections of paraffin-embedded trephine biopsy specimens (Fig. 2.8).

A distinctive appearance has been reported in patients in whom parenteral iron has previously been administered, with there being finely granular, often curvilinear, arrays of Perls-positive material [13]. Practice differs between laboratories as to

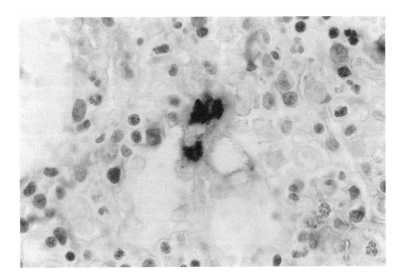

Fig. 2.7 Section of normal BM: macrophage containing iron. Resin-embedded, Perls' stain ×100.

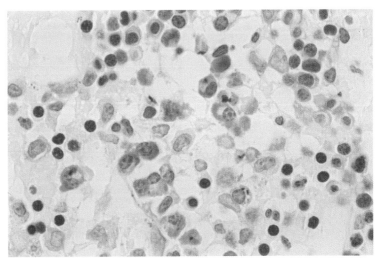

Fig. 2.8 Section of trephine biopsy specimen from a child with iron overload associated with congenital sideroblastic anaemia showing a number of plasma cells containing large haemosiderin deposits. Paraffin-embedded, Perls' stain ×100.

whether a Perls' stain for haemosiderin is performed routinely. If a bone marrow aspirate containing adequate fragments is available then iron staining on trephine biopsy sections is redundant. We no longer perform an iron stain routinely but reserve its use for those cases where it is likely to give information of specific diagnostic use.

Problems and pitfalls The amount of iron that is leached out when a paraffin-embedded biopsy specimen is decalcified is variable and unpredictable. The amount of stainable iron is reduced and sometimes all stainable iron is removed. Loss of stainable iron is less with ethylene diamine tetra-

acetic acid (EDTA) decalcification than with other methods. Because of the unpredictable leaching out of iron it is not possible to quantify iron accurately on a decalcified biopsy specimen. It is only possible to say that iron is present or increased but not that it is decreased or absent.

There are conflicting reports of the comparability of iron stains performed on aspirates and biopsy specimens, not all of which are readily explicable by the factors already mentioned. Lundin *et al.* [4] found that in 8% of cases iron was detectable in a biopsy specimen and not in an aspirate, and that in another 8% the reverse was true; by assessing other factors they were not able to establish that one or other method was more valid. Fong *et al.* [5] found that in 8% of patients iron was present in an aspirate but was not detectable in a biopsy sample; however, this was not due to the process of decalcification since it was noted with regard to sections of marrow fragments as well as for trephine biopsy sections. Conflicting findings were reported by Krause *et al.* [14] who found that iron was always detectable in a biopsy when it was present in an aspirate but that two thirds of patients with absent iron in an aspirate had detectable iron in a biopsy specimen. It is clear that minor variations in technique may be critical. Our own observations are that when specimens are decalcified using manual processing techniques there may be a failure to detect iron in a trephine biopsy specimen when it is clearly present in an aspirate [12]. Iron stains performed on aspirates and biopsy specimens should clearly be regarded as complementary.

Reticulin and collagen stains

Histological sections, either from particle preparations or trephine biopsy specimens, can be stained for reticulin using a silver-impregnation technique and also for collagen using a trichrome stain. We have found a Martius scarlet blue stain superior to a van Gieson stain for the identification of collagen. Reticulin and collagen deposition can be quantified as shown in Table 2.2 [15] and illustrated in Figs 2.9–2.13. An alternative grading proposed by Thiele *et al.* [16] has been accepted in the World Health Organization (WHO) classification of tumours of haematopoietic and lymphoid tissues (see page 240); it does not have any clear advantages over that of

Table 2.2 Quantification of bone marrow reticulin and collagen [15]. (Reprinted by permission of *Am J Clin Path*, **56**, 24–31, 1970.)

0	No reticulin fibres demonstrable
1	Occasional fine individual fibres and foci of a fine fibre network
2	Fine fibre network throughout most of the section; no coarse fibres
3	Diffuse fibre network with scattered thick coarse fibres but no mature collagen
4	Diffuse often coarse fibre network with areas of collagenization

Bauermeister [15] shown in Table 2.2, although these authors make the important point that reticulin deposition should be assessed in relation to haemopoietic tissue, not in fatty areas of marrow. The majority of haematologically normal subjects have a reticulin grade of 0 or 1 but occasional subjects have a grade of 2. There is a tendency for more reticulin to be detected in iliac crest biopsies than in sections of particles aspirated from the sternum. Reticulin is concentrated around blood vessels and close to bone trabeculae and these areas should be disregarded in grading reticulin deposition.

The term myelofibrosis is used to indicate deposition of collagen in the marrow and sometimes also to indicate increased reticulin deposition. To avoid any ambiguity it is preferable to either grade reticulin/collagen deposition as shown in Table 2.2 or to use the term 'reticulin fibrosis' for grade 3 fibrosis and 'myelofibrosis' for grade 4. The term myelosclerosis has also been used in various senses; it is best regarded as a synonym for myelofibrosis.

A reticulin stain should be performed on every trephine biopsy specimen. It has two major roles. Firstly, increased reticulin deposition provides nonspecific evidence of an abnormality of the bone marrow. Secondly, focal abnormality in the pattern of reticulin deposition can be very useful in detecting abnormalities that might be overlooked in an H&E-stained section. Abnormal infiltrates may show an associated increase in reticulin deposition or, less often, there may be a general increase in reticulin but with an absence of reticulin in an area that is heavily infiltrated by non-haemopoietic cells. Focal abnormalities that may be highlighted by a localized increase in reticulin deposition include granulomas and infiltrates of carcinoma or lymphoma cells. In addition to its two major roles, a reticulin stain shows bone structure clearly, e.g. the mosaic pattern of Paget's disease. Occasionally a reticulin stain highlights the presence of fungi, silver being deposited on the microorganisms [17].

Problems and pitfalls To avoid confusion, pathologists should refer to reticulin and collagen deposition in a precise manner. Increased reticulin deposition provides evidence of a bone marrow abnormality but should not be over-interpreted since the causes are multiple. The causes of collagen deposition are fewer and this abnormality is

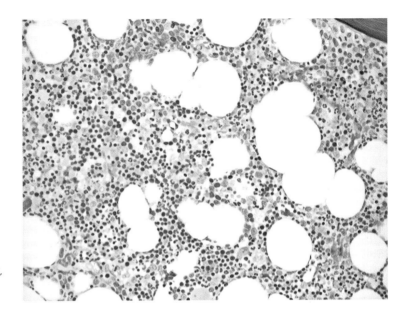

Fig. 2.9 Section of normal BM: reticulin grade 0, showing no stainable fibres. Paraffin-embedded, Gomori's reticulin stain with nuclear fast red counterstain ×20.

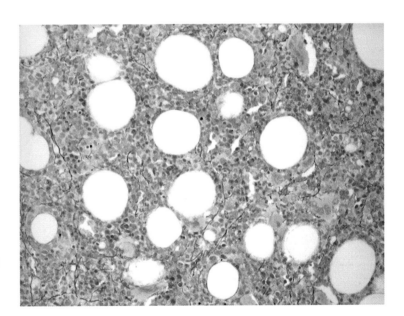

Fig. 2.10 Section of normal BM: reticulin grade 1, showing scattered fine fibres. Paraffin-embedded, Gomori's reticulin stain with nuclear fast red counterstain ×20.

therefore of more diagnostic significance. The significance of reticulin and collagen deposition is discussed in Chapter 3 (see pages 153–156).

Other histochemical stains
Other potentially useful histochemical stains and their roles in diagnosis are shown in Table 2.3. A

chloroacetate esterase (Leder) stain is illustrated in Fig. 2.14.

Problems and pitfalls The reactivity of histochemical stains is influenced by the choice of fixative, the method of embedding and the process of decalcification employed. Fixation in either Bouin's or

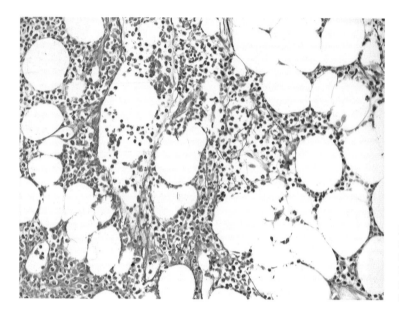

Fig. 2.11 Section of normal BM: reticulin grade 2, showing a fine fibre network but no coarse fibres. Paraffin-embedded, Gomori's reticulin stain with nuclear fast red counterstain ×20.

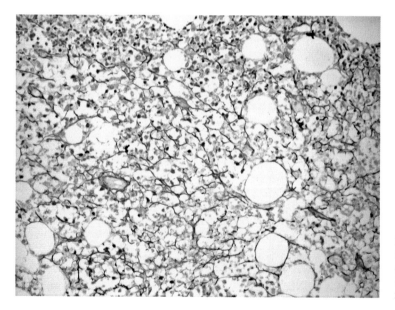

Fig. 2.12 Section of abnormal BM: reticulin grade 3, showing thick coarse fibres. Paraffin-embedded, Gomori's reticulin stain with nuclear fast red counterstain ×20.

Zenker's solution leads to reduced metachromatic staining of mast cells with a Giemsa stain and also reduces or abolishes chloroacetate esterase activity. Other common histochemical stains are satisfactory with fixation in formalin or Bouin's or Zenker's solution. However, it should be noted that prolonged storage of formalin at high ambient temperatures can lead to formic acid production; if the

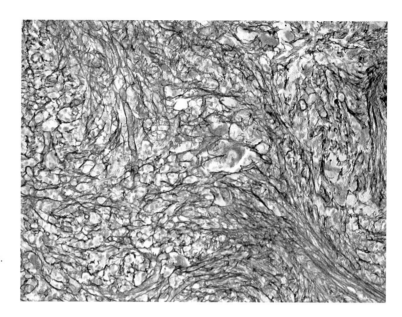

Fig. 2.13 Section of abnormal BM: reticulin grade 4, showing a coarse fibre network; collagen was present. Paraffin-embedded, Gomori's reticulin stain with nuclear fast red counterstain ×20.

Table 2.3 Cytochemical and histochemical stains and their indications.

Cytochemical stain	Role
Chloroacetate esterase (Leder)	Identification of granulocytic differentiation and mast cells
Periodic acid–Schiff (PAS)*	Staining of complex carbohydrates: identification of plasma cells and megakaryocytes (staining is variable); identification of some tumour cells; identification of fungi
Toluidine blue	Identification of mast cells
Alcian blue	Identification of cryptococci and some tumour cells; staining of stromal mucins
Grocott's methenamine silver (GMS) stain	Identification of fungi
Congo red stain	Identification of amyloid
Ziehl–Neelsen (ZN) stain	Identification of mycobacteria
Martius scarlet blue (MSB)	Staining of collagen and fibrin/fibrinoid

*Neutrophils are also PAS positive.

formalin is unbuffered, inadvertent decalcification may occur during the process of fixation with resultant adverse effects on staining. Histochemical stains are satisfactory with both paraffin and resin embedding. Acid decalcification impairs chloro-acetate esterase activity whereas EDTA decalcification does not. Over-exposure to EDTA reduces or abolishes Giemsa staining.

We have found that many of the proprietary combined fixation–decalcification solutions, which

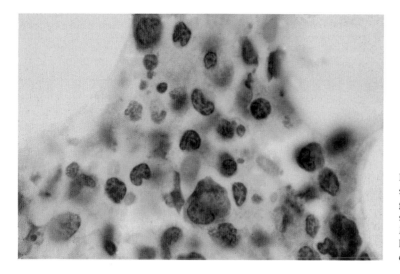

Fig. 2.14 Section of trephine biopsy specimen from a patient with large granular lymphocyte leukaemia stained for chloroacetate esterase. Myeloid precursors are positive and lymphocytes are negative. Resin-embedded, Leder's stain ×100.

are sometimes used to achieve rapid processing, impair histochemical stains. For example, haematoxylin staining may be impaired so that nuclear detail and cytoplasmic basophilia are not apparent. Giemsa staining may be severely impaired.

Immunophenotyping

Antigens may be expressed on the surface of cells, within the cytoplasm or within the nucleus. Depending on the techniques applied for immunophenotyping, there may be detection of only surface membrane antigens or cytoplasmic and nuclear antigens may also be detected. Detection of antigens may be by means of polyclonal antibodies, raised in animals such as rabbits, but monoclonal antibodies produced by hybridoma technology are now predominantly used. Many monoclonal antibodies, reactive with lymphoid or myeloid antigens, have been characterized at a series of international workshops and are described by cluster of differentiation (CD) numbers. A CD number refers to a group of antibodies that recognize the same antigen and also refers to the antigen expressed. It is important to note that monoclonal antibodies may recognize specific epitopes on antigens so that not all antibodies with the same CD number have exactly the same reactivity with normal and abnormal cells. A complete list of CD numbers is given in reference 18. Some important

monoclonal antibodies have not yet been assigned a CD number, e.g. FMC7.

Immunophenotyping by immunofluorescence flow cytometry

If there are significant numbers of circulating abnormal cells, it is most convenient to perform flow cytometric immunophenotyping on a peripheral blood sample. Otherwise this procedure can be performed on a bone marrow aspirate or, alternatively, on cerebrospinal fluid, a serous exudate or a suspension of cells from a lymph node or other tissue. When peripheral blood is used, the procedure can be applied to either a mononuclear cell preparation or to whole blood in which the red cells have been lysed [19]. The latter technique minimizes cell loss and potential artefacts that can be induced by exposure to Ficoll and density gradient separation. It also increases the speed and convenience of the procedure. Choice of appropriate proprietary lysis solutions is important to avoid the reduction of expression of certain antigens [20].

The principle of flow cytometry is that cells bearing specific antigens are identified by means of a monoclonal antibody (or, occasionally, a polyclonal antiserum) labelled with a fluorochrome (Fig. 2.15). The flow cytometer permits classification of cells according to their light-scattering characteristics and the intensity of their fluorescence upon activation by laser light, detected after passing through an appropriate filter for the particular

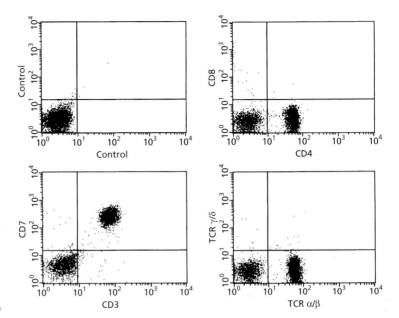

Fig. 2.15 Scatter plot showing flow cytometry immunophenotyping in a case of T-lineage prolymphocytic leukaemia. The leukaemic cells are positive for CD4, CD7 and TCRαβ; they are negative for CD8. (By courtesy of Mr R. Morilla, London.)

fluorochrome employed. Three or more fluorochromes can be used so that the simultaneous expression of two, three or more antigens can be studied. If permeabilization techniques are employed, cytoplasmic and nuclear antigens can be detected as well as those expressed on cell surfaces. Techniques are also available for the quantification of antigen expression.

Flow cytometry immunophenotyping is applicable to diagnosis and classification of haematological neoplasms. When expression of three or four antigens is assessed simultaneously it is also applicable to the detection of minimal residual disease.

Problems and pitfalls
Flow cytometry has the disadvantage that the immunophenotype cannot be related directly to cytology. Results must always be interpreted in the light of the cytological features of the cells being studied.

When there are large numbers of circulating neoplastic cells, results of peripheral blood analysis are generally reliable. However, a low frequency of abnormal cells may not be detected. When flow cytometry is performed on cell suspensions from bone marrow or other tissues, results may be misleading in two circumstances. Firstly, an abnormal infiltrate may not be represented in the aspirate to any significant extent. This is often the case in follicular lymphoma with paratrabecular infiltration, but may also occur in any lymphoma in which reticulin deposition is increased in the infiltrated area, interfering with aspiration of abnormal cells. Secondly, if neoplastic cells are outnumbered by reactive cells, as in Hodgkin lymphoma and in T-cell-rich B-cell lymphoma, the immunophenotyping may relate only to reactive T lymphocytes, not to the minor population of neoplastic cells. In both of these circumstances immunohistochemistry is superior. It has been suggested that immunophenotyping by flow cytometry may not be cost effective in comparison with histology supplemented by immunohistochemistry in lymphoma diagnosis. In one investigation a monoclonal population was detected in only 49 of 59 patients with bone marrow histologically involved by lymphoma, and in patients with normal histology only five of 116 had a monoclonal population detected [21]. If detection of bone marrow infiltration is crucial for patient management we would nevertheless advise the use of flow cytometry. Whether immunohistochemistry is also needed when an abnormal population has been detected by flow cytometry can be decided on a case by case basis.

Correct techniques are of critical importance. For example, if gating techniques (see below) are used in order to determine the immunophenotype of a subpopulation of cells, it is essential to ensure that the gated cells are the neoplastic population.

Caution is required in interpreting flow cytometry findings during post-treatment follow-up of acute lymphoblastic leukaemia (ALL). Normal immature lymphoid cells, known as haematogones, express CD10, CD34 and terminal deoxynucleotidyl transferase (TdT) and can thus be confused with residual leukaemic cells [22] unless the strength of expression of antigens is also considered. The detection of persisting cells with an aberrant combination of antigens is more reliable, as is polymerase chain reaction (PCR) analysis for rearranged immunoglobulin heavy chain or T-cell receptor loci (see below).

Immunocytochemistry

By convention, the term immunocytochemistry refers to the study of the antigen expression of cells by means of polyclonal antisera or monoclonal antibodies applied to fixed cells on glass slides. The material investigated may be either a blood or bone marrow film or a cytocentrifuged preparation of washed mononuclear cells isolated from blood or bone marrow. The reaction of antibodies with cells carrying a specific antigen is detected by either (i) direct labelling of the primary antibody with an enzyme such as peroxidase or alkaline phosphatase, or (ii) an indirect method using a second, labelled antibody that recognizes the first (e.g. a secondary antibody reactive with mouse immunoglobulins when the primary antibody is murine). A variety of indirect methods are available. Indirect labelling techniques offer the advantage of increased sensitivity but are more time-consuming to perform than direct labelling, which is increasingly used.

The use of washed, separated cells in cytocentrifuge preparations is necessary for immunocytochemistry to detect surface membrane immunoglobulins, including κ and λ light chains. Plasma immunoglobulins interfere with the staining if blood films or films of bone marrow aspirates are used. For the detection of most other antigens, either cytocentrifuge preparations or wedge-spread films are satisfactory. If there are significant numbers of abnormal cells in the circulating blood then a peripheral blood sample is very satisfactory

for immunocytochemistry. Otherwise study of a bone marrow aspirate is necessary.

Immunocytochemistry can also be used to demonstrate the product of an oncogene or a cancer-suppressing gene. For example, PML protein, the product of the gene that is rearranged and dysregulated in acute promyelocytic leukaemia can be demonstrated with a fluorochrome-labelled monoclonal antibody and an abnormal pattern of distribution can be shown in this type of leukaemia. Similarly, a labelled antibody can be used to demonstrate increased expression of p53 protein when the gene is mutated or dysregulated; p53 protein is below the level of detection when only normal wild-type expression is present.

Problems and pitfalls

Immunocytochemistry has the advantage that reactivity with an antibody can be related to cell morphology. However, it should be noted that cytocentrifugation introduces artefactual changes, such as nuclear lobulation. It is useful to examine an MGG-stained cytocentrifuge preparation in parallel with the immunocytochemical stains and wedge-spread films.

Cytochemistry is slow and labour intensive and thus is not suitable for large workloads or for producing rapid results. Interpretation is subjective and, because only a small number of cells can be assessed, results are imprecise. Some useful antibodies, for example FMC7, cannot be used successfully for immunocytochemistry although they are very reliable with flow cytometry.

Relative advantages of flow cytometry and immunocytochemistry

Flow cytometry has the following considerable advantages over immunocytochemistry and is therefore the preferred technique:

1 It is rapid and less labour intensive.

2 It permits large numbers of cells to be analysed so that the percentage of cells bearing a specific antigen is estimated much more precisely and minor populations of cells may be identified.

3 Multiple directly-labelled antibodies can be used to study the coexpression of two, three, four or even more antigens.

4 It is possible to 'gate' for cells having particular characteristics in order to investigate antigen expression by a defined population ('gating' or selection of a subpopulation may be based on light-scattering characteristics of cells or on expression of a specific antigen).

5 The amount of antigen expressed on a specific population of cells can be quantified, whereas immunocytochemistry is *not* quantitative.

These advantages of flow cytometry mean that it can be used to identify minor normal populations, such as CD34-positive haemopoietic stem cells, and minor abnormal populations showing atypical combinations of antigen expression, as in the detection of minimal residual disease in patients treated for haematological neoplasms.

There are two potential disadvantages of flow cytometry in comparison with immunocytochemistry:

1 Without modification, the technique detects only surface membrane antigens and not antigens expressed within the cytoplasm or in the nucleus.

2 Cytological features of the cells studied cannot be appreciated.

The first disadvantage can be overcome readily by the use of techniques for permeabilizing cells so that antigens expressed in the nucleus or in the cytoplasm can be detected. The second defect cannot be overcome easily but assessment of light-scattering characteristics of cells permits recognition of granular cells with high sideways light scatter and determination of whether specific antigens are expressed on large or small cells, deduced from forward light scatter. Results of flow cytometry should not be interpreted in isolation; the cytological features of the cells being studied must be taken into account.

Immunocytochemistry has the advantage over flow cytometry that the precise cytological features of cells bearing a certain antigen can be recognized. As mentioned above, however, it is very labour intensive and more time-consuming than flow cytometry and the results are not quantitative. Double or multiple antigen combinations on individual cells cannot be demonstrated routinely. Although techniques exist for sequential immunocytochemical staining of several antigens in the same preparation, these are largely restricted to use as research tools at present because of their practical difficulties.

Antibodies for flow cytometry and immunocytochemistry

Antibodies to be used in flow cytometry are selected depending upon the purpose of the investigation. There are relatively few circumstances in which a single antibody is used in isolation. Specific combinations are used for the investigation of suspected acute leukaemia or possible lymphoproliferative disorders. Suggested panels are provided in Tables 2.4 and 2.5.

In addition, flow cytometry can be used for the following:

1 Detection of minimal residual disease in acute leukaemia (using a panel of antibodies and four-colour flow cytometry permits detection of a leukaemia-related immunophenotype in more than 90% of childhood cases [23]).

2 Detection of phenotypes associated with adverse prognosis, e.g. in chronic lymphocytic leukaemia (CLL).

3 Quantification of CD34-positive haemopoietic stem cells for stem cell harvesting and transplantation.

4 Quantification of CD4-positive lymphocytes for assessment of immune status in human immunodeficiency virus (HIV) infection.

5 Quantification of DNA for cell cycle and ploidy studies, e.g. for detection of hyperdiploidy in acute lymphoblastic leukaemia.

Problems and pitfalls

Because many immunophenotypic markers are not lineage-specific it is always necessary to use a panel of antibodies rather than relying on reactivity with a single antibody. Specific panels are selected, depending on the disease that is suspected. Immunophenotypic markers showing good lineage specificity include CD19 and CD22 for the B lineage, CD3 for the T lineage and myeloperoxidase for myeloid cells. Expression of CD79a is less specific for the B lineage since it also occurs in some cases of T-lineage ALL [24]. Rarely, carcinoma cells express CD45 or neoplastic cells in non-Hodgkin lymphoma or ALL express keratin [25]. Commonly used immunophenotypic markers with poor lineage specificity, but used for other reasons, include TdT, human leukocyte antigen DR (HLA-DR), CD7 and CD10.

Table 2.4 Monoclonal and other antibodies useful in immunocytochemistry and flow cytometry immunophenotyping in suspected acute leukaemia.

Primary panel	
For detection of myeloid differentiation	CD13*, CD33, CD65, CD117, anti-MPO
For detection of B-lymphoid differentiation	CD19, CD22*, CD79a
For detection of T-lymphoid differentiation	CD2, CD3*, anti-TCR$\alpha\beta$, anti-TCR$\gamma\delta$
For detection of immature cells	Anti-TdT, CD34, HLA-DR
For gating on leucocyte subpopulations	CD45
Secondary panel	
For further investigation of myeloid differentiation	Anti-glycophorin (CD235a, CD236R) for erythroid differentiation; CD41 (or CD61) for megakaryocyte differentiation; CD11c, CD14, CD36, CD64, lysozyme for monocytic differentiation; CD11b for granulocytic or monocytic maturation
For further investigation of B-lineage differentiation	CD10, CD20, cytoplasmic μ chain, surface membrane immunoglobulin
For further investigation of T-lineage differentiation	CD1a, CD4, CD5, CD7, CD8
For diagnosis of blastic plasmacytoid dendritic cell neoplasm	CD4, CD56, CD123

HLA, human leukocyte antigen; TCR, T-cell receptor; TdT, terminal deoxynucleotidyl transferase.
*Testing is more sensitive if cytoplasmic rather than surface membrane antigen is tested for, either by 'permeabilizing' cells or by using immunocytochemistry rather than flow cytometry.

Immunohistochemistry

Immunohistochemistry is a technique for the demonstration of antigens in histological tissue sections. It has advantages and disadvantages in relation to flow cytometry and immunocytochemistry. For practical purposes, flow cytometry and immunohistochemistry should be regarded as complementary investigations.

In flow cytometry, a wider range of antibodies can be used and quantification of antigen expression can be achieved. There is also less likelihood of non-specific staining in flow cytometry than in immunohistochemistry. However, immunohistochemistry has the advantage that immunophenotypic information can be obtained and assessed in association with preserved information regarding the spatial organization of labelled and unlabelled cells. Immunohistochemistry also permits assessment of the cytological features of cells expressing particular antigens, in a context which is often more familiar than that offered by immunocytochemistry (particularly cytocentrifuge prepara-

tions, in which significant morphological artefacts are induced by the centrifugation technique itself).

Because a large number of antigens can be stained individually in adjacent thin tissue sections, the lack of easy techniques for double-staining is not a major problem in immunohistochemistry performed for diagnostic and staging purposes. In a complex infiltrate it is relatively easy to demonstrate a variety of cell types differing in morphological and immunophenotypic characteristics. For example, in T-cell/histiocyte-rich B-cell lymphoma, the large, neoplastic cells can be shown to have a B-cell phenotype while the more numerous T cells are seen to be cytologically normal small lymphocytes.

Immunohistochemistry can permit the identification and characterization of an abnormal bone marrow infiltrate not represented in the patient's aspirate sample. This situation usually arises when there is significant reticulin fibrosis associated with an infiltrate, which hinders aspiration of cells from

Table 2.5 Monoclonal and other antibodies useful in flow cytometric immunophenotyping in suspected chronic lymphoproliferative disorders.

Primary panel	
To establish lineage	A pan-B marker such as CD79a, CD19 or CD20 and a pan-T marker such as CD2 or CD3
To establish clonality of B-lineage lymphoproliferative disorders and to establish the strength of expression of surface membrane immunoglobulin	Anti-κ and anti-λ
To distinguish B-lineage chronic lymphocytic leukaemia from other less common B- and T-lineage disorders	CD79b (or CD22), CD5, CD23, FMC7 (CLL cells are usually CD5 and CD23 positive, CD22, CD79b and FMC7 weak or negative, and show weak expression of SmIg; the reverse pattern is usual in most types of B-lineage non-Hodgkin lymphoma)
Secondary panel	
For further investigation of suspected or demonstrated B-lineage lymphoproliferative disorder	CD10 (more often positive in follicular lymphoma); CD11c, CD25, CD103, CD123 (for suspected hairy cell leukaemia); anti-cyclin D1 (suspected mantle cell lymphoma); CD38, CD79a, CD138, cIg (for suspected plasma cell or lymphoplasmacytoid neoplasm); ZAP70 (B-cell expression) in CLL
For further investigation of suspected or demonstrated T-lineage lymphoproliferative disorder	CD4, CD8 (usually positive in large granular lymphocyte leukaemia), CD7 (usually positive in T-prolymphocytic leukaemia), CD25 (usually positive in adult T-cell leukaemia/lymphoma); CD11b, CD16, CD56, CD57 (for suspected large granular lymphocyte or NK cell leukaemia/lymphoma)
To distinguish lymphocyte precursors (in ALL or lymphoblastic lymphoma) from mature lymphocytes	Terminal deoxynucleotidyl transferase
For planning of therapy	Antibodies reactive with any antigens that might be a target of monoclonal antibody therapy (e.g. CD20, if not included in primary panel, and CD52)

ALL, acute lymphoblastic leukaemia; c, cytoplasmic; CLL, chronic lymphocytic leukaemia; NK, natural killer.

the involved area or areas of bone marrow. Such reticulin fibrosis occurs frequently in follicular lymphoma and almost invariably accompanies bone marrow infiltration by Hodgkin lymphoma.

When immunohistochemistry first gained widespread use in histopathology during the 1970s, it was commonly assumed that decalcification, particularly with methods involving exposure to acids, led to the destruction of many antigens. This has proved to be untrue and the procedure can be performed very successfully with acid or EDTA-decalcified trephine biopsies as well as with non-decalcified samples embedded in methacrylate resins. A few important technical modifications were required to overcome the different performance of bone marrow trephine biopsy specimens relative to other formalin-fixed tissues. For example, early antigen retrieval techniques, involving tissue digestion by proteolytic enzymes, to reverse protein–protein binding induced by formalin fixation, were responsible for many initial poor results of immunohistochemistry in bone marrow trephine biopsy specimens as a consequence of degradation of the antigenic target. Prior exposure to acid appears to render formalin-fixed tissue more susceptible to proteolysis and leads to degradation of some antigenic targets during incubation with the enzyme. In general, considerably short-

Table 2.6 Antigens expressed by myeloid cells and demonstrable by immunohistochemistry in fixed, decalcified bone marrow trephine biopsy specimens.

Antigen	Antibody*	Specificity	Comments
CD34	QBEnd/10	Primitive haemopoietic cells, granular cytoplasmic staining	Endothelial cells also positive; they show homogeneous membrane staining and are spindle shaped; megakaryocytes may be positive in both reactive and neoplastic conditions [26]
CD45	PD7/26, RP2/18, RP2/22	Lymphoid, granulocytic and monocytic cells	Proteolytic pre-treatment abolishes granulocytic and monocytic reactivity
Lysozyme (muramidase)	Polyclonal antisera	Granulocytic and monocytic cells	
Myeloperoxidase	Polyclonal antisera	Granulocytic and monocytic cells	May be less specific than McAb [27]
	2C7	Neutrophil lineage	
Alpha-1-antitrypsin	Polyclonal antisera	Granulocytic and monocytic cells	
CD66e (carcinoembryonic antigen – CEA)	85A12, 12-140-10, II-7	Granulocytic cells	Many metastases of epithelial origin also positive
CD68 (broad specificity)	KP1	Granulocytic and monocyte-lineage cells, including osteoclasts	Mast cells and cells of malignant melanoma are positive
CD68R (monocyte restricted)	PG-M1	Monocyte-lineage cells including osteoclasts	Mast cells also positive and cells of malignant melanoma are positive
CD163	10D6, BerMAC3	Monocyte-lineage cells including osteoclasts	
CD14	NCL-CD14-223	Monocytic cells	Developing monocytes strongly positive; macrophages weak or negative
Neutrophil elastase	NP57	Neutrophil-lineage cells	Promyelocytes and myelocytes strongly positive; metamyelocytes and mature neutrophils stain weakly or are negative
CD15	LeuM1, BY87, C3D-1, Carb-3	Monocytic and granulocytic cells, especially late granulocyte precursors	Membrane and cytoplasmic staining but membranes negative after proteolytic pre-treatment; expressed by neoplastic cells of Hodgkin lymphoma
Calprotectin (previously called calgranulin)	Mac387	Late granulocyte precursors and monocytic cells	Macrophages weakly stained or negative
Eosinophil peroxidase	ICR10	Eosinophil lineage	
Eosinophil major basic protein	BMK13	Eosinophil lineage	
Basogranulin [28]	BB1	Basophil lineage	
Mast cell tryptase	AA1	Mast cells	Avoidance of problems with diffusion of reaction product and non-specific background staining needs careful pre-treatment†

Table 2.6 (continued)

Antigen	Antibody*	Specificity	Comments
Mast cell chymase	CC1 or B7	Mast cells	Detects normal mast cells and those in reactive conditions but negative in the majority of mast cells in the myelodysplastic syndrome and systemic mastocytosis
CD117	57A5D8	Mast cells (strong)	Some haemopoietic progenitor cells (more weakly), the population overlapping with that stained by CD34; expressed by some promyelocytes and proerythroblasts; aberrantly expressed in some cases of myeloma
CD123	6H6	Plasmacytoid dendritic cells, hairy cells	
Glycophorin A (α-sialoglycoprotein) (CD235a)	JC159, BRIC101	Erythroid cells	Very early proerythroblasts not stained
Glycophorin C (β-sialoglycoprotein) (CD236R)	Ret40f	Erythroid cells	Expression seen in earlier proerythroblasts than α-sialoglycoprotein; cross-reactivity with myeloblasts is seen in some cases of acute myeloid leukaemia
Spectrin	Polyclonal antisera [29]	Erythroid cells	No commercially available antibody at present
Haemoglobin A	Polyclonal antisera	Haemoglobinized erythroid cells	Early erythroid precursors weak or negative
An epitope on the ABO blood group H glycoprotein	BNH9	Erythroid cells	Expressed from earliest recognizable stages of erythroid differentiation; also expressed by endothelial cells, megakaryocytes and cells of some large cell lymphomas
CD42b	MM2/174	Megakaryocytes	Strong, uniform cytoplasmic staining, including early and dysplastic forms
CD61	Y2/51, NCL-CD61-308	Megakaryocytes	Variable staining between cells; some early or dysplastic megakaryocytes may be unstained
Von Willebrand factor (previously known as factor VIII-related antigen)	F8/86, 36B11 and various polyclonal antisera	Megakaryocytes	Strong cytoplasmic staining; variable results with early and dysplastic forms; endothelial cells also positive
CD31	JC70A, 1A10	Megakaryocytes and monocytes	Endothelial cells also positive
CD1a	MTB1, JPM30, O10	Langerhans cells	Few, if any, such cells are normally present; used in diagnosis of Langerhans cell histiocytosis

McAb, monoclonal antibody.

*The list of monoclonal antibodies is not exhaustive. New clones are continually being developed.

†Some mast cell tryptase activity in leukaemic myeloblasts has been demonstrated using McAb G3 [30].

ened incubation times have therefore been found to be beneficial with these antigen retrieval methods. The major advance, however, has come through development of wet heat methods for antigen retrieval, exposing tissue sections to acid or alkaline solutions in combination with microwave oven or pressure cooker heating. This has been as important for immunohistochemistry as a general tool in histopathology as it has been for bone marrow trephine biopsy specimens. It has encouraged a huge expansion in the development of new monoclonal antibodies for diagnosis in addition to making possible excellent results using many existing antibodies that were previously unsuccessful.

The second technical modification required for successful immunohistochemistry in bone marrow biopsy specimens was necessary to minimize non-specific staining due to endogenous enzyme activity. Most methods employ indirect labelling techniques with either peroxidase or alkaline phosphatase conjugated to the secondary antibody. The enzyme generates an insoluble, coloured product from a chromogenic substrate to permit visualization of the primary antigen–antibody interaction. Cells of the granulocyte series, particularly eosinophils, are rich in endogenous peroxidase and bone marrow stroma contains dendritic cells that are rich in alkaline phosphatases. When performing immunohistochemistry on bone marrow trephine biopsy specimens, additional steps are required to block such endogenous enzyme activities and minimize non-specific staining. To compound this problem, highly efficient amplification steps are included in many current immunohistochemistry methods, increasing sensitivity by exploiting the extremely high binding affinity of avidin or streptavidin for biotin. Endogenous biotin activity, particularly in mast cells, may also therefore require specific blockade to avoid false-positive staining.

In practice, the necessary technical modifications are easy to incorporate to achieve excellent results in bone marrow trephine biopsy samples with a range of primary antibodies. While this range is somewhat limited compared with that used in flow cytometry, it is nonetheless extensive. Moreover, since much bone marrow trephine biopsy immunohistochemistry is performed in the investigation of lymphoproliferative disorders, it is valuable that

the antibodies that can be used successfully are also entirely suitable for use with other formalin-fixed tissue samples such as biopsied lymph nodes. Most histopathology laboratories now have fully automated immunostaining systems, some including automation of other steps in the procedure such as antigen retrieval.

Immunohistochemistry can be used to demonstrate surface membrane, cytoplasmic and nuclear antigens. It can be used specifically to provide molecular genetic information, e.g. by demonstration of the protein product of oncogenes, such as *ALK*, *CCND1* (*BCL1*) and *BCL2*, or of cancer-suppressing genes, such as *TP53*.

Tables 2.6 and 2.7 [26–33] give details of useful antibodies for the immunohistochemical detection of antigen expression on haemopoietic and lymphoid cells in bone marrow trephine biopsy sections. Immunohistochemical stains are illustrated in Figs 2.16–2.19. Monoclonal antibodies useful in the detection of microorganisms are shown in Table 3.1 and those for use in the diagnosis of non-haemopoietic malignancy in Tables 10.1 and 10.2. Monoclonal antibodies can also be used to identify: bone marrow blood vessels (CD31 and CD34); stromal fibroblasts (CD10, low affinity nerve growth factor receptor); and follicular dendritic cells (CD21 and CD23).

Problems and pitfalls

Lack of lineage specificity of antigens   There is a tendency to regard antigen expression as being lineage-specific, whereas expression is more accurately considered as lineage-associated or lineage-restricted. It is important to be familiar with the full range of cellular expression of different antigens, including that by non-haemopoietic tumour cells. Otherwise, misinterpretation can lead to serious diagnostic error. Many antigens familiar in the context of their expression by T cells, B cells or both in lymphoid tissues are also expressed by myeloid lineages (Fig. 2.20). This is particularly the case with T-cell-associated antigens, which are widely expressed by cells of granulocytic and monocytic lineages. CD43 should be avoided as a T-cell marker in bone marrow since it is expressed on many other types of cell. Antibodies reactive with CD45RO

Table 2.7 Antigens expressed by lymphoid cells (B, T and NK lineages) and demonstrable by immunohistochemistry in fixed, decalcified bone marrow trephine biopsy specimens.*†

Antigen	Antibody*	Specificity	Comments
CD45	PD7/26, RP218, RP2/22	Lymphoid, granulocytic and monocytic cells	Proteolytic pre-treatment minimizes granulocytic and monocytic staining
Terminal deoxynucleotidyl transferase (TdT)	NPT26, SEN28	Primitive lymphoid cells and some primitive myeloid cells	In addition to ALL, up to 15% of AML are positive
CD10	56C6	Subsets of B cells	Expressed in common and pre-B ALL, Burkitt' lymphoma, follicular lymphoma and most DLBCL of germinal centre type; also expressed by haematogones, some neutrophils and a subset of marrow stromal cells; renal cell carcinoma may be positive
CD20	L26, 7D1, MJ1	Most B cells	Some early B-lineage lymphoid cells and cells showing plasmacytic differentiation are negative
CD79a	Mb1, HM47/A9, JCB117, 11E3, 11D10	Most B cells	Includes early B-lineage lymphoid cells and those with plasmacytic differentiation; often reduced or absent in neoplastic plasma cells; megakaryocytes may be weakly positive
CD75	LN-1	B cells	Preferential staining of large, transformed B cells (e.g. centroblasts and immunoblasts)
CD45RA	4KB5	B cells and a subset of T-lineage lymphoid cells	Small, mature B cells stain preferentially
Immunoglobulin light chains – κ and λ	Polyclonal antisera are usually used	Plasma cells; demonstrable in some B-cell NHL when expression level is high	Expression by other B cells usually too weak to be detected; excessive background staining may occur due to plasma immunoglobulins within the tissue; detection of κ and λ mRNA by *in situ* hybridization is preferred in some laboratories
Immunoglobulin heavy chains – γ, α, μ, ε, δ	Polyclonal antisera are usually used	Plasma cells; demonstrable in some B-cell NHL when expression level is high	Expression by other B cells usually too weak to be detected; excessive background staining may occur due to plasma immunoglobulins within the tissue
Rough endoplasmic reticulum-associated antigen (p63)	VS38c	Plasma cells	Osteoblasts and a subset of stromal cells also stain
CD138 (syndecan)	B-B4, 5F7, MI15	Plasma cells	Some carcinomas and large cell NHL are positive
CD38	AT13/5, SPC32	Plasma cells	Also expressed by thymocytes, early B cells, germinal centre B cells, and some erythroid cells and neutrophils
MUM1/IRF4	MUM1p	Normal and neoplastic plasma cells, occasional T cells and germinal centre B cells	Neoplastic cells of classical and NLPHL and some NHL are positive

continued

Table 2.7 (continued)

Antigen	Antibody*	Specificity	Comments
PAX5	Clone 24, A452, 1EW	Pan-B cell-associated; down-regulated with plasma cell differentiation	May be expressed in neuroendocrine tumours, other carcinomas (rarely) and some acute myeloid leukaemias, e.g. associated with t(8;21)
CD72	DBA.44	B cells	Relative specificity for hairy cell leukaemia; red cell membranes and some macrophages may also stain
Tartrate-resistant acid phosphatase	9C5, 14G6, 26E5	Hairy cell leukaemia	Mast cells, Langerhans cells, macrophages and osteoclasts also stain [31]
CD23	1B12, MHM6	Subset of B cells: only rare lymphocytes positive in normal bone marrow	Small lymphocytic lymphoma/CLL positive; mantle cell, lymphoplasmacytic and follicular lymphomas negative; follicular dendritic cells in reactive nodules and in some nodular neoplastic B-cell infiltrates are positive
CD5	4C7, CD5/54/F6	Subset of B cells, most T cells	Small lymphocytic lymphoma/CLL and mantle cell lymphoma positive; lymphoplasmacytic and follicular lymphomas negative
BCL2	Bcl-2/100/D5, BCL2/124, 3.1	Widely expressed: T cells, mantle zone B lymphocytes, neoplastic follicles of follicular lymphoma, proliferation centres of CLL; often expressed by neoplastic cells of classical Hodgkin lymphoma but not those of NLPHL	Non-neoplastic germinal centre cells are negative; other B-cell lymphomas and some haemopoietic cells are positive; it is difficult to interpret positive staining of subtle interstitial infiltrates in the bone marrow
Cyclin D1	DCS-6, P2D11F11	Mantle cell lymphoma (nuclear expression)	Apoptotic nuclei and nuclei of stromal cells, including endothelial cells, are positive; expressed by other neoplasms with t(11;14), e.g. myeloma and (more weakly) by hairy cells [32]
BCL6	PG/B6p, LN22, P1F6	Positive in lymphomas of germinal centre origin and in some anaplastic large cell lymphomas and T-lymphoblastic lymphomas; positive in neoplastic cells in NLPHL but not those of classical Hodgkin lymphoma [32]	
BCL10	151	Detectable in nucleus of neoplastic cells in some extranodal marginal zone lymphomas of MALT type	

Table 2.7 (continued)

Antigen	Antibody*	Specificity	Comments
CD2	AB75, 11F11	Most T cells, neoplastic mast cells	Also expressed by some monocytes
CD3	CD3-12, PS1, LN10, F7.2.38 and polyclonal antisera	Most T cells	More specific than CD2; monoclonal antibodies are superior in performance to polyclonal antisera
CD3ε	F-2-2-38 and polyclonal antisera	Most T cells, in association with other CD3 components; expressed without other CD3 components in the cytoplasm of NK cells	
CD7	CD7-272, LP15, CBC.32	Most normal and reactive T cells; often reduced or absent expression by neoplastic T cells	Nucleolar staining may occur with CD7-272 but specific reactivity is at cell membrane
T-cell receptor β chain	βF1	Major subset of T cells expressing αβ T-cell receptor	The majority of non-neoplastic CD3-positive T cells and cells of many T-lineage neoplasms
CD45RO – broad specificity	UCHL1	Antigen-experienced T cells (membrane expression)	Granulocytes, monocytes and macrophages are also positive (cytoplasmic expression); excessive decalcification may lead to non-specific nuclear staining
CD45RO – T-cell restricted	OPD4	Antigen-experienced T cells (membrane expression)	Less reactivity than UCHL1 with non-lymphoid lineage cells
CD43	MT1, DFT1	Most T cells and a subset of B cells; lymphocytic lymphoma/CLL and mantle cell lymphoma are usually positive; follicular lymphoma, lymphoplasmacytic lymphoma and marginal zone lymphomas are negative	Strong expression by granulocytic and monocytic cells; expressed by mast cells
CD4	1F6, 4B12	T-cell subset, blastic plasmacytoid dendritic cell neoplasm	There is often poor localization of reaction product to individual cells; macrophages are also positive
CD8	4B11, 1A5	T-cell subset	

continued

Table 2.7 (continued)

Antigen	Antibody*	Specificity	Comments
CD279 (PD1)	NAT	Germinal centre-associated T cells; expressed by neoplastic cells in many cases of angioimmunoblastic T-cell lymphoma	
CD25	4C9	Subset of T cells; strongly positive in adult T-cell leukaemia/lymphoma	Neoplastic mast cells and hairy cells also positive
CD56	1B6, CD564, 123C3	NK cells and some cytotoxic T cells; blastic plasmacytoid dendritic cell neoplasm	Nerve fibres. neuro-ectodermal tumours including small cell carcinoma of lung, some leukaemic myeloblasts and cells of some cases of myeloma are positive; marrow stromal matrix at trabecular margins is strongly positive
CD57	Leu7, NC-1, NK-1, TB01	NK cells and some cytotoxic T cells	Some nerve fibres and neuro-ectodermal tumours are positive
TIA-1	266A19FS	Cytotoxic T cells and NK cells	Neutrophils often strongly positive [33]
Granzyme B	GRB-7, 11F1	Cytotoxic T cells and NK cells	Neutrophils also positive
Perforin	5B10	Cytotoxic T cells and NK cells	
CD30	BerH2, 1G12, 15B3	Reed–Sternberg cells and mononuclear Hodgkin cells, cells of anaplastic large cell lymphoma and some other pleomorphic large cell lymphomas	Plasma cells and some erythroid precursors positive if proteolytic pre-treatment is used; wet-heat antigen retrieval is preferred; some carcinomas, especially embryonal, are positive
CD15	LeuM1, BY87, C3D-1, Carb-3	Neoplastic cells in classical Hodgkin lymphoma (but may be negative in up to 15% of cases); negative in NLPHL	Granulocytic and monocytic cells positive, particularly late granulocyte precursors
BOB.1	TG14	B-cell transcriptional coactivation protein expressed by normal B cells and neoplastic cells in most B-cell NHL and NLPHL; absent from neoplastic cells of classical Hodgkin lymphoma	Should be investigated in parallel with OCT-2

Table 2.7 (continued)

Antigen	Antibody*	Specificity	Comments
OCT-2	Oct-207	B-cell transcription factor expressed by normal B cells and neoplastic cells in most B-cell NHL and NLPHL; absent from neoplastic cells of classical Hodgkin lymphoma	Should be investigated in parallel with BOB.1
Epithelial membrane antigen (EMA)	GP1.4	Cells of anaplastic large cell lymphoma	Some plasma cell are positive; neoplastic cells in some cases of Hodgkin lymphoma and many carcinomas are positive; some cases of anaplastic large cell lymphoma are negative
CD246	ALK1, ALKc, 5A4	Cells of anaplastic large cell lymphoma, ALK-positive subtype; subcellular distribution reflects associated gene translocation	Positive in inflammatory myofibroblastic tumour and occasionally in neuroblastoma and rhabdomyosarcoma [32]
Ki-67 antigen	Ki-67, MM1, MIB1	Proliferating cells (nuclear expression)	Useful for assessing grade of lymphoma from infiltrates in bone marrow; proliferating haemopoietic cells are also positive
ZAP70	ZAP70-LR, L453R, 2F3.2	Expressed by T cells, NK cells and some B-cell neoplasms	Expression of ZAP70 in CLL correlates with unmutated *IGVH* genes and predicts an adverse prognosis

ALL, acute lymphoblastic leukaemia; AML, acute myeloid leukaemia; CLL, chronic lymphocytic leukaemia; DLBCL, diffuse large B-cell lymphoma; MALT, mucosa-associated lymphoid tissue; NHL, non-Hodgkin lymphoma; NK, natural killer; NLPHL, nodular lymphocyte predominant Hodgkin lymphoma.
*The list of monoclonal antibodies is not exhaustive. New clones are continually being developed.
†In addition to the antibodies in this table, antibodies detecting viral products (e.g. Epstein–Barr virus, human herpesvirus 8) are also relevant in the diagnosis of lymphoma, as are antibodies reactive with p53 and p21 (see Table 10.1).

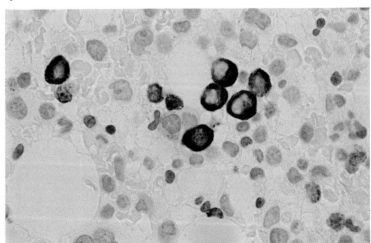

Fig. 2.16 Section of trephine biopsy specimen from a patient with a myelodysplastic syndrome showing elastase-positive granulocyte precursors. Paraffin-embedded; immunoperoxidase technique with anti-elastase McAb NP57 ×100.

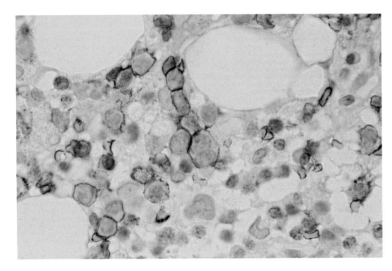

Fig. 2.17 Section of trephine biopsy specimen from a patient with French–American–British (FAB) M6 AML showing erythroblasts, one of which is binucleated. Paraffin-embedded, immunoperoxidase technique with anti-glycophorin antibody McAb Ret40f (CD236R) ×100.

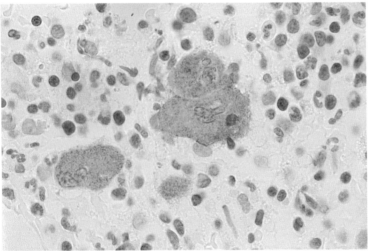

Fig. 2.18 Section of trephine biopsy specimen from a patient with myelodysplastic syndrome showing a cluster of megakaryocytes. Paraffin-embedded, immunoperoxidase technique with CD61 McAb ×100.

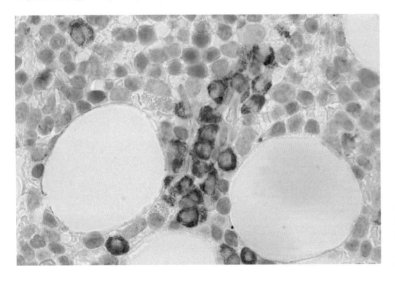

Fig. 2.19 Section of trephine biopsy specimen showing pericapillary plasma cells. Paraffin-embedded, immunoperoxidase technique with McAb VS38c ×100.

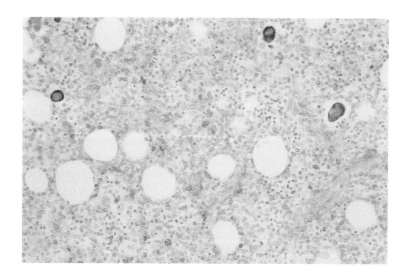

Fig. 2.20 BM trephine biopsy section from a patient with diffuse large B-cell lymphoma; there is heavy interstitial lymphoid infiltration by lymphoma cells showing moderate activity for CD79a (clone Mb1) whereas three megakaryocytes show strong cross reactivity. Paraffin-embedded, immunoperoxidase, CD79a ×20.

should be selected with care; the clone OPD4 stains T cells preferentially, with little granulocytic and monocytic reactivity, while UCHL1 often stains cells of the latter types strongly. Expression of CD45RO by granulocytes and monocytes can be distinguished from that shown by T cells since the former is cytoplasmic, whereas T cells show membrane staining. Bone marrow stromal macrophages express CD4 and, because of the poor localization of a rather weak signal that is often seen with the currently available antibodies, accurate assessment of CD4-positive T cells may not be possible. Monoclonal antibodies reactive with CD3 are currently the most specific T-cell markers for use with bone marrow trephine biopsy sections. It should be noted that antibodies in the CD3 cluster include some recognizing the CD3ε epitope, an epitope that is not T-cell-restricted, since it is also expressed on natural killer (NK) cells. Although less specific than CD3, CD2 monoclonal antibodies are also very useful.

For B cells, we recommend use of both CD20 and CD79a. CD20 is a reliable antigenic target for B cells although in certain circumstances it is down-regulated, e.g. after treatment with rituximab. Some CD79a clones recognize epitopes expressed by vascular smooth muscle and megakaryocytes; these reactivities rarely cause problems in interpretation. Antibodies directed against CD5 and BCL2 react with T cells as well as subsets of normal and neoplastic B cells; results should be interpreted with

care in bone marrow lymphoid infiltrates, in which non-neoplastic T cells frequently predominate.

The specificity of CD45 antibodies for lymphoid cells can be improved if myeloid reactivity is reduced by proteolysis (performed as for antigen retrieval). CD30 antibodies may react positively with plasma cells and occasionally with erythroid cells. Expression in these cell types is cytoplasmic whereas in Reed–Sternberg cells and cells of anaplastic large cell lymphoma it is in the Golgi zone or membrane-associated. This reactivity is unlikely to cause difficulty in the interpretation of possibly lymphoid infiltrates. However, it can be abolished by use of wet heat for antigen retrieval, rather than proteolysis.

Endothelial cell expression of CD34 can mimic reactivity in haemopoietic cells if tiny capillaries are viewed in cross-section. However, the granular nature of haemopoietic cell CD34 expression can be distinguished from the homogeneous pattern seen in endothelium.

Problems relating to fixation and decalcification Use of proprietary combined fixative/decalcifier solutions can lead to extensive loss of immunoreactivity within tissues, as can excessive decalcification by EDTA. Even in optimally fixed and decalcified tissues, some antigens are difficult to demonstrate. Cyclin D1 and CD4 remain problematical in this regard for some laboratories; careful attention to clone selection and technical detail is needed to obtain consistently good results. Non-specific nuclear staining may occur with a variety of antibodies in tissues that are poorly fixed, excessively decalcified or both. In our experience, the antibodies UCHL1 (CD45RO), BER-H2 (CD30) and NB84 are particularly prone to this problem.

Technical problems due to endogenous enzyme activity and non-specific or unwanted antibody binding Endogenous enzyme activity and unwanted antibody binding can both lead to technical problems. When immunostaining trephine biopsy sections with detection systems based on horseradish peroxidase, particular attention must be paid to the blockade of endogenous peroxidase activity. Granulocytes have strong peroxidase activity that is not destroyed by fixation or processing. Use of methanolic hydrogen peroxide is satisfactory but longer incubation (e.g. 30 minutes, compared with 15 minutes for most other tissues) is helpful. Because the solution oxidizes rapidly, replacement with freshly prepared methanol/H_2O_2 at intervals during incubation is helpful. Addition of sodium azide to the final chromogenic substrate provides additional peroxidase blockade in difficult cases.

When using an alkaline phosphatase–anti-alkaline phosphatase detection system there is rarely any problem from endogenous alkaline phosphatase activity, since the enzyme is largely destroyed during processing. A weak background blush may be seen in some cases, due to residual activity in stromal cells. This can be inhibited by adding levamisole to the chromogenic substrate.

Occasionally, endogenous biotin expression can cause non-specific staining when avidin–biotin or streptavidin–biotin detection systems are used. This is found particularly when using antibody AA1 to demonstrate mast cell tryptase. Such activity can be blocked by sequential incubation of sections with saturating solutions of avidin and biotin prior to immunostaining.

Unwanted binding of antibodies to unrelated epitopes, which may be a particular problem with polyclonal antisera, can be blocked by pre-incubation of sections with bovine serum albumin or normal human serum. Background staining of immunoglobulins in plasma and tissue fluid by anti-immunoglobulin light and heavy chain antibodies may be reduced by the use of wet heat methods for antigen retrieval rather than proteolysis.

Weak reactions Sometimes, immunocytochemical reactions are weak or apparently negative although the cells can be shown, by flow cytometry, to express the relevant antigen. This may occur with CD5 expression on neoplastic B cells [34]. In addition CD34 and TdT expression may be positive by flow cytometry and negative by immunohistochemistry [34] or vice versa as antibodies in current use for the two techniques recognize different epitopes.

Problems of interpretation Other problems in interpretation can occur. As mentioned above, immunostaining for antigens such as CD4 and cyclin D1 can be suboptimal and results need to be interpreted with care. Positive controls, with known reactivity, should always be performed to ensure that the technique has worked satisfactorily. It may be necessary to repeat the staining in some cases. It should be noted that cyclin D1 expression in mantle cell lymphoma is nuclear (and only a proportion of cells are positive). This nuclear staining should not be confused with non-specific weak cytoplasmic staining that is sometimes observed in other neoplastic lymphocytes.

Expression of CD5 by neoplastic B cells in CLL and mantle cell lymphoma is much weaker than the constitutive expression of this antigen by T cells. For this reason it is important to ensure that the dilution of the antibody used is optimal for the detection of weakly expressed antigens on neoplastic cells. Similarly, it is important to use for comparison a positive control that represents one of these lymphomas, rather than normal tissue. The detection of neoplastic B cells in CD5-immunostained bone marrow trephine biopsy sections requires careful evaluation of sections since such cells are often present among a background population that contains numerous, strongly stained, non-neoplastic T cells.

Detection of BCL2 expression by cells in B-cell lymphoid infiltrates in bone marrow is seldom useful because of the abundance of non-neoplastic, BCL2-positive T cells, the rarity of follicle formation and the positive reactions that are observed not only in follicular lymphoma but also in other B-cell lymphomas.

Cytogenetic analysis

Specific, non-random chromosomal abnormalities are a common finding in haematological neoplasms and often play a central role in pathogenesis. In addition, some haematological neoplasms are defined more precisely by the presence of specific chromosomal abnormalities than by haematological or histological features. For example, a specific subtype of acute myeloid leukaemia (AML), which can be designated M4Eo/inv(16)(p13.1q22)/*CBFB-MYH11* fusion AML, is better defined by the presence of inversion of chromosome 16 than by the cytological or histological features of acute myelomonocytic leukaemia with eosinophilia. The presence of certain chromosomal abnormalities also offers prognostic information. For example, in AML the presence of t(8;21)(q22;q22), t(15:17) (q22;q12) or inv(16)(p13.1q22) is indicative of a better prognosis. Cytogenetic analysis can also help in distinguishing a neoplastic from a reactive process, as when the demonstration of a clonal cytogenetic abnormality provides evidence that a case of 'idiopathic' hypereosinophilic syndrome is actually eosinophilic leukaemia.

Classical cytogenetic analysis can be performed only on cell suspensions such as those obtained from peripheral blood or bone marrow [35]. Cytogenetic analysis for investigation of suspected haematological neoplasms involves the examination of metaphase spreads which can be prepared from blood or from bone marrow aspirates either as direct preparations, in tumours with a high proliferative fraction, or after a preliminary period of culture either with or without mitogens. Cells are arrested in metaphase by exposure to a spindle poison such as colcemid. After cell lysis the chromosomes are visualized with stains such as Giemsa or quinacrine mustard (a fluorescent agent). Individual chromosomes are identified by their size, by the position of the centromere and by their banding pattern (the sequence of light and dark bands apparent after staining). The findings may be illustrated by a karyogram, an ordered array of chromosomes (Fig. 2.21). Alternatively, they may be expressed as a karyotype. For example, the karyotype 47,XY,+8[18],46,XY[2] from the bone marrow of a male patient indicates the presence of a clone of cells with trisomy 8; of the 20 metaphases examined, two were normal.

Cytogenetic analysis has a major role in haematological diagnosis. Applications include:

1 Confirmation of diagnosis, e.g. by demonstration of t(15;17)(q22;q12) in acute promyelocytic leukaemia.

2 Detection of chromosomal rearrangements that are indicative of good or bad prognosis and should be considered in the choice of treatment, e.g. dem-

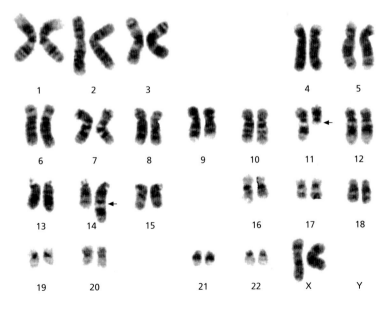

Fig. 2.21 A karyogram showing t(11;14)(q13;q32) in mantle cell lymphoma. (By courtesy of Dr Fiona Ross, Salisbury.)

onstration of hyperdiploidy, indicative of good prognosis in ALL.

3 Confirmation of a neoplastic process when this is otherwise difficult, e.g. in patients with hypereosinophilia or in lymphocytosis with large granular lymphocytes.

4 Monitoring treatment, e.g. by estimation of the number of Philadelphia chromosome-positive metaphases when a patient with chronic granulocytic leukaemia is being treated with interferon.

5 Post-transplant monitoring, e.g. by study of sex chromosomes in a sex-mismatched allogeneic stem cell or bone marrow transplant recipient.

6 Diagnosis of therapy-related AML and MDS.

7 Confirmation of a constitutional abnormality that may underlie the development of a haematological malignancy, e.g. detection of trisomy 21 in a child with acute megakaryoblastic leukaemia in whom Down's syndrome is suspected or demonstration of sensitivity to clastogenic agents, confirming a diagnosis of underlying Fanconi anaemia in a patient presenting with AML.

Problems and pitfalls

Metaphase spreads in leukaemias are often of poor quality so that the characterization of an abnormality can be difficult. In addition, some specific chromosomal rearrangements, e.g. t(12;21) (p13;q22) in ALL, are very difficult to detect by karyotypic analysis while others are impossible; for these rearrangements, molecular genetic techniques are required.

Cytogenetic analysis fails or yields too few metaphases for adequate analysis in a proportion of cases of acute leukaemia. Inappropriate techniques may mean that there is selection for residual normal cells, e.g. if direct examination rather than preliminary culture is used for the investigation of acute promyelocytic leukaemia.

When there is only partial replacement of the marrow by a neoplastic clone, e.g. in MDS, a cytogenetically abnormal clone may be present but may not be identified if insufficient metaphases are examined.

In some slowly growing tumours it is not possible to obtain suitable metaphase preparations and metaphases may represent residual normal cells rather than neoplastic cells. This is often the case, for example, in CLL.

Molecular genetic analysis

Cytogenetic analysis has been part of the diagnostic assessment of haematological neoplasms for many years. More recently, techniques such as Southern blot analysis, PCR and reverse transcriptase PCR (RT-PCR) have allowed molecular genetic events associated with such chromosomal abnormalities to be studied. These techniques have also led to the detection of additional genetic abnormalities in haematological diseases. They are being used increasingly for diagnosis and follow-up of patients on a routine basis.

In addition, molecular genetic analysis can be used to establish clonality; this is particularly valuable in lymphoid neoplasms, where antigen receptor gene rearrangements provide unique clonal markers for neoplastic cell populations. Molecular genetic techniques are most readily applicable to peripheral blood or bone marrow aspirates but modified techniques suitable for application to trephine biopsy specimens are being developed currently. *TCR* (T-cell receptor) and *IGH* (immunoglobulin heavy chain) locus rearrangements are not lineage-specific and, when testing for clonality is indicated, both should be studied. The most useful *TCR* loci are *TCRB* and *TCRG*, encoding TCR-β and TCR-γ, respectively. The *TCRA* locus, encoding TCR-α, is too large for easy analysis by PCR and *TCRD*, encoding TCR-δ, is sometimes lost when *TCRA* is rearranged. *TCRB* analysis requires many primer sets whereas *TCRG* has less allelic variation and is therefore easier to analyse.

New concepts with regard to somatic hypermutation of antigen receptor (*IGH* and *TCR*) variable region genes in lymphoid cell maturation are emerging currently from molecular genetic analysis. Knowledge of such mechanisms in T-cell maturation is much less advanced than it is for the B-cell lineage. Basic understanding of the somatic mutation processes underlying affinity maturation of immunoglobulin molecules, which occur within germinal centres, allows distinction between lymphomas derived from pre-germinal centre (non-mutated), germinal centre (hypermutated with evidence of ongoing acquisition of additional mutations) and post-germinal centre (hypermutated with no ongoing mutation) lymphoid cells. For example, subcategories of CLL have been described which differ by virtue of showing pre-germinal centre (60%) and post-germinal centre (40%) patterns of *IGH* hypermutation, the latter being associated with a better prognosis.

Molecular analysis can also be used to identify viral DNA or RNA in blood or bone marrow (see page 113).

Fluorescence and other *in situ* hybridization techniques

In situ hybridization (ISH) is a molecular genetic technique although it can also be regarded as an extension of conventional cytogenetics. It is based on the hybridization of a labelled probe to interphase nuclei or metaphase spreads. The technique can employ fluorescence labelling (fluorescence *in situ* hybridization or FISH), or an enzymatic [36–38] or radioactive label. Probes, consisting of synthetic DNA in various forms, visualized with the aid of fluorochromes, enzymes or radioisotopes, can be used to detect numerical abnormalities of chromosomes or the presence of various chromosomal rearrangements. Target DNA may be identified by means of a probe conjugated to a fluorochrome. Alternatively, binding of the probe to target DNA can be identified by means of hybridization of the primary probe to complementary bases in a second complementary probe that also contains a reporter molecule [35]. Following stringency washes, performed to remove excess probe, binding of the probe to its target DNA is detected by means of complexing of the reporter molecule in the second probe with a reporter-binding molecule conjugated either to a fluorochrome or to an enzyme such as peroxidase or alkaline phosphatase. By using different fluorochromes or two enzymes it is possible to identify simultaneously multiple (typically two or three) specific DNA sequences in a single preparation of cells. Direct fluorescence methods are more rapid than indirect and give less non-specific background staining, whereas indirect fluorescence methods generally give a stronger signal. Enzymatic methods are currently less used but have the advantage that a fluorescence microscope is not needed and the preparations are permanent.

Fluorescence and other *in situ* hybridization techniques are applicable to films of blood or bone marrow cells, to imprints of trephine biopsy speci-

mens, to cytocentrifuge preparations and to films of cells that have been cultured with or without mitogens. To a more limited extent, FISH is applicable to trephine biopsy sections (see below). These techniques have the particular advantage over classical cytogenetic analysis that they can be applied not only to metaphase spreads but also to interphase nuclei. Chromosome abnormalities can therefore be detected in neoplastic cells that do not readily enter mitosis, such as the neoplastic cells of CLL and myeloma. The technique can also be important in detecting a molecular abnormality that is not associated with a visible cytogenetic abnormality, e.g. deletion of the intervening *CHIC2* gene during formation of the *FIP1L1-PDGFRA* fusion gene in eosinophilic leukaemia. In addition, ISH can be applied to blood or bone marrow films previous stained with a Romanowsky stain or by immunocytochemistry, thus permitting correlation of cytological and immunophenotypic features with karyotypic information. Obviously, unlike cytogenetic analysis, ISH permits visualization of only restricted areas of individual chromosomes rather than giving a global view of the entire chromosome complement within a cell.

The probes available for ISH techniques include: (i) repetitive sequence centromeric probes for individual chromosomes (available for all chromosomes and applicable to cells in interphase or metaphase), repetitive sequence pan-centromeric probes, repetitive sequence pan-telomeric probes and repetitive sequence telomeric or subtelomeric probes for individual chromosomes; (ii) whole chromosome paints (available for all chromosomes but applicable only to cells in metaphase) or short arm or long arm or region-specific paints; and (iii) specific sequence probes, including those identifying oncogenes, cancer-suppressing genes and the breakpoints of recurring translocations (applicable to cells in interphase or metaphase).

Numerical abnormalities of chromosomes can be detected either with centromeric probes or with whole chromosome paints. When such probes are used, normal cells have two separate fluorescent signals. If there is an abnormality of chromosome number, the number of signals varies from normal. For example, in trisomy 12 FISH with a centromeric probe for chromosome 12 shows three signals per cell, whereas in monosomy 7 FISH with a cen-

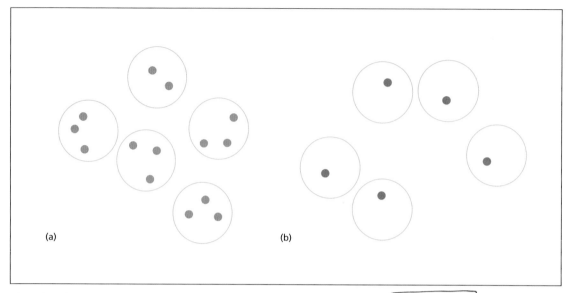

(a)   (b)

Fig. 2.22 Diagrammatic representation illustrating the principles of FISH, using a centromeric probe for the identification of trisomy or monosomy. (a) Centromeric probe for chromosome 12 in chronic lymphocytic leukaemia showing four trisomic cells and one disomic cell. (b) Centromeric probe for chromosome 7 in myelodysplastic syndrome showing all cells to have monosomy 7.

tromeric probe for chromosome 7 shows only one signal per cell (Fig. 2.22). If using centromeric probes, rather than whole chromosome paints, care must be taken in making assumptions that the gain or loss of a signal represents gain or loss of an entire chromosome target.

Several strategies can be used for detecting specific translocations or other rearrangements. Use of a single probe spanning a specific chromosomal breakpoint is useful when multiple chromosomal partners can disrupt a gene of interest, as is the case with *MLL* and *BCL6*. When both partner chromosomes are predictable a variety of techniques can be used. Whole chromosome paints can be used for the two chromosomes of interest. Alternatively, two probes can be selected that bind to specific oncogenes or bind to the two chromosomes of interest at a site close to the expected breakpoint. The two probes are labelled with different fluorochromes. In normal cells there will be two separate signals of different colours whereas, in cells in which a translocation has occurred, the two colours come together on a single chromosome (Fig. 2.23). Alternatively, probes spanning the expected break-

point on each chromosome can be used so that, if a translocation has occurred, the signals are split. Each abnormal chromosome then has two adjacent signals of different colours (which appear fused so that red-green fusion signals are seen as yellow), while the two remaining normal chromosomes have a single colour signal (Fig. 2.24); this technique is sometimes referred to as D-FISH, signifying double fusion FISH. It is also possible to combine one probe spanning an expected breakpoint with another that is adjacent to the second breakpoint. A single probe spanning one of the breakpoints can also be used, a split signal being consistent with a translocation. In this case it is sometimes be necessary to demonstrate that three signals represent a normal and a split signal rather than trisomy (Fig. 2.25). Triple colour FISH permits the use of a single probe identifying a sequence on one of the chromosomes implicated together with two separate probes identifying genes on either side of the breakpoint on the second chromosome. The latter two signals are dissociated when the relevant translocation occurs (Fig. 2.26).

Probes spanning specific breakpoints are also

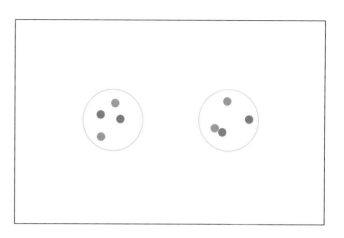

Fig. 2.23 Diagrammatic representation illustrating the principles of FISH, using two oncogene probes to detect a translocation. Probes for *BCR* (red) and *ABL1* (green) have been used. In the normal cell (left) there are four separate signals. In the cell from a patient with t(9;22)(q34;q11.2) associated with chronic granulocytic leukaemia (right) there are single normal *BCR* and *ABL1* signals and a double red plus green signal where the two oncogenes have been juxtaposed.

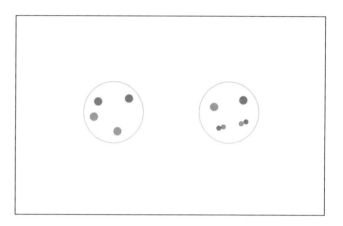

Fig. 2.24 Diagrammatic representation illustrating the principles of FISH, using two oncogene probes, both of which are split in a given translocation, to detect the translocation. Probes spanning *BCR* (red) and *ABL1* (green) have been used. In the normal cell (left) there are four separate signals. In the cell from a patient with t(9;22)(q34;q11.2) associated with chronic granulocytic leukaemia (right) there are single normal *BCR* and *ABL1* signals and two double red plus green signals representing *BCR–ABL1* and *ABL1–BCR*.

useful for detecting isochromosome formation (Fig. 2.27) and chromosomal inversion. For example, inversion of chromosome 16 can be detected by using a probe that spans one of the breakpoints. When a pericentric inversion has occurred, the signal is split and appears on both the long and short arms of the chromosome in a metaphase spread (Fig. 2.28).

Fluorescence *in situ* hybridization can also be used to identify deletion or amplification of chromosomal material. For example, specific probes can be used to show deletion of a cancer-suppressing gene such as *RB1* or *TP53* or amplification of an oncogene such as *MYC*.

The ISH technique has the following advantages over classical cytogenetics:

1 Living cells are not required.

2 Some abnormalities can be recognized in interphase nuclei, making the technique particularly useful for neoplasms, such as CLL, with a low proliferative rate.

3 A suspected abnormality can be confirmed when morphology of the chromosomes is poor.

4 Chromosomal rearrangements, such as inversion(16), which have only subtle alterations in the chromosome banding pattern and are therefore difficult to recognize on classical cytogenetic analysis if preparations are suboptimal, can be detected.

5 Large numbers of cells can be scanned so that a low frequency abnormal population can be recognized.

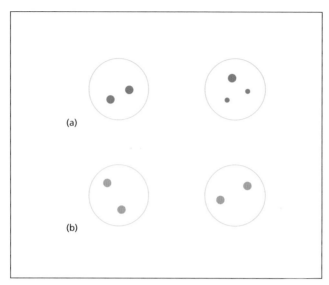

Fig. 2.25 Diagrammatic representation illustrating the principles of FISH, using a whole chromosome paint to detect a translocation. (a) In this case, a paint for chromosome 11 has been used. A normal cell (left) shows two signals whereas a cell from a patient with t(11;14)(q13;q32) associated with mantle cell lymphoma (right) shows three signals representing, respectively, one normal chromosome and two signals from the chromosome that has participated in the translocation. (b) To ensure that the three signals do not represent trisomy for chromosome 11, FISH can also be performed with a centromeric probe for chromosome 11; since the centromere is not split in the translocation this shows two signals in both the normal cell (left) and the cell with the translocation (right).

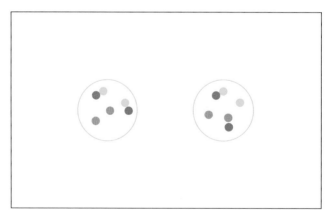

Fig. 2.26 Diagrammatic representation of triple colour FISH, a technique used to reduce the probability of false-positive results, utilizing an *ABL1* probe (red), a *BCR* probe (green) and a probe for the *ASS* gene (yellow) which is just proximal to *ABL1*. A normal cell (left) has two green *BCR* signals and two fused yellow–red signals representing *ABL1* plus *ASS*. A cell from a patient with t(9;22)(q34;q11.2) (right) has one normal *BCR* signal (green) and one normal *ASS* plus *ABL1* signal (yellow plus red); the translocation has separated *ASS* from *ABL1* so that there is a separate *ASS* signal (yellow) and a *BCR–ABL1* fusion signal (red plus green).

Fig. 2.27 Diagrammatic representation of the demonstration of an isochromosome by FISH. A normal cell (left) is compared with a cell from a patient with T-lineage prolymphocytic leukaemia (right) showing an isochromosome of the long arm of chromosome 8. A centromeric probe (red) has been combined with a probe for the *MYC* oncogene (green) which is located on 8q. The normal cell shows two chromosomes, each with a red signal and a green signal. The lymphoma cell shows, in addition, an isochromosome with two green (*MYC*) signals on either side of the centromeric (red) signal.

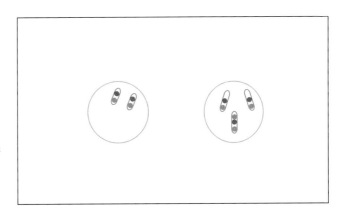

Fig. 2.28 Diagrammatic representation of the use of FISH to demonstrate chromosomal inversion showing a normal cell (left) and cell from a patient with M4Eo AML and inv(16) (p13.1q22) (right). A chromosome paint for the short arm of chromosome 16 has been used. In the normal cell there are two chromosomes, each with a single red signal. In the cell with an inversion there is one normal chromosome (with a single signal) and one abnormal chromosome (with a split signal). The inversion is pericentric and the inverted telomeric part of the short arm is now fused with the telomeric part of the long arm.

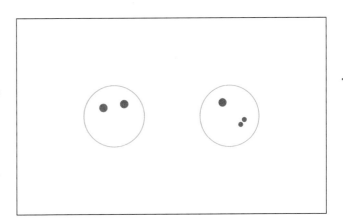

6 Deletion of cancer-suppressing genes or amplification of oncogenes can be demonstrated.

Fluorescent immunophenotyping and interphase cytogenetics (FICTION) is a technique combining immunophenotyping with FISH. It can be used, for example, to demonstrate that trisomy 12 in CLL can occur in only a proportion of the clonal lymphocytes.

A further development of FISH is spectral karyotyping (SKY) in which a complex panel of probes applied simultaneously permits the identification of all chromosomes in metaphase preparations. This technique is particularly useful for investigating complex chromosomal abnormalities. Because expensive equipment, reagents and software are required the technique is currently mainly used in research rather than in routine diagnosis. Multicolour FISH (M-FISH), using five fluoro-

chromes, filters and computer software, can similarly permit the identification of all 24 chromosomes and the elucidation of complex chromosomal abnormalities [39]. Further modifications of FISH technology are cross-species colour banding (Rx-FISH), multicolour FISH of telomeric regions (M-TEL) [38] and primed *in situ* hybridization (PRINS). PRINS is a technique for identifying specific chromosomes by means of primers, which are annealed to target α satellite chromosome-specific repetitive DNA sequences, followed by *in situ* primer extension using Taq DNA polymerase and incorporating fluorochrome-labelled dUTP; this technique is applicable, for example, to the detection of monosomy 7 or trisomy 8.

Fluorescence *in situ* hybridization is applicable to a more limited extent to trephine biopsy sections, but at present is best restricted to analysis of potential chromosomal gains and some translocations. For mathematical reasons, analysis of chromosomal loss in tissue sections (in which many nuclei are only partly represented) is complex. Spatial resolution of FISH signals in histological sections is sufficient to permit application of dual colour techniques to demonstrate translocations; a fusion signal resulting from a translocation [40] and split signals from a probe spanning an expected breakpoint can be resolved. Gentle decalcification techniques, e.g. using EDTA, facilitate FISH on trephine biopsy sections [41]. Some of the limitations of the application of FISH to histological sections can be overcome by applying FISH to cytocentrifuge preparations from intact nuclei or whole cells extracted by proteolysis from thick sections. As for immunohistochemistry, pre-treatments are required to unmask target DNA sequences. Because these vary considerably with different fixation and decalcification protocols, FISH applied to bone marrow trephine biopsy specimens is still predominantly a research tool although its utility for diagnostic and prognostic use is increasing.

It should be noted that ISH techniques to detect messenger RNA (mRNA) targets can also be applied to cytological and histological bone marrow preparations. Either enzymes or fluorochromes can be used to identify the target mRNA. Double labelling with two different fluorochromes is possible, e.g. for either κ or λ mRNA and for either tumour necrosis factor α (TNFα) or interleukin 1β (IL1β) mRNA, in order to demonstrate whether neoplastic light-chain-restricted plasma cells are capable of synthesizing these cytokines. In diagnostic practice, ISH for the detection of mRNA is useful for the demonstration of κ- or λ-expressing plasma cells (Fig. 2.29). It is also applicable to the detection of expression of genes relevant to oncogenesis, e.g. *CCND1* (encoding cyclin D1) [42]. Other roles are likely to emerge.

ISH techniques can be used for the detection of viral mRNA, such as EBERs of Epstein–Barr virus (EBV) (in Hodgkin lymphoma, non-Hodgkin lymphoma and post-transplant lymphoproliferative disorders), human herpesvirus 8 DNA (in Castleman's disease and primary effusion lymphoma) and parvovirus B19 DNA (in pure red cell aplasia). ISH can also be used for the detection of the DNA of bacteria; e.g. a whole genome probe can be used for the detection of *Mycobacterium tuberculosis*.

Problems and pitfalls

Fluorescence *in situ* hybridization and other ISH techniques have various disadvantages:

1 In any single preparation, it is only possible to identify the specific abnormality for which relevant probes are being employed; for example, if cells are being investigated for the presence of t(8;21), other leukaemia-associated translocation such as t(15;17) or t(9;11) will not be detected.

2 Secondary abnormalities are not recognized; for example, if the proportion of Philadelphia-positive metaphases were being evaluated in a case of chronic granulocytic leukaemia, the presence of an isochromosome of 17q (which might be associated with impending acute transformation) would not be detected.

3 The use of whole chromosome paints does not permit the detection of rearrangements within a single chromosome, such as an inversion, or small deletions.

4 In screening for trisomies and monosomies there are some false-positive findings, caused by accidental co-localization of signals, so that a low frequency of the abnormality being sought cannot be detected reliably.

5 If neoplastic cells are present in the bone marrow but cannot be aspirated because of associated fibrosis there will be a failure to detect any relevant cytogenetic abnormality.

The first two of these disadvantages can be circumvented to some extent by the use of multicolour FISH or spectral karyotyping [36].

Southern blot analysis

In this technique DNA is extracted from a fresh, unfixed tissue sample and digested with a panel of restriction endonucleases. Sometimes, when the bone marrow is cellular, unfixed bone marrow films on glass slides may yield sufficient material for analysis. The restriction endonucleases used are enzymes that recognize specific nucleotide sequences between 4 and 10 base pairs in length and cut the DNA molecule wherever their target sequences occur. This results in DNA fragments of variable length that can be separated, according to

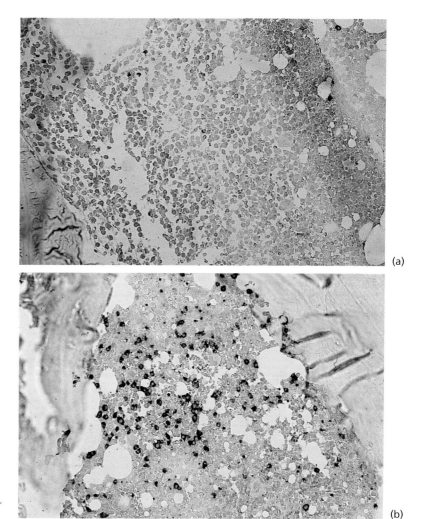

(a)

(b)

Fig. 2.29 *In situ* hybridization showing (a) κ and (b) λ light chain messenger RNA. There are only occasional κ-positive cells but λ-positive cells are numerous. Paraffin-embedded, immunoperoxidase-labelled probes ×20.

their size, by gel electrophoresis. These are then transferred by capillary action onto a more solid nitrocellulose membrane to create a Southern blot. Fragments containing the DNA sequences of interest can then be identified by hybridization with a radiolabelled DNA probe followed by autoradiography. One of the major breakthroughs that Southern blot analysis allowed was the detection of clonality in B- and T-lymphoid neoplasms (see below). In addition, rearrangement of a gene arising from translocation or some other acquired chromosomal rearrangement can be detected. This technique is used, for example, for detecting rearrangement of

the *MLL* or *BCL6* genes since rearrangement can result from a considerable number of different translocations, not all of which can be detected by alternative techniques. The Southern blot technique is also applicable for the detection of translocations in which there is considerable heterogeneity of breakpoints, which precludes use of a simple PCR technique.

Southern blot analysis can be used to demonstrate clonal integration of human T-cell lymphotropic virus I (HTLV-I) proviral DNA and integration of defective HTLV-I in adult T-cell leukaemia/lymphoma [43].

Problems and pitfalls

The major drawbacks of Southern blot analysis as a diagnostic tool are the requirement for radioactive materials, long turnaround times and the need for relatively large quantities of high molecular weight DNA in the diagnostic sample, which limits the sensitivity of the method. The latter feature greatly limits its applicability to trephine biopsy specimens [44].

The polymerase chain reaction

The polymerase chain reaction [45,46] is a method of *in vitro* amplification of a defined DNA target that is flanked by regions of known sequence. The development of this technique has greatly expanded the diagnostic potential of molecular genetics as a result of its ability to generate almost limitless copies of selected target DNA sequences. The technique is 400–4000 times more sensitive than Southern blot analysis. It consists of a repeating cycle of three basic steps (denaturation, primer annealing and elongation), with each cycle potentially leading to a doubling of the amount of the target DNA sequence.

The first step (denaturation) involves heating the DNA sample to around 90 °C, which causes the double-stranded DNA molecule to separate into two complementary single strands. The next stage (primer annealing) requires short DNA primer sequences that are complementary to the ends of the target DNA segment that is to be amplified. The primer is added to the denatured single-stranded DNA and the sample is cooled. As cooling occurs, the primers anneal (link via the complementary nucleotide sequences) to the single-stranded target DNA. The third step (elongation) requires addition of free nucleotides to the ends of the primer DNA segments producing complementary copies of each of the two single-stranded target DNA sequences. This is achieved using a thermostable DNA polymerase. The strands of DNA thus generated are separated from their complementary strands by elevating the temperature again. The cycle is repeated by elevating and lowering the temperature of the container in which the reaction takes place. This process is performed in an automated thermal cycling instrument pre-set with specific temperatures and times that are optimized for each primer pair. The cycles of denaturing, annealing and elongation are repeated 10–40 times. Amplification is initially exponential since each cycle doubles the amount of DNA template present. In later cycles the rate of increase in the quantity of DNA is closer to linear than to exponential. Nevertheless, very large quantities of the target DNA sequence are generated. The size of the DNA segment can be estimated by electrophoresis, by comparison with known standards (Fig. 2.30). The DNA generated can be directly visualized by staining with ethidium bromide and viewing under ultraviolet light. This technique has many advantages over Southern blot analysis for diagnostic use, principally the short turnaround time, the lack of a requirement for radioisotopes, the ability to amplify very small quantities of target DNA and its applicability to fixed tissue, including archival samples and even stained or unstained blood or bone marrow films scraped off glass slides. Stained slides are, however, less satisfactory than paraffin-embedded tissue because DNA degradation is greater. Techniques are available for use with decalcified paraffin-embedded trephine biopsy specimens [47]; EDTA decalcification rather than formic acid decalcification is required to minimize DNA degradation [48]. The amplification achieved by PCR makes the technique very sensitive. The DNA fragments produced are suitable for sequencing. Because of these advantages PCR, or its modification RT-PCR, has replaced Southern blot analysis for most diagnostic applications. To distinguish it from RT-PCR, PCR is sometimes referred to as genomic PCR or DNA-PCR.

In situ PCR is a modification of the PCR technique performed on tissue sections pre-treated with a proteinase to facilitate entry of primers [49]. It remains largely a research technique.

The polymerase chain reaction can be used for the following:

1 Investigation of clonality (by amplification of *IGH*, *IGK*, *IGL* (encoding immunoglobulin κ and λ chains), *TCRB*, *TCRG* or *TCRD*).

2 Detection of rearrangement of genes resulting from acquired cytogenetic abnormalities.

3 Detection of bacterial or viral sequences (for example, sequences of the *Mycobacterium tuberculosis* genome in a bone marrow aspirate).

It can also be used to demonstrate clonality of lymphoid cells by the amplification of EBV DNA.

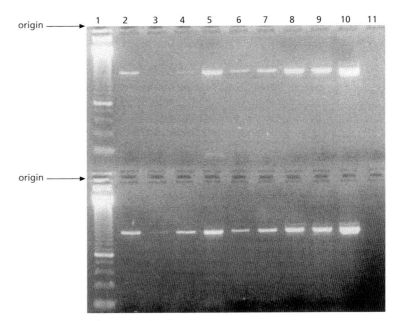

Fig. 2.30 Polyacrylamide gel stained with ethidium bromide and visualized with ultraviolet light showing PCR amplification of the 643 base pair BRCA1 exon 11A (top panel) and 482 base pair BRCA2 exon 11B (bottom panel). Lane 1 contains size standards and lanes 2–10 contain amplified samples of DNA extracted from EDTA-decalcified bone marrow trephine biopsy specimens. (By courtesy of Mrs Caroline Wickham, Exeter.)

Because of a variable number of terminal repeats in the circular episomal forms of the virus, a polyclonal lymphoid population with a variety of forms of the virus can be distinguished from a monoclonal population with a single form. This can be useful for establishing clonality of EBV-induced natural killer cell lymphomas for which there are usually no alternative techniques for demonstrating clonality.

Problems and pitfalls
Great care is required to avoid contamination during PCR analysis as even the smallest quantity of DNA with a sequence complementary to the primers will be amplified. Meticulous technique is required.

Although PCR is applicable to archival material, poor preservation of DNA can lead to negative results [44]; amplification of a constitutional gene, for example *G6PD*, *BCR*, *ABL1* or *HBB* (the β globin gene), can be used to control for DNA degradation. Preservation of DNA is determined by the fixative used and the method of processing. Formalin fixation has been found to give optimal results but other fixatives, e.g. B5, can be used [44]. As noted above, DNA from archival glass slides is often of inferior quality. A higher success rate may be achieved with frozen biopsy specimens and splitting a biopsy specimen in two and fixing only half has therefore been recommended [50].

Negative results can result from sampling error when tissue infiltration is focal. Variant breakpoints may be missed if appropriate primers are not used. For example, in testing for *BCL2* rearrangement in follicular lymphoma it is usual to screen for breakpoints in the minor cluster region, intermediate cluster region and major breakpoint region and even this will not detect all possible breakpoints.

In some neoplasms PCR to amplify fusion genes is an insensitive diagnostic technique, because of the wide scatter of breakpoints. For example, in mantle cell lymphoma, even with optimized primer sets for breakpoints throughout the major translocation cluster, *CCND1-IGH* will only be detected in 50–60% of cases [46,51].

Reverse transcriptase polymerase chain reaction

The polymerase chain reaction is applied to genomic DNA. Because of the presence of introns, a gene may be very large so that satisfactory amplification is difficult. This problem can be circumvented by the use of mRNA as the starting material since the

Table 2.8 Modifications of the polymerase chain reaction (PCR) and reverse transcriptase PCR (RT-PCR) techniques.

Modification	Principle
Nested PCR	A second pair of primers, recognizing sequences internal to those recognized by the first pair, increase sensitivity and specificity
Multiplex PCR	A number of pairs of primers permit the recognition of two or three unrelated gene rearrangements in a single procedure
Quantitative PCR Real-time quantitative PCR (RQ-PCR) Competitive PCR Limiting dilution PCR Co-amplification of target and control genes	The PCR procedure becomes quantitative rather than merely qualitative, permitting quantification of minimal residual disease
Long-range PCR	A process in which fragments up to 10kb are generated, using modified polymerases
5′-RACE (rapid amplification of cDNA ends)	A technique for the identification of unknown translocation partners when one partner is well characterized but the other is not
LA-PCR (long and accurate PCR)	A technique for the identification of precise translocation breakpoints using forward primers complementary to RACE-determined gene partners and reverse primers complementary to introns of the known translocation partner
Long distance inverse PCR	A technique for detecting various translocation partners when the breakpoints of one partner are clustered; particularly useful for detecting translocations involving the *IGH* locus
Allele-specific PCR	PCR that distinguishes between two alleles of a gene, e.g. wild type and a mutant with a single nucleotide substitution

introns will have been excised and the segment to be amplified is shorter. The mRNA must first be transcribed into complementary DNA by means of reverse transcriptase. Amplification can then proceed, as in PCR of genomic DNA. RT-PCR is now very commonly employed for the detection of leukaemia and lymphoma-related fusion genes. RT-PCR can also be used for the detection of viral mRNA.

Modifications of PCR and RT-PCR techniques

Modifications of PCR and RT-PCR techniques (Table 2.8) can increase sensitivity, specificity and usefulness and permit an approximate quantification of the number of copies of the fusion gene present. Among these modifications is multiplex PCR, in which a number of sets of primers are used to amplify simultaneously two or three different fusion genes. This makes it possible, for example, to screen simultaneously for the three fusion genes found in the three subtypes of AML associated with a better prognosis: *RUNX1-RUNX1T1* (previously known as *AML1-ETO*), *PML-RARA* and *CBFB-MYH11*. The development of various techniques for quantification of the amount of target DNA or mRNA present means that PCR and RT-PCR are now becoming useful for the detection of minimal residual disease and for monitoring the response to therapy. One application of quantitative methods is in monitoring *BCR-ABL1* during imatinib therapy or following transplantation for chronic granulocytic leukaemia. In real-time quantitative PCR (RQ-PCR) the PCR technique results in displacement of a fluorogenic product-specific probe, which is degraded during the reaction generating a fluorescent signal. Nested PCR is a technique that achieves greater sensitivity so is particularly useful in T- and B-cell clonality studies and in the detection of *FIP1L1-PDGFRA* fusion. Allele-specific PCR allows simultaneous detection of wild type and mutant DNA; its most important application is in the detection of *JAK2* V617F in myeloproliferative disorders.

Problems and pitfalls

Reverse transcriptase PCR requires intact RNA and is therefore not a suitable technique for use with most archival material. False-negative results can occur if there is degradation of RNA and amplification of a control mRNA sequence is therefore advised.

As for genomic PCR, the high sensitivity of the technique means that there is a risk of false-positive results if contamination is permitted to occur. Multicentre studies have sometimes shown a high rate of false-positive reactions so that inclusion of a negative control in each assay is considered to be critical [52]. RT-PCR techniques are poorly standardized and quality control is not optimal so that different laboratories produce divergent results in a significant proportion of cases [46].

Since RT-PCR uses a small tissue sample, negative results can occur when infiltration, e.g. of a trephine biopsy specimen, is focal. Sometimes microscopy permits the detection of infiltration by lymphoma when results of RT-PCR are negative [44].

It must also be noted that sensitive techniques have detected gene rearrangements typical of leukaemia and lymphoma in people who do not have an identifiable neoplastic condition. This has been noted for *BCR-ABL1*, *NPM1-ALK*, *MLLT2-MLL* (*AF4-MLL*) and the *BCL2* rearrangement, characteristic respectively of chronic granulocytic leukaemia, large cell anaplastic lymphoma, acute lymphoblastic/biphenotypic leukaemia of infants and follicular lymphoma.

There are also problems in knowing when the detection of minimal residual disease is clinically significant. Detection of a residual clonal abnormality for a year or more after cessation of treatment is sometimes compatible with continued disease-free survival. This has been noted for *RUNX1-RUNX1T1*, *MYH11-CBFB* and *TCF3-PBX1* (*E2A-PBX1*)

fusion genes and for *IGH* locus rearrangements [45,53].

Microarray analysis

Microarray analysis is a technique for determining the expression of dozens, hundreds or even thousands of genes by means of hybridizing fluorescence-labelled patient DNA with an array of known DNA sequences [54]. Automated detection of fluorescent signals is followed by computer analysis of the results, which can be either supervised or unsupervised. Supervised analysis means that cases are classified into disease entities – e.g. AML with t(8;21), AML with t(15;17), ALL – according to a recognized system and differences in gene expression are then sought between different categories; these differences can then be used for 'class prediction' of future cases. Unsupervised analysis means that the programme seeks clusters of genes being expressed together, which may identify new disease categories, a process of 'class discovery'. For example, large B-cell lymphomas were found to fall into two or three different classes that differed in prognosis [54]. Microarray analysis is currently mainly a research tool but there is potential to use it for: (i) diagnosis; (ii) determining prognosis; (iii) stratifying patients for treatment; and (iv) identifying targets for molecule-directed treatment.

Other molecular genetic techniques

Other molecular genetic techniques are rarely used in routine diagnosis but have research uses. They include:

1 Northern blot analysis for the investigation of RNA.

2 Western blot analysis for the investigation of proteins including the 'oncoproteins' that are the products of fusion genes.

3 Comparative genomic hybridization (CGH) and array CGH to detect segments of chromosomes that are under- or over-represented in leukaemic cells.

4 Single nucleotide polymorphism (SNP) analysis, which is somewhat similar to array CGH and can define smaller areas of genetic gain and loss.

5 Gene expression microarray analysis and related methods such as multiplexed quantum dot-based ISH analysis.

6 DNA sequencing, which is necessary for the cloning of new genes.

The application of molecular genetic techniques in the investigation of leukaemia and lymphoma

Molecular genetic techniques have two principal applications in the investigation of haematological neoplasms. Firstly, they can be used to demonstrate that a monoclonal population is present and can give information on the nature of the lymphoid cell in which a mutation occurred (see below). Secondly, they can be used to demonstrate the presence of fusion genes or fusion RNA transcripts that are known to be associated with specific neoplasms. Demonstration of clonality is mainly done by investigation of the *IGH* or *TCR* gene loci, although demonstration of rearrangement or mutation of any gene could be used as a marker of clonality.

Detecting clonal immunoglobulin and T-cell receptor gene rearrangements

Clonal populations of B or T lymphocytes can be detected by demonstrating clonal rearrangements of the *IGH* or *TCR* gene loci using Southern blot analysis or PCR. The basic principle underlying the technique is similar since genes at the *TCR* and *IGH* loci are made up of a number of variable (V), diversity (D) and joining (J) regions, present in germline DNA, which rearrange during lymphocyte development to produce a functioning gene. During rearrangement single V, D and J regions are combined with a constant (C) region and simultaneously nucleotides (known as N) are added and removed between the V, D and J regions. This results in a unique DNA sequence in a cell and its progeny. Rearrangement of *IGK* (κ) and *IGL* (λ) loci is similar except that a D region is lacking.

Using Southern blot analysis, probes that detect either part of the immunoglobulin heavy chain J region or *TCRB* or *TCRG* are used to detect clonal rearrangements. In polyclonal populations of lymphocytes there are a large number of different rearrangements and no single discrete band can be visualized. In a clonal population, since all the cells share the same rearrangement, there is a single discrete band on electrophoresis, which is separate from the germline band. However, Southern blot analysis has now been largely replaced by PCR.

The technique for detecting clonal rearrangements using PCR is somewhat different from that used for Southern blot analysis. Primers with sequences complementary to segments of the immunoglobulin heavy chain V and J regions that are relatively constant are used to amplify part of the rearranged *IGH* locus. Differences in the numbers of nucleotides (N) inserted between the V and J regions during rearrangement result in multiple, different-sized segments of DNA being amplified in polyclonal populations so that no discrete band is visualized. In clonal populations, there is amplification of a single rearranged fragment which appears as a discrete band separate from the germline band on electrophoresis. The same principle underlies detection of *IGK* and *IGL* rearrangement for B-cell clonality analysis and detection of rearranged *TCRG* and *TCRB* in T-cell clonality analysis.

Molecular genetic analysis has led to new concepts with regard to somatic hypermutation of antigen receptor (*IGH* and *TCR*) variable region genes in lymphoid cell maturation, with potential relevance to our understanding of the origins and behaviour of all lymphomas. Knowledge of such mechanisms in T-cell maturation is much less advanced than it is for the B-cell lineage. Basic understanding of the somatic mutation processes underlying affinity maturation of immunoglobulin molecules, which occur within germinal centres, allows distinction between lymphomas derived from pre-germinal centre, germinal centre and post-germinal centre lymphoid cells.

Problems and pitfalls   Although PCR is more sensitive than Southern blotting at detecting small clonal populations it will not detect all rearrangements. Approximately 80% of B-cell neoplasms will show clonal rearrangements on PCR using primers for *IGHV* regions, whereas the great majority will have a rearrangement detectable by Southern blot analysis. Hence caution is required in interpreting negative PCR results. The likelihood of detecting *IGH* rearrangement by PCR varies between different types of lymphoma, in one study ranging from around 40% with follicular lymphoma to around 80% with mantle cell and small lymphocytic lymphomas [46]. The negative results in follicular and certain other lymphomas are consequent on the high rate of somatic mutation, which is responsible for a failure of consensus primers to bind to rearranged genes [44]. In one study, PCR was found to be less sensitive than flow cytometry for the detection of a clonal population in bone marrow in the case of B-cell neoplasms but was more sensitive than flow cytometry in the case of T-cell neoplasms [55].

It should also be noted that rearrangement of *IGH* and *TCR* genes is not entirely lineage-specific. Inappropriate gene rearrangement is quite frequently seen in ALL and occurs, although less often, in lymphomas of mature T and B cells. In addition, *IGH* or *TCR* rearrangement is sometimes found in AML. Rearrangement of *IGK* or *IGL* is much more specific for the B-lymphocyte lineage than *IGH* rearrangement.

It is likewise important to recognize that, although the detection of a clonal rearrangement usually indicates a neoplastic process, clonal *IGH* and *TCR* rearrangements have been detected in some reactive conditions. Interpretation of results in a clinical context is essential.

Detection of leukaemia/lymphoma-associated fusion genes

As discussed earlier, many haematological neoplasms are associated with a specific non-random chromosomal abnormality. The genes involved in many of these rearrangements have been identified, permitting the use of molecular genetic techniques for their detection. Some translocations can be detected by PCR, by employing specific primers with sequences complementary to segments of DNA that flank the chromosomal breakpoints. The intervening segment across the breakpoint will only be amplified if the translocation is present. However, this technique is only applicable if the breakpoint occurs in a relatively constant position and the fusion gene is not too long. Many more translocations can be detected by RT-PCR. Translocations that can detected by PCR or RT-PCR include t(9:22)(q34;q11.2) in chronic granulocytic leukaemia and some acute lymphoblastic leukaemias; t(14:18)(q32;q21) in follicular lymphoma; t(2:5)(p23;q35) in anaplastic large cell lymphoma; and various translocations or inversions associated with AML including t(8:21)(q22;q22), t(15:17)(q22;q12) and inv(16)(p13.1q22).

Advantages of PCR and RT-PCR are that they give a more rapid result than conventional cytogenetic analysis and do not require viable cells for metaphase preparations. The highly sensitive nature of the PCR analysis also means that this technique can be used to detect very small numbers of neoplastic cells; consequently the method can be used for the detection of minimal residual disease and early relapse. However it should be noted that, using these sensitive techniques, fusion genes characteristic of leukaemia or lymphoma are sometimes detected in normal tissues or tissues showing only reactive changes. For example the rearrangement characteristic of follicular lymphoma has been detected in tonsils removed surgically for reactive conditions.

Problems and pitfalls   Disadvantages, other than the possibility of contaminating DNA being amplified, include the fact that not all rearrangements can be detected. This is because of the necessity for a chromosomal abnormality to have been fully characterized so that specific primers for each breakpoint can be designed. It should also be noted that, in contrast to standard cytogenetic analysis, molecular genetic techniques permit the detection only of those abnormalities that are being specifically sought. Nevertheless many chromosomal rearrangements can be detected by PCR and RT-PCR and some such rearrangements are sufficiently common that these techniques are very practical for the rapid and precise categorization of cases of acute leukaemia and for confirming the diagnosis of certain categories of lymphoma. It has already been noted that there may be low level amplification of a number of fusion genes in healthy subjects.

Ultrastructural examination

Ultrastructural examination, in which the structure of cells is studied by electron microscopy, can be applied to peripheral blood and bone marrow but is little used in routine diagnostic haematology. Advances in immunophenotyping have rendered electron microscopy redundant in identifying French–American–British (FAB) M0 and M7 categories of AML. It remains of some use in identifying small Sézary cells (Fig. 2.31) and in making a

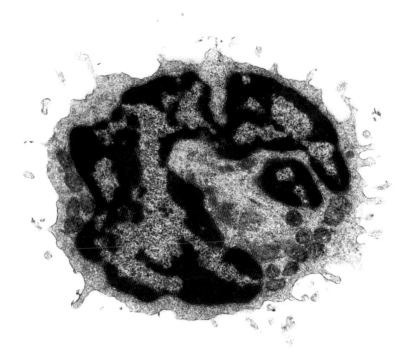

Fig. 2.31 Ultrastructural examination in Sézary syndrome showing a Sézary cell with a highly irregular nuclear outline. (By courtesy of Dr Estella Matutes, London.)

precise diagnosis in congenital dyserythropoietic anaemia.

Ultrastructural examination can also be applied to trephine biopsy specimens but it is rarely necessary for diagnosis. It can be used for the detection of Birbeck's granules to confirm the diagnosis of Langerhans cell histiocytosis but immunohisto-chemistry, including the application of a CD1a monoclonal antibody, is an alternative more readily available confirmatory technique.

Bone marrow culture for assessment of haemopoietic progenitor cell numbers

Short- and long-term culture techniques for hae-mopoietic cells have found extensive use in research and, although they are not yet widely used in diag-nostic practice, they have been incorporated into WHO criteria for the diagnosis of several haemato-logical neoplasms.

Short-term culture

The major current use of short-term culture in clinical practice is for assessment of harvested bone marrow or peripheral blood stem cells prior to their use for engraftment.

Short-term haemopoietic cultures are performed using cells suspended at a known starting concen-tration in methyl cellulose or agar supplemented with culture medium, fetal bovine serum and growth-promoting substances such as granulocyte–macrophage colony-stimulating factor (GM-CSF), erythropoietin and thrombopoietin. They are then incubated at 37 °C for 14 days, in a humidified atmosphere containing 5% carbon dioxide. Depending upon the precise conditions of the assay, multipotential cells in the patient's (or donor's) sample will form colonies containing vari-able proportions of differentiating cells of various haemopoietic lineages. The starting cells are seeded at a sufficiently low concentration that individual colonies localized around each single multipoten-tial parent cell can be visualized separately from any neighbouring colonies. The colonies can then be counted at low power magnification by standard light microscopy.

The most primitive multipotential cell type usually assayed in such a culture system is the mixed colony-forming unit (CFU-mix), which can generate erythroid bursts and colonies of granulocytic and monocytic cells. More commonly, however, GM-CSF, in the absence of other added growth factors, is used to supplement the culture medium and these conditions permit growth of mixed granulocyte and monocyte colonies without any erythroid growth. This culture system constitutes the granulocyte/monocyte CFU (CFU-GM) assay and is the usual assay of haemopoietic cell growth potential in harvested marrow or mobilized peripheral blood stem cell collections prior to transplantation. Colony number correlates only loosely with CD34-positive cell counts in such collections. The CFU-GM provides an independent predictor of engraftment.

Occasionally, the erythropoietic potential of primitive haemopoietic cells requires assessment. This is done using the erythroid burst-forming unit (BFU-E) assay, in which erythropoietin is used to supplement the culture medium in the absence of granulocyte and monocyte growth-promoting factors. Primitive erythroid cells produce multiple, rather than single colonies, radiating as a so-called 'burst' around the progenitor cell (BFU-E), with each individual colony representing the offspring of a more mature erythroid precursor, the erythroid CFU (CFU-E). Erythroid colonies are readily seen by light microscopy because of the orange/red colour of their cytoplasmic haemoglobin.

Apart from the use of culture systems as assays for predicting haemopoietic function in transplantation, spontaneous colony formation (i.e. colony formation with no growth factor supplementation) is used by some laboratories to assist in diagnosing chronic myeloproliferative neoplasms and juvenile myelomonocytic leukaemia. Spontaneous megakaryocyte CFU (CFU-Meg) activity, spontaneous BFU-E activity or both is demonstrable in peripheral blood or bone marrow cells from many patients with essential thrombocythaemia. Spontaneous BFU-Es also develop from peripheral blood and bone marrow cells of patients with polycythaemia vera and this is a supplementary diagnostic criterion in the WHO classification. Blood or marrow cells from normal individuals and patients with reactive thrombocytosis or secondary polycythaemia do not usually show spontaneous BFU-E activity. However, they may occasionally give rise to CFU-Meg. This potential for false-positive results and a relatively high false-negative rate in true cases of essential thrombocythaemia and polycythaemia vera, together with the cumbersome nature of the assays, has limited the diagnostic application of short-term colony-forming assays. *In vitro* hypersensitivity of myeloid progenitors to GM-CSF is a supplementary WHO criterion for the diagnosis of juvenile myelomonocytic leukaemia.

Long-term culture

Long-term cultures, in which haemopoietic precursor cells are seeded onto layers of pre-grown marrow stroma, can potentially assess the activity of stem cells even more primitive than those that survive in short-term cultures. Assay of seeded cells is achieved, once they have adhered to the stroma, by replacing liquid medium with methylcellulose or agar-containing semi-solid medium and assessing colony formation as above. This system is known as the long-term culture-initiating cell (LTC-IC) assay. It is mainly employed in research, despite its possible value in predicting engraftment. Long-term cultures have also been used for *ex vivo* purging and expansion of haemopoietic cells for engraftment but these approaches have yet to find widespread clinical application.

Bone marrow culture for microorganisms

Bone marrow culture for microorganisms, for example mycobacteria, *Leishmania donovani* or *Histoplasma capsulatum*, can be of use in diagnosis and will be discussed in the next chapter.

References

1 Hughes DA, Stuart-Smith S and Bain BJ (2004) How should stainable iron in bone marrow films be assessed? *J Clin Pathol*, **57**, 1038–1040.
2 Rath CE and Finch CA (1948) Sternal marrow hemosiderin; a method for determining available iron stores in man. *J Lab Clin Med*, **33**, 81–86.

3 Gale E, Torrance J and Bothwell T (1963) The quantitative estimation of total iron stores in human bone marrow. *J Clin Invest*, **42**, 1076–1082.

4 Lundin P, Persson E and Weinfeld A (1964) Comparison of hemosiderin estimation in bone marrow sections and bone marrow smears. *Acta Med Scand*, **175**, 383–390.

5 Fong TP, Okafor LA, Thomas W and Westerman MP (1977) Stainable iron in aspirated and needle-biopsy specimens. *Am J Hematol*, **2**, 47–51.

6 Douglas AS and Dacie JV (1953) The incidence and significance of iron-containing granules in human erythrocytes and their precursors. *J Clin Pathol*, **6**, 307–313.

7 Bainton DF and Finch CA (1964) The diagnosis of iron deficiency anemia. *Am J Med*, **37**, 62–70.

8 Hansen HA and Weinfeld A (1965) Hemosiderin estimations and sideroblast counts in the differential diagnosis of iron deficiency and other anemias. *Acta Med Scand*, **165**, 333–356.

9 Wulfhekel U and Düllman J (1999) Storage iron in bone marrow plasma cells. *Acta Haematol*, **101**, 7–15.

10 Hayhoe FGJ and Quaglino D (1988) *Haematological Cytochemistry*, 2nd edn. Churchill Livingstone, Edinburgh.

11 Bain BJ (2003) *Leukaemia Diagnosis*, 3rd edn. Blackwell Publishing, Oxford.

12 Stuart-Smith SE, Hughes DA and Bain BJ (2005) Are routine iron stains on bone marrow trephine biopsy specimens necessary? *J Clin Pathol*, **58**, 269–272.

13 Thomason RW, Lavelle J, Nelson D, Lin K and Uherova P (2007) Parenteral iron therapy is associated with a characteristic pattern of iron staining on bone marrow aspirate smears. *Am J Clin Pathol*, **128**, 590–593.

14 Krause JR, Brubaker D and Kaplan S (1979) Comparisons of stainable iron in aspirated and needle biopsy specimens of bone marrow. *Am J Clin Pathol*, **72**, 68–70.

15 Bauermeister DE (1971) Quantification of bone marrow reticulin – a normal range. *Am J Clin Pathol*, **56**, 24–31.

16 Thiele J, Kvasnicka HM, Facchetti F, Franco V, van der Walt J and Orazi A (2005) European consensus on grading bone marrow fibrosis and assessment of cellularity. *Haematologica*, **90**, 1128–1132.

17 Ahluwalia J, Garewal G, Das R and Vaiphet K (2003) The reticulin stain in bone marrow biopsies: beyond marrow. *Br J Haematol*, **123**, 378.

18 Bain BJ (1999) *Interactive Haematology Imagebank*. Blackwell Science, Oxford.

19 Gratama JW, Bolhuis RLH and Van 't Veer MB (1999) Quality control of flow cytometric immunophenotyping of haematological malignancies. *Clin Lab Haematol*, **21**, 155–160.

20 Bain BJ, Barnett D, Linch D, Matutes E and Reilly JT (2002) Revised guideline on immunophenotyping in acute leukaemias and chronic lymphoproliferative disorders. *Clin Lab Haematol*, **24**, 1–13.

21 Hanson CA, Kurtin PJ, Katzmann JA, Hoyer JD, Li C-Y, Hodnefield JM et al. (1999) Immunophenotypic analysis of peripheral blood and bone marrow in the staging of B-cell malignant lymphoma. *Blood*, **94**, 3889–3896.

22 Kallakury BVS, Hartmann D-P, Cossman J, Gootenberg JE and Bagg A (1999) Posttherapy surveillance of B-cell precursor acute lymphoblastic leukemia: value of polymerase chain reaction and limitations of flow cytometry. *Am J Clin Pathol*, **111**, 759–766.

23 Coustan-Smith E, Sancho J, Hancock ML, Boyett JM, Behm FG, Raimondi SC et al. (2000) Clinical importance of minimal residual disease in childhood acute lymphoblastic leukemia. *Blood*, **96**, 2691–2696.

24 Pileri SA, Ascano S, Milani M, Visani G, Piccioli M, Orcioni CF et al. (1999) Acute leukaemia immunophenotyping in bone-marrow routine sections. *Br J Haematol*, **105**, 394–401.

25 Foucar K (2001) *Bone Marrow Pathology*, 2nd edn. ASCP Press, Chicago.

26 O'Malley DP, Czader MB and Orazi A (2003) CD34 immunoreactivity of megakaryocytes in reactive conditions. *Am J Clin Pathol*, **120**, 442.

27 Arber DA, Snyder DS, Fine M, Dagis A, Niland J and Slovak ML (2001) Myeloperoxidase immunoreactivity in adult acute lymphoblastic leukemia. *Am J Clin Pathol*, **116**, 25–33.

28 Agis H, Krauth MT, Bohm A, Mosberger I, Mullauer L, Simonitsch-Klupp I et al. (2006) Identification of basogranulin (BB1) as a novel immunohistochemical marker of basophils in normal bone marrow and patients with myeloproliferative disorders. *Am J Clin Pathol*, **125**, 273–281.

29 Sadahira Y, Kanzaki A, Wada H and Yawata Y (1999) Immunohistochemical identification of erythroid precursors in paraffin embedded bone marrow biopsy sections: spectrin is a superior marker to glycophorin. *J Clin Pathol*, **52**, 919–921.

30 Sperr WR, Jordan J-H, Baghestanian M, Kiener H-P, Samorapoompichit P, Semper H et al. (2001) Expression of mast cell tryptase by myeloblasts in a group of patients with acute myeloid leukemia. *Blood*, **98**, 2200–2209.

31 Janckila AJ, Walton SP and Yam LT (1998) Species specificity of monoclonal antibodies to human tartrate-resistant acid phosphatase. *Biotech Histochem*, **73**, 316–324.

32 Falini B and Mason DY (2001) Proteins encoded by genes involved in chromosomal alterations in lymphoma and leukemia: clinical value of their detection by immunocytochemistry. *Blood*, **99**, 409–426.

33 Morice WG, Kurtin PJ, Tefferi A and Hanson CA (2002) Distinct bone marrow findings in T-cell granular lymphocytic leukemia revealed by paraffin section immunoperoxidase stains for CD8, TIA-1, and granzyme B. *Blood*, **99**, 268–274.

34 Nguyen D and Diamond L (2000) *Diagnostic Hematology: A pattern approach*. Butterworth-Heinemann, Oxford.

35 Fonatsch C and Streubel B (1998) Classical and molecular cytogenetics. In: Huhn D (ed) *New Diagnostic Methods in Oncology and Hematology*. Springer, Berlin.

36 Kearney L (1999) The impact of the new FISH technologies on the cytogenetics of haematological malignancies. *Br J Haematol*, **104**, 648–658.

37 Fletcher JA (1999) DNA in situ hybridization as an adjunct to tumor diagnosis. *Am J Clin Pathol*, **112** (Suppl. 1), S11–S18.

38 Kearney L (2001) Molecular cytogenetics. *Bailliere's Clin Haematol*, **14**, 645–558.

39 Jalal SM, Law ME, Stamberg J, Fonseca R, Seely JR, Myers WH and Hanson CA (2001) Detection of diagnostically critical, often hidden, anomalies in complex karyotypes of haematological disorders using multicolour fluorescence in situ hybridization. *Br J Haematol*, **112**, 975–980.

40 Le Maitre CL, Byers RJ, Yin JAL, Hoyland JA and Freemont AJ (2001) Dual colour FISH in paraffin wax embedded bone trephines for identification of numerical and structural chromosomal abnormalities in acute myeloid leukaemia and myelodysplasia. *J Clin Pathol*, **54**, 730–733.

41 Korać P, Jones M, Dominis M, Kušec R, Banham AH and Ventura RA (2006) Application of the FICTION technique for the simultaneous detection of immunophenotype and chromosomal abnormalities in routinely fixed, paraffin wax embedded bone marrow trephines. *J Clin Pathol*, **58**, 1336–1338.

42 Athanasiou E, Kaloutsi V, Kotoula V, Hytiroglou P, Kostopoulos I, Zervas et al. (2001) Cyclin D1 overexpression in multiple myeloma. *Am J Clin Pathol*, **116**, 535–542.

43 Tsukasaki K, Imaizumi Y, Tawara M, Fujimoto T, Fukushima T, Hata T et al. (1999) Diversity of leukaemic cell morphology in ATL correlates with prognostic factors, aberrant immunophenotype and defective HTLV-1 genotype. *Br J Haematol*, **105**, 369–375.

44 Pittaluga S, Tierens A, Dodoo YL, Delabie J and de Wolf-Peeters C (1999) How reliable is histologic examination of bone marrow trephine biopsy specimens for the staging of non-Hodgkin lymphoma? A study of hairy cell leukemia and mantle cell lymphoma involvement of the bone marrow trephine specimen by histologic, immunohistochemical, and

45 Neubauer A, Thiede C and Nagel S (1998) Molecular biology. In: Huhn D (ed) *New Diagnostic Methods in Oncology and Hematology*. Springer, Berlin.

46 Bagg A and Kallakury BVS (1999) Molecular pathology of leukemia and lymphoma. *Am J Clin Pathol*, **112** (Suppl. 1), S76–S92.

47 Wickham CI, Boyce M, Joyner MV, Sarsfield P, Wilkins BS, Jones DB and Ellard S (2000) Amplification of PCR products in excess of 600 base pairs using DNA extracted from decalcified, paraffin wax embedded bone marrow trephine biopsies. *J Clin Pathol Mol Pathol*, **53**, 19–23.

48 Sarsfield P, Wickham CL, Joyner MV, Ellard S, Jones DB and Wilkins BS (2000) Formic acid decalcification of bone marrow trephines degrades DNA: alternative use of EDTA allows the amplification and sequencing of relatively long PCR products. *J Clin Pathol Mol Pathol*, **53**, 336.

49 Evans PAS and Morgan GJ (1999) Molecular diagnostics in haemato-oncology. *CME Bull Haematol*, **2**, 94–99.

50 Parrens M, Carrere N, Bouabdallah K, Fitoussi O, Goussot J-F, Dubus et al. (2006) Splitting bone marrow trephines into frozen and fixed fragments allows parallel histological and molecular detection of B cell malignant infiltrates. *J Clin Pathol*, **59**, 1111–1113.

51 van Dongen JJ, Langerak AW, Brüggemann M, Evans PA, Hummel M, Lavender FL et al. (2003) Design and standardization of PCR primers and protocols for detection of clonal immunoglobulin and T-cell receptor gene recombinations in suspect lymphoproliferations: reports of the BIOMED-2 Concerted Action BMH4-CT98-3936. *Leukemia*, **17**, 2257–2317.

52 Yee K, Anglin P and Keating A (1999) Molecular approaches to the detection and monitoring of chronic myeloid leukemia: theory and practice. *Blood Rev*, **13**, 105–126.

53 Foroni L, Harrison CJ, Hoffbrand AV and Potter MN (1999) Investigation of minimal residual disease in childhood and adult acute lymphoblastic leukaemia by molecular analysis. *Br J Haematol*, **105**, 7–24.

54 Rosenwald A, Wright G, Chan WC, Connors JM, Campo E, Fisher RI et al., for the Lymphoma/Leukemia Molecular Profiling Group (2002) The use of molecular profiling to predict survival after chemotherapy for diffuse large B-cell lymphoma. *N Engl J Med*, **346**, 1937–1947.

55 Crotty PL, Smith BR and Tallini G (1998) Morphologic, immunophenotypic, and molecular evaluation of bone marrow involvement in non-Hodgkin's lymphoma. *Diagn Mol Pathol*, **7**, 90–95.

polymerase chain reaction techniques. *Am J Clin Pathol*, **111**, 179–184.

THREE

INFECTION AND REACTIVE CHANGES

Infection

The response of the bone marrow to infection is very variable, depending on the nature and chronicity of the infection, the age of the subject and the presence of any associated diseases. The response differs according to whether the infection is bacterial, rickettsial, viral or fungal. The peripheral blood and bone marrow responses to infection are non-specific and similar changes occur in many other conditions, including trauma and other tissue damage, administration of growth factors, carcinoma, Hodgkin lymphoma, non-Hodgkin lymphoma and autoimmune disorders such as systemic lupus erythematosus. Only a minority of patients with an infection show peripheral blood or bone marrow changes suggestive of a particular microorganism.

Bacterial and rickettsial infection

Peripheral blood

In adults, the usual haematological response to an acute bacterial infection is neutrophil leucocytosis with a left shift (an increase of band forms and possibly the appearance of neutrophil precursors in the peripheral blood) (Fig. 3.1). The neutrophils usually show toxic granulation and sometimes Döhle bodies and cytoplasmic vacuolation. When there is very severe bacterial infection and in neonates, alcoholics and patients with reduced bone marrow reserve, neutrophilia does not occur but there is a left shift with the above 'toxic' changes in neutrophils. Some bacterial infections,

specifically typhoid, paratyphoid, tularaemia and brucellosis, are characterized by neutropenia rather than neutrophilia. Typhoid fever can also cause isolated thrombocytopenia, anaemia, bicytopenia or pancytopenia and brucellosis can cause thrombocytopenia.

In severe infection, particularly if there is shock or hypoxia, nucleated red blood cells may appear in the blood, the presence of both granulocyte precursors and nucleated red cells being referred to as leucoerythroblastosis. The lymphocyte count is reduced but a few atypical lymphocytes, including plasmacytoid lymphocytes, may be present; plasma cells are sometimes seen. The eosinophil count is reduced during acute infection but eosinophilia can occur during recovery.

Children may respond to bacterial infection with lymphocytosis rather than neutrophilia, and certain bacterial infections, particularly whooping cough and sometimes brucellosis, are characterized by lymphocytosis. In bacterial infection, the platelet count is often reduced but sometimes increased.

Certain bacterial infections can be complicated by haemolytic anaemia. Infection by *Escherichia coli* or shigella species can be followed by a microangiopathic haemolytic anaemia as part of a haemolytic–uraemic syndrome. Sepsis due to *Clostridium welchii* can be complicated by acute haemolysis with spherocytic red cells. Mycoplasma infection is commonly associated with the production of cold autoantibodies so that red cell agglutinates are present in blood films made at room temperature and haemolytic anaemia sometimes occurs.

Rarely, neutrophils contain phagocytosed bacteria. The presence of bacteria, either extracellularly or within neutrophils, is usually only seen in overwhelming infections, particularly when there is associated hyposplenism. In relapsing fever,

Bone Marrow Pathology. By Barbara Bain, David Clark and Bridget Wilkins. © 2010, Blackwell Publishing.

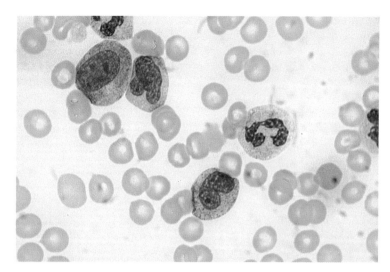

Fig. 3.1 Peripheral blood (PB), bacterial infection, left shift and toxic granulation. May–Grünwald–Giemsa (MGG) ×100.

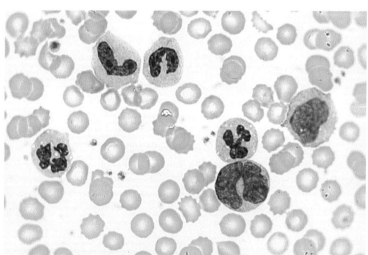

Fig. 3.2 PB, bacterial infection, monocytosis and neutrophilia. MGG ×100.

however, the characteristic spiral organisms of borrelia species appear episodically in the bloodstream and are seen lying free between red cells. In ehrlichia and anaplasma infections, organisms are often detectable within monocytes or granulocytes. They are detected in monocytes in human monocytic ehrlichiosis (caused by *Ehrlichia chaffeensis*) and in neutrophils in human granulocytic anaplasmosis (caused by *Anaplasma phagocytophilum*, previously known both as *Ehrlichia phagocytophila* and *E. equi*) and in ehrlichiosis ewingii (caused by *E. ewingii* – closely related to *E. canis*) [1]. The detection of organisms within leucocytes is facilitated by examination of buffy coat films.

In more chronic infections, there may be anaemia, increased rouleaux formation, increased background staining and monocytosis (Fig. 3.2). Anaemia is initially normocytic and normochromic but, as the infection becomes increasingly chronic, the anaemia develops the characteristics of the anaemia of chronic disease with the cells produced being hypochromic and microcytic.

Pulmonary tuberculosis characteristically causes anaemia, increased rouleaux formation and, when severe, neutrophilia. Monocytosis occurs in a minority of patients, monocytopenia actually being more common. In miliary tuberculosis, leucocytosis and leucopenia both occur; similarly, both neutropenia and neutrophilia can occur [2]. The lymphocyte count is reduced. There may be either thrombocytosis or thrombocytopenia [2]. Pancytopenia can occur but is uncommon [2]; sometimes it is a consequence of haemophagocytosis and, less often, it is associated with bone marrow necrosis.

Rickettsial infections cause varied haematological effects, which may include neutrophilia, neutropenia, lymphocytosis, the presence of atypical lymphocytes and thrombocytopenia which is sometimes severe.

Periodic acid–Schiff (PAS)-positive monocytes have been detected in the peripheral blood in Whipple's disease [3] and, rarely, organisms associated with erythrocytes are present [4].

Occasionally, severe infections are associated with a haematological picture that simulates leukaemia, designated a leukaemoid reaction (see below).

Bone marrow cytology

In severe bacterial infection, the bone marrow features reflect those of the peripheral blood. There is granulocytic hyperplasia with associated toxic changes (Fig. 3.3). In overwhelming infection, the marrow sometimes shows an increase of granulocyte precursors but with few maturing cells. Erythropoiesis is depressed and erythroblasts show reduced siderotic granulation. When there is thrombocytosis, megakaryocytes may be increased.

Macrophages are increased and, in a minority of patients with severe infection, prominent haemophagocytosis occurs. When infection is chronic, an increase of iron stores is apparent.

Microscopy or bone marrow culture occasionally provides evidence of a specific infection. In Whipple's disease, the causative organisms, *Tropheryma whipplei* (previously *Tropheryma whippelii*), may be seen within PAS-positive bone marrow macrophages [5]. In human monocytic ehrlichiosis, organisms can be detected in bone marrow monocytes whereas in human granulocytic ehrlichiosis they are present in granulocytes [6]. Bacteria visible within macrophages have also been reported in bacterial endocarditis. In typhoid fever, the bone marrow aspirate shows only nonspecific features but bone marrow culture can be useful since it increases the detection rate by 50% in comparison with peripheral blood culture [7]; overall, stool cultures are positive in about 30% of patients, blood cultures in 60–80% and bone marrow cultures in 80–95% [8]. In brucellosis, the bone marrow is usually hypercellular with prominent haemophagocytosis and increased eosinophils and plasma cells [9] but occasional patients have pancytopenia associated with a hypocellular marrow [10]. Bone marrow culture is more often positive than blood culture, about 90% in comparison with about 70% [11], but, since the diagnosis can be made serologically, bone marrow aspiration is not indicated for this purpose. Reversible bone

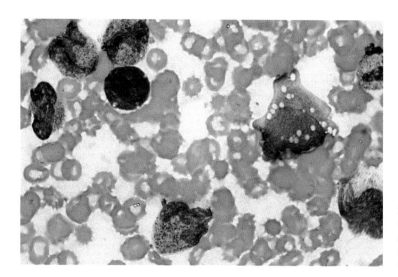

Fig. 3.3 Bone marrow (BM) aspirate film from a patient with severe infection showing heavy toxic granulation and vacuolation of neutrophil precursors. MGG ×100.

marrow hypoplasia leading to severe pancytopenia has been reported in Legionnaires' disease [12].

In tuberculosis, the bone marrow aspirate shows non-specific features such as increased iron stores and an increase in macrophages, often with hae-mophagocytosis. Mycobacteria may be detected in a minority of cases using appropriate stains (Ziehl–Neelsen (ZN) or auramine). Rarely, in atypical mycobacterial infection, organisms may be appar-ent in Romanowsky-stained films as negative rod-shaped images within bone marrow macrophages [13,14] (Fig. 3.4) or as beaded red refractile rods

[13]. Cultures should always be performed when this diagnosis is suspected. Negative images of bacilli within macrophages can also be apparent in lepromatous leprosy [15].

Bone marrow histology

Severe bacterial infection leads to an increase in marrow cellularity due to granulocytic hyperplasia. There is often a left shift of the granulocytic series, i.e. an increase in the numbers of immature precur-sors (myelocytes and promyelocytes) in relation to mature polymorphonuclear neutrophils (Fig. 3.5).

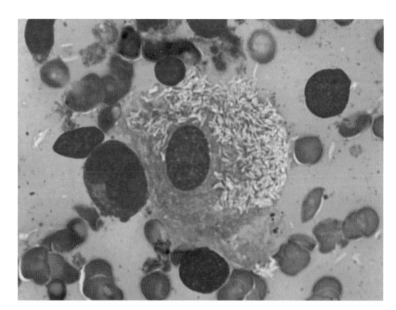

Fig. 3.4 BM aspirate from a patient with HIV infection showing numerous atypical mycobacteria (negative images) within a macrophage and free between cells. MGG ×100.

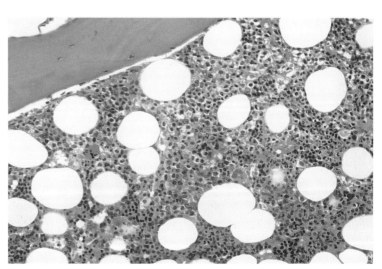

Fig. 3.5 BM trephine biopsy section, bacterial infection with leukaemoid reaction: there is increased cellularity and granulocytic hyperplasia with left shift; note emperipolesis of a mature neutrophil by a megakaryocyte. Paraffin-embedded, haematoxylin and eosin (H&E) ×20.

However, the normal topographical arrangement of granulopoiesis is retained, with the more immature cells (mainly promyelocytes) found predominantly in the paratrabecular region [16]. Megakaryocytes are often increased in number [17]; they are morphologically normal, but there may be an increase in 'bare' megakaryocyte nuclei and increased emperipolesis. Erythropoiesis is often reduced although morphologically normal.

In more chronic bacterial infections, changes in other lineages become apparent. Bone marrow plasmacytosis is a common but non-specific response [18]. Very rarely, there may be up to 50% plasma cells in the marrow in reactive conditions including infections. The differential diagnosis of increased numbers of plasma cells in the marrow is discussed on page 134. In infections, plasma cells are distributed through the marrow in an interstitial manner, often with focal pericapillary accentuation. This may be accompanied by plasma cell satellitosis, in which a central macrophage is surrounded by three or more plasma cells. The plasma cells have mature nuclear and cytoplasmic characteristics although there are often occasional binucleate forms and cells containing Russell bodies. Chronic infection is also associated with an increased frequency of reactive lymphoid aggregates (see page 132). Macrophages may be increased and commonly contain ingested granulocytes (Fig. 3.6). Varying degrees of haemophagocytosis are common in infections by a wide variety of agents, including

bacteria. When severe, this can lead to a haemophagocytic syndrome (see page 140). Stromal changes related to infection include oedema, prominent sinusoids, focal reticulin fibrosis, red cell leakage into the interstitial space and rarely, in very severe chronic infections, gelatinous change (see page 152). A decrease in marrow cellularity and loss of fat spaces usually accompany gelatinous transformation [19].

Features that can be seen in Whipple's disease include granuloma formation (cells within the granuloma often being PAS positive), PAS-positive macrophages and intra- and extracellular PAS-positive bacillary bodies [20]. In one reported patient, megakaryocytes showed prominent PAS-positive inclusions [20].

In anaplasmosis, the bone marrow can be hypocellular with reduced granulocytic cells and megakaryocytes or hypercellular with both granulocytic and megakaryocytic hyperplasia; erythrophagocytosis has been reported in one patient [21]. *Anaplasma phagocytophilum* has the capacity to infect granulocytic precursors and suppress bone marrow function [22]. Granulomas are often present. In human monocytic ehrlichiosis, inclusions (morulae) can be identified in macrophages [23] (Fig. 3.7). They are PAS negative. Their identity can be confirmed immunocytochemically [23].

Mycobacterial infections can cause the same reactive changes as infection by other bacteria. However, haemophagocytosis and granuloma for-

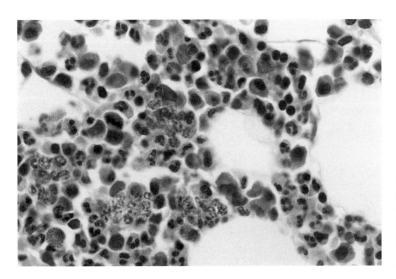

Fig. 3.6 Section of BM trephine specimen showing neutrophil shadows within macrophages in a patient with Hodgkin lymphoma; similar features are seen in bacterial infection. Paraffin-embedded, H&E ×100.

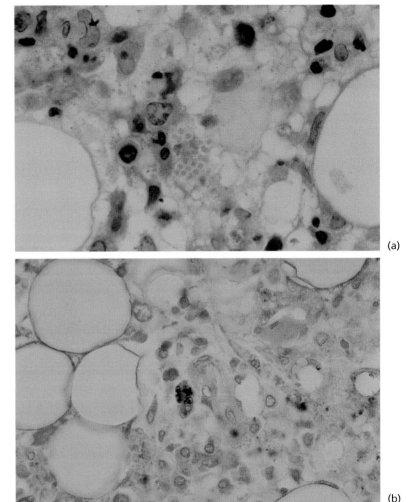

(a)

(b)

Fig. 3.7 Intracellular ehrlichiae in a bone marrow trephine biopsy section. (a) Paraffin-embedded, PAS stain with haematoxylin counterstain. (b) Paraffin-embedded, immunoperoxidase stain with anti-ehrlichial immunoglobulin G antibody. (By courtesy of Dr C. D. Paddock, Dr R. L. Kerschmann and Dr B. G. Herndier, San Francisco; reprinted by permission of the *New England Journal of Medicine*, **329**, 1164, 1993.)

mation are particularly common. The bone marrow is usually hypercellular but a markedly hypocellular bone marrow can also occur [24]. There may be dyserythropoiesis. In miliary tuberculosis, the majority of patients have granulomas and, in about half of them, caseation is present [2]. Occasionally bone marrow culture is positive in the absence of granulomas although positive cultures are obtained in only a minority of those with granulomas [2]. Whenever granulomas are present it is necessary to perform stains such as a ZN or auramine, in the

latter instance mycobacteria being detected by fluorescence microscopy. In one study, immunohistochemistry with a polyclonal antibody to mycobacteria was found to be more sensitive than an acid-fast stain [25] but this has not found widespread use. Occasional patients with mycobacterial infection have extensive necrosis, which is indicative of poor prognosis. In those with impaired immunity, there may be a generalized increase in interstitial macrophages rather than granuloma formation. Macrophages may appear foamy.

Mycobacterium leprae infection may cause granuloma formation and, in lepromatous leprosy, numerous foamy macrophages. Patients have also been reported in whom interstitial lepra bacilli were found in bone marrow sections, stained with a Fite stain, in the absence of any macrophage proliferation or granulomas [26].

Granuloma formation can also occur in riskettsial infections such as Q fever (infection by *Coxiella burnetti*) and Rocky Mountain spotted fever (infection by *Rickettsia rickettsii*).

Problems and pitfalls

Negative ZN or auramine stains do not exclude a diagnosis of tuberculosis. These stains are often negative in patients with haemophagocytosis or granulomas caused by miliary tuberculosis. Cultures are more sensitive than microscopy.

Overwhelming infection can be associated with a leukaemoid reaction, simulating either acute myeloid leukaemia (AML) or chronic myelomonocytic leukaemia (CMML). In a leukaemoid reaction, anaemia and thrombocytopenia are common. The white cell count is sometimes low with neutropenia and sometimes high; the blood film may show granulocyte precursors or be leucoerythroblastic. Leukaemoid reactions are most often seen in association with very severe bacterial infection, particularly when there is coexisting megaloblastic anaemia. The bone marrow response to miliary tuberculosis can also simulate leukaemia.

Toxic changes such as toxic granulation and neutrophil vacuolation are useful clues to the correct diagnosis. If necessary, a bone marrow examination makes the distinction. In severe infection there may be the appearance of maturation arrest with increased promyelocytes and a lack of maturing cells; there is no significant increase in blasts and the promyelocytes differ from those of acute hypergranular promyelocytic leukaemia in having prominent Golgi zones and no Auer rods.

The blood and bone marrow features of severe chronic infection may be difficult to distinguish from those of CMML since 'toxic' changes may be lacking. Consideration of the clinical features facilitates the distinction. It is imprudent to make a diagnosis of CMML in a patient with a significant infection unless there are dysplastic features of a type showing a strong association with the myelodysplastic syndromes (MDS).

Viral infection

Peripheral blood

Viral infections usually provoke lymphocytosis. Often the cells that are produced are morphologically fairly normal but sometimes they have atypical features. Infectious mononucleosis consequent on infection by the Epstein–Barr virus (EBV) is characterized by the production of large numbers of atypical lymphocytes, often referred to as atypical mononuclear cells (Fig. 3.8). These are pleo-

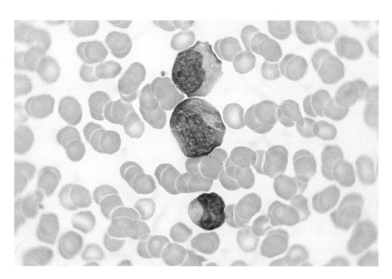

Fig. 3.8 PB, infectious mononucleosis, atypical lymphocytes. MGG ×100.

morphic, usually large, and often have abundant basophilic cytoplasm; some have nuclei with a diffuse chromatin pattern and nucleoli. The presence of large numbers of atypical mononuclear cells is not specific for EBV infection; this may also be a feature of primary infection by other viruses (cytomegalovirus (CMV), human immunodeficiency virus (HIV), hepatitis A and adenovirus) and of toxoplasmosis, as well as being seen in hypersensitivity reactions to drugs. Smaller numbers of similar atypical lymphocytes are seen in a wider variety of infective (and non-infective) conditions. Viral infections that may be associated with marked lymphocytosis without many atypical features include those due to Coxsackie virus, various adenoviruses and HIV; other haematological abnormalities produced by HIV are discussed below (see page 144). In immunosuppressed hosts, e.g. following bone marrow transplantation, CMV infection can cause neutropenia, thrombocytopenia and pancytopenia. CMV infection in such patients may be associated with very large virus-infected cells, which are probably endothelial in origin, in the feathered edge of the film [27]. Human herpesvirus 6 (HHV6) can be responsible for transient erythroblastopenia of childhood (see page 480). Viral infections, particularly those due to herpesviruses, may be associated with a haemophagocytic syndrome (see page 140) with the peripheral blood showing resultant pancytopenia. In a few individuals, hepatitis, particularly non-A non-B non-C hepatitis (of suspected but not proven viral origin), is followed in a period of a few weeks or months by pancytopenia caused by aplastic anaemia. In certain subjects who are unable to mount a normal immune response to EBV, infection by this virus may also be followed by chronic pancytopenia due to bone marrow aplasia. Parvovirus commonly causes transient pure red cell aplasia but, unless red cell survival is reduced, this may go unnoticed; less often, it is a cause of neutropenia or thrombocytopenia.

In patients with viral infections, the haemoglobin concentration can be reduced as a result of bone marrow suppression, haemorrhage or haemolysis (see below for immune mechanisms). Occasionally in patients with a severe capillary leak syndrome, e.g. in meningococcal septicaemia or hantavirus cardiopulmonary syndrome, the haemoglobin concentration is increased. Thrombocytopenia, result-

ing from increased platelet consumption, is a characteristic feature of viral haemorrhagic fevers caused by a wide range of viruses.

Viral infections may be complicated by cytopenias consequent on either damage to cells by immune complexes or autoantibody production. Rubella and, less often, other viral infections may be followed by transient thrombocytopenia caused by damage to platelets by immune complexes. Infectious mononucleosis may be complicated by either autoimmune thrombocytopenia or autoimmune haemolytic anaemia due to a cold antibody with anti-i specificity; in these cases, there are red cell agglutinates and occasional spherocytes. Rarely, viral infections, particularly measles, are followed by acute haemolysis due to an autoantibody with anti-P specificity ('paroxysmal' cold haemoglobinuria); in these cases, the blood film usually shows only occasional spherocytes and subsequently polychromasia. Contrary to what might be anticipated from the name, there is only a single episode of haemolysis.

Chronic hepatitis C infection can cause immunologically-mediated thrombocytopenia. Some patients develop mixed cryoglobulinaemia with associated haematological features (see pages 449–451). A single case has also been reported of pure red cell aplasia associated with hepatitis C infection [28].

An association has been reported between hepatitis B vaccination and pancytopenia (associated with bone marrow infiltration by cytotoxic T lymphocytes and hypoplasia of myeloid cells) [29].

In patients with impaired immunity, EBV infection may be associated with a spectrum of lymphoproliferative disorders, including lymphoma (see page 399). Patients with a *SHD2D1A* (*SAP*) mutation, leading to X-linked lymphoproliferative disorder, can develop not only EBV-related lymphomas but also fatal infectious mononucleosis [30].

If fresh tissue is available, molecular techniques can be used for the detection of viral infection. For example, in suspected EBV infection reverse transcriptase polymerase chain reaction (RT-PCR) can be used to detect mRNA for EBNA-1 and -2, LMP-1, -2A and -2B, BZLF1 (ZEBRA 'protein') and BCRF1 (viral IL10).

Bone marrow cytology
In viral infection, the bone marrow shows an increase of lymphocytes, either typical or atypical.

In EBV and CMV infection, atypical lymphoid cells, morphologically identical to those in the peripheral blood, can be seen in the marrow. In some infections, particularly by herpesviruses, haemophagocytosis is prominent. In immunosuppressed hosts, CMV [31] and HHV8 [32] infection can also cause marked bone marrow hypocellularity with suppression of all lineages. HHV8 is also responsible for multicentric Castleman's disease in HIV-positive patients (see pages 110–111). Fatal infectious mononucleosis in X-linked lymphoproliferative disorder is associated with haemophagocytosis and bone marrow infiltration by activated T cells, immunoblasts and plasma cells; there is progression to bone marrow necrosis and hypoplasia [30]. When a viral infection causes haemolytic anaemia, e.g. in infectious mononucleosis, erythroid hyperplasia will be apparent.

The bone marrow is hypocellular in dengue fever with cells of all lineages being reduced [33]. There may be dyserythropoiesis and haemophagocytosis [34].

Parvovirus-induced pure red cell aplasia that is clinically apparent usually occurs only in individuals with a shortened red cell survival or immune deficiency. In other patients the aplasia is too brief for anaemia to be symptomatic. In parvovirus-induced pure red cell aplasia there are prominent, very large proerythroblasts with a striking lack of more mature cells. These cells may have PAS-positive cytoplasmic inclusions representing glycogen. In one patient with parvovirus-induced pancytopenia there were also large atypical cells of granulocyte lineage, which were shown to contain viral antigens [35]. Rarely parvovirus infection has been associated with transient pure red cell aplasia leading to anaemia in haematologically and immunologically normal subjects [36], transient severe dyserythropoiesis [37], recurrent pure granulocytic aplasia with neutropenia [38] or pure megakaryocyte hypoplasia or aplasia with thrombocytopenia [36,39]. Uncommonly, in apparently immunologically normal people, there is persistent infection leading to chronic red cell aplasia. Parvovirus infection is usually confirmed by serology but in patients with an impaired antibody response it may be necessary to use *in situ* DNA hybridization or immunofluorescence to detect either a capsid antigen [35] or a nuclear antigen.

When viral infections are complicated by thrombocytopenia due to increased platelet destruction, megakaryocytes are present in normal or increased numbers. Occasionally platelets are visible within bone marrow macrophages (Fig. 3.9).

Bone marrow histology

Viral infections may lead to an increase of bone marrow lymphocytes, plasma cells and macrophages, with or without haemophagocytosis. In EBV (Figs 3.10–3.13) and CMV infection the bone marrow may show extensive infiltration by atypical

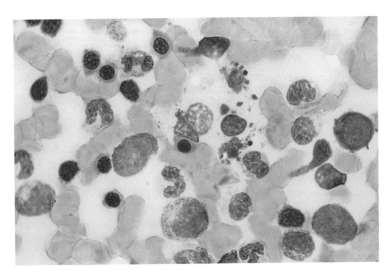

Fig. 3.9 BM aspirate: platelets within a macrophage in a patient with severe thrombocytopenia during acute cytomegalovirus infection. MGG ×100.

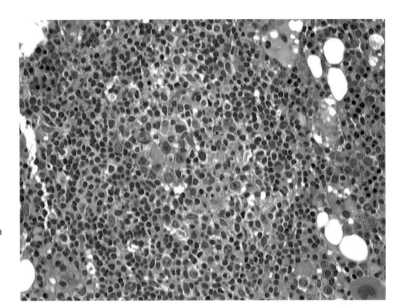

Fig. 3.10 BM trephine biopsy section from a patient with infectious mononucleosis. There is a germinal centre including some large cells (shown to be B cells) with prominent nucleoli, which resemble mononuclear Hodgkin cells. Paraffin-embedded, H&E ×20.

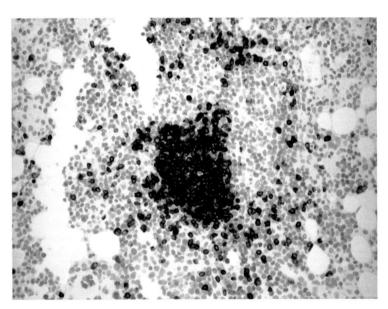

Fig. 3.11 BM trephine biopsy section from a patient with infectious mononucleosis (same patient as Fig. 3.10) demonstrating that the large cells in the germinal centre are predominantly B cells. Paraffin-embedded, immunoperoxidase for CD20 ×10.

lymphoid cells. In CMV infection, eosinophilic intranuclear inclusions may be seen, albeit rarely, in endothelial cells and in cells, probably macrophages, within granulomas or interspersed among haemopoietic cells [40]. A hypocellular marrow with some areas of gelatinous transformation and a diffuse increase in reticulin has been reported in a patient with pancytopenia associated with acute EBV infection [41]. Atypical lymphoid cells with intranuclear viral inclusions have also been detected in HHV6 infection [42]. In the post-transplant setting, CMV [31], HHV6 [43] and HHV8 [32] infection can cause severe bone marrow hypoplasia. In bone marrow hypoplasia associated with HHV8 infection, interstitial plasmacytosis has also been noted [32]. In HIV-positive patients with HHV8-associated diseases, such as Kaposi's sarcoma or primary effusion lymphoma, there are scattered

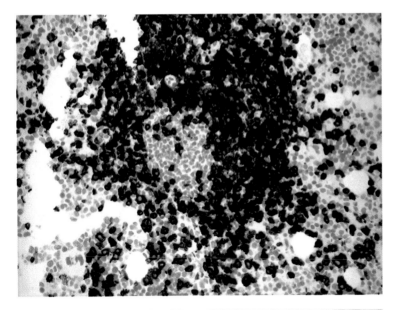

Fig. 3.12 BM trephine biopsy section from a patient with infectious mononucleosis (same patient as Fig. 3.10) showing T cells surrounding the germinal centre. Paraffin-embedded, immunoperoxidase for CD3 ×10.

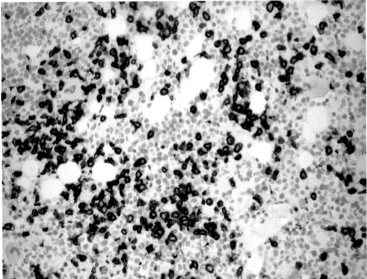

Fig. 3.13 BM trephine biopsy section from a patient with infectious mononucleosis (same patient as Fig. 3.10) showing a marked interstitial increase in T cells. Paraffin-embedded, immunoperoxidase for CD3 ×10.

plasmacytoid cells in the marrow showing nuclear expression of HHV8-latent nuclear antigen [44]. In HIV-positive patients with multicentric Castleman's disease, the bone marrow sometimes shows lymphoid follicles with depleted or hyalinized germinal centres and mantle zones in which there are scattered HHV8-positive plasmablasts [44] (Figs 3.14 and 3.15); these plasmablasts are CD20 positive, CD79a positive and CD138 negative and express

monotypic λ light chain (Fig. 3.16), whereas interstitial, pericapillary and perisinusoidal plasma cells and plasmablasts are polytypic. The presence of CMV (Fig. 3.17), EBV and HHV8 (Fig. 3.15) can be confirmed by immunohistochemistry using monoclonal antibodies [45–49] (Table 3.1). However, it should be noted that, even in patients with generalized CMV infection, it is unusual for virus-infected cells to be detectable in the bone marrow. *In situ*

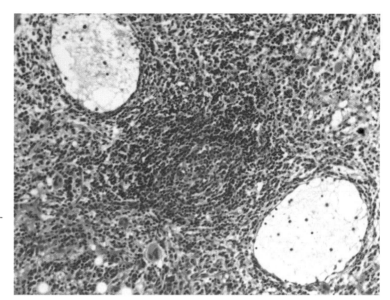

Fig. 3.14 BM trephine biopsy section from an HIV-positive patient with HHV8-associated multicentric Castleman's disease showing a lymphoid follicle. Paraffin-embedded, H&E ×10.
(By courtesy of Dr Ahmet Dogan, Rochester, Minnesota.)

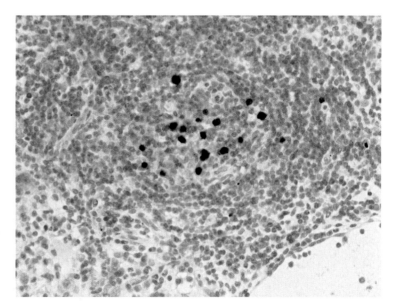

Fig. 3.15 BM trephine biopsy section from an HIV-positive patient with HHV8-associated multicentric Castleman's disease showing that plasmablasts in the germinal centre express HHV8 latent membrane antigen 1. Paraffin-embedded, immunoperoxidase ×20. (By courtesy of Dr Ahmet Dogan, Rochester, Minnesota.)

hybridization (ISH) techniques can also be used for the detection of viral RNA. The detection of EBER (EBV early RNA) in lymphoma cells has been found to be a useful and sensitive technique for the demonstration of bone marrow infiltration in EBV-related lymphomas [50].

Pure red cell aplasia is characteristically seen in infection by parvovirus B19 and is readily detected in trephine biopsy sections; giant proerythroblasts are readily apparent (Fig. 3.18). Very occasionally, parvovirus has been associated with erythroid hyperplasia, sometimes with marked dyserythropoiesis [51]. Parvovirus B19 capsid antigens may be detectable by immunohistochemistry although this technique is less sensitive than PCR [52]; curiously, in one study, the positive cells were among the few late erythroid cells while the giant proerythroblasts were negative [52].

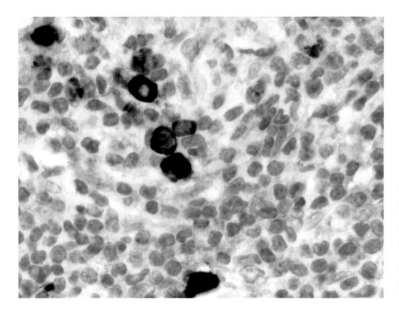

Fig. 3.16 BM trephine biopsy section from an HIV-positive patient with HHV8-associated multicentric Castleman's disease showing that plasmablasts in the germinal centre express λ light chain. Paraffin-embedded, immunoperoxidase ×40. (By courtesy of Dr Ahmet Dogan, Rochester, Minnesota.)

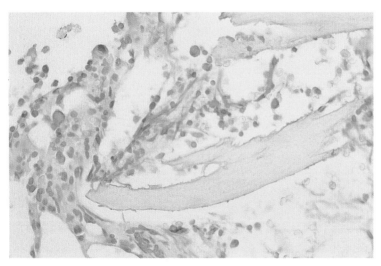

Fig. 3.17 BM trephine biopsy section from a renal transplant patient with cytomegalovirus infection showing one positive cell (top left). Paraffin-embedded, immunoperoxidase with Dako-CMV McAb ×100.

Viral infections, particularly herpesvirus infections, can lead to the formation of small non-caseating granulomas (Fig. 3.19; see Table 3.3). Chronic hepatitis B and hepatitis C infection may be associated with the presence of reactive lymphoid nodules [53] (Fig. 3.20). Hepatitis C infection can also be complicated by the development of low grade B-cell lymphoma, often supervening in a patient with mixed type II cryoglobulinaemia; the lymphoid infiltrate is then monoclonal and more extensive.

As already noted, immunohistochemistry is useful in the diagnosis of viral infections. The techniques applicable to trephine biopsies for confirmation of infection by specific viruses are summarized in Table 3.1.

Problems and pitfalls

Lymphocytosis with atypical lymphocytes can be confused with a lymphoproliferative disorder, particularly with mantle cell lymphoma and the less common cases of chronic lymphocytic leukaemia

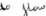

Table 3.1 Immunohistochemical (IHC), *in situ* hybridization (ISH) and Southern blot (SB) techniques applicable to trephine biopsy specimens for confirmation of certain viral infections.

Virus	Technique and component	Monoclonal antibody or probe
Epstein–Barr virus (EBV)	IHC for detection of latent membrane protein 1 (LMP-1)* or Epstein–Barr nuclear antigen 2 (EBNA-2) in latent infection; negative in acute EBV infection and insufficiently sensitive for detection of expression in some lymphoproliferative disorders in immunocompromised patients	CS1-4, a cocktail of four clones directed at LMP-1 (Dakopatts, Novocastra or Serotec); PE2 directed at EBNA-2 (Dako and Novocastra)
	IHC for EBV early lytic antigens	G3-E31 (Novocastra) directed at 50–52 kDa diffuse early antigen; W1-F2 (Novocastra) directed at 85 kDa restricted early antigen
	IHC for detection of BZLF ('ZEBRA' protein) in lytic EBV infection	Clone βZ.1 directed at βZLF1 (Dako)
	ISH for detection of nuclear Epstein–Barr virus early RNA (EBER) in active and latent EBV infection; more sensitive than IHC	EBER-1 PNA probe/FITC kit (Dako) or EBER-probe ISH kit (Novocastra)
	SB analysis to detect EBV clonality (dependent on the number of terminal repeats) [45]	
Cytomegalovirus (CMV)	IHC	AAC10 (Dako) directed at CMV lower matrix protein pp65; QB1/42 (Novocastra) directed at CMV early antigen in nucleus; QB1/06 (Novocastra) directed at CMV late antigens in nucleus and cytoplasm
	ISH for detection of viral RNA or DNA	CMV probe ISH kit (Novocastra) for viral early gene RNA; CMV BioProbe (ENZO Diagnostics) for CMV DNA [46]
Human herpesvirus 8 (HHV8)	IHC for HHV8 latent nuclear antigen 1 in lymphoid cells or tumour cells of Kaposi's sarcoma [47]	ORF73 (Advanced Biotechnologies); 13B10 (Leica Microsystems)
	ISH for viral RNA in nucleus	NCL-HHV8
Herpes simplex	Immunohistochemistry for detection of various shared and type-specific antigens	Rabbit polyclonal antiserum (Dako)
Parvovirus B19	IHC with detection of a nuclear antigen or a viral capsid antigen	R92F6 (Novocastra) directed at capsid proteins VP1 and VP2
	ISH for detection of viral DNA	Digoxigenin-labelled parvovirus B19 DNA probe [48]
Human immunodeficiency virus (HIV)	IHC for p24 capsid protein	Kal-1 (Dako)

*LMP-1 is detected by a cocktail of clones (CS1–4). Cross-reaction with normal early myeloid and erythroid precursors, leukaemic myeloblasts and leukaemic lymphoblasts has been reported [49] but this has not been our experience when using formalin fixation and formic acid or ethylene diamine tetra-acetic acid (EDTA) decalcification. We have observed no false-positive staining in normal bone marrow or in acute myeloid leukaemia and in acute lymphoblastic leukaemia we have observed weak nuclear staining only, whereas the specific product would be cytoplasmic.

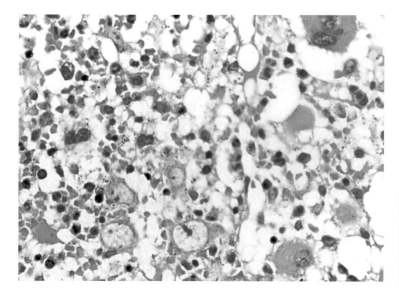

Fig. 3.18 BM trephine biopsy section from a patient with parvovirus B19 infection showing giant proerythroblasts with inclusion-like nucleoli and a striking lack of maturing erythroblasts. Paraffin-embedded, H&E ×100.

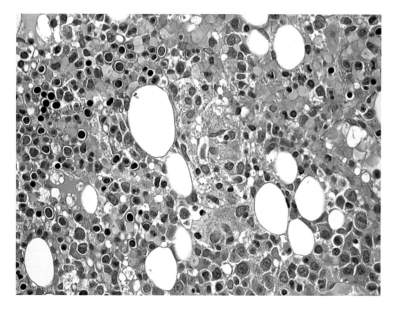

Fig. 3.19 BM trephine biopsy section from a patient with infectious mononucleosis (same patient as Fig. 3.10). The bone marrow is hypercellular and there is a poorly formed granuloma associated with a polymorphous population of activated lymphoid cells. Paraffin-embedded, H&E ×40.

in which neoplastic cells are pleomorphic. When there is diagnostic difficulty, immunophenotyping is indicated to demonstrate or exclude a clonal proliferation of B lymphocytes.

Virus-induced haemophagocytic syndrome can be confused with malignant histiocytosis. The latter is a very rare condition and the diagnosis should be made with caution. It is characterized by proliferation of very immature cells of monocyte–macro-phage lineage which, in contrast to the cells of virus-induced haemophagocytic syndrome, usually show little phagocytic activity. Marked haemophagocytosis therefore suggests that the process is reactive. Virus-induced haemophagocytosis can also be confused with other reactive haemophagocytic syndromes, including those associated with some T-cell and natural killer (NK) cell lymphomas.

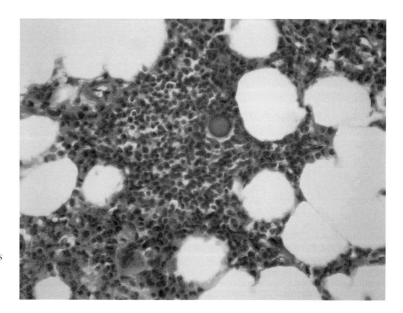

Fig. 3.20 BM trephine biopsy section from a patient with hepatitis C infection showing a lymphoid aggregate and a single Russell body. Paraffin-embedded, H&E ×40.

Fungal infections

Fungal infections are seen in otherwise healthy people but they are much more common in immunodeficiency, e.g. in patients with the acquired immune deficiency syndrome (AIDS) and following intensive chemotherapy.

Peripheral blood

Fungal infections have no specific haematological features. Pancytopenia sometimes occurs [54]. Some fungal diseases, for example actinomycosis and coccidioidomycosis, are associated with neutrophilia. Aspergillus and other fungi may evoke an allergic response and be associated with eosinophilia. When systemic fungal infections occur in immunocompromised hosts fungi, such as candida or histoplasma, are occasionally seen in the peripheral blood. Candida may also be seen in blood films when there is infection originating from a colonized indwelling venous line.

Bone marrow cytology

Fungi are rarely seen in the bone marrow aspirate in immunologically normal subjects. Histoplasma is an exception, organisms sometimes being detected within bone marrow macrophages. In South American blastomycosis (paracoccidioidomycosis) also, aspirate films from immunologically normal

hosts may show occasional yeast forms of *Paracoccidioides brasiliensis* [55]. Fungi are much more often detected in bone marrow aspirates from severely immunocompromised patients such as those with HIV infection or following bone marrow transplantation, when *Candida albicans, Aspergillus fumigatus, Histoplasma capsulatum* (Fig. 3.21), *Cryptococcus neoformans* (Fig. 3.22), *Penicillium marneffei* (Fig. 3.23) [56], *Blastomyces dermatitidis* and *Coccidioides immitis* may be seen. *Rhodotorula rubra*, which is usually non-pathogenic, has been observed in an immunosuppressed renal transplant patient [54]. Fungi may be found within macrophages or lying free. Although organisms may be seen in bone marrow aspirate films, trephine biopsy is usually more sensitive for the detection of fungal infection. Fungi may also be cultured from the bone marrow, sometimes when peripheral blood culture and other cultures are negative.

Bone marrow histology

In systemic fungal infections, particularly in immunocompromised patients such as those with AIDS, organisms can sometimes be identified in the marrow (Figs 3.24–3.26). Usually fungi are within macrophages, including the altered macrophages comprising granulomas, or are associated with necrotic tissue. Rarely they are detectable

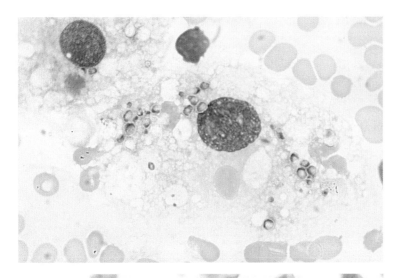

Fig. 3.21 BM aspirate. Histoplasmosis in a patient with AIDS, showing numerous organisms within a macrophage. MGG ×100.

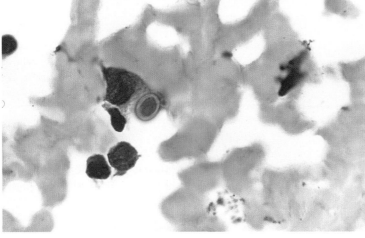

(a)

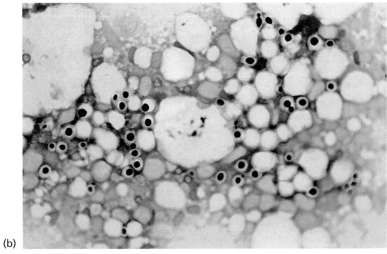

(b)

Fig. 3.22 BM aspirate. (a) Budding cryptococcus in an HIV-positive man. MGG ×100. (b) Budding cryptococcus in another HIV-positive man. Grocott's methenamine silver (GMS) ×100. (By courtesy of Dr Christine Costello, London.)

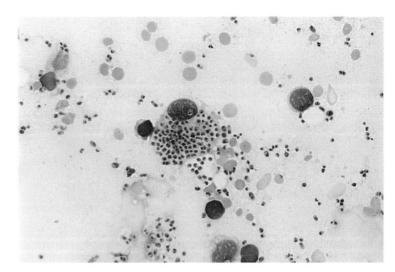

Fig. 3.23 BM aspirate. *Penicillium marneffei* in an HIV-positive man. MGG ×100. (By courtesy of Dr K. F. Wong, Hong Kong.)

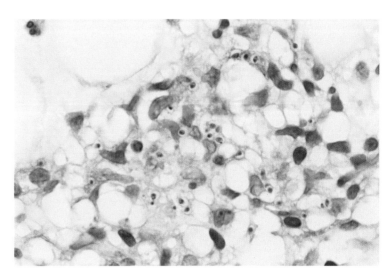

Fig. 3.24 BM trephine biopsy section from a patient with AIDS showing *Histoplasma capsulatum*. Paraffin-embedded, PAS-diastase ×100.

only within megakaryocytes [57]. The presence of a 'capsule' helps to identify *Histoplasma capsulatum*, although this appearance is actually an artefact resulting from cytoplasmic shrinkage. *Paracoccidioides brasiliensis* has been associated with granuloma formation, bone marrow and bone necrosis, and fibrosis (mainly reticulin but occasionally collagen) [55].

The morphological features of clinically important fungi that can be seen in histological sections of bone marrow are summarized in Table 3.2 [58–60]. Cases of disseminated infection caused by fungi not previously known to be pathogenic con-

tinue to be recognized in immunocompromised patients [54,61].

Problems and pitfalls

Diagnosis of fungal infection does not present any difficulty when organisms are detectable in the bone marrow. However, when there are granulomas without detectable microorganisms or if there are only reactive changes, diagnosis can be difficult. Detection can also be difficult in severely hypocellular or necrotic marrows following cytotoxic chemotherapy when there is no cellular reaction. Bone marrow culture is more sensitive than micro-

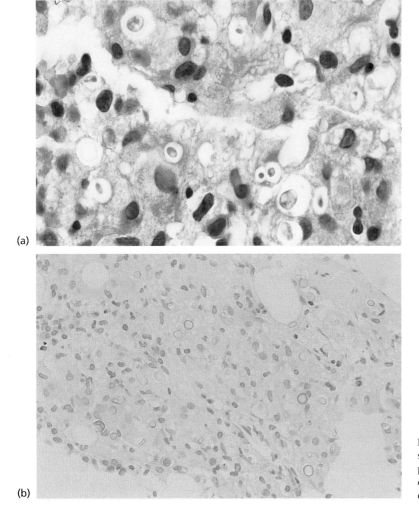

(a)

(b)

Fig. 3.25 BM trephine biopsy section, *Cryptococcus neoformans* in a patient with AIDS. (a) Paraffin-embedded, H&E ×100. (b) Paraffin-embedded, Alcian blue ×40.

scopy for the detection of fungi and can be employed when bone marrow examination is performed for investigation of fever, particularly in immunosuppressed patients. For example, bone marrow cultures are positive in 90% of patients with disseminated histoplasmosis, whereas the detection rate with microscopy of bone marrow aspirates is considerably lower and the proportion of patients with granulomas is lower still [62,63]. However it should be noted that peripheral blood cultures for histoplasma have almost as high a success rate as bone marrow cultures [63]. Supplementary tests, such as testing urine or serum for cryptococcal or histoplasma antigens, can also be useful. Testing for histoplasma antigen in the urine is highly sensitive and in endemic areas can avoid the need for a bone marrow examination [64]. PCR for the detection of aspergillus DNA can also be useful.

Parasitic diseases

Peripheral blood

Parasites that may be recognized in blood films include plasmodium, babesiae, microfilariae, trypanosomes, leishmaniae (uncommonly) and toxoplasma (rarely) [65].

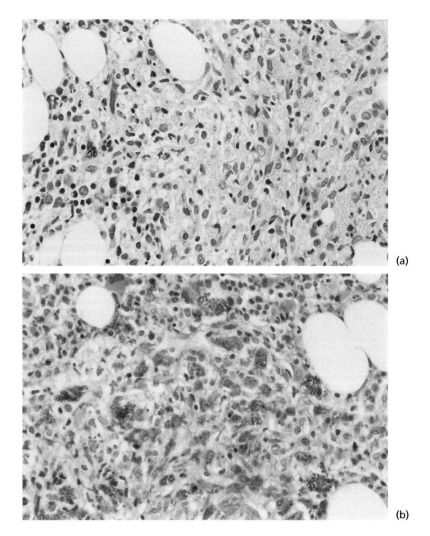

(a)

(b)

Fig. 3.26 Section of BM trephine biopsy specimen in a patient with AIDS with *Penicillium marneffei* infection. (a) Paraffin-embedded, H&E ×40. (b) Paraffin-embedded, PAS ×40.

The presence of parasites within the bowel may lead to blood loss with consequent iron deficiency anaemia. Similarly, schistosomiasis affecting the urinary bladder can lead to chronic blood loss and iron deficiency. Chronic parasitic infections can also cause the anaemia of chronic disease. Eosinophilia is common in patients with helminth infections. In malaria and babesiosis, parasites are seen within red cells. Malaria is associated with haemolytic anaemia, leucocytosis, neutrophilia, lymphocytosis, monocytosis and sometimes thrombocytopenia; the reticulocyte count may be inappropriately low as a result of bone marrow suppression. Pancytopenia has also been reported [66]. Atypical lymphocytes are present both in malaria and in some patients with hyper-reactive malarial splenomegaly. Toxoplasmosis can be associated with lymphocytosis and the presence of considerable numbers of atypical lymphocytes. Leishmaniasis can cause a normocytic normochromic anaemia, leucopenia or pancytopenia and increased rouleaux formation. Phagocytosed parasites are occasionally detectable within peripheral blood monocytes or neutrophils. Hypersplenism

Table 3.2 Differential diagnosis of fungal and protozoal pathogens.

Species	Tissue forms	Special stains
Fungi		
Candida albicans	Non-branching pseudohyphae and small (2–4 μm) budding yeast forms	PAS* and GMS
Cryptococcus neoformans	Yeast forms (5–10 μm), thick capsule, narrow-based unequal buds	PAS*, GMS and mucicarmine
Histoplasma capsulatum	Small (2–5 μm) yeast forms†	PAS* and GMS
Penicillium marneffei	Small (2–6 μm), round or oval to sausage-shaped containing reddish-purple dot-like structures and sometimes septae	PAS* and GMS
Pneumocystis jiroveci [58] (previously *Pneumocystis carinii*)		GMS or IHC
Protozoa		
Toxoplasma gondii	Tachyzoites (ovoid 3 × 6 μm, tiny nucleus, 'single-dot' appearance); occasionally cysts with numerous small bradyzoites	Giemsa, PAS‡ and IHC
Leishmania donovani	Small (3 μm) intracellular amastigote, nucleus and paranuclear kinetoplast gives 'double-dot' appearance	Giemsa

GMS, Grocott's methenamine silver stain; IHC, immunohistochemistry; PAS, periodic acid–Schiff.
*Pre-treatment with diastase to remove glycogen considerably reduces positive staining of neutrophils and megakaryocytes and facilitates the detection of microorganisms.
†*Histoplasma capsulatum* var. *duboisii*, which is the cause of African histoplasmosis, is a larger organism, 12–15 μm in diameter [59].
‡Tachyzoites are PAS negative, cysts and bradyzoites are usually PAS positive [60].

leading to pancytopenia can occur in hyper-reactive malarial splenomegaly, leishmaniasis and schistosomiasis. Cryoglobulinaemia and paraproteinaemia can occur.

Bone marrow cytology

A bone marrow aspirate is very useful in the diagnosis of leishmaniasis (Fig. 3.27) and is a recommended diagnostic method when this is suspected. Macrophages are increased and contain organisms. These are characterized by a small paranuclear basophilic body, known as the kinetoplast, giving the organism a characteristic 'double-dot' appearance. Leishmaniasis usually results from *Leishmania donovani* infection but in India may be due to *L. tropica* [67]; both can be detected by bone marrow examination. Leishmaniasis is usually associated with a conspicuous increase in plasma cells and there may also be prominent dyserythropoiesis. Trypanosomes are sometimes detected in the bone

marrow, but less often than leishmaniae. Detection is more common in immunosuppressed patients. [68].

The unstained bone marrow films of patients who have had repeated bouts of malaria may appear slate grey or black because of the accumulation of phagocytosed malaria pigment [69]. Malaria parasites are sometimes detected, in red cells or neutrophils, in a bone marrow aspirate (Fig. 3.28), although bone marrow aspiration is not a recommended diagnostic method if malaria is suspected. In acute falciparum malaria the bone marrow may be hypocellular, normocellular or mildly hypercellular. Erythropoiesis is reduced. In chronic falciparum malaria there is hypercellularity with erythroid hyperplasia. Other features of the bone marrow in falciparum malaria include dyserythropoiesis, giant metamyelocytes and increased eosinophils, lymphocytes, plasma cells and macrophages [69–71]. There may be haemophagocytosis and

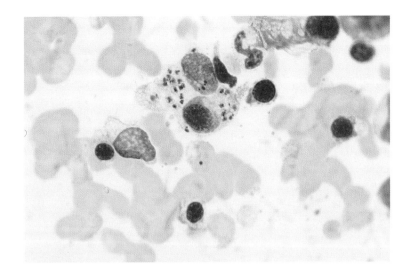

Fig. 3.27 BM aspirate, leishmaniasis, showing a macrophage containing numerous organisms which, in addition to a nucleus, have a small paranuclear kinetoplast giving them a characteristic 'double-dot' appearance. MGG ×100.

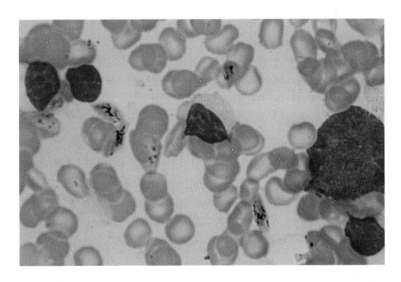

Fig. 3.28 BM aspirate from a patient with falciparum malaria showing gametocytes. MGG ×100. (By courtesy of Dr D. Swirsky, Leeds.)

macrophages can also contain malarial pigment. The bone marrow in *Plasmodium vivax* malaria is also characterized by dyserythropoiesis, increased macrophages (some showing haemophagocytosis), increased plasma cells and sometimes increased eosinophils [69]. In hyper-reactive malarial splenomegaly. there may be a marked increase in bone marrow lymphocytes [72].

Microfilaria are occasionally observed in a bone marrow aspirate in immunologically normal hosts (Fig. 3.29) and are more often seen in immuno-compromised patients [73]. Toxoplasma (Fig. 3.30)

have also sometimes been found in immunodeficient patients.

Features useful in distinguishing leishmaniasis and toxoplasmosis from fungal infections are shown in Table 3.2.

An increased number of bone marrow eosinophils and their precursors are often seen in helminth infection.

Bone marrow histology

In visceral leishmaniasis, there may be granuloma formation. In more severe cases there is a diffuse

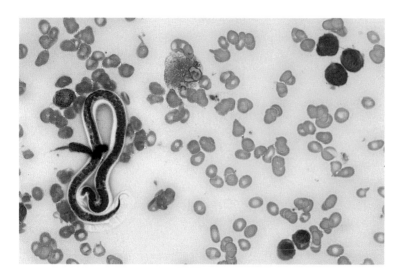

Fig. 3.29 BM aspirate from a patient with filariasis showing a microfilaria. MGG ×50. (By courtesy of Mrs Seema M. Zainal, Bahrein.)

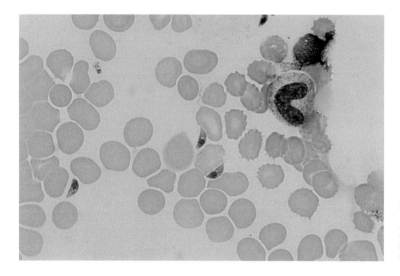

Fig. 3.30 BM aspirate showing *Toxoplasma gondii*, in a patient who had had a renal transplant. MGG ×100. (By courtesy of Dr R. Cobcroft, Brisbane.)

increase of macrophages. The organisms are often seen within macrophages (Fig. 3.31); their small size (3 μm) sometimes leads to their being confused with the fungus *Histoplasma capsulatum*. However, leishmaniae fail to stain with PAS or silver stains and a Giemsa stain will demonstrate the 'double-dot' of nucleus and kinetoplast (less apparent than in the aspirate).

A bone marrow biopsy in malaria usually shows increased cellularity and increased macrophage activity, often with haemophagocytosis. During acute attacks of malaria, sinusoids may be packed with parasitized red cells [71]. In patients who have suffered recurrent attacks of malaria, the bone marrow may be slate grey or black due to deposition of malaria pigment. It is important to distin-

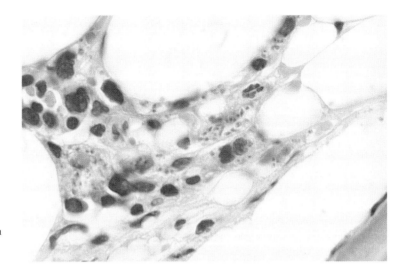

Fig. 3.31 BM trephine biopsy section from an HIV-positive man showing *Leishmania donovani* within macrophages. Paraffin-embedded, H&E ×100.

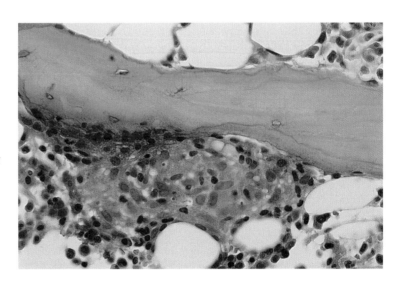

Fig. 3.32 BM trephine biopsy section, toxoplasmosis, showing a small granuloma in a paratrabecular position containing several small organisms with a single nucleus consistent with the tachyzoites of *Toxoplasma gondii*. Fungal stains were negative and the patient had raised serum IgM antibodies to *Toxoplasma*. Resin-embedded, H&E ×40.

guish malaria pigment (haemozoin) from formalin pigment. Haemozoin is found not only in macrophages but also within erythroid and granulocytic precursors, possibly contributing to dyserythropoiesis and erythroid suppression [74].

Granulomas are also seen in toxoplasmosis; rarely, in immunosuppressed individuals, organisms are seen in the marrow (Fig. 3.32). These usually take the form of tachyzoites, which are 3–6 μm in diameter and have a tiny single nucleus.

Occasionally, cysts containing numerous bradyzoites are present. Bradyzoites are of a similar size to tachyzoites and also have a single nucleus; the lack of a kinetoplast helps to distinguish them from leishmaniae. Toxoplasma can be identified by immunohistochemistry.

Extrapulmonary infection with *Pneumocystis jiroveci* (previously *Pneumocystis carinii*) is rare; it is invariably secondary to pulmonary disease, and appears to be more common in those patients who have received aerosolized pentamidine therapy. Approximately a third of patients with extrapulmonary infection have marrow involvement [75]. There are areas of 'frothy' exudate which is pink in a haematoxylin and eosin (H&E)-stained section; Grocott's methenamine silver stain demonstrates the cysts, which are 4–6 μm in diameter and often have a crumpled or cup-shaped appearance. Diagnosis is aided by immunohistochemistry.

Microsporidiosis rarely involves the bone marrow but involvement has been reported at autopsy in a patient with AIDS [76].

Problems and pitfalls

The trephine biopsy can be critical in the diagnosis of visceral leishmaniasis. Patients not uncommonly present with hepatosplenomegaly and B symptoms and either acute leukaemia or lymphoma may be suspected. In non-endemic areas the diagnosis may not have been considered and it is incumbent on the laboratory haematologist/histopathologist to detect such cases. Macrophages should be examined carefully for microorganisms in patients with unexplained hepatosplenomegaly and reactive changes in the bone marrow.

Bone marrow granulomas

A granuloma is a compact aggregate of macrophages. These may include a major component of epithelioid macrophages, which have large amounts of pale pink cytoplasm and ovoid or elongated nuclei with a dispersed chromatin pattern. Often several epithelioid cells fuse to form a giant cell. Two common types of giant cell are recognized in granulomas: Langhans type with numerous nuclei arranged around the periphery of the cell and foreign body type with nuclei scattered throughout the cell. Other cells including lymphocytes, plasma cells, neutrophils, eosinophils and fibroblasts may be found within granulomas, but these are not a constant feature.

A wide range of aetiological agents are associated with marrow granulomas [20,55,77–97] (Table 3.3). It should be noted that patients with immunodeficiency, such as AIDS, may fail to produce granulomas in response to infection with organisms that stimulate granuloma formation in normal individuals; this is probably consequent on the lack of important T-cell functions that facilitate the formation of some types of granuloma.

Peripheral blood

There are no specific peripheral blood findings associated with the presence of bone marrow granulomas. The blood film may show features associated with the primary disease or, if bone marrow disease is extensive, there may be anaemia or pancytopenia with a leucoerythroblastic blood film. Lymphopenia is also common [81].

Table 3.3 Bone marrow granulomas [20,55,77–97].

Infection
Tuberculosis
Atypical mycobacterial infection
Disseminated bacillus Calmette–Guérin (BCG) infection, following vaccination [78] or intravesical therapy for bladder cancer [79]
Brucellosis
Leprosy
Syphilis
Typhoid fever
Paratyphoid [80]
Legionnaire's disease

Table 3.3 (continued)

Tularaemia [81]
Ehrlichiosis [82]
Q fever
Lyme disease (*Borrelia burgdorferi* infection) [83]
Rocky Mountain spotted fever [81]
Whipple's disease [20]
Leishmaniasis
Toxoplasmosis
Histoplasmosis
Cryptococcosis
Saccharomyces cerevisiae infection [81]
Blastomycosis
Coccidioidomycosis [84]
Paracoccidioidomycosis [55]
Herpesvirus infection (Epstein–Barr virus, cytomegalovirus, herpes zoster)
Hantaan virus infection (Korean haemorrhagic fever) [85]
Cat scratch disease [85]

Sarcoidosis

Malignant disease
Hodgkin lymphoma*
Multiple myeloma [86]
Non-Hodgkin lymphoma*
Chronic natural killer cell lymphocytosis [87]
Mycosis fungoides [81]
Acute lymphoblastic leukaemia [81,85,88]
Myelodysplastic syndrome [88]
Polycythaemia vera [89]
Metastatic carcinoma (breast or colon) [90,91]

Drug hypersensitivity
Phenytoin
Procainamide
Phenylbutazone [81]
Chlorpropamide
Sulphasalazine [92]
Ibuprofen [81]
Indomethacin [91]
Allopurinol
Carbamazepine [93]
Amiodarone [94]

Associated with eosinophilic interstitial nephritis

Reaction to foreign substances
Anthracosis and silicosis [85,88,95]
Talc [96]
Berylliosis [97]

*With or without bone marrow infiltration.

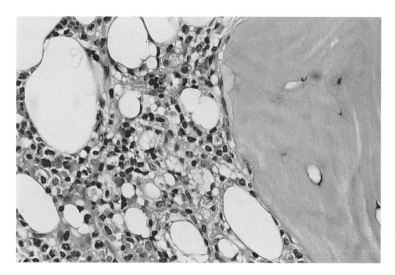

Fig. 3.33 BM trephine biopsy section, lipid granuloma. Paraffin-embedded, H&E ×40.

Bone marrow cytology

There are no specific features in the bone marrow aspirate in patients with bone marrow granulomas. Occasionally it is possible to recognize epithelioid cells.

Bone marrow histology

Lipid granulomas Lipid granulomas (Fig. 3.33) have been reported to be the most common type of granuloma seen in the marrow, being present in up to 9% of biopsies [98]. In our experience, they are less common than this. They are of no clinical importance and must be distinguished from epithelioid granulomas which they can some-times resemble. Similar lesions may be seen in the liver, spleen and lymph nodes and some of these cases have been reported to be associated with ingestion of mineral oil [99]. In the marrow they are usually located close to sinusoids or lymphoid nodules and measure from 0.2 to 0.8 mm in diameter. They contain fat vacuoles, which vary in size but are usually smaller than the vacuoles in marrow fat cells and may be multiple. Lipid granulomas usually have plasma cells, eosinophils and lymphocytes within them, and approximately 5% contain giant cells. Occasionally, the fat vacuoles may be small and easily overlooked, giving the granulomas a sarcoid-like appearance.

Other granulomas Unless a specific organism can be demonstrated within a granuloma, there are usually no histological features that allow a definitive diagnosis to be made [100]. Because of this, it is important for the pathologist to be aware of all relevant clinical details, in order to be able to suggest an appropriate differential diagnosis. All biopsy specimens with granulomas should have appropriate stains for acid-fast bacilli and fungi performed. Ideally, in those cases in which marrow granulomas with an infective aetiology are possible, for example in patients with a pyrexia of unknown origin, this should be anticipated and part of the marrow aspirate should be cultured for mycobacteria and fungi.

Granulomas are found on marrow biopsy in 15–40% of patients with miliary tuberculosis (Fig. 3.34). Tuberculous granulomas usually contain Langhans type giant cells and caseation is present in approximately half of cases with marrow involvement [100]. Acid-fast bacilli cannot be demonstrated in most cases and, when seen, they are usually scanty (Fig. 3.35).

Approximately 50% of patients with disseminated *Mycobacterium avium intracellulare* infection have marrow granulomas (Figs 3.36 and 3.37), ranging from small, ill defined lymphohistiocytic aggregates to larger, more solid lymphohistiocytic lesions and small, well-formed epithelioid granulomas [101]. Giant cells are only present in a minority

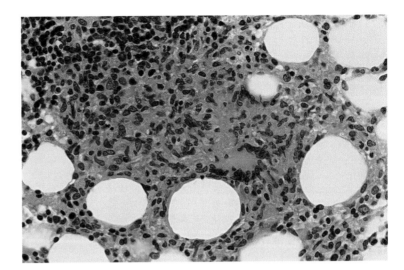

Fig. 3.34 trephine biopsy section, miliary tuberculosis, showing an epithelioid granuloma containing a Langhans giant cell; there are numerous lymphocytes at the periphery of the granuloma. Paraffin-embedded, H&E ×40.

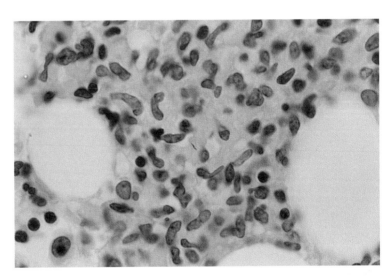

Fig. 3.35 BM trephine biopsy section, miliary tuberculosis, showing a granuloma containing an acid-fast bacillus. Paraffin-embedded, ZN stain ×100.

of lesions and necrosis is not usually seen. When organisms are very numerous, the macrophages containing them may appear foamy (Fig. 3.37a) or may resemble Gaucher cells. Occasionally, organisms are recognizable on a Giemsa stain (Fig. 3.37b). Atypical mycobacteria may be demonstrated by PAS and ZN stains, sometimes in large numbers; they tend to be longer, more curved and more coarsely beaded than tubercle bacilli. They are PAS positive, whereas *M. tuberculosis* is PAS negative.

Marrow granulomas containing foamy macrophages are occasionally seen in patients with leprosy; a Fite stain will demonstrate the acid-fast bacilli of *M. leprae* [15]. Foamy macrophages may also be a feature of granulomas due to typhoid. Bone marrow granulomas in Whipple's disease may contain distinctive PAS-positive bacilli [102]. Small, poorly formed epithelioid granulomas are found in the bone marrow in most cases of brucellosis.

Disseminated infection by the fungus *Histoplasma capsulatum* usually involves the bone marrow; in normal hosts there are numerous granulomas, often with Langhans giant cells and necrosis. Discrete granulomas are present in only a minority of immunodeficient hosts; more commonly such patients have ill-defined lymphohistiocytic aggre-

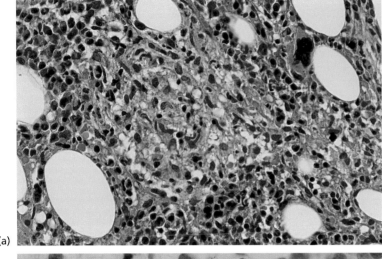

(a)

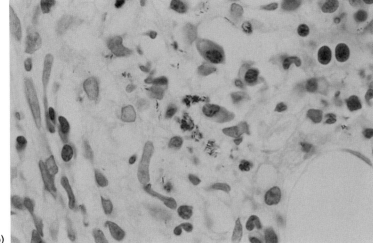

(b)

Fig. 3.36 BM trephine biopsy section from a patient with AIDS and disseminated *Mycobacterium avium intracellulare* infection. (a) Poorly formed granuloma made up of epithelioid macrophages, many of which have vacuolated cytoplasm. Paraffin-embedded, H&E ×40. (b) Large numbers of acid-fast bacilli; note the coarse beading of the organisms. Paraffin-embedded, ZN stain ×100.

gates or sheets of macrophages infiltrating between haemopoietic cells [103] (see Fig. 3.24). Tiny yeast forms, 2–5 μm in diameter, some of which show unequal budding, are present within macrophages. Fungi may be seen with an H&E stain, but are best visualized using a silver stain (e.g. Gomori's methenamine silver or Grocott) or a PAS stain. *Cryptococcus neoformans* infection can also cause granulomas. The organisms seen in tissue sections are yeasts (5–10 μm in diameter) with a wide capsular halo and narrow-based, unequal budding (Fig. 3.38); with a mucicarmine stain the capsule

of the yeast is red. The capsule is also well stained with Alcian blue (see Fig. 3.25b) and with PAS (Fig. 3.38a). Infection with the protozoans *Leishmania donovani* and *Toxoplasma gondii* may involve the marrow and provoke granuloma formation (see Figs 3.31 and 3.32).

In up to 60% of patients with infectious mononucleosis, small epithelioid granulomas are seen in histological sections of bone marrow; Langhans type giant cells and necrosis are not seen. Marrow granulomas are seen less commonly in other viral infections.

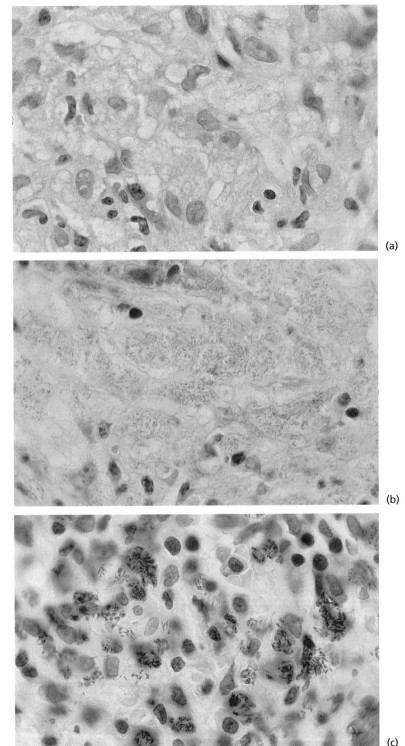

Fig. 3.37 BM trephine biopsy section from a patient with AIDS and *Mycobacerium avium intracellulare* infection showing foamy macrophages packed with microorganisms. Paraffin-embedded ×100: (a) H&E; (b) Giemsa; (c) ZN stain.

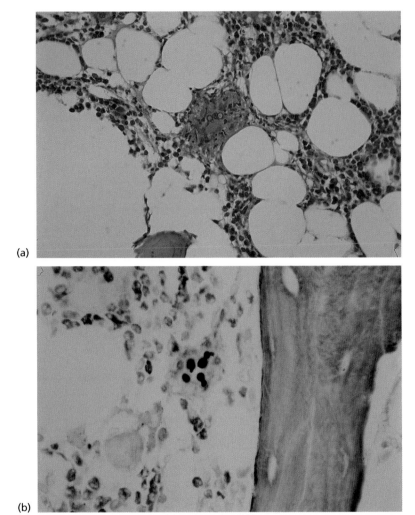

(a)

(b)

Fig. 3.38 BM trephine biopsy sections from a patient with Cryptococcus neoformans infection. (a) A small epithelioid granuloma containing large yeast forms with narrow-based unequal budding. Paraffin-embedded, PAS ×20. (b) Budding yeast forms. Paraffin-embedded, GMS ×40.

Granulomas may be seen in Hodgkin lymphoma [104], non-Hodgkin lymphoma (Fig. 3.39) and multiple myeloma [86] (Fig. 3.40) in association with neoplastic infiltration of the marrow. In both Hodgkin lymphoma and non-Hodgkin lymphoma, granulomas also occur in the absence of marrow involvement; these are usually small, well-formed epithelioid granulomas although larger, poorly formed lymphohistiocytic lesions have also been reported [105]. Since patients with lymphoma have an increased susceptibility to many of the infections associated with marrow granulomas,

these should always be excluded before attributing the granulomas to the underlying neoplastic disease. Bone marrow granulomas, in the absence of any apparent infection, have also been reported in single cases of hairy cell leukaemia treated with 2-chlorodeoxyadenosine (cladribine) [106], AML treated with interleukin (IL) 2 and lymphokine-activated killer cells [107] and in a total of four cases of chronic NK cell lymphocytosis [108,109].

The bone marrow is commonly involved in sarcoidosis; granulomas were seen in nine out of 21 patients in a biopsy series [100]. Often patients

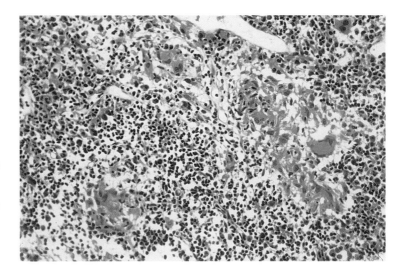

Fig. 3.39 BM trephine biopsy section showing a reactive granuloma in a patient with diffuse bone marrow involvement by low grade non-Hodgkin lymphoma (follicular lymphoma). No evidence of an infective cause of the granuloma was found in this patient. Paraffin-embedded, H&E ×20.

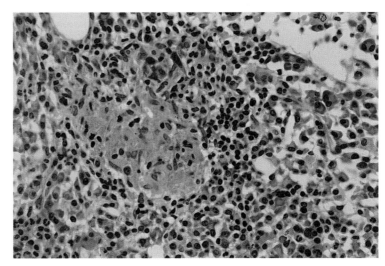

Fig. 3.40 BM trephine biopsy, multiple myeloma, showing large numbers of plasma cells and an epithelioid granuloma (centre). No evidence of an infective cause for the granuloma was found in this patient. Paraffin-embedded, H&E ×40.

with marrow granulomas have evidence of multisystem involvement, such as hepatosplenomegaly, although chest radiography may be normal [110]. Typically there are numerous, well-formed epithelioid granulomas which, in approximately a third of cases, contain Langhans type giant cells; necrosis is seen very rarely. Sarcoid granulomas usually lack a surrounding zone of inflammatory cells. They are associated with prominent reticulin fibrosis and sometimes collagen formation, which may encircle the individual granulomas. Giant cells in sarcoid granulomas may contain cytoplasmic asteroid and Schaumann bodies (Fig. 3.41) but these are not specific.

Granulomas associated with drug hypersensitivity are often poorly circumscribed lymphohistiocytic lesions, which may contain eosinophils. Rarely, they are accompanied by a systemic vasculitis, which may involve marrow vessels.

Distinctive 'doughnut type' or ring granulomas may be seen in the marrow in Q fever [111] although they do not appear to be specific for this disease [40]. They have also been reported, for example, in CMV infection in immunodeficient subjects [112] and in brucellosis [113], infectious mononucleosis [114], typhoid fever, Lyme disease [83], T-lineage non-Hodgkin lymphoma [115] and Hodgkin lymphoma. This type of granuloma often

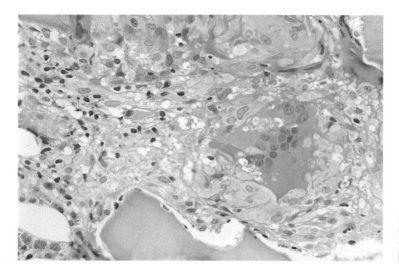

Fig. 3.41 BM trephine biopsy, sarcoidosis, showing a granuloma with a giant cell containing asteroid bodies. Resin-embedded, H&E ×40.

has a central empty space, surrounded by neutrophils, lymphocytes, histiocytes and concentrically arranged, laminated fibrinoid material; more haphazardly arranged lesions without a central space also occur, as do small areas of fibrinoid necrosis [111].

Problems and pitfalls
Determining the cause of bone marrow granulomas requires careful clinicopathological correlation, including a detailed drug history. Despite this, no cause is found in many cases. Conditions that can simulate granulomas include mastocytosis and metastases. Failure to detect organisms on ZN and auramine stains does not exclude mycobacterial infection.

Reactive lymphoid aggregates and polymorphous lymphoid hyperplasia

An increase in interstitial lymphocytes can occur in infection, inflammation, non-haemopoietic malignancy, autoimmune disease and persistent polyclonal lymphocytosis. Reactive lymphoid aggregates, sometimes referred to as 'benign lymphoid aggregates', are commonly present in the bone marrow, their incidence increasing with age. An increased frequency has been reported in association with infection, inflammation, haemolysis, myeloproliferative disorders and autoimmune diseases such as

rheumatoid arthritis and thyrotoxicosis. They are common in patients with chronic myelogenous leukaemia treated with imatinib [116]. Their frequency is increased in Castleman's disease [44,117]. Bone marrow lymphoid aggregates, assessed histologically as benign, have been associated with the subsequent development of low grade lymphoma [118].

Peripheral blood
There are no specific peripheral blood features associated with the presence of reactive lymphoid aggregates in the bone marrow.

Bone marrow cytology
The bone marrow aspirate is usually normal but may show an increase in normal, mature lymphocytes.

Bone marrow histology
Reactive lymphoid aggregates are usually few in number, not paratrabecular and well circumscribed. They are composed predominantly of small mature lymphocytes interspersed with some plasma cells, macrophages and sometimes occasional eosinophils, mast cells and immunoblasts [118,119] (Fig. 3.42). Reactive lymphoid aggregates may be associated with small blood vessels. The lymphocytes show more pleomorphism than those in most neoplastic lymphoid aggregates. Occasionally germinal centres are seen [44,120] (Fig. 3.43).

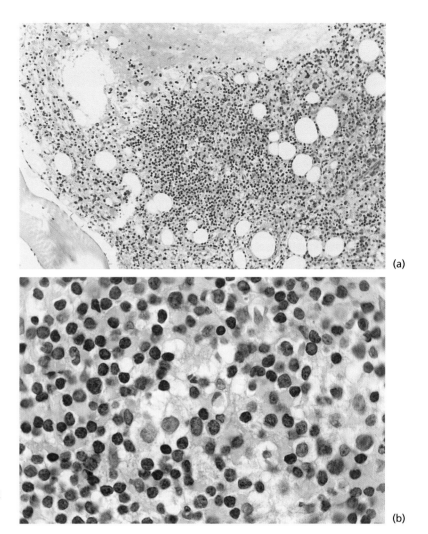

(a)

(b)

Fig. 3.42 Section of BM trephine biopsy. (a) A reactive lymphoid nodule and surrounding normal haemopoietic cells. H&E ×10. (b) The centre of a lymphoid nodule containing several macrophages and an occasional immunoblast, in addition to normal small lymphocytes. Paraffin-embedded, H&E ×100.

Reticulin fibres are increased within the nodule. Bone marrow biopsy sections showing reactive lymphoid aggregates have an increased incidence of lipid granulomas and plasmacytosis.

Demonstration of a mixture of T and B cells may be helpful in confirming the reactive nature of a lymphoid nodule [121,122]. However, it should be noted that, although lymphoid aggregates composed of homogeneous B cells are likely to be neoplastic and most reactive lymphoid aggregates contain a mixture of T and B cells [121,122], there may also be admixed reactive T cells in infiltrates of low grade B-cell lymphoma.

Unusual causes of reactive lymphoid infiltrates are thymoma, which has been associated with a nodular and interstitial infiltrate of polyclonal T cells [123], and persistent polyclonal B-cell lymphocytosis of middle-aged, mainly cigarette-smoking, females which has been associated with a nodular (and intravascular) infiltrate of B cells [124].

Occasional paratrabecular infiltrates have been reported in apparently healthy people [125] but this is very rare and a paratrabecular infiltrate is unlikely to be reactive. We advocate follow-up of such patients.

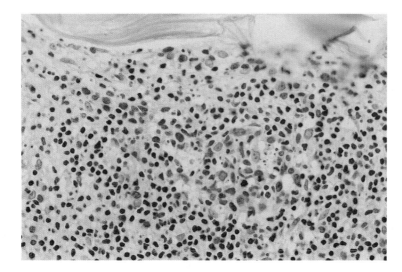

Fig. 3.43 Section of BM trephine biopsy showing a secondary lymphoid follicle in a patient with rheumatoid arthritis. Paraffin-embedded, H&E ×20. (By courtesy of Dr R. Brunning, Minnesota.)

More extensive lymphoid infiltrates, often with admixed eosinophils, macrophages including epithelioid cells, endothelial cells, plasma cells and immunoblasts, are common in AIDS (see Figs 3.54 and 3.55) and may also be seen in congenital immunodeficiency, angioimmunoblastic lymphadenopathy, following bone marrow transplantation and occasionally in association with autoimmune diseases such as rheumatoid arthritis. An extensive polymorphous lymphoid infiltrate can also be seen in the lymphoproliferative disorder associated with phenytoin therapy [126]. It is sometimes not possible to distinguish polymorphous reactive lymphoid hyperplasia from T-cell lymphoma, T-cell/histiocyte-rich diffuse large B-cell lymphoma or even Hodgkin lymphoma on the basis of histology alone.

Problems and pitfalls

Making a distinction between reactive and neoplastic infiltrates is not always possible on histological grounds. Clinicopathological correlation, immunophenotyping and molecular analysis may be needed.

Plasmacytosis and cytological abnormalities in plasma cells

A reactive increase of polyclonal plasma cells is common and is associated with a variety of conditions including HIV infection, leishmaniasis and other infections, chronic inflammatory diseases (particularly rheumatoid arthritis), haemopoietic and non-haemopoietic malignant disease, angioimmunoblastic lymphadenopathy, systemic Castleman's disease, cirrhosis, diabetes mellitus, iron deficiency, megaloblastic anaemia and haemolytic anaemia [18,127]. A reactive increase in plasma cells needs to be distinguished from bone marrow infiltration by neoplastic plasma cells such as occurs in multiple myeloma and in many cases of immunocyte-derived amyloidosis, systemic light chain disease, and monoclonal gammopathy of undetermined significance.

Peripheral blood

Patients with reactive bone marrow plasmacytosis commonly show non-specific abnormalities in the peripheral blood consequent on the underlying disease. There is often anaemia, which may have the features of anaemia of chronic disease (either a normochromic, normocytic anaemia or, if the inflammatory process is severe, a hypochromic, microcytic anaemia). Rouleaux formation is commonly increased as a consequence of an increased concentration of polyclonal immunoglobulins and other reactive changes in plasma proteins. Occasional patients with reactive plasmacytosis have plasma cells in the peripheral blood, usually in small numbers.

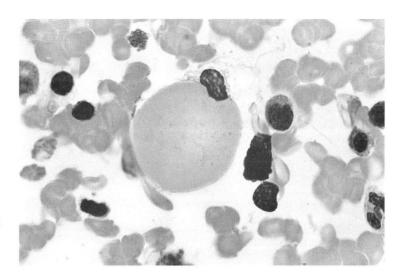

Fig. 3.44 BM aspirate film showing a Russell body in a plasma cell in a patient with reactive plasmacytosis. MGG ×100.

Bone marrow cytology

In reactive plasmacytosis the bone marrow shows an increased number of plasma cells, not usually exceeding 10–20% of nucleated cells but in rare cases 50% or more. Prominent plasmacytosis, in one case 51%, is common in angioimmunoblastic T-cell lymphoma [128]. In one exceptional patient with an adverse drug reaction more than 90% of bone marrow cells were plasma cells [129]. The plasma cells are predominantly mature (see Fig. 1.50) although occasional cells may have nucleoli, a diffuse chromatin pattern or some degree of nucleocytoplasmic asynchrony. Small numbers of bi- or trinucleated forms can be present. The plasma cells may contain cytoplasmic vacuoles or inclusions. Large homogeneous hyaline inclusions, often single, 2–3 μm in diameter and displacing the nucleus, are designated Russell bodies. They are occasionally identified in bone marrow aspirates (Fig. 3.44). Cells containing multiple weakly basophilic spherical inclusions are referred to as Mott cells, grape cells or morular cells; the inclusions within the Mott cell may also be referred to as Russell bodies [130,131]. Plasma cells can also contain cytoplasmic crystals. They may have a pyknotic nucleus and voluminous pale-staining cytoplasm as a result of greatly dilated endoplasmic reticulum; such cells are sometimes designated thesaurocytes, mistakenly suggesting that they are storing the products they have synthesized. Cells that synthesize carbohydrate can have flaming pink cytoplasm ('flaming cells'). All these inclusions and unusual tinctorial qualities result from increased immunoglobulin synthesis within the rough endoplasmic reticulum. Apparent intranuclear inclusions have been described in reactive plasmacytosis but they are more characteristic of neoplastic plasma cells. These inclusions, known as Dutcher bodies, are actually consequent on cytoplasmic invagination. Cells of these various types are characteristic of conditions with immune stimulation but neoplastic plasma cells often show similar features. Plasmacytic satellitism (a central macrophage surrounded by plasma cells) and increased mast cells, eosinophils and megakaryocytes favour reactive rather than neoplastic plasmacytosis [18].

Occasionally plasma cells contain haemosiderin inclusions, which are irregular in shape, relatively large and stain greenish-black with a May–Grünwald–Giemsa (MGG) stain (see Fig. 2.4). Their presence is associated with iron overload (e.g. haemochromatosis and transfusion siderosis), copper deficiency [132,133] and chronic alcoholism [134].

Bone marrow histology

A trephine biopsy section in reactive plasmacytosis shows an interstitial infiltrate of plasma cells, particularly adjacent to capillaries (see Fig. 1.51). Plasma cells are sometimes clustered around

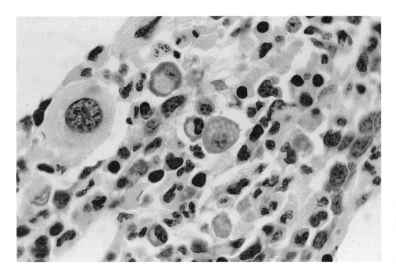

Fig. 3.45 BM trephine biopsy section, myelodysplastic syndrome, showing prominent plasma cells including one with multiple cytoplasmic vacuoles (Mott cell). Resin-embedded, H&E ×100.

macrophages. A minority of cases have small clusters of plasma cells but large homogeneous nodules, which are a feature of multiple myeloma, are not seen. The variety of inclusions described above may also be apparent in histological sections (Fig. 3.45) and some degree of cellular immaturity may be noted. Russell bodies and Dutcher bodies stain pink with an H&E stain, blue-green to dark blue with a Giemsa stain and show variable PAS staining. In reactive plasmacytosis immunohistochemistry or ISH shows that κ- and λ-expressing plasma cells are present in a ratio of approximately 2:1. Approximately half of the plasma cells express γ heavy chain, about a third α and the remainder μ [135].

Plasmacytosis may be associated with other reactive changes such as granulocytic hyperplasia, lymphoid aggregates and increased numbers of macrophages. The macrophages may have enhanced haemophagocytic activity and an increased iron content.

Mast cells

Small numbers of mast cells are present in normal bone marrow aspirates. However, it should be noted that the normal number of mast cells in the trephine biopsy sections of healthy subjects has not been defined. Mast cells are increased as a reactive

change in association with a variety of pathological processes. Increased numbers have been noted in infection, inflammation, renal failure, sarcoidosis, hyperparathyroidism, Paget's disease, reactive lymphocytosis and lymphoproliferative disorders (particularly lymphoplasmacytic lymphoma but also chronic lymphocytic leukaemia, hairy cell leukaemia and Hodgkin lymphoma), aplastic anaemia, paroxysmal nocturnal haemoglobinuria, myeloproliferative neoplasms, MDS and AML [89,136–140]. Mast cells accumulate in areas of connective tissue proliferation, for example in fracture callus and in zones of osteitis fibrosa in patients with renal failure. They are increased in a rare inherited disorder associated with a constitutional *KIT* mutation. Increased numbers of mast cells are present also in systemic mastocytosis but these neoplastic mast cells are usually morphologically abnormal (see pages 269–278).

Peripheral blood
There are no specific peripheral blood features associated with a reactive increase of bone marrow mast cells.

Bone marrow cytology
The cytological features of bone marrow mast cells have been described on pages 26–27. Lymphocytosis and plasmacytosis may coexist with a reactive increase in mast cells.

Bone marrow histology

The characteristics of mast cells in histological sections have been described on pages 26–27 and the features of systemic mastocytosis will be described on pages 273–278. In histological sections, normal and reactive mast cells are not readily identified with an H&E stain but are easily recognized with a Giemsa or other metachromatic stain, which highlights the numerous granules packing the cytoplasm. Normal and reactive mast cells are round or, less often, spindle-shaped.

When mast cells are increased, there may be an associated increase in plasma cells and lymphocytes.

Problems and pitfalls

Increased numbers of cytologically normal mast cells should not be confused with infiltration in systemic mastocytosis. Neoplastic mast cells are more often spindle-shaped and are usually hypogranular, to the extent that they can be confused with fibroblasts or macrophages. They are also present as clusters, whereas reactive mast cells are dispersed among other cells. Lesions of systemic mastocytosis often show associated fibrosis but it should be noted that reactive paratrabecular mast cells can also be associated with a slight increase of reticulin.

Histiocytosis

A diffuse increase in macrophages (histiocytes) is common in a variety of infective and inflammatory conditions and whenever there is bone marrow hyperplasia, ineffective haemopoiesis or increased breakdown of blood cells. All of the conditions capable of causing granuloma formation and haemophagocytic syndromes can also cause an increase of macrophages in the absence of granuloma formation or prominent haemophagocytosis. Macrophages present may range from relatively immature cells showing little phagocytic activity to mature cells which may be foamy or contain cellular debris, haemosiderin or a few haemopoietic cells, erythrocytes, neutrophils or platelets.

Increased bone marrow macrophages may be seen after granulocyte–macrophage colony-stimulating factor (GM-CSF) therapy when they may constitute as many as 90% of bone marrow cells [141]. They have been prominent in patients with failure to engraft after bone marrow transplantation particularly, but not only, when GM-CSF has been given [142]. A marked increase in macrophages has been reported at presentation of acute lymphoblastic leukaemia in a patient without any apparent infection [143].

Reactive macrophages, including haemophago-

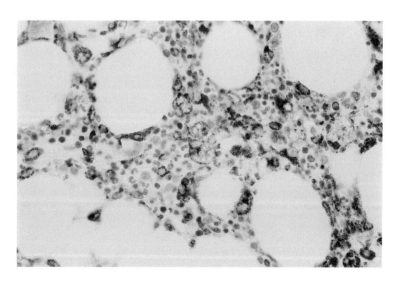

Fig. 3.46 BM trephine biopsy section showing a reactive increase in macrophages. Paraffin-embedded, immunoperoxidase CD68 (McAb PG-M1) ×40.

cytic forms, can be highlighted by immunohisto-chemical staining with CD68R or CD163 (Fig. 3.46).

Increased macrophages are also seen in storage diseases (see Chapter 9).

Haemophagocytic syndromes

Haemophagocytic syndromes result from macro-phage activation with increased numbers of

Table 3.4 Conditions associated with a haemophagocytic syndrome [77,144–200].

Malignant histiocytosis

Reactive haemophagocytic syndromes
Induced by viral infection
  Herpesviruses:
    Epstein–Barr virus (including fatal infectious mononucleosis in X-linked lymphoproliferative syndrome)*
    herpes simplex
    varicella/zoster virus
    human herpesvirus 6 [144]
    human herpesvirus 7 [145]
    human herpesvirus 8 [146,147]
    cytomegalovirus
  Other viruses:
    adenovirus
    measles (vaccine virus)
    influenza A [148]
    para-influenza
    vaccinia
    rubella (congenital)
    parvovirus B19 [149]
    respiratory syncytial virus [150]
    Kyasanur forest disease
    dengue [151]
    hepatitis A virus [152]
    hepatitis B virus [153]
    hepatitis C virus [153]
    coxsackievirus A9 [153]
    echovirus II [153]
    swine influenza virus [153]
    hantavirus [154]
    Crimean-Congo haemorrhagic fever [155]

Induced by bacterial infection
  Brucellosis
  Staphylococcal, streptococcal, *Escherichia coli*, *Haemophilus influenzae*, acinetobacter species, *Bacteroides fragilis*, pseudomonas, klebsiella species, *Borrelia burgdorfer*, brucella species, *Salmonella typhi*, salmonella species and serratia species infections [151–153,156–159]
  Legionnaires' disease (*Legionella pneumophila*)
  Mycobacterium tuberculosis infection
  Atypical mycobacterial infection
  Psittacosis [151]
  Mycoplasma pneumoniae infection [160]
  Human granulocytic anaplasmosis and human monocytic ehrlichiosis [161,162]

Induced by rickettsiae
  Rocky Mountain spotted fever
  Q fever [163]
  Rickettsia tsutsugamushi infection [151]

Table 3.4 (continued)

Induced by protozoan and other parasites
  Toxoplasmosis
  Leishmaniasis (kala azar)
  Malaria, mainly *Plasmodium falciparum* but sometimes *P. vivax* [164,165]
  Babesiosis [166]
  Strongyloidiasis [153]

Induced by fungi
  Histoplasmosis
  Candidiasis [158]
  Trichosporonosis [167]
  Penicilliosis [153,168]
  Cryptococcosis [169]
  Pneumocystis jiroveci (previously *Pneumocystis carinii*) infection [153]

Associated with certain lymphomas and other lymphoid neoplasms, particularly T-cell lymphomas [170–172],
  including subcutaneous panniculitis T-cell lymphoma [173], T-cell large granular lymphocytic lymphoma [174]
  and adult T-cell leukaemia/lymphoma [175] and anaplastic large T-cell lymphoma [176] but occasionally NK cell
  lymphoma [177], B-cell lymphoma [178] including the Asian variant of intravascular lymphoma [179], Hodgkin
  lymphoma [180] and multiple myeloma [181]
Sinus histiocytosis with massive lymphadenopathy [182]
Erdhein–Chester syndrome [183]
Kawasaki's disease
Kikuchi's disease [184]
Sickle cell disease [185]
Anticonvulsant lymphadenopathy
Sarcoidosis [172]
Systemic lupus erythematosus [151], juvenile onset rheumatoid arthritis [186] and other autoimmune diseases [187]
  ('macrophage activation syndrome')
Graft-versus-host disease [188]
Following long-acting G-CSF [189], GM-CSF [190] or IL3 [191] administration
Cytophagic histiocytic panniculitis [192]
Lysinuric protein intolerance [193]
Retinoic acid syndrome in acute promyelocytic leukaemia [194]
Hereditary fructose intolerance [186]
Multiple sulphatase deficiency [186]
Type 2 Griscelli syndrome [195]
Following liver transplantation [196]
As a complication (often terminal) in patients with various immunodeficiencies and malignant conditions (ALL,
  CLL, Hodgkin disease, NHL, hairy cell leukaemia, AML, carcinoma, Chédiak–Higashi syndrome, Langerhans cell
  histiocytosis [197]) – probably as a complication of infection

Familial haemophagocytic lymphohistiocytosis [198,199]
Mutation in *PERF1* gene
Mutation in *UNC13D* encoding Munc13-4
Mutation in *STX11* encoding syntaxin 11
Linked to 9q21.3-22

ALL, acute lymphoblastic leukaemia; AML, acute myeloid leukaemia; CLL, chronic lymphocytic leukaemia; G-CSF, granulocyte colony-stimulating factor; GM-CSF, granulocyte–macrophage colony-stimulating factor; IL3, interleukin 3; NHL, non-Hodgkin lymphoma; NK, natural killer.
*Epstein–Barr virus-associated haemophagocytic syndrome may result from proliferation of a neoplastic clone of T lymphocytes or NK cells [200].

haemophagocytic macrophages and cytopenia. Common clinical features are hepatomegaly, splenomegaly and fever. Haemophagocytic syndromes result from a variety of underlying disorders [77,144–200] (Table 3.4). A lesser degree of haemophagocytosis without cytopenia is common in many of the same conditions. Haemophagocytic syndromes are often secondary to bacterial or viral infection, occurring either in previously healthy subjects or as a terminal complication in patients with a defective immune response. They are relatively common when viral or mycobacterial infections occur in patients with AIDS or with haemopoietic or other malignancy. Haemophagocytosis can also be prominent in patients with lymphoma, particularly T-cell lymphoma, when there is no evidence of infection; it is likely that in these cases there is increased proliferation of macrophage precursors and enhanced phagocytic activity in response to lymphokines secreted by the lymphoma cells.

Haemophagocytic lymphohistiocytosis can also be a primary familial condition [198,199]. This familial syndrome is an autosomal recessive condition of early childhood with NK cell dysfunction and helper T-cell and macrophage activation [201]. Presentation is usually at 2–6 months of age but congenital cases are recognized [199]. The condition is genetically heterogeneous but 20–40% of cases result from a mutation in the perforin gene (*PRF1*) at 10q21-22 [202] and others to mutations in *UNC13D*, *STX11* or an unidentified gene at 9q21.3-22. Since the haemophagocytosis may be triggered by infection and since cytological and histological features cannot be distinguished from those of infection-induced haemophagocytosis, the diagnosis must rest on clinical differences [198]. Small family size may lead to familial cases not being recognized as such unless one of the causative gene mutations is demonstrated.

There are other well-defined inherited immune deficiency syndromes with a propensity to infection-related haemophagocytic syndromes; these include the Chédiak–Higashi and Griscelli syndromes [203], purine nucleoside phosphorylase deficiency [204], type II Hermansky–Pudlak syndrome [205], lysinuric protein intolerance [193] and the X-linked lymphoproliferative disorder (Duncan's syndrome), resulting from mutation in either the *SH2D1A* gene [206] or the *BIRC4* gene [207]. In lysinuric protein intolerance there is phagocytosis by myeloid precursors as well as by mature macrophages [208].

It should be noted that the term 'erythrophagocytosis' refers to phagocytosis of mature erythrocytes whereas haemophagocytosis refers to phagocytosis of nucleated cells. Erythrophagocytosis can occur in haemophagocytic syndromes but can also be consequent on the presence of antibody-coated or abnormal erythrocytes.

Hyperlipidaemia, hyperferritinaemia and hypofibrinogenaemia are common in the haemophagocytic syndromes [153,186]. There are often markedly increased serum levels of various cytokines including interferon γ, soluble IL2 receptor, macrophage colony-stimulating factor, IL6 and tumour necrosis factor α [153]. Soluble CD25 and CD178 are also increased [186]. Liver dysfunction is usual and disseminated intravascular coagulation sometimes occurs.

Peripheral blood
The haemophagocytic syndromes are characterized by pancytopenia. Phagocytic macrophages are rarely present in the peripheral blood although in malignant histiocytosis there may be small numbers of monoblasts. The blood film may also show features of the primary condition, for example atypical lymphocytes in patients with familial lymphohistiocytosis (Fig. 3.47) or EBV or other viral infection.

Bone marrow cytology
In haemophagocytic syndromes there are increased numbers of macrophages and haemophagocytosis is usually prominent, with many macrophages having ingested numerous cells of various haemopoietic lineages (Figs 3.48 and 3.49). The macrophages are mainly mature and lack atypical features. However, phagocytic macrophages may initially be infrequent and repeated bone marrow examination may be needed to establish the diagnosis; abnormalities may be detected at presentation in less than a third of patients [186,198]. The bone marrow aspirate may also show other abnormalities due to the primary disease. For example, in

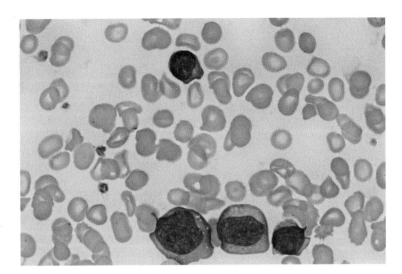

Fig. 3.47 PB film from a child with familial lymphohistiocytosis showing atypical lymphoid cells. MGG ×100.

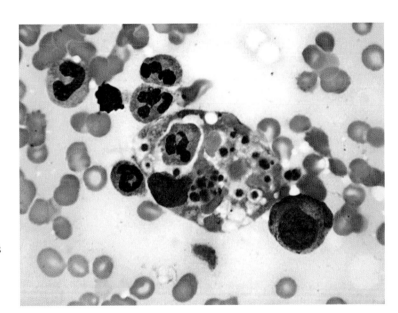

Fig. 3.48 BM aspirate, reactive haemophagocytosis, in a patient with both staphylococcal and HHV8 infection showing a macrophage that has ingested a neutrophil, erythrocytes and platelets. MGG ×100.

viral infections there is usually an increase of lymphocytes, which may be immature or atypical, and in bacterial infection there is granulocytic hyperplasia with toxic changes in the neutrophil lineage. Dyserythropoiesis may be prominent with features such as nuclear lobulation or fragmentation, bi- and trinuclearity and basophilic stippling [209]. In familial haemophagocytic lymphohistiocytosis, the bone marrow findings (Fig. 3.50) are identical to those of infection-induced haemophagocytosis.

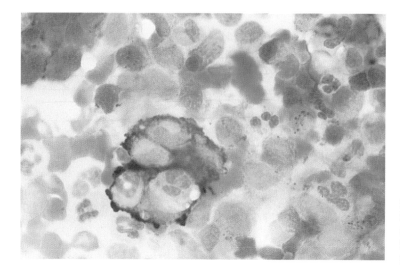

Fig. 3.49 BM aspirate, reactive haemophagocytosis, showing an iron-laden macrophage that has ingested neutrophils and neutrophil precursors. Perls' stain ×100.

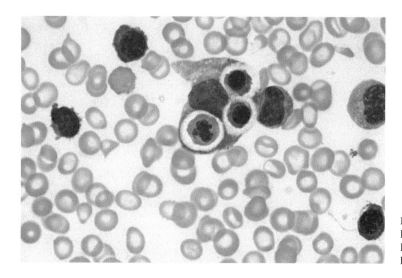

Fig. 3.50 BM aspirate, familial lymphohistiocytosis, showing haemophagocytosis and atypical lymphoid cells. MGG ×100.

When haemophagocytosis is secondary to a T-cell lymphoma the marrow may show closely inter-mingled lymphoma cells and macrophages, but cases have also been reported in which the bone marrow shows only haemophagocytosis with the lymphomatous infiltrate being confined to other tissues [171].

Bone marrow histology

In early cases of reactive haemophagocytic syn-drome (e.g. virus-induced) there is a hypercellular bone marrow with few macrophages [158]. Later there are more macrophages with hypoplasia of erythroid and myeloid lines; megakaryocyte numbers are either normal or increased. The degree of macrophage infiltration is variable (Fig. 3.51); in some cases it is inconspicuous while in others there is diffuse replacement of the marrow by mature macrophages with a low nucleocytoplasmic ratio, dispersed chromatin, inconspicuous nucleoli and

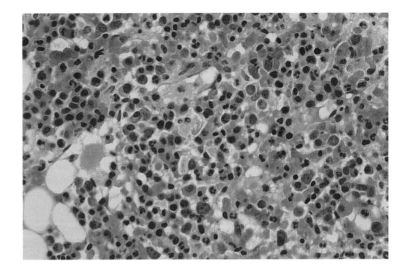

Fig. 3.51 BM trephine biopsy section, AIDS, showing increased cellularity, dyserythropoiesis and numerous macrophages, some of which contain erythrocytes and apoptotic normoblasts (haemophagocytosis). Paraffin-embedded, H&E ×40.

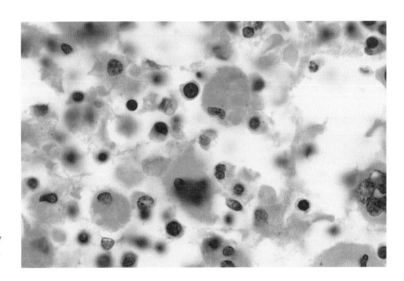

Fig. 3.52 BM sections from an autopsy on a child with terminal haemophagocytic syndrome as a complication of Chédiak–Higashi syndrome showing macrophages stuffed with red cells. Paraffin-embedded, H&E ×100. (By courtesy of Dr Wendy Erber and Dr L. Matz, Perth, Western Australia.)

abundant cytoplasm which is often vacuolated. Haemophagocytosis is often less apparent than in marrow films [158,210]; however, in some cases it is striking (Fig. 3.52). Features of the underlying disease may be present. Atypical lymphoid cells are seen in some cases of EBV infection. Lymphoma cells may be detected (see Fig. 6.67) but it should be noted that there may be no detectable neoplastic cells in the bone marrow in cases of lymphoma-associated haemophagocytic syndrome. Granulomas may be present in tuberculosis [211] and a variety

of other infections associated with a haemophago-cytic syndrome.

If haemophagocytic lymphohistiocytosis is sus-pected, a trephine biopsy is recommended because clusters or sheets of macrophages may be detected in cases in which the bone marrow aspirate shows no significant abnormality [212].

Problems and pitfalls

The major problems in assessing haemophagocytic syndromes are: (i) distinguishing reactive conditions from malignant histiocytosis; and (ii) determining the nature of the underlying condition. In the past, reactive haemophagocytosis was often misdiagnosed as malignant histiocytosis, which is actually a very rare disease. The latter is characterized by primitive cells with limited phagocytosis.

Vigorous efforts should be made to identify an infective cause. Immunohistochemistry and ISH techniques (see Table 3.1) are useful for demonstrating underlying CMV or EBV infection [213] and stains and cultures for mycobacteria may be positive. Most childhood cases of haemophagocytic lymphohistiocytosis, both sporadic and familial, are infection-related. However, some sporadic cases in children have atypical, large, granular lymphocytes; since T cells in such cases are sometimes shown to be clonal it is possible that there is an underlying T-cell neoplasm [214]. Demonstration of rearrangement of *IGH* or *TCR* loci provides presumptive evidence of an underlying lymphoid neoplasm but does not give definite evidence of the lineage involved. Molecular evidence of clonality is lacking when the associated neoplasm is of NK lineage.

Iron overload

Iron overload can result either from genetic haemochromatosis and other rare inherited abnormalities or from a haematological disorder. The haematological conditions leading to iron overload are characterized either by ineffective erythropoiesis, leading to increased iron absorption, or by anaemia that leads to transfusion dependence and transfusional iron overload; in some patients both mechanisms operate.

Peripheral blood
The peripheral blood is normal unless the iron overload results from a haematological abnormality.

Bone marrow cytology
In genetic haemochromatosis there is an increase in sideroblast iron and storage iron within bone marrow macrophages but the bone marrow is otherwise normal. When iron overload results from a haematological abnormality the features of that disorder will be apparent in the bone marrow

aspirate. When iron accumulation results from thalassaemia, the erythroblasts show siderotic granules that are increased in number and size; there are occasional ring sideroblasts. When iron overload results from sideroblastic anaemia, ring sideroblasts are much more numerous and other abnormal sideroblasts are also present. Haemosiderin inclusions may be apparent in plasma cells in patients with iron overload.

Bone marrow histology
When bone marrow storage iron is increased it is usually apparent in sections of decalcified paraffin-embedded trephine biopsy specimens but only resin-embedded specimens permit its reliable detection and quantification. Such sections show not only increased macrophage iron but also iron in sinus endothelial cells, in endosteal cells, in osteoid seams and in osteocytic lacunae [89]. Resin embedding also permits the detection of ring sideroblasts. Haemosiderin inclusions in plasma cells may be detected in sections of both resin-embedded and paraffin-embedded biopsy specimens. Trephine biopsy sections showing iron overload may also show osteoporosis.

HIV infection and the acquired immune deficiency syndrome

In some HIV-infected patients the initial presentation is haematological, e.g. autoimmune thrombocytopenia, thrombotic thrombocytopenic purpura or lymphoma. In patients presenting with lymphoma, a trephine biopsy may be the initial diagnostic procedure. Other important indications for examination of the bone marrow are pyrexia of unknown origin and various cytopenias. Biopsy may also be required as a staging procedure in patients with an established diagnosis of lymphoma. A trephine biopsy is very often useful, particularly in patients with a hypocellular aspirate. Part of any aspirate from a febrile patient should be submitted for microbiological culture. In addition to routine stains, biopsied tissues should be stained, when appropriate, for acid-fast bacilli and fungi.

Peripheral blood
The earliest haematological manifestations of HIV infection occur at the time of primary infection

when atypical lymphocytes appear in the peripheral blood, often in association with a febrile illness, which clinically can resemble infectious mononucleosis. Primary HIV infection also occasionally causes transient pancytopenia. Patients with established infection may have lymphocytosis, consequent on an increase in CD8-positive lymphocytes, or isolated thrombocytopenia resulting from autoimmune destruction. Less often thrombocytopenia is a feature of a syndrome resembling thrombotic thrombocytopenic purpura and, in such cases, red cell fragments are present [215]. Late in the course of the disease, there is usually pancytopenia with very marked lymphopenia. Red cells may show anisocytosis and poikilocytosis. The reticulocyte count is reduced. Neutrophils may be dysplastic. Because of the frequency of opportunistic infections, the peripheral blood may also show non-specific reactive changes such as increased rouleaux formation, left shift and toxic changes in neutrophils, and the presence of immature monocytes and reactive lymphocytes. The haematological effects of the HIV infection itself, and the associated opportunistic infections, may be compounded by the effects of therapy; patients taking zidovudine, particularly in the higher doses used in single-agent anti-retroviral therapy, usually have marked macrocytosis and there may be marked dysplastic changes in blood cells.

Bone marrow cytology

Early in the course of HIV infection the bone marrow is of normal cellularity or, during the course of intercurrent infection, shows granulocytic hyperplasia. When there is immune thrombocytopenia, megakaryocyte numbers are normal or increased. Common non-specific changes are infiltration by lymphocytes and plasma cells and an increase of macrophages or eosinophils. Erythropoiesis may show mild dysplastic features such as nuclear irregularity and fragmentation. In patients taking zidovudine, erythropoiesis is megaloblastic and dyserythropoiesis is more marked; dysplastic changes such as nuclear fragmentation are also noted in the granulocytic series. Giant metamyelocytes are quite common, their presence correlating with the occurrence of detached nuclear fragments in granulocytes [216]. Apoptosis is increased. With advancing disease, the bone

marrow becomes progressively more hypocellular and aspiration becomes difficult due to increased reticulin deposition. Gelatinous transformation is very common, being greatest in cachectic patients. Bone marrow necrosis is sometimes seen. In patients with advanced disease, the bone marrow aspirate may provide evidence of miliary tuberculosis, atypical mycobacterial infection or disseminated fungal or parasitic infection. A microfilaria of *Mansonella perstans* has been noted in an aspirate of a patient with HIV infection [73]. Because of the deficient host response, mycobacterial infection may be associated with the presence of numerous bacteria within macrophages which may appear foamy or resemble Gaucher cells. Haemophagocytic syndromes secondary to tuberculosis or other infections are relatively common in patients with AIDS. Bone marrow involvement is common when lymphoma, particularly Burkitt lymphoma or Hodgkin lymphoma, complicates AIDS. The former is often detected in a bone marrow aspirate but in Hodgkin lymphoma the aspirate is often negative, even when bone marrow infiltration is detected on trephine biopsy.

Flow cytometry often shows an increase in haematogones (see page 310) [217].

Bone marrow histology

A wide variety of non-specific reactive changes are commonly seen in HIV infection [218–220]. The cellularity is increased in approximately 40% of cases, and decreased in 20–40%; hypocellularity is more common in patients on zidovudine therapy and in those with advanced disease. Frequently the haemopoietic marrow has an oedematous appearance with cells being separated by clear spaces. Focal gelatinous transformation is seen in up to 20% of cases. Dyserythropoiesis is common; the erythroblastic islands are often large and poorly organized, and megaloblastic change may be present, particularly in patients taking zidovudine. Granulocytic hyperplasia with left shift is seen in some patients, usually in response to infection. Megakaryocytes are usually present in normal or increased numbers, apparently bare nuclei are a frequent finding and, occasionally, dysplastic forms are seen. Clustering of megakaryocytes may occur (Fig. 3.53). Haemopoietic cells may be present within vessels [221]. Plasma cells are increased in

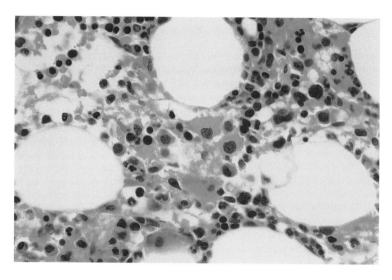

Fig. 3.53 BM trephine biopsy section, AIDS, showing clustering of megakaryocytes and a bare megakaryocyte nucleus. Paraffin-embedded, H&E ×40.

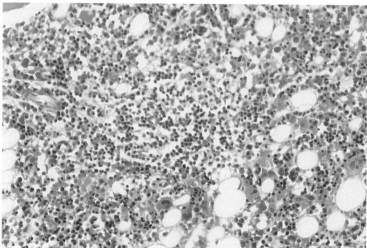

Fig. 3.54 BM trephine biopsy section, AIDS, showing increased cellularity and a polymorphous lymphoid aggregate (centre). Paraffin-embedded, H&E ×20.

50–60% of biopsy specimens and lymphoid aggregates are seen in approximately a third. The lymphoid aggregates are often large and poorly circumscribed. They consist mainly of small lymphocytes, with variable numbers of plasma cells, macrophages and eosinophils (Figs 3.54 and 3.55); sometimes there is proliferation of small vessels within the lesion. In some cases with a mixed infiltrate of lymphocytes and inflammatory cells the lesions may resemble infiltration by a peripheral T lymphoma [40]. Increased reticulin is seen in the majority of cases (Fig. 3.56). As a consequence there may be 'streaming' of haemopoietic cells and open sinusoids (in paraffin-embedded specimens),

both features being apparent in H&E-stained sections. Rarely, the combination of marked marrow hypercellularity, severe reticulin fibrosis and increased numbers and clustering of megakaryocytes may closely resemble the appearance of a myeloproliferative neoplasm.

In all cases, a careful search should be made for evidence of opportunistic infections [222], in particular tuberculosis and atypical mycobacterial infection (see page 129), fungal infection (see Table 3.2), *Pneumocystis jiroveci* infection and protozoal diseases (leishmaniasis and toxoplasmosis) (see page 123). Approximately 15% of biopsy specimens contain granulomas: the commonest cause is atypi-

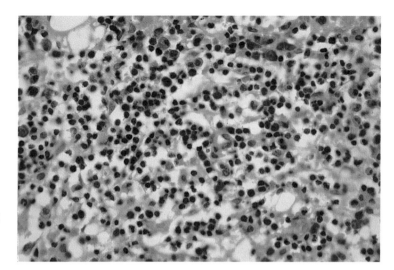

Fig. 3.55 BM trephine biopsy section, AIDS, showing a polymorphous lymphoid aggregate, composed of lymphocytes and small numbers of macrophages, eosinophils and plasma cells. Paraffin-embedded, H&E ×40.

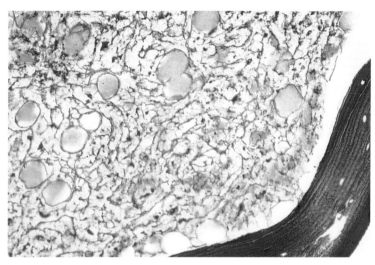

Fig. 3.56 BM trephine biopsy section, AIDS, showing reticulin fibrosis (grade 3). Paraffin-embedded, Gordon and Sweet stain ×20.

cal mycobacterial infection; other causes include tuberculosis, histoplasmosis, cryptococcal infection, leishmaniasis and, in endemic areas, coccidioid-omycosis [223]. In patients with AIDS, granuloma formation in response to fungal and protozoal infections is often poor. Associated changes in toxo-plasmosis include interstitial oedema and focal necrosis with both free forms and pseudocysts being found within granulocytes, macrophages and meg-akaryocytes [60]. Atypical mycobacteria can be cul-tured from the marrow in up to 20% of patients with AIDS who require a bone marrow biopsy. Granulomas are present in approximately 50% of culture-positive cases and acid-fast bacilli can be seen with appropriate stains in 60%. Atypical mycobacteria may be seen in biopsies in the absence of granulomas, usually within macrophages scat-tered throughout the marrow; occasionally cells which morphologically resemble Gaucher cells are seen. Culture of the bone marrow and examination of sections for acid-fast bacilli has been found to be less sensitive than peripheral blood culture in the diagnosis of atypical mycobacterial infection in AIDS but, when bacilli can be found in a stained aspirate film, diagnosis is much more rapid than when it is dependent on culture [224]. Focal areas of epithelioid angiomatosis have been observed in the marrow of HIV-positive patients with bacillary angiomatosis or disseminated cat scratch disease, conditions consequent on infection by organisms of the rochalimaea genus or the related *Afipia felis* [225,226]; a Warthin–Starry stain may demonstrate the causative organisms [226].

Bone marrow involvement by multicentric Castleman's disease has been reported in several HIV-positive patients who were also positive for HHV8 [44,227] (see Figs 3.14–3.16).

The incidence of non-Hodgkin lymphoma is greatly increased in HIV infection [228]. The incidence of Hodgkin lymphoma is increased to a lesser extent and is almost always EBV-associated. Marrow involvement is common in non-Hodgkin lymphoma associated with AIDS. These are almost always high grade lymphomas, either Burkitt lymphoma (with plasmacytoid differentiation) or diffuse large B-cell lymphoma (sometimes immunoblastic with plasmacytoid features). Bone marrow infiltration is much more common in Burkitt lymphoma than in diffuse large B-cell lymphomas. In Hodgkin lymphoma there is a propensity to involve the bone marrow early in the course of the illness so that trephine biopsy may provide the first evidence of the disease [229].

Plasma cell tumours also occur as AIDS-related neoplasms. Although initial presentation is often at extramedullary sites, the bone marrow may also be infiltrated [230].

Kaposi's sarcoma has a greatly increased incidence in AIDS and, in the rare instances when spread to the bone marrow occurs, this may be detected by trephine biopsy.

Bone marrow necrosis

The term 'bone marrow necrosis' is conventionally used to describe necrosis of haemopoietic cells or necrosis of neoplastic cells that have replaced normal bone marrow cells. Bone marrow stromal cells may also be necrotic. There is usually associated death of bone cells. Bone marrow necrosis usually results from impairment of the blood supply, often in association with a hypercellular marrow. Causes are multiple [30,77,231–246] (Table 3.5). A high concentration of tumour necrosis factor in the blood may act as a mediator of necrosis [243]. Anti-phospholipid antibodies may

also cause, or contribute to, bone marrow necrosis [237,244]. Necrosis is followed by ingrowth of small blood vessels accompanied by fibroblasts and macrophages followed by haemopoietic regeneration, either with or without small fibrotic scars, or occasionally by extensive fibrosis. Bone marrow necrosis commonly occurs at multiple sites. Clinical features include bone pain and fever. Fatal fat embolism can occur [247]. Bone marrow necrosis in patients with acute leukaemia or non-Hodgkin lymphoma correlates with a worse prognosis [248].

Peripheral blood
If bone marrow necrosis is extensive, pancytopenia occurs. The blood film shows leucoerythroblastic, and sometimes microangiopathic [249], features. Recovery is associated with a rise in the reticulocyte count and recovery of the haemoglobin concentration and platelet and white cell counts.

Bone marrow cytology
A bone marrow aspirate is often macroscopically abnormal. It is sometimes opaque and whitish and sometimes reddish-purple. The stained film shows amorphous pink-staining material in which the faint outlines of necrotic cells can be seen (Fig. 3.57). Necrotic nuclei appear as darker-staining smudges. Some intact cells may also be present.

Bone marrow necrosis is more often noted in bone marrow trephine biopsy sections than in aspirates. This may be partly because a larger volume is sampled and partly because necrotic cells mixed with intact cells in an aspirate are often dismissed as an artefact.

Bone marrow histology
The appearances depend to some extent on the condition underlying the necrosis. In cases in which the necrosis is secondary to infiltration by leukaemia or lymphoma (Fig. 3.58), low power examination may reveal hypercellularity and loss of fat cells. In the early stages there is nuclear pyknosis and the cells have granular cytoplasm with indistinct margins. Later, there is nuclear karyorrhexis and complete loss of cell outlines. Necrosis of sinusoids and capillaries leads to extravasation of erythrocytes. Finally, all that remains is amorphous eosinophilic debris. Marrow necrosis is often accompanied by necrosis of the adjacent bone.

Table 3.5 Causes of bone marrow necrosis [30,77,231–246].

Relatively common associations
Sickle cell anaemia and sickle cell/haemoglobin C disease (particularly during pregnancy)
Acute myeloid leukaemia (sometimes following administration of G-CSF) [231]
Acute lymphoblastic leukaemia
Metastatic carcinoma (sometimes in association with carcinoma-related thrombotic thrombocytopenic purpura) [232]
Caisson disease

Less common associations
Chronic granulocytic leukaemia
Essential thrombocythaemia [233]
Lymphoma (mainly high grade non-Hodgkin lymphoma but also Hodgkin lymphoma)*
Chronic lymphocytic leukaemia
Multiple myeloma
Post-transplant lymphoproliferative disorder [234]
Malignant histiocytosis
Myelofibrosis
Other haemoglobinopathies (S/D, S/β thalassaemia and sickle cell trait)
Megaloblastic anaemia plus infection
Acute haemolytic anaemia
Embolism of the bone marrow, e.g. by vegetations from cardiac valves or tumour embolism [235]
Disseminated intravascular coagulation
Hyperparathyroidism
Systemic lupus erythematosus [236]
Primary anti-phospholipid syndrome [237]
Diclofenac overdose [238]
Imatinib therapy (for gastrointestinal stromal cell tumour) [239]
Infections:
  Typhoid fever
  Gram-positive infections, e.g. streptococcal, staphylococcal infection
  Gram-negative infections, e.g. *Escherichia coli*
  Diphtheria
  Miliary tuberculosis
  Cytomegalovirus infection [240]
  Q fever
  Mucormycosis
  Histoplasmosis
  Fusobacterium necrophorum infection [241]
  Parvovirus infection [242]
  HIV infection (AIDS)
  Fatal infectious mononucleosis in X-linked lymphoproliferative syndrome [30]

AIDS, acquired immune deficiency syndrome; G-CSF, granulocyte colony-stimulating factor; HIV, human immunodeficiency virus.
*Necrosis of bone marrow infiltrated by low grade lymphoma has been observed following fludarabine [245] and rituximab [246] therapy.

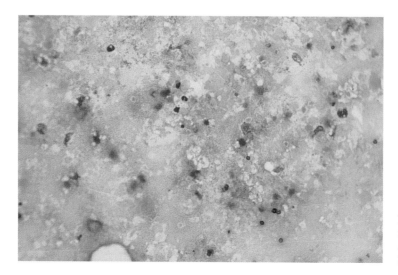

Fig. 3.57 BM aspirate, bone marrow necrosis, showing amorphous debris containing karyorrhectic nuclei. MGG ×100.

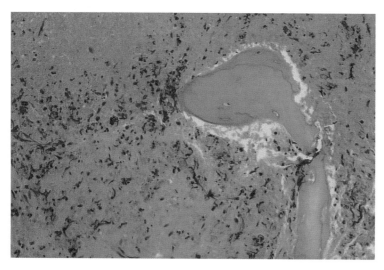

Fig. 3.58 BM trephine biopsy section showing necrosis in a marrow infiltrated by high grade lymphoma. Note the necrosis of both the lymphoma cells infiltrating the marrow and of osteocytes within the bone trabecula. Paraffin-embedded, H&E ×20.

Osteocytes disappear. In the early reparative phase there are increased numbers of macrophages in loosely fibrotic stroma. There is new bone formation, appositional and to a lesser extent metaplastic (Figs 3.59 and 3.60). Seams of new bone cover the surface of infarcted trabeculae and are progressively remodelled from woven into mature lamellar bone. The marrow cavity is eventually repopulated with haemopoietic cells. The only signs of previous necrosis may be small areas of fibrous scarring around bony trabeculae that have lost osteocytes [250]. Occasionally there is extensive fibrosis (Fig. 3.61).

In some patients, the necrosis is very extensive and biopsy of several different sites may be necessary before a sample diagnostic of the underlying disease is obtained.

Problems and pitfalls

Immunohistochemistry may be very misleading if used in an attempt to identify neoplastic cells within necrotic areas, as a consequence both of the tendency of antibodies to adhere in a non-specific way to necrotic tissue and of loss of some antigens by necrotic cells. However it is sometimes possible

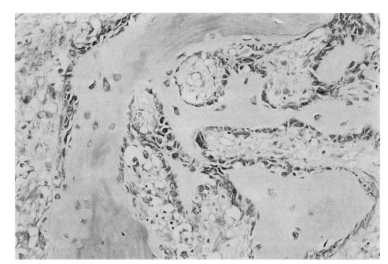

Fig. 3.59 BM trephine biopsy section showing new bone formation in an area of previous bone marrow necrosis. Paraffin-embedded, Giemsa ×20.

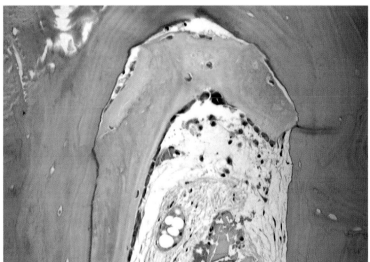

Fig. 3.60 BM trephine biopsy section from a patient with AML in remission following induction chemotherapy; the patient had extensive bone marrow necrosis at presentation. There is now a seam of reparative new bone forming on the surface of bone that has undergone necrosis. There are no osteocytes within the lacunae of the previously infarcted bone whereas the new bone has both osteocytes and a layer of osteoblasts. Loose fibrous tissue has replaced the adjacent marrow. Paraffin-embedded, H&E ×10.

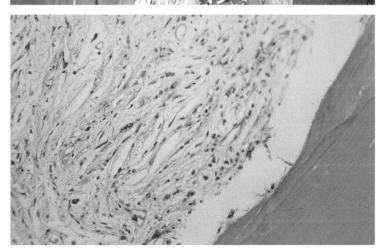

Fig. 3.61 BM trephine biopsy section, repair following marrow necrosis, showing collagen fibrosis. Paraffin-embedded, H&E ×20.

to identify B-lineage neoplasms using immunohistochemistry for CD20.

Gelatinous transformation

Gelatinous transformation, also known as serous degeneration or serous atrophy, is a condition in which there is loss of fat cells and haemopoietic cells from the bone marrow with replacement by an increased amount of extracellular matrix. Common causes include anorexia nervosa and cachexia due to chronic debilitating illnesses such as AIDS, carcinoma, lymphoma and tuberculosis or other chronic infection. It has been reported in association with renal failure, coeliac disease [251], severe hypothyroidism [252], alcoholism [253] and chronic heart failure [253]. In one patient a strictly starch-free diet was causative [254]. Gelatinous transformation can also develop rapidly as is seen in acute infection and in other acute illnesses with multiple organ failure [19]. It occurs at sites exposed to high dose X-irradiation.

Peripheral blood
The peripheral blood shows variable cytopenia, often pancytopenia. In patients with anorexia nervosa, acanthocytes are seen but their presence has not been noted in other patients with gelatinous transformation.

Bone marrow cytology
The aspirate may not spread normally when a film is prepared. It contains amorphous matrix material, sometimes fibrillar or finely granular, which is composed of acid mucopolysaccharide with a high content of hyaluronic acid. With Romanowsky stains it is pink or pinkish-purple (Fig. 3.62). This abnormal matrix material is positive with a PAS stain, the reaction being diastase-resistant. Positive staining also occurs with Alcian blue; this reaction is stronger at pH 2.5 than pH 1.0 [19]. A toluidine blue stain is weakly positive.

Bone marrow histology
The changes are usually patchy; less commonly the whole of a biopsy section is affected. There is atrophy of fat cells, which are both reduced in number and of variable size. In the affected areas there is a mild to marked hypoplasia of haemopoietic cells. Both fat and haemopoietic cells are replaced by amorphous material which, with H&E staining, has a light blue to pale pink colour and a finely granular appearance (Fig. 3.63). With Giemsa staining it is pink [253]. Its other staining characteristics are identical to those seen in marrow films (see above). Alcian blue positivity distinguishes areas of gelatinous transformation from oedema fluid which is also pink on H&E staining and weakly PAS positive [253].

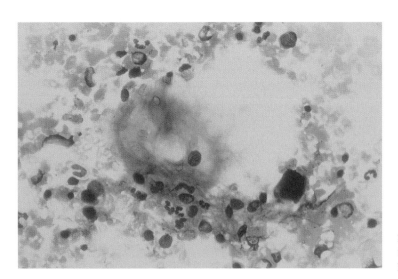

Fig. 3.62 BM aspirate, gelatinous transformation, showing amorphous purplish-pink material. MGG ×40.

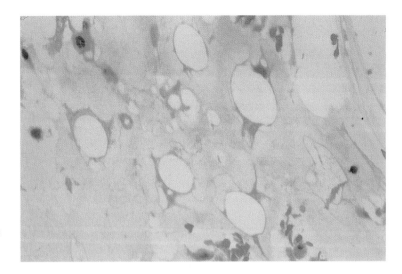

Fig. 3.63 BM trephine biopsy, gelatinous transformation, showing replacement of haemopoietic marrow and fat cells by amorphous pink material. Paraffin-embedded, H&E ×40.

Amyloid deposition

Deposition of amyloid in the bone marrow is seen not only in light chain-associated amyloidosis (see page 445) but also, less often, in secondary amyloidosis in patients with familial Mediterranean fever and chronic inflammatory conditions such as rheumatoid arthritis. Bone marrow amyloid is most often in vessel walls but is sometimes interstitial. The haemopoietic bone marrow shows increased atypical monotypic plasma cells in light chain-associated amyloidosis. In secondary amyloidosis there may be an increase of polyclonal plasma cells and other features of chronic inflammation. The appearance of amyloid in aspirates and trephine biopsy sections and its staining characteristics are discussed further on pages 445–448.

Bone marrow fibrosis

Bone marrow fibrosis indicates an increase of reticulin or of reticulin and collagen in the bone marrow [255]. Such fibrosis may be focal or generalized. Reticulin and collagen deposition are graded 0 to 4 as shown in Table 2.2 (page 60). Some patients with grade 4 fibrosis also have osteosclerosis. Increased reticulin formation and even collagen deposition can revert to normal if the causative condition is amenable to treatment. It should be noted that a different system for grading

fibrosis has been adopted in the World Health Organization (WHO) classification of tumours of haematopoietic and lymphoid tissues (see page 240).

An increase in bone marrow reticulin is common and is a useful non-specific indication that the marrow is abnormal. It is also of some use in differential diagnosis; for example, it may be increased in hypoplastic AML and hypoplastic MDS but is not increased in aplastic anaemia. Conditions characteristically associated with increased reticulin deposition, but with little if any collagen formation, include hairy cell leukaemia and HIV infection. Reticulin deposition may also be a feature of myeloproliferative neoplasms, such as polycythaemia vera and early primary myelofibrosis, and occurs in some patients with acute leukaemia (lymphoblastic as well as myeloid), MDS and multiple myeloma. The increase in reticulin in uncomplicated polycythaemia vera is not marked.

A focal increase in reticulin may have a different significance from a general increase, often indicating the presence of a focal infiltrate. Collagen deposition is uncommon and of greater diagnostic significance than an increase in reticulin. It is therefore useful to distinguish between these two degrees of abnormality, either by grading the fibrosis or by using the terms 'reticulin fibrosis' for a grade 3 abnormality and 'fibrosis' or 'myelofibrosis' for a grade 4 abnormality. Causes of bone marrow fibrosis are shown in Table 3.6 [77,256–264].

Table 3.6 Causes of grade 4 bone marrow fibrosis [77,256–264].

Generalized myelofibrosis
Inherited
Autosomal recessive in young children [257]
Malignant disease:
   Primary (idiopathic) myelofibrosis* (myelofibrosis with myeloid metaplasia)
   Myelofibrosis secondary to essential thrombocythaemia or polycythaemia vera*
   Chronic granulocytic leukaemia*
   Transitional myeloproliferative syndrome
   Acute megakaryoblastic leukaemia*
   Other acute myeloid leukaemias
   Acute lymphoblastic leukaemia [258]
   Systemic mastocytosis*
   Myelodysplastic syndromes (particularly therapy-related MDS)
   Paroxysmal nocturnal haemoglobinuria
   Hodgkin lymphoma
   Non-Hodgkin lymphoma
   Multiple myeloma
   Waldenström's macroglobulinaemia
   Secondary carcinoma*
Bone and connective tissue diseases:
   Marble bone disease – osteopetrosis
   Primary and secondary hyperparathyroidism
   Nutritional and renal rickets (vitamin D deficiency)
   Osteomalacia
   Primary hypertrophic osteoarthropathy [259]
   Pachydermoperiostosis (one case) [260]
Miscellaneous:
   Tuberculosis
   Other granulomatous diseases
   Grey platelet syndrome
   Systemic lupus erythematosus
   Systemic sclerosis
   Sjögren's syndrome [261]
   Primary autoimmune myelofibrosis [262]
   Antiphospholipid antibodies [263]
   Other autoimmune myelofibrosis [264]
   Thorium dioxide exposure

Focal or localized
Osteomyelitis
Paget's disease
Following bone marrow necrosis
Following irradiation of the bone marrow
Adult T-cell leukaemia/lymphoma
Healing fracture
Site of previous trephine biopsy

*Osteosclerosis may also occur.

Increased reticulin deposition has also been reported in association with pulmonary hypertension, both primary and secondary to connective tissue disease; the great majority, but not all, reported patients were being treated with epoprostenol; some patients had anaemia or thrombocytopenia but a leucoerythroblastic blood film and teardrop poikilocytes were not features [265,266].

Peripheral blood

Bone marrow fibrosis is commonly associated with a leucoerythroblastic anaemia; red cells show anisocytosis and poikilocytosis with teardrop poikilocytes often being prominent. When fibrosis is extensive, there may also be thrombocytopenia and leucopenia. The blood may also show abnormalities related to the primary disease that has caused the fibrosis. When bone marrow fibrosis has developed acutely, as in acute megakaryoblastic leukaemia, there may be little anisocytosis and poikilocytosis and the blood film is not necessarily leucoerythroblastic.

Bone marrow cytology

Bone marrow fibrosis often leads to failure of bone marrow aspiration or to aspiration of peripheral blood or a diluted marrow specimen. Otherwise the aspirate may show carcinoma cells or the specific features of the primary disease that has led to the fibrosis. If there is associated osteosclerosis, the aspirate may contain increased numbers of osteoblasts and osteoclasts.

Bone marrow histology

The appearances of primary myelofibrosis (often still referred to as idiopathic myelofibrosis and less often as myelofibrosis with myeloid metaplasia) are described on pages 262–264. In secondary fibrosis, findings range from a mild increase of fibroblasts and the presence of scattered collagen fibres to a dense fibrosis that obliterates normal haemopoietic tissue. An increase of reticulin can be suspected from an H&E stain by the distortion and angularity of fat cells and by the 'streaming' of haemopoietic cells held between parallel reticulin fibres. Fibrosis may also be suspected when sinusoids, which are normally collapsed in paraffin-embedded specimens, are held open. Increased reticulin deposition is confirmed by a silver impregnation technique such as the Gomori stain. Collagen fibres are detected as eosinophilic fibres, which may be in bundles. The oval nuclei of fibroblasts are apparent in relation to these collagen fibres. It is important not to confuse either mast cells or endothelial cells of collapsed capillaries with fibroblasts. The presence of collagen is confirmed by a trichrome stain such as Martius scarlet blue (Fig. 3.64). The distribution of reticulin and collagen within the marrow depends on the causative condition. In renal osteodystrophy and primary hyperparathyroidism,

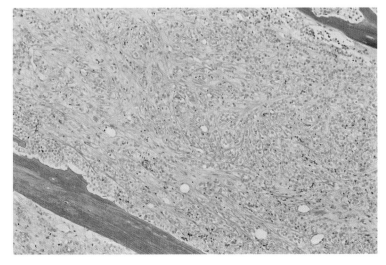

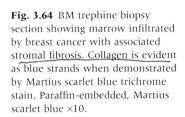

Fig. 3.64 BM trephine biopsy section showing marrow infiltrated by breast cancer with associated stromal fibrosis. Collagen is evident as blue strands when demonstrated by Martius scarlet blue trichrome stain. Paraffin-embedded, Martius scarlet blue ×10.

fibrosis is usually paratrabecular. In Paget's disease, it is often preferentially paratrabecular. When associated with a myeloproliferative neoplasm or with the grey platelet syndrome, fibrosis may be spatially related to megakaryocytes.

The biopsy specimen may show features of the causative condition, e.g. infiltrating carcinoma or lymphoma. In autoimmune myelofibrosis, there may be interstitial or aggregated lymphocytes, both T and B cells [264].

Problems and pitfalls

When the bone marrow is very fibrotic, any bone marrow aspirate is likely to be very unrepresentative. No attempt should be made to assess cellularity. However, it is always worth looking for tumour cells or dysplastic haemopoietic cells, regardless of the quality of the aspirate. If no aspirate can be obtained, a trephine biopsy imprint can yield useful information as to the nature of any abnormal cells present.

Due weight must be given to the presence of focal reticulin deposition and the corresponding area in the H&E-stained sections should be examined carefully. A generalized increase in reticulin is an indication of an abnormal bone marrow and an explanation should be sought by reviewing clinical, haematological and histological features.

When fibrosis is very pronounced, it may be difficult to distinguish residual haemopoietic cells, particularly megakaryocytes, from tumour cells. Immunohistochemistry is useful in this situation.

References

1 Goodman JL (1999) Ehrlichiosis – ticks, dogs and doxycycline. *N Engl J Med*, **341**, 195–197.
2 Maartens G, Willcox PA and Benatar SR (1990) Miliary tuberculosis: rapid diagnosis, hematologic abnormalities, and outcome in 109 treated adults. *Am J Med*, **89**, 291–196.
3 Invernizzi R, Travaglino E and Perfetti V (2003) PAS positive monocytes in Whipple's disease. *Haematologica*, **88**, EIM16.
4 Lowsky R, Archer GL, Fyles G, Minden M, Curtis J, Messner H *et al.* (1994) Brief report: diagnosis of Whipple's disease by molecular analysis of peripheral blood. *N Engl J Med*, **331**, 1343–1346.
5 Rausing A (1973) Bone marrow biopsy in the diagnosis of Whipple's disease. *Acta Med Scand*, **193**, 5–8.
6 Barenfanger J, Patel PG, Dumler JS and Walker DH (1996) Clinical and pathology rounds: identifying human ehrlichiosis. *Lab Med*, **27**, 372–374.
7 Farooqui BJ, Khurshid M, Ashfaq MK and Khan MA (1991) Comparative yield of *Salmonella typhi* from blood and bone marrow cultures in patients with fever of unknown origin. *J Clin Pathol*, **44**, 258–259.
8 Parry CM, Hien TT, Dougan G, White NJ and Farrar JJ (2002) Typhoid fever. *N Engl J Med*, **347**, 1770–1782.
9 Al-Eissa YA, Assuhaimi SA, Al-Fawaz IM, Higgy KE, Al-Nasser MN and Al-Mobaireek KF (1993) Pancytopenia in children with brucellosis: clinical manifestations and bone marrow findings. *Acta Haematol*, **89**, 132–136.
10 Yildirmak Y, Palanduz A, Telhan L, Arapoglu M and Kayaalp N (2003) Bone marrow hypoplasia during brucella infection. *J Pediatr Hematol Oncol*, **25**, 63–64.
11 Artac M and Sari R (2007) Brucellosis in febrile neutropenia. *Leuk Lymphoma*, **48**, 827–828.
12 Martinez E, Domingo P and Ruiz D (1991) Transient aplastic anaemia associated with Legionnaires' disease, *Lancet*, **338**, 264.
13 Torlakovic E, Clayton F and Ames ED (1992) Refractile mycobacteria in Romanowsky-stained bone marrow smears. A comparison of acid-fast stained tissue sections and Romanowsky-stained smears. *Am J Clin Pathol*, **97**, 318–321.
14 Bañas Llanos MH and Anton CS (2001) Disseminated *Mycobacterium avium intracellulare* infection in a patient with AIDS. *Br J Haematol*, **113**, 566.
15 Lawrence C and Schreiber AJ (1979) Leprosy's footprints in bone marrow macrophages. *N Engl J Med*, **300**, 834–835.
16 Schmid C, Frisch B, Beham A, Jager K and Kettner G (1990) Comparison of bone marrow histology in early chronic granulocytic leukaemia and in leukaemoid reaction. *Eur J Haematol*, **44**, 154–158.
17 Thiele J, Holgado S, Choritz H and Georgii A (1983) Density distribution and size of megakaryocytes in inflammatory reaction of the bone marrow (myelitis) and chronic myeloproliferative disorders. *Scand J Haematol*, **31**, 329–341.
18 Hyun BH, Kwa D, Gabaldon H and Ashton JK (1976) Reactive plasmacytic lesions of the bone marrow. *Am J Clin Pathol*, **65**, 921–928.
19 Amos RJ, Deane M, Ferguson C, Jeffries G, Hinds CJ and Amess JAL (1990) Observations on the haemopoietic response to critical illness. *J Clin Pathol*, **43**, 850–856.
20 Walter R, Bachmann SP, Schaffner A, Rüegg R and Schoedon G (2001) Bone marrow involvement in Whipple's disease: rarely reported, but really rare? *Br J Haematol*, **112**, 677–679.

21 Case Records of the Massachusetts General Hospital (2001) Case 37-2001: a 76-year-old man with fever, dyspnea, pulmonary infiltrates, pleural effusions, and confusion. *N Engl J Med*, **345**, 1627–1635.

22 Gaines P, Thomas V, Fikrig E and Berliner N (2005) Infection with *Anaplasma phagocytophilum* inhibits proliferation and differentiation of myeloid progenitors: new insights into infection-related pancytopenia. *Blood*, **106**, 858a.

23 Paddock CD, Suchard DP, Grumbach KL, Hadley WK, Kerschmann RL, Abbey NW *et al.* (1993) Brief report: fatal seronegative Ehrlichiosis in a patient with HIV infection. *N Engl J Med*, **329**, 1164–1167.

24 Demiroğlu H, Ozcebe OI, Ozdemir L, Sungur A and Dundar S (1994) Pancytopenia with hypocellular bone marrow due to miliary tuberculosis: an unusual presentation. *Acta Haematol*, **91**, 49–51.

25 Wiley EL, Perry A, Nightingale SD and Lawrence J (1994) Detection of *Mycobacterium avium-intracellulare* complex in bone marrow specimens of patients with acquired immunodeficiency syndrome. *Am J Clin Pathol*, **101**, 446–451.

26 Suster S, Cabello-Inchausti B and Robinson MJ (1990) Nongranulomatous involvement of the bone marrow in lepromatous leprosy. *Am J Clin Pathol*, **92**, 797–801.

27 Pooley RJ, Peterson L, Finn WG and Kroft SH (1999) Cytomegalovirus-infected cells in routinely prepared peripheral blood films of immunosuppressed patients. *Am J Clin Pathol*, **112**, 108–112.

28 Davidovitz Y, Halpern Z, Vardi J, Ballin A and Meytes D (1998) Pure red cell aplasia responsive to interferon-α in a patient with hepatitis C infection. *Acta Haematol*, **100**, 213–215.

29 Villiard J-F, Boiron J-M, Parrens M, Moreau J-F, Ranchin V, Reiffers J *et al.* (2000) Severe pancytopenia triggered by recombinant hepatitis B vaccine. *Br J Haematol*, **110**, 230–233.

30 Gaspar HB, Sharifi R, Gilmour KC and Thrasher AJ (2002) X-linked lymphoproliferative disease: clinical diagnostic and molecular perspective. *Br J Haematol*, **119**, 585–595.

31 Bilgrami S, Almeida GD, Quinn JJ, Tuck D, Bergstrom S, Dainiak N *et al.* (1994) Pancytopenia in allogeneic marrow transplant recipients: role of cytomegalovirus. *Br J Haematol*, **87**, 357–362.

32 Luppi M, Barozzi P, Schulz TF, Setti G, Staskus K, Trovato R *et al.* (2000) Bone marrow failure associated with human herpesvirus 8 infection after transplantation. *N Engl J Med*, **343**, 1378–1386.

33 Srichaikul T and Nimmannitya S (2000) Haematology of dengue fever and dengue haemorrhagic fever. *Bailliere's Clin Haematol*, **13**, 261–176.

34 Lu PL, Hsiao HH, Tsai JJ, Chen TC, Feng MC, Chen TP and Lin SF (2005) Dengue-virus associated hemo-

35 Kobayashi S, Maruta A, Yamamoto T, Katayama N, Higuchi R, Sakano Y *et al.* (1998) Human parvovirus B19 capsid antigen in granulocytes in parvovirus-B19-induced pancytopenia after bone marrow transplantation. *Acta Haematol*, **100**, 195–199.

36 Nagai K, Morohoshi T, Kudoh T, Yoto Y, Suzuki N and Matsunaga Y (1992) Transient erythroblastopenia of childhood with megakaryocytopenia associated with human parvovirus B19 infection. *Br J Haematol*. **80**, 131–132.

37 Yeh SP, Chiu CF, Lee CC, Peng CT, Kuan CY and Chow KC (2004) Evidence of parvovirus B19 infection in patients of pre-eclampsia and eclampsia with dyserythropoietic anaemia. *Br J Haematol*, **126**, 428–433.

38 Pont J, Puchhammer-Stockl E, Chott A, Popow-Kraupp T, Kienzer H, Postner G and Honetz N (1992) Recurrent granulocytic aplasia as clinical presentation of a persistent parvovirus B19 infection. *Br J Haematol*, **80**, 160–165.

39 Bhattacharyya J, Kumar R, Tyagi S, Kishore J, Mahapatra M and Choudhry VP (2005) Human parvovirus B19-induced acquired pure amegakaryocytic thrombocytopenia. *Br J Haematol*, **128**, 128–129.

40 Brunning RD (1989) Bone marrow. In: Rosai J (ed) *Ackerman's Surgical Pathology*, 7th edn, vol. 2. Mosby, St Louis.

41 Politano S, Maselli D, Zenali MJ, Nguyen A, Quintás-Cardama A (2008) Bone marrow fibrosis and gelatinous atrophy associated with acute Epstein-Barr virus infection. *Am J Hematol*, **83**, 606–607.

42 Prezioso PJ, Cangiarella J, Lee M, Nuovo GJ, Borkowsky W, Orlow SJ and Greco MA (1992) Fatal disseminated infection with human herpes virus-6. *J Pediatr*, **120**, 921–923.

43 Johnston RE, Geretti A-M, Prentice HG, Clark AD, Wheeler AC, Potter M and Griffiths PD (1999) HHV-6-related secondary graft failure following allogeneic bone marrow transplantation. *Br J Haematol*, **105**, 1041–1043.

44 Bacon CM, Miller RF, Noursadeghi M, McNamara C, Du MQ and Dogan A (2005) Pathology of bone marrow in human herpes virus-8 (HHV8)-associated multicentric Castleman disease. *Br J Haematol*, **127**, 585–591.

45 Cleary ML, Nalesnik MA, Shearer WT and Sklar J (1988) Clonal analysis of transplant-associated lymphoproliferations based on the structure of genetic termini of the Epstein–Barr virus. *Blood*, **72**, 349–352.

46 Rimsza LM, Vela EE, Frutiger YM, Rangel CS, Solano M, Richter LC *et al.* (1996) Rapid automated combined in situ hybridization and immunohistochemistry for sensitive detection of virus in paraffin-

embedded tissue biopsies. *Am J Clin Pathol*, **106**, 544–548.

47 Patel RM, Goldblum JR and His ED (2002) Immunohistochemical detection of human herpes virus-8 latent nuclear antigen-1 is useful in the diagnosis of Kaposi sarcoma. *Mod Pathol*, **17**, 456–460.

48 Liu W, Ittman M, Liu J, Schoentag R, Tierno P, Greco MA *et al.* (1997) Human parvovirus in bone marrows from adults with acquired immunodeficiency syndrome: a comparative study using in situ hybridization and immunohistochemistry. *Hum Pathol*, **28**, 760–766.

49 Hammer RD, Scott M, Shahab I, Carey TT, Cousar JB and Macon WR (1996) Latent membrane protein antibody reacts with normal hematopoietic precursor cells and leukemic blasts in tissues lacking Epstein–Barr virus genome by polymerase chain reaction. *Am J Clin Pathol*, **106**, 469–474.

50 Wong K-F, Chan JKC, Cheung MMC and So JCC (2001) Bone marrow involvement by nasal NK cell lymphoma at diagnosis is uncommon. *Am J Clin Pathol*, **115**, 266–270.

51 Rinn R, Chow WS and Pinkerton PH (1995) Transient acquired myelodysplasia associated with parvovirus B19 infection in a patient with congenital spherocytosis. *Am J Hematol*, **50**, 71–72.

52 Dorvault C, Raikow R and Contis L (1998) Evaluation of a monoclonal antibody to human parvovirus in B5-fixed bone marrow biopsy specimens. *Am J Clin Pathol*, **110**, 540–541.

53 Thiele J, Zirbes TK, Kvasnicka HM and Fischer R (1999) Focal lymphoid aggregates (nodules) in bone marrow biopsies: differentiation between benign hyperplasia and malignant lymphoma-a practical guide. *J Clin Pathol*, **52**, 294–300.

54 Navarro JT, Lauzurica R and Gimenez M (2001) *Rhodotorula rubra* infection in a kidney transplant patient with pancytopenia. *Haematologica*, **86**, 111.

55 Resende LSR, Mendes RP, Bacchi MM, Marques SA, Barraviera B, Souza LR *et al.* (2006) Infiltrative myelopathy by paracoccidioidomycosis. A review and report of nine cases with emphasis on bone marrow morphology. *Histology*, **48**, 377–386.

56 Wong KF, Tsang DNC and Chan JKC (1994) Bone marrow diagnosis of penicilliosis. *N Engl J Med*, **330**, 717–718.

57 Ferry JA, Pettit CJ, Rosenberg AE and Harris NL (1991) Fungi in megakaryocytes. An unusual manifestation of fungal infection of the bone marrow. *Am J Clin Pathol*, **96**, 577–581.

58 Grimes MM, La Pook JD, Bar MH, Wasserman HS and Dwork A (1987) Disseminated *Pneumocystis carinii* infection in a patient with acquired immunodeficiency syndrome. *Hum Pathol*, **18**, 307–308.

59 Strauchen JA (1996) *Diagnostic Histopathology of the Bone Marrow*. Oxford University Press, Oxford.

60 Brouland JP, Audouin J, Hofman P, Le Tourneau A, Basset D, Rio B *et al.* (1996) Bone marrow involvement by disseminated toxoplasmosis in acquired immunodeficiency syndrome: the value of bone marrow trephine biopsy and immunohistochemistry for the diagnosis. *Hum Pathol*, **27**, 302–306.

61 Piehl MR, Kaplan RL and Haber MH (1988) Disseminated penicilliosis in a patient with acquired immunodeficiency syndrome. *Arch Pathol Lab Med*, **112**, 1262–1264.

62 Wheat LJ, Connolly-Stringfield PA, Baker RL, Curfman MF, Eads ME, Israel KS *et al.* (1990) Disseminated histoplasmosis in the acquired immune deficiency syndrome: clinical findings, diagnosis and treatment, and review of the literature, *Medicine*, **69**, 361–374.

63 McKinsey DS, Gupta MR, Riddler SA, Driks MR, Smith DL and Kurtin PJ (1989) Long-term amphotericin B therapy for disseminated histoplasmosis in patients with acquired immunodeficiency syndrome (AIDS). *Ann Intern Med*, **111**, 655–659.

64 Wheat LJ, Connolly-Stringfield P, Kohler RB, Frame PT and Gupta MR (1989) Histoplasma capsulatum polysaccharide antigen detection in diagnosis and management of disseminated histoplasmosis in patients with acquired immunodeficiency syndrome. *Am J Med*, **87**, 396–400.

65 Bain BJ (2006) *Blood Cells: A practical guide*, 4th edn. Blackwell Publishing, Oxford.

66 Gupta SK, Jain D and Singh T (2008) *Plasmodium falciparum* in trephine biopsy. *Am J Hematol*, **83**, 602.

67 Sacks DL, Kenney RT, Kreutzer RD, Jaffe CL, Gupta AK, Sharma MC *et al.* (1995) Indian kala-azar caused by *Leishmania tropica*. *Lancet*, **345**, 959–961.

68 Kirchhoff LV (1993) American trypanosomiasis (Chagas' disease) – a tropical disease now in the United States. *N Engl J Med*, **329**, 639–644.

69 Wickramasinghe SN and Abdalla SH (2000) Blood and bone marrow changes in malaria. *Bailliere's Clin Haematol*, **13**, 277–299.

70 Abdalla SH (1991) Hematopoiesis in human malaria. *Blood Cells*, **16**, 401–416.

71 Phillips RE and Pavsol G (1992) Anaemia of *Plasmodium falciparum* malaria. *Baillière's Clin Haematol*, **5**, 315–330.

72 Bates I, Bedu-Addo G, Bevan DH and Rutherford TR (1991) Use of immunoglobulin gene rearrangements to show clonal lymphoproliferation in hyper-reactive malarial splenomegaly. *Lancet*, **337**, 505–507.

73 Molina MA, Cabezas MT and Gimenez MJ (1999) *Mansonella perstans* filariasis in a HIV patient: finding in bone marrow. *Haematologica*, **84**, 861.

74 Casals-Pascual C, Kai O, Cheung JO, Williams S, Lowe B, Nyanoti M *et al.* (2006) Suppression of erythropoiesis in malarial anemia is associated with

hemozoin in vitro and in vivo. *Blood*, **108**, 2569–2577.

75 Telsak EE, Cote RJ, Gold JMW, Campbell SW and Armstrong D (1990) Extrapulmonary *Pneumocystis carinii* infections. *Rev Infect Dis*, **12**, 380–386.

76 Yachnis AT, Berg J, Martinez-Salazar A, Bender BS, Diaz L, Rojiani AM *et al.* (1996) Disseminated microsporidiosis specially infecting the brain, heart, and kidneys. Report of a newly recognized pansporoblastic species in two symptomatic AIDS patients. *Am J Clin Pathol*, **106**, 535–543

77 Bain BJ and Wickramasinghe SNW (1986) Pathology of the bone marrow: general considerations. In: Wickramasinghe SNW (ed), Symmers W St C (series ed) *Systemic Pathology, Blood and Bone Marrow.* Churchill Livingstone, Edinburgh.

78 Epstein HD and Kruskall MS (1988) Spurious leukopenia due to *in vitro* granulocyte aggregation. *Am J Clin Pathol*, **89**, 652–655.

79 Mooren FC, Lerch MM, Ukkeruch HH, Bürger H and Domschke W (2000) Systemic granulomatous disease after intravesical BCG installation. *BMJ*, **320**, 219.

80 Lee WS, Kim JH and Choi TY (2004) Bone marrow granulomas in *Salmonella paratyphi* A infection. *Br J Haematol*, **127**, 242.

81 Bodem CR, Hamory BH, Taylor HM and Kleopfer L (1983) Granulomatous bone marrow disease. A review of the literature and clinicopathological analysis of 58 cases. *Medicine (Baltimore)*, **62**, 372–383.

82 Dumler JS, Dawson JE and Walker DH (1993) Human ehrlichiosis: hematopathology and immunohistologic detection of *Ehrlichia chaffeensis*. *Hum Pathol*, **24**, 391–396.

83 Kvasnicka HM, Thiele J and Ahmadi T (2003) Bone marrow manifestation of Lyme disease (Lyme borreliosis). *Br J Haematol*, **120**, 723.

84 Ampel NM, Ryan KJ, Carry PJ, Wieden MA and Schifman RB (1986) Fungemia due to Coccidioides immitis. An analysis of 16 episodes in 15 patients and a review of the literature. *Medicine (Baltimore)*, **65**, 312–321.

85 Hyun BH (1986) *Colour Atlas of Clinical Hematology.* Igaku-Shoin Med US, New York.

86 Falini B, Tabilio A, Velardi A, Cernetti C, Aversa F and Martelli MF (1982) Multiple myeloma with a sarcoidosis-like reaction. *Scand J Haematol*, **29**, 211–216.

87 Rabbani GR, Phyliky RL and Tefferi A (1999) A long-term study of patients with chronic natural killer cell lymphocytosis, *Br J Haematol*, **106**, 960–966.

88 Vilalta-Castel E, Váldes-Sanchez MD, Guerra-Vales JM, Teno-Esteban C, Garzón A, Lopéz JI *et al.* (1988) Significance of granulomas in bone marrow: a study of 40 cases. *Eur J Haematol*, **41**, 12–14.

89 Frisch B and Bartl R (1999) *Biopsy Interpretation of Bone and Bone Marrow: Histology and immunohistology in paraffin and plastic*, 2nd edn. Arnold, London.

90 Bhargava V and Farhi DC (1988) Bone marrow granulomas: clinicopathologic findings in 72 cases and review of the literature. *Hematol Pathol*, **2**, 43–50.

91 Kettle P and Allen DC (1997) Bone marrow granulomas in infiltrating lobular breast cancer. *J Clin Pathol*, **50**, 166–168.

92 Poland GA and Love KR (1986) Marked atypical lymphocytosis, hepatitis, and skin rash in sulfasalazine drug allergy. *Am J Med*, **81**, 707–708.

93 Case Records of the Massachusetts General Hospital (1996) A seven-year-old boy with fever, lymphadenopathy, hepatosplenomegaly, and prominent eosinophilia. *N Engl J Med*, **335**, 577–586.

94 Mukhopadhyay S, Mukhopadhyay S, Abraham NZ, Jones LA, Howard L and Gajra A (2004) Unexplained bone marrow granulomas: is amiodarone the culprit? A report of 2 cases. *Am J Hematol*, **75**, 110–112.

95 Pelstring RJ, Kim K, Lower EE and Swerdlow SH (1988) Marrow granulomas in coal workers' pneumoconiosis. *Am J Clin Pathol*, **89**, 553–556.

96 Lewis JH, Sundeen JT, Simon GL, Schulof RS, Wand GS, Gelfand RL *et al.* (1985) Disseminated talc granulomatosis: acquired immunodeficiency syndrome and fatal cytomegalovirus infection. *Arch Pathol Lab Med*, **109**, 147–150.

97 Davis S and Trubowitz S (1982) Pathologic reactions involving the bone marrow. In: Trubowitz S and Davis S (eds) *The Human Bone Marrow: Anatomy, physiology and pathophysiology*, vol. 2. CRC Press, Boca Raton.

98 Rywlin AM and Ortega R (1971) Lipid granulomas of the bone marrow. *Am J Clin Pathol*, **57**, 457–462.

99 Hudson P and Robertson GM (1966) Demonstration of mineral oil in splenic lipid granulomas. *Lab Invest*, **15**, 1134–1135.

100 Pease GL (1956) Granulomatous lesions in bone marrow. *Blood*, **11**, 720–734.

101 Farhi DC, Mason UG and Horsburgh CR (1984) The bone marrow in disseminated *Mycobacterium avium intracellulare* infection. *Am J Clin Pathol*, **83**, 463–468.

102 Jarolim DR, Parker GA and Sheehan WW (1991) Bone marrow involvement by Whipple bacillus. *J Infect Dis*, **163**, 1169–1170.

103 Kurtin PJ, McKinsey DS, Gupta MR and Driks M (1989) Histoplasmosis in patients with acquired immunodeficiency syndrome. Hematologic and bone marrow manifestation. *Am J Clin Pathol*, **93**, 367–372.

104 Kadin ME, Donaldson SS and Dorfman RF (1970) Isolated granulomas in Hodgkin's disease. *N Engl J Med*, **283**, 859–861.

105 Yu NC and Rywlin AM (1982) Granulomatous lesions of the bone marrow in non-Hodgkin's lymphoma. *Hum Pathol*, **13**, 905–910.

106 Franco V, Florena AM, Quintini G and Musso M (1994) Bone marrow granulomas in hairy cell leukaemia following 2 chlorodeoxyadenosine therapy. *Histopathology*, **24**, 271–273.

107 O'Brien DV, Boon AP and Boughton BJ (1992) Bone marrow granulomas in acute myeloid leukaemia following interleukin 2 and lymphokine-activated killer cells. *Histopathology*, **20**, 271–272.

108 Amodie LA and Tefferi A (1996) Bone marrow granulomas and fevers of unknown origin associated with chronic natural killer cell lymphocytosis. *Br J Haematol*, **93** (Suppl. 2), 108.

109 Tefferi A and Li CY (1997) Bone marrow granulomas associated with chronic natural killer cell lymphocytosis. *Am J Hematol*, **54**, 258–262.

110 Browne PM, Sharma OP and Salkin D (1978) Bone marrow sarcoidosis. *JAMA*, **240**, 2654–2655.

111 Okun DB, Sun NCJ and Tanaka KR (1979) Bone marrow granulomas in Q-fever. *Am J Clin Pathol*, **71**, 117–121.

112 Young JF and Goulian M (1993) Bone marrow fibrin ring granulomas and cytomegalovirus infection. *Am J Clin Pathol*, **99**, 65–68.

113 Foucar K (2001) *Bone Marrow Pathology*, 2nd edn. ASCP Press, Chicago.

114 Blanco P, Viallard J-F, Parrens M, Mercié P and Pellegrin J-L (2003) Bone-marrow fibrin-ring granuloma. *Lancet*, **362**, 1234.

115 Raya Sanchez JM, Arguelles HA, Brito Barroso ML and Nieto LH (2001) Bone marrow fibrin-ring (doughnut) granulomas and peripheral T-cell lymphoma: an exceptional association. *Haematologica*, **86**, 112.

116 Braziel RM, Launder TM, Druker BJ, Olson SB, Magenis RE, Mauro MJ *et al.* (2002) Hematopathologic and cytogenetic findings in imatinib mesylate-treated chronic myelogenous leukemia patients: 14 months experience. *Blood*, **100**, 435–441.

117 Frizzera G, Banks PM, Massarelli G and Rosai J (1983) A systemic lymphoproliferative disorder with morphologic features of Castleman's disease. Pathological findings in 15 patients. *Am J Surg Pathol*, **7**, 211–231.

118 Faulkner-Jones BE, Howie AJ, Boughton BJ and Franklin IM (1988) Lymphoid aggregates in bone marrow: study of eventual outcome. *J Clin Pathol*, **41**, 768–775.

119 Rywlin AM, Ortega RS and Dominguez CJ (1974) Lymphoid nodules of bone marrow. *Blood*, **43**, 389–400.

120 Farhi DC (1989) Germinal centres in the bone marrow. *Hematol Pathol*, **3**, 133–136.

121 Horny HD, Wehrmann M, Griessner H, Tiemann M, Bultman B and Kaiserling E (1993) Investigation of bone marrow lymphocyte subsets in normal, reactive and neoplastic states using paraffin-embedded biopsy specimens. *Am J Clin Pathol*, **99**, 142–149.

122 Bluth RF, Casey TT and McCurley TL (1993) Differentiation of reactive from neoplastic small-cell lymphoid aggregates in paraffin-embedded marrow particle preparations using L26 (CD20) and UCHL-1 (CD45 RO) monoclonal antibodies. *Am J Clin Pathol*, **99**, 150–156.

123 Smith GP, Perkins SL, Segal GH and Kjeldsberg CR (1994) T-cell lymphocytosis associated with invasive thymomas. *Am J Clin Pathol*, **102**, 447–453.

124 Agrawal S, Matutes E, Voke J, Dyer MJS, Khokhar T and Catovsky D (1994) Persistent polyclonal B-cell lymphocytosis. *Leuk Res*, **18**, 791–795.

125 Harris NL and Ferry JA (1992) Follicular lymphoma and related disorders. In: Knowles DW (ed) *Neoplastic Hematopathology*. Williams & Wilkins, Baltimore.

126 Gatter K and Brown D (1997) *An Illustrated Guide to Bone Marrow Diagnosis*. Blackwell Science, Oxford.

127 Klein H and Block M (1953) Bone marrow plasmacytosis. *Blood*, **8**, 1034–1041.

128 Grogg KL, Morice WG and Macon WR (2007) Spectrum of bone marrow findings in patients with angioimmunoblastic T-cell lymphoma. *Br J Haematol*, **137**, 416–422.

129 Breier DV, Rendo P, Gonzalez J, Shilton G, Stivel M and Goldztein S (2001) Massive plasmocytosis due to methimazole-induced bone marrow toxicity. *Am J Hematol*, **67**, 259–261.

130 Russell W (1890) An address on an organism of cancer. *BMJ*, **ii**, 1356–1360.

131 Bain BJ (2009) Russell bodies and Mott cells. *Am J Hematol*, in press. PMID 19384941.

132 Gregg KT, Reddy V and Prchal JT (2002) Copper deficiency masquerading as myelodysplastic syndrome. *Blood*, **100**, 1493–1495.

133 Mangles SE, Abdalla SH, Gabriel CM and Bain B (2007) Case report 37: neutropenia and macrocytosis in a middle-aged man. *Leuk Lymphoma*, **48**, 1846–1848.

134 Wulfhekel U and Dullmann J (1999) Storage of iron in bone marrow plasma cells. Ultrastructural characterization, mobilization, and diagnostic significance. *Acta Haematol*, **101**, 7–15.

135 Crocker J and Curran RC (1981) Quantitative study of the immunoglobulin-containing cells in trephine samples of bone marrow. *J Clin Pathol*, **34**, 1080–1082.

136 Peart KM and Ellis HA (1972) Quantitative observations on iliac crest bone marrow mast cells in chronic renal failure. *J Clin Pathol*, **28**, 947–955.

137 Yoo D, Lessin LS and Jensen WN (1978) Bone marrow mast cells in lymphoproliferative disorders. *Ann Intern Med*, **88**, 753–757.

138 Prokimer M and Polliack A (1980) Increased bone marrow mast cells in preleukemic syndromes, acute leukaemia, and lymphoproliferative disorders. *Am J Clin Pathol*, **75**, 34–38.

139 Natkunam Y and Rouse RV (2000) Utility of paraffin section immunohistochemistry for C-KIT (CD117) in the differential diagnosis of systemic mast cell disease involving the bone marrow. *Am J Surg Pathol*, **24**, 81–91.

140 Horny H-P and Valent P (2001) Diagnosis of masto-cytosis: general histopathological aspects, morpho-logical criteria, and immunohistochemical findings. *Leuk Res*, **25**, 543–551.

141 Wilson PA, Ayscue LH, Jones GR and Bentley SA (1993) Bone marrow histiocytic proliferation in association with colony-stimulating factor therapy. *Am J Clin Pathol*, **99**, 311–313.

142 Rosenthal NS and Fahri DC (1994) Failure to engraft after bone marrow transplantation; bone marrow morphologic findings. *Am J Clin Pathol*, **102**, 821–824.

143 Hirayama Y, Yoshioka K and Shiozaki N (1995) Histiocytosis and two classes of M-proteinemia in pre-treated Ph positive ALL. *Am J Hematol*, **49**, 358–359.

144 Huang LM, Lee CY, Lin KH, Chuu WM, Lee PI, Chen RL *et al.* (1990) Human herpesvirus-6 associated with fatal haemophagocytic syndrome. *Lancet*, **336**, 60–61.

145 Kawa-Ha K, Tanaka K, Inoue M, Sakata N, Okada S, Kurata T *et al.* (1993) Isolation of human herpesvirus 7 from a child with symptoms mimicking chronic Epstein–Barr virus infection. *Br J Haematol*, **84**, 545–548.

146 Low P, Neil F, Rascu A, Steininger H, Manger B, Fleckenstein B *et al.* (1998) Suppression of HHV-8 viremia by foscarnet in an HIV-infected patient with Kaposi's sarcoma and HHV-8 associated hemophago-cytic syndrome. *Eur J Med Res*, **3**, 461–464.

147 Grossman WJ, Radhi M, Schauer D, Gerday E, Grose C and Goldman FD (2005) Development of hemo-phagocytic lymphohistiocytosis in triplets infected with HHV-8. *Blood*, **106**, 1203–1206.

148 Potter MN, Foot ABM and Oakhill A (1991) Influenza A and virus-associated haemophagocytic syndrome: cluster of three cases in children with acute leukae-mia. *J Clin Pathol*, **44**, 297–299.

149 Komp DM, Buckley PJ, McNamara J and van Hoff J (1989) Soluble interleukin-2 receptors in hemo-phagocytic histiocytosis. *Pediatr Hematol Oncol*, **6**, 253–264.

150 Lelong F (1993) Syndrome d'activation macrophag-ique. *Les Mercredis Cytologiques de Necker*, No. 5.

151 Wong K-F and Chan JKC (1992) Reactive haemo-phagocytic syndrome – a clinico-pathologic study of 40 patients in an Oriental population. *Am J Med*, **93**, 177–180.

152 Tsuda H and Fujisao S (1999) Th1/Th2 milieu in adult hemophagocytic syndrome. *Acta Haematol*, **101**, 157–160.

153 Risdall R (1998) Haemophagocytic syndrome twenty years after. *23rd E. T. Bell Pathology symposium*. Update in Pathology, Minneapolis, Minnesota.

154 Baty V, Schuhmacher H, Bourgoin C, Latger V, Buisine J, May T and Canton P (1998) Syndrome hèmophagocytaire e fièvre hèmororrhagique avec syndrome rénal. *Presse Med*, **27**, 1577.

155 Fisgin NT, Fisgin T, Tanyel E, Doganci L, Tulek N, Guler N and Duru F (2008) Crimean-Congo hemor-rhagic fever: five patients with hemophagocytic syndrome. *Am J Hematol*, **83**, 73–76.

156 Woda BA and Sullivan J (1993) Reactive histiocytic disorders. *Am J Clin Pathol*, **99**, 460–463.

157 Manoharan A and Catovsky D (1981) Histiocytic medullary reticulosis revisited. In: Schmalzl F, Huhn D and Schaefer HE (eds) *Haematology and Blood Transfusion , vol. 27, Disorders of the Monocyte Macrophage System*. Springer-Verlag, Berlin.

158 Risdall RJ, Brunning RD, Hernandez JI and Gordon DH (1984) Bacteria associated hemophagocytic syn-drome. *Cancer*, **54**, 2968–2972.

159 Bourquelot P, Bouscary D, Paul G, Picard F, Varet B, Dreyfus F and Tulliez M (1996) Hemophagocytic syndrome associated with Bacteroides fragilis infec-tion in a patient with acute monoblastic leukemia. *Leuk Lymphoma*, **22**, 177–179.

160 Gill K and Marrie TJ (1987) Hemophagocytosis secondary to *Mycoplasma pneumoniae* infection. *Am J Med*, **82**, 668–670.

161 Abbott KC, Vukelja ST, Smith CE, McAllister CK, Konkol KA, O'Rourke TJ, Holland CJ and Ristic M (1991) Hemophagocytic syndrome: a cause of pan-cytopenia in human Ehrlichiosis. *Am J Hematol*, **38**, 230–234.

162 Walker DH and Dumler JS (1997) Human monocytic and granulocytic ehrlichioses. Discovery and diagno-sis of emerging tick-borne infections and the critical role of the pathologist. *Arch Pathol Lab Med*, **121**, 785–791.

163 Estrov Z, Bruck R, Shtalrid M, Berrebi A and Resnitzky P (1983) Histiocytic hemophagocytosis in Q-fever. *Arch Pathol Lab Med*, **108**, 7.

164 Shome DK, Rakheja D and Sonkar S (1997) Haemophagocytosis in bone marrow aspirates, *Acta Haematol*, **98**, 173–174.

165 Aouba A, Noguera ME, Clauvel JP and Quint L (2000) Haemophagocytic syndrome associated with *Plasmodium vivax* infection. *Br J Haematol*, **108**, 832–833.

166 Auerbach M, Haubenstock A and Soloman G (1980) Systemic babebiosis. Another cause of the hemophagocytic syndrome. *Am J Med*, **80**, 301–303.

167 Higgins EM, Layton DM, Arya R, Salisbury J and du Vivier AWP (1994) Disseminated *Trichosporon beigelii* infection in an immunosuppressed child. *J Roy Soc Med*, **87**, 292–293.

168 Chim CS, Fong CY, Ma SK, Wong SS and Yuen KY (1998) Reactive hemophagocytic syndrome associated with *Penicillium marneffei* infection. *Am J Med*, **104**, 196–197.

169 Numata K, Tsutsumi H, Wakai S, Tachi N and Chiba S (1998) A child case of haemophagocytic syndrome associated with cryptococcal meningoencephalitis. *J Infect*, **36**, 118–119.

170 Jaffe ES, Costa J and Fauci AS (1981) Erythrophagocytic T lymphoma. *N Engl J Med*, **305**, 103–104.

171 Chan E, Pi D, Chan GT, Todd D and Ho FC (1989) Peripheral T-cell lymphoma presenting as hemophagocytic syndrome. *Hematol Oncol*, **7**, 275–285.

172 Sonneveld P, van Lom K, Kappers-Klunne M, Prins MER and Abels J (1990) Clinico-pathological diagnosis and treatment of malignant histiocytosis. *Br J Haematol*, **75**, 511–516.

173 Gonzalez CL, Medeiros LJ, Braziel RM and Jaffe ES (1991) T cell lymphoma involving subcutaneous tissue. A clinicopathologic entity commonly associated with haemophagocytic syndrome. *Am J Surg Pathol*, **15**, 17–27.

174 Noguchi M, Kawano Y, Sato N and Oshimi K (1997) T-cell lymphoma of CD3+CD4+CD56+granular lymphocytes with hemophagocytic syndrome. *Leuk Lymphoma*, **26**, 349–358.

175 Aouba A, Lambotte O, Vasiliu V, Divine M, Valensi F, Varet B *et al.* (2004) Hemophagocytic syndrome as a presenting sign of transformation of smoldering to acute adult T-cell leukemia/lymphoma: efficacy of anti-retroviral and interferon therapy. *Am J Hematol*, **76**, 187–189.

176 Sevilla DW, Chie JK and Gonz JZ (2007) Mediastinal adenopathy, lung infiltrates, and hemophagocytosis: unusual manifestation of pediatric anaplastic large cell lymphoma: report of two cases. *Am J Clin Pathol*, **127**, 458–464.

177 Okuda T, Sakamoto S, Deguchi T, Misawa S, Kashimi K, Yoshihara T *et al.* (1991) Hemophagocytic syndrome associated with natural killer cell leukemia. *Am J Hematol*, **38**, 321–323.

178 Takeshita M, Kikuchi M, Ohshima K, Nibu K, Suzumiya J, Hisano S *et al.* (1993) Bone marrow findings in malignant histiocytosis and/or malignant lymphoma with concurrent hemophagocytic syndrome. *Leuk Lymphoma*, **12**, 79–89.

179 Narimatsu H, Morishita Y, Saito SA, Shimada K, Ozeki K, Kohno A *et al.* (2004) Usefulness of bone marrow aspiration for definite diagnosis of Asian variant of intravascular lymphoma: four autopsied cases. *Leuk Lymphoma*, **45**, 1611–1616.

180 Chim CS and Hui PK (1997) Reactive hemophagocytic syndrome and Hodgkin's disease. *Am J Hematol*, **55**, 49–50.

181 Venizelos LD, Garipidou V and Perifanis V (2002) Hemophagocytic syndrome associated with multiple myeloma, *Leuk Lymphoma*, **43**, 897–899.

182 Sakai Y, Atsumi T, Itoh T and Koike T (2003) Uveitis, pancarditis, haemophagocytosis, and abdominal masses. *Lancet*, **361**, 843.

183 Rao RN, Chang C-c, Uysal N, Presberg K, Shidham VB and Tomashefski JF (2005) Fulminant multisystem non-Langerhans cell histiocytic proliferation with haemophagocytosis: a variant form of Erdheim–Chester disease. *Arch Path Lab Med*, **129**, e39–e43.

184 Mahadeva U, Allport T, Bain B and Chan WK (2000) Haemophagocytic syndrome with histiocytic necrotizing lymphadenitis (Kikuchi's disease). *J Clin Pathol*, **53**, 636–638.

185 Kio E, Onitilo A, Lazarchick J, Hanna M, Brunson C and Chaudhary U (2004) Sickle cell crisis associated with hemophagocytic lymphohistiocytosis. *Am J Hematol*, **77**, 229–232.

186 Janka GE and Schneider EM (2004) Modern management of children with haemophagocytic lymphohistiocytosis. *Br J Haematol*, **124**, 4–14.

187 Kumakura S, Ishikura H, Umegae N, Yamagata S and Kobayashi S (1997) Autoimmune-associated hemophagocytic syndrome. *Am J Med*, **102**, 113–115.

188 Janka GE (1989) Familial hemophagocytic lymphohistiocytosis: diagnostic problems and differential diagnosis. *Pediatr Hematol Oncol*, **6**, 219–226.

189 Glasser L, Legolvan M and Horwitz HM (2007) Florid histiocytic hemophagocytosis following therapy with long acting G-CSF (pegfilgrastim). *Am J Hematol*, **82**, 753–757.

190 Urabe AU (1994) Colony-stimulating factor and macrophage proliferation. *Am J Clin Pathol*, **101**, 116.

191 Hurwitz N, Probst A, Zufferey G, Tichelli A, Pless M, Kappos L *et al.* (1996) Fatal vascular leak syndrome with extensive hemorrhage, peripheral neuropathy and reactive erythrophagocytosis: an unusual complication of recombinant IL-3 therapy. *Leuk Lymphoma*, **20**, 337–340.

192 Cheah PL, Looi LM, Tan PE, Bosco J and Kuperan P (1992) Cytophagic histiocytic panniculitis: a diagnostic dilemma. *Hematol Oncol*, **10**, 331–337

193 Van den Bos C, de Konig TJ, Bierings MB, Poll-The BT, Zegers BJM, Rijkers GT and Révész T (1998) Hemopoietic and imunological abnormalities in two patients with lysinuric protein intolerance. *Br J Haematol*, **102**, 314.

194 García-Suárez J, Bañas H, Krsnik I, de Miguel D, Reyes E and Burgaleta C (2004) Hemophagocytic syndrome associated with retinoic acid syndrome in acute promyelocytic leukemia. *Am J Hematol*, **76**, 172–175.

195 Çetin M, Hiçsönmez G and Gögüs S (1998) Myelodysplastic syndrome associated with Griscelli syndrome. *Leuk Res*, **22**, 859–862.

196 Barnardo A, Lim ZY, Ramasamy K, Devereux S, Ho AYL, Heaton N *et al.* (2006) Haemophagocytic lymphohistiocytosis (HLH) following orthoptic liver transplantation: a single centre report of 37 cases. *Br J Haematol*, **133** (Suppl. 1), 34.

197 Case Records of the Massachusetts General Hospital (2003) Case 13-2003: a 14-month-old boy with hepatomegaly, perianal lesions, and a bony lump on the forehead. *N Engl J Med*, **348**, 1692–1701.

198 Aricó M, Caselli D and Burgio GR (1989) Familial hemophagocytic lymphohistiocytosis: clinical features. *Pediatr Hematol Oncol*, **6**, 247–251.

199 Lipton JM, Westra S, Haverty CE, Roberts D and Harris NL (2004) Case 28-2004: newborn twins with thrombocytopenia, coagulation defects, and hepatosplenomegaly. *N Engl J Med*, **351**, 1120–1130.

200 Imashuku S, Hibi S, Tabata Y, Itoh E, Hashida T, Tsunamoto K *et al.* (2000) Outcome of clonal hemophagocytic lymphohistiocytosis: analysis of 32 cases. *Leuk Lymphoma*, **37**, 577–584.

201 Ohadi M, Lalloz MR, Sham P, Zhao J, Dearlove AM, Shiach C *et al.* (1999) Localization of a gene for familial hemophagocytic lymphohistiocytosis at chromosome 9q21.3-22 by homozygosity mapping. *Am J Hum Genet*, **64**, 165–171.

202 Stepp S, Dufourcq-Lagelouse R, Le Deist F, Bhawan S, Certain S, Mathew P *et al.* (2000) Perforin gene defects in familial hemophagocytic lymphohistiocytosis. *Science*, **286**, 1957–1960.

203 Klein C, Philippe N, Le Deist F, Fraitag S, Prost C, Durandy A *et al.* (1994) Partial albinism with immunodeficiency (Griscelli syndrome). *J Pediatr*, **125**, 886–895.

204 Wakefield R, McClean P, Gooi HC, Batcup G and Richards M (2001) Fatal haemophagocytic lymphohistiocytosis (HLH) associated with measles infection and purine nucleoside phosphorylase deficiency. *Br J Haematol*, **113** (Suppl. 1), 43.

205 Enders A, Zieger B, Schwarz K, Yoshimi A, Speckmann C, Knoepfle E-M *et al.* (2006) Lethal hemophagocytic lymphohistiocytosis in Hermansky–Pudlak syndrome type II. *Blood*, **108**, 81–87.

206 Arico M, Imashuku S, Clementi R, Hibi S, Teramura T, Danesino C *et al.* (2001) Hemophagocytic lymphohistiocytosis due to germline mutation in *SH2D1A*, the X-linked lymphoproliferative disease gene. *Blood*, **97**, 1131–1133.

207 Rigaud S, Fondaneche M-C, Lambert N, Pasquier B, Mateo V, Soulas P *et al.* (2006) XIAP deficiency in humans causes an X-linked lymphoproliferative syndrome. *Nature*, **444**, 110–114.

208 Gordon WC, Gibson B, Leach MTJ and Robinson P (2007) Haemophagocytosis by myeloid precursors in lysinuric protein intolerance. *Br J Haematol*, **138**, 1.

209 Maceta M, Will AM, Houghton JB and Wynn RF (2001) Prominent dyserythropoiesis in four cases of haemophagocytic lymphohistiocytosis. *J Clin Pathol*, **54**, 961–963.

210 Risdall RJ, McKenna RW, Nesbitt ME, Krivit W, Balfour HH, Simmons RL and Brunning RD (1979) Virus-associated hemophagocytic syndrome: a benign histiocytic proliferation distinct from malignant histiocytosis. *Cancer*, **44**, 993–1002.

211 Campo E, Condom E, Miro M-J, Cid M-C and Romagosa V (1986) Tuberculosis associated haemophagocytic syndrome. *Cancer*, **58**, 2640–2645.

212 Hirst WJR, Layton DM, Singh S, Mieli-Vergani G, Chessells JM, Strobel S and Pritchard J (1994) Haemophagocytic lymphohistiocytosis; experience in two U.K. centres. *Br J Haematol*, **88**, 731–739.

213 Han K, Kim Y, Kahng J, Lee J, Moon Y, Kang C and Shim S (1996) In situ hybridization studies of cytomegalovirus and Epstein–Barr virus in reactive histiocytic hyperplasia with hemophagocytosis. *Acta Haematol*, **96**, 140–145.

214 Imashuku S, Hibi S, Morinaga S, Takagi K, Chen J, Mugishima H *et al.* (1997) Haemophagocytic lymphohistiocytosis in association with granular lymphocyte proliferative disorders in early childhood: characteristic bone marrow morphology. *Br J Haematol*, **96**, 708–714.

215 Nair JMG, Bellevue R, Bertoni M and Dosik H (1988) Thrombotic thrombocytopenia in patients with the acquired immunodeficiency syndrome (AIDS)-related complex: a report of two cases. *Ann Intern Med*, **109**, 242–243.

216 Bain BJ (1997) The haematological features of HIV infection. *Br J Haematol*, **99**, 1–8.

217 McKenna RW, Washington LT, Aquino DB, Picker LJ and Kroft SH (2001) Immunophenotypic analysis of hematogones (B-lymphocyte precursors) in 662 consecutive bone marrow specimens by 4-color flow cytometry). *Blood*, **98**, 2498–2507.

218 Oshorne BM, Guarda LA and Butler JJ (1984) Bone marrow biopsies in the acquired immunodeficiency syndrome. *Hum Pathol*, **15**, 1048–1053.

219 Scheider DR and Picker LJ (1985) Myelodysplasia in the acquired immunodeficiency syndrome. *Am J Clin Pathol*, **84**, 144–152.

220 Castella A, Croxson TS, Mildvan D, Witt DH and Zalusky R (1985) The bone marrow in AIDS. *Am J Clin Pathol*, **84**, 425–432.

221 Mehta K, Gascoyne P and Robboy S (1992) The gelatinous bone marrow (serous atrophy) in patients with acquired immunodeficiency syndrome. *Arch Pathol Lab Med*, **116**, 504–508.

222 Bain BJ (1998) The haematologist and the infective complications of HIV infection. *Haematology*, **3**, 153–164.

223 Nguyen D and Diamond L (2000) *Diagnostic Hematology: A pattern approach*. Butterworth-Heinemann, Oxford.

224 Hussong J, Peterson LR, Warren JR and Peterson L-AC (1998) Detecting disseminated *Mycobacterium avium* complex infections in HIV-positive patients. *Am J Clin Pathol*, **110**, 806–809.

225 Relman DA, Loutit JS, Schmidt TM, Falkow S and Tompkins LS (1990) The agent of bacillary angiomatosis – an approach to the identification of uncultured pathogens. *N Engl J Med*, **323**, 1573–1580.

226 Milam MW, Balerdi MJ, Toney JF, Foulis PR, Milam CP and Behnke RH (1990) Epithelioid angiomatosis secondary to disseminated cat scratch disease involving the bone marrow and skin in a patient with acquired immune deficiency syndrome: a case report. *Am J Med*, **88**, 180–183.

227 Zietz C, Bogner JR, Goebel F-D and Lohrs U (1999) An unusual cluster of Castleman's disease during highly active antiretroviral therapy for AIDS. *N Engl J Med*, **340**, 1923–1924.

228 Bain BJ (1998) Lymphomas and reactive lymphoid lesions in HIV infection. *Blood Reviews*, **12**, 154–162.

229 Karcher DS (1993) Clinically unsuspected Hodgkin disease presenting initially in the bone marrow of patients infected with the human immunodeficiency virus. *Cancer*, **71**, 1235–1238.

230 Kumar S, Kumar D, Schnadig VJ, Selvanayagam P and Slaughter DP (1994) Plasma cell myeloma in patients who are HIV-positive. *Am J Clin Pathol*, **102**, 633–639.

231 Katayama Y, Deguchi S, Shinagawa K, Teshima T, Notohara K, Taguchi K *et al.* (1998) Bone marrow necrosis in a patient with acute myeloblastic leukemia during administration of G-CSF and rapid hematologic recovery after allotransplantation of peripheral blood stem cells. *Am J Hematol*, **57**, 238–240.

232 González N, Ríos E, Martín-Noya A and Rodríguez JM (2002) Thrombotic thrombocytopenic purpura and bone marrow necrosis as a complication of gastric neoplasm. *Haematologica*, **87**, ECOR1.

233 Majumdar G, Phillips JK and Pearson TC (1994) Massive bone marrow necrosis and post-necrotic myelofibrosis in a patient with primary thrombocythaemia. *J Clin Pathol*, **47**, 674–676.

234 Rossi D, Ramponi A, Fransecchetti S, Stratta P and Giadano G (2008) Bone marrow necrosis complicating post-transplant lymphoproliferative disorder: resolution with rituximab. *Leuk Res*, **32**, 829–834.

235 Laso F-J, González-Diaz M, Paz J-I and De Castro S (1983) Bone marrow necrosis associated with tumor emboli and disseminated intravascular coagulation. *Arch Intern Med*, **143**, 2220.

236 Upchurch KS (1988) Case records of the Massachusetts General Hospital. Case 38–1988. *N Engl J Med*, **319**, 768–781.

237 Paydas S, Kocak R, Zorludemir S and Baslamisli F (1997) Bone marrow necrosis in antiphospholipid syndrome. *J Clin Pathol*, **50**, 261–262.

238 Ayogdu I, Erkurt MA, Ozhan O, Kaya E, Kuku I, Yitmen E and Aydin NE (2006) Reversible bone marrow necrosis in a patient due to overdosage of diclofenac sodium. *Am J Hematol*, **81**, 298.

239 Vanel D, Bonvalot S, Pechoux CL, Cioffi A, Domont J and Cesne AL (2007) Imatinib-induced bone marrow necrosis detected on MRI examination and mimicking bone metastases. *Skeletal Radiol*, **36**, 895–898.

240 Rustgi VK, Sacher RA, O'Brien P and Garagusi VF (1983) Fatal disseminated cytomegalovirus infection in an apparently normal adult. *Arch Intern Med*, **143**, 372–373.

241 Epstein M, Pearson ADJ, Hudson SJ, Bray R, Jaylor M and Beesley J (1992) Necrobacillosis with pancytopenia. *Arch Dis Child*, **67**, 958–959.

242 Petrella T, Bailly F, Mugneret F, Caillot D, Chavanat P, Guy H *et al.* (1992) Bone marrow necrosis and human parvovirus associated infection preceding a Ph1 acute lymphoblastic leukemia. *Leuk Lymphoma*, **8**, 415–419.

243 Knupp C, Pekela PH and Cornelius P (1988) Extensive bone marrow necrosis in patients with cancer and tumor necrosis factor activity in plasma. *Am J Hematol*, **29**, 215–221.

244 Murphy PT, Sivakumaran M, Casey MC, Liddicoat A and Wood JK (1998) Lymphoma associated bone marrow necrosis with raised anticardiolipin antibody. *J Clin Pathol*, **51**, 407–409.

245 Aboulafia DM and Demirer T (1995) Fatal bone marrow necrosis following fludarabine administration in a patient with indolent lymphoma. *Leuk Lymphoma*, **19**, 181–184.

246 Ramamoorthy SK, Marangolo M, Durrant E, Akima S and Gottlieb DJ (2006) Unusual reaction to rituximab with intravascular hemolysis, rhabdomyolysis, renal failure and bone marrow necrosis. *Leuk Lymphoma*, **47**, 747–775.

247 Case Records of the Massachusetts General Hospital (1998) Tachycardia, changed mental status, and pancytopenia in an elderly man with treated lymphoma, *N Engl J Med*, **339**, 254–261.

248 Forrest D, Mack BJ, Nevill TJ, Couban SH, Zayed E and Foyle A (2000) Bone marrow necrosis in adult acute leukemia and non-Hodgkin's lymphoma. *Leuk Lymphoma*, **38**, 627–632.

249 Bermejo A, Gonzalez FA, Villegas A and Alarcon C (1995) Bone marrow necrosis. *Am J Hematol*, **50**, 65–66.

250 Kiraly JF and Wheby MS (1976) Bone marrow necrosis. *Am J Med*, **60**, 361–368.

251 Clarke BE, Brown DJ and Xipell JM (1983) Gelatinous transformation of the bone marrow. *Pathology*, **15**, 85–88.

252 Savage RA and Sipple C (1987) Marrow myxedema: gelatinous transformation of marrow ground substance in patient with severe hypothyroidism. *Arch Pathol Lab Med*, **111**, 375–377.

253 Böhm J (2000) Gelatinous transformation of the bone marrow: the spectrum of underlying diseases. *Am J Surg Pathol*, **24**, 56–65.

254 Wang C, Amato D and Fernandes B (2001) Gelatinous transformation of bone marrow from a starch-free diet. *Am J Hematol*, **68**, 58–59.

255 Kuter D, Bain B, Mufti G, Bagg A and Hasserjian RP (2007) Bone marrow fibrosis: pathophysiology and clinical significance of increased bone marrow stromal fibres. *Br J Haematol*, **139**, 351–262.

256 McCarthy DM (1985) Fibrosis of the bone marrow: content and causes. *Br J Haematol*, **59**, 1–7.

257 Rossbach HC (2006) Familial infantile myelofibrosis as an autosomal recessive disorder: preponderance among children from Saudi Arabia. *Pediatr Hematol Oncol*, **23**, 453–454.

258 Hann IM, Evans DIK, Marsden HB, Jones PM and Palmer MK (1978) Bone marrow fibrosis in acute lymphoblastic leukaemia of childhood. *J Clin Pathol*, **31**, 313–315.

259 Fontenay-Roupie M, Dupuy E, Berrou E, Tobelem G and Bryckaert M (1995) Increased proliferation of bone-marrow derived fibroblasts in primitive hypertrophic osteoarthropathy with severe myelofibrosis. *Blood*, **85**, 3229–3238.

260 Moellmann AC, Corrêa Bt, Dobbin JA and Maia RC (2003) Familial (primary) pachydermoperiostosis and severe myelofibrosis. *Leuk Lymphoma*, **44** (Suppl.), S83–S84.

261 Terzic T, Shahgoli B, Boricic J, Vidovic A, Stojanovic R, Radojevic S *et al.* (2002) Autoimmune myelofibrosis with juvenile primary Sjogren syndrome: a case report. *Histology*, **41** (Suppl. 1), 94.

262 Pullarkat VA, Bass RD, Gong JZ, Feinstein DI and Brynes RK (2001) Primary autoimmune myelofibrosis: a distinct clinicopathological syndrome. *Blood*, **98**, 280b.

263 Webster JA, Humble SD and Polski JM (2003) Bone marrow necrosis and fibrosis associated with primary antiphospholipid antibodies. *Am J Clin Pathol*, **120**, 470.

264 Bass RD, Pullarkat V, Fienstein DI, Kaul A, Winberg CD and Brynes RK (2001) Pathology of autoimmune myelofibrosis: a report of three cases and a review of the literature. *Am J Clin Pathol*, **116**, 211–216.

265 Popat U, Frost A, Liu E, May R, Bagg R, Reddy V and Prchal JT (2005) New onset of myelofibrosis in association with pulmonary arterial hypertension. *Ann Intern Med*, **143**, 466–467.

266 Popat U, Frost A, Liu E, Guan Y, Durette A, Reddy V and Prchal JT (2006) High levels of circulating CD34 cells, dacrocytes, clonal hematopoiesis, and *JAK2* mutation differentiate myelofibrosis with myeloid metaplasia from secondary myelofibrosis associated with pulmonary hypertension. *Blood*, **107**, 3486–3488.

FOUR

ACUTE MYELOID LEUKAEMIA, MIXED PHENOTYPE ACUTE LEUKAEMIA, THE MYELODYSPLASTIC SYNDROMES AND HISTIOCYTIC NEOPLASMS

Acute myeloid leukaemia (AML) is a disease resulting from the neoplastic proliferation of a clone of myeloid cells, characterized by uncoupling of proliferation and maturation. The leukaemic clone may be derived from a pluripotent haemopoietic stem cell (capable of giving rise to both myeloid and lymphoid lineages), from a multipotent myeloid stem cell (capable of giving rise to more than one myeloid lineage) or from a committed precursor cell (for example, one capable of giving rise only to cells of granulocyte and monocyte lineages). Normal haemopoietic marrow is largely replaced by immature myeloid cells, mainly blast cells, which show a limited ability to differentiate into mature cells of the different myeloid lineages. Pancytopenia is common, as a result both of the replacement of normal bone marrow and of the defective capacity for maturation of the leukaemic clone.

The myelodysplastic syndromes (MDS) resemble AML in that normal polyclonal haemopoietic bone marrow is largely replaced by cells of a neoplastic clone, usually derived from a multipotent stem cell. The neoplastic clone is characterized by defective maturation so that haemopoiesis is usually both morphologically dysplastic and functionally ineffective. In the great majority of patients with MDS, the bone marrow is hypercellular but there is increased intramedullary death of haemopoietic precursors leading to defective production of mature cells of one or more haemopoietic lineages. This process, which leads to various combinations

of anaemia, neutropenia and thrombocytopenia, is designated ineffective haemopoiesis. In MDS, as in AML, there is imbalance between proliferation and maturation but the degree of abnormality is less than in AML so that the proportion of blast cells is lower. The neoplastic cells in MDS show a tendency to clonal evolution; emergence of a subclone with more 'malignant' characteristics may be manifest clinically as transformation to acute leukaemia. The myelodysplastic syndromes may therefore be regarded as preleukaemic conditions.

Acute myeloid leukaemia

Acute myeloid leukaemia is a heterogeneous disease. In different patients cells of the leukaemic clone show various patterns of differentiation and maturation. From 1976 onwards, an international co-operative group, the FAB (French–American–British) group, published a series of papers on the classification of AML. This classification [1,2] became widely accepted and was subsequently incorporated into other systems of classification. It is based on the pattern of differentiation shown (for example: granulocytic, monocytic, erythroid, megakaryocytic) and the extent of maturation (for example: myeloblast, promyelocyte, granulocyte). Both differentiation and maturation are assessed and the predominant cell types in peripheral blood and bone marrow are determined. The FAB classification is summarized in Table 4.1 [1,2]. This classification contributed to the evolution of the World Health Organization (WHO) classification,

Bone Marrow Pathology. By Barbara Bain, David Clark and Bridget Wilkins. © 2010, Blackwell Publishing.

Table 4.1 The French–American–British (FAB) classification of acute myeloid leukaemia (AML) [1,2].

Criteria for diagnosis of AML	FAB category	Criteria for classification as specific FAB subtype of AML	Equivalent name
	M1	• Blasts ≥90% of BM NEC • ≥3% of blasts MPO or SBB positive • Maturing monocytic component in bone marrow ≤10% • Maturing granulocytic component in bone marrow ≤10%	Acute myeloblastic leukaemia without maturation
	M2	• Blasts 30–89% of BM NEC • BM maturing granulocytic component >10% NEC • BM monocytic component <20% of NEC and other criteria of M4 not met	Acute myeloblastic leukaemia with maturation
	M3	• Characteristic morphology	Acute promyelocytic leukaemia
Blasts ≥30% of bone marrow cells*	M3v	• Characteristic morphology	Variant form of acute promyelocytic leukaemia
≥3% of blasts SBB or MPO positive†	M4	• Blasts ≥30% of BM NEC • Granulocytic component ≥20% of BM NEC • Monocytic component ≥20% of BM NEC and *either* PB monocytes ≥5 × 10^9/l *or* BM like M2 but PB monocytes ≥5 × 10^9/l and cytochemical proof of monocytic differentiation	Acute myelomonocytic leukaemia
	M5a	• Blasts ≥30% of NEC • BM monocytic component ≥80% of NEC • Monoblasts ≥80% of BM monocytic component	Acute monoblastic leukaemia
	M5b	• Blasts ≥30% of NEC • BM monocytic component monocytic component • Monoblasts <80% of BM monocytic component	Acute monocytic leukaemia
	M6	• Erythroid cells ≥50% of BM cells • BM blasts ≥30% of NEC	Acute erythroleukaemia
	M7	• Blasts shown to be predominantly megakaryoblasts	Acute megakaryoblastic leukaemia
	M0	• <3% of blasts MPO or SBB positive • Lymphoid markers negative • Immunological or ultrastructural evidence of myeloid differentiation	Acute myeloid leukaemia with minimal evidence of myeloid differentiation

BM, bone marrow; MPO, myeloperoxidase, NEC, non-erythroid cells; PB, peripheral blood; SBB, Sudan black B.
*Except in some M3 and some M6.
†Except in M0 and some M5a.

and continues to be used in parallel with it to provide a largely morphological classification. The WHO classification is based to a considerable extent on cytogenetic and molecular categories of AML. In addition it separates *de novo* cases from therapy-related disease and cases arising in MDS. The 2008 update of the WHO classification is summarized in Table 4.2 [3]. The major aim of this classification is to recognize subtypes of AML that differ in their pathogenesis, clinical and haematological features

Table 4.2 The 2008 WHO classification of acute myeloid leukaemia (AML)[3].

AML with recurrent genetic abnormalities
  AML with t(8;21)(q22;q22); *RUNX1-RUNX1T1*
  AML with inv(16)(p13.1q22) or t(16;16)(p13;q22); *CBFB-MYH11*
  AML with t(15;17)(q22;q12); *PML-RARA*
  AML with t(9;11)(p22;q23); *MLLT3-MLL*
  AML with t(6;9)(p23;q34); *DEK-NUP214*
  AML with inv(3)(q21q26.2) or t(3;3)(q21;q26.2); *RPN1-EVI1*
  AML with t(1;22)(p13;q13); *RBM15-MKL1*
  Provisional entity: AML with mutated *NPM1*
  Provisional entity: AML with mutated *CEBPA*
AML with myelodysplasia-related changes
Therapy-related myeloid neoplasms
AML not otherwise categorized
  AML with minimal differentiation
  AML without maturation
  AML with maturation
  Acute myelomonocytic leukaemia
  Acute monoblastic/monocytic leukaemia
  Acute erythroid leukaemia
    Pure erythroid leukaemia
    Erythroleukaemia, erythroid/myeloid
  Acute megakaryoblastic leukaemia
  Acute basophilic leukaemia
  Acute panmyelosis with myelofibrosis
Myeloid sarcoma
Myeloid proliferation related to Down's syndrome
  Transient abnormal myelopoiesis
  Myeloid leukaemia associated with Down's syndrome
Blastic plasmacytoid dendritic cell neoplasm

and prognosis. The classification is hierarchical, so cases are assigned, in order, to: (i) therapy-related AML; (ii) AML with recurrent genetic abnormalities; (iii) AML with myelodysplasia-related changes; and (iv) AML, not otherwise specified. In addition there are specific categories for myeloid sarcoma, myeloid proliferations related to Down's syndrome and blastic plasmacytoid dendritic cell neoplasms. An important difference from the FAB classification is that cases with between 20% and 30% of bone marrow blasts are classified as AML rather than as MDS, as are cases with 20% or more peripheral blood blast cells. In addition, cases with

an even lower blast percentage are accepted as AML if they have certain specific cytogenetic abnormalities – t(8;21), t(15;17), inv(16) or t(16;16).

Acute myeloid leukaemia occurs at all ages but becomes increasingly common with advancing age. The incidence rises from one to 10 per 100 000 per year between the ages of 20 and 70 years and is somewhat higher in men than in women.

The different categories of AML have many clinical features in common but also differences. Some degree of hepatomegaly and splenomegaly is common, particularly in those categories with a prominent monocytic component (FAB M5 and, to a lesser extent, M4 subtypes). Lymphadenopathy and infiltration of the skin, gums and tonsils are also more common in AML with a prominent monocytic component. As a consequence of pancytopenia, patients commonly exhibit pallor and bruising and show susceptibility to infection. A more marked bleeding tendency is usual in acute promyelocytic leukaemia (FAB M3 AML, WHO AML associated with t(15;17) and *PML-RARA* fusion), in which disseminated intravascular coagulation (DIC) is a frequent feature.

The different categories of AML have certain haematological features in common although the morphological features of the predominant leukaemic cells differ. Normocytic normochromic anaemia, neutropenia and thrombocytopenia are common. The total white blood cell count (WBC) is usually elevated, as a result of the presence of circulating leukaemic cells, but some patients have a normal or low WBC with few circulating immature cells. A normal or low count is most often observed in acute promyelocytic leukaemia, acute megakaryoblastic leukaemia and acute panmyelosis with myelofibrosis. In adults, acute megakaryoblastic leukaemia commonly presents with the features of acute myelofibrosis, i.e. with pancytopenia, few circulating immature cells and a bone marrow which, as a result of bone marrow fibrosis, cannot be aspirated. (However, it should be noted that not all cases of 'acute myelofibrosis' are examples of acute megakaryoblastic leukaemia.)

The blood film and bone marrow aspirate features are of prime importance in the diagnosis of AML. The bone marrow trephine biopsy is of secondary importance except in those cases in which an adequate aspirate cannot be obtained. Assignment to FAB and WHO categories is more readily done on the basis of the blood and bone marrow aspirate findings and is not always straightforward from tissue sections. It may also be impossible, in tissue sections, to distinguish AML with little maturation (FAB M1 and M0 AML) from acute lymphoblastic leukaemia (ALL) unless immunohistochemistry is employed.

Cytochemistry

Cytochemistry permits the confirmation of a diagnosis of AML in all cases except those with minimal evidence of myeloid differentiation (FAB M0 AML) and acute megakaryoblastic leukaemia (FAB M7 AML). It has declined in importance since immunophenotyping became widely available but retains a role when flow cytometric immunophenotyping is not readily and rapidly accessible. Immunophenotyping can be important to distinguish AML without maturation (FAB M1 AML) from ALL and to distinguish acute monoblastic leukaemia (FAB M5a AML) from high grade lymphoma. Recommended cytochemical stains are either myeloperoxidase (MPO) or Sudan black B (SBB) (for identification of granulocytic differentiation) and a non-specific esterase (NSE) stain such as α-naphthyl acetate esterase (ANAE) for identification of monocytic differentiation [4]. Auer rods are also stained with MPO or SBB. A naphthol AS-D chloroacetate esterase (chloroacetate esterase, CAE) stain is very specific for granulocytic differentiation but is less useful than MPO/SBB for the identification of Auer rods.

Flow cytometric immunophenotyping

When facilities permit, immunophenotyping is now widely applied in the diagnosis and classification of AML [5] (Table 4.3). It is essential for distinguishing AML with minimal evidence of myeloid differentiation (FAB M0 AML) and acute megakaryoblastic leukaemia (FAB M7 AML) from ALL. It can also be essential for the recognition of pure erythroleukaemia since the primitive cells may be cytologically unrecognizable. It is also necessary for the recognition of mixed phenotype acute leukaemia. In addition, flow cytometry provides a means of identifying minimal residual disease during fol-

Table 4.3 Monoclonal antibodies useful for flow cytometry immunophenotyping in the diagnosis of acute myeloid leukaemia.

Specificity	Antibodies
Panmyeloid	CD13, CD33, CD65, CD117, anti-myeloperoxidase
Markers of maturation	CD15, CD11b
Markers of monocytic differentiation	CD14, CD11b, CD64
Erythroid markers	Anti-glycophorin A (CD235a, JC159) or glycophorin C (CD236R, Ret40f)
Megakaryocytic markers	CD41, CD42a, CD42b, CD61
Markers of immaturity	CD34, anti-terminal deoxynucleotidyl transferase

low-up if a specific leukaemia-associated phenotype is demonstrated at diagnosis.

Bone marrow histology

Bone marrow histology [6–9] is often a supplementary investigation in AML. However, when the peripheral blood features are not diagnostic and bone marrow aspiration is difficult or impossible it can be essential for diagnosis. This is most likely to occur when there is either a hypocellular bone marrow or fibrosis. Hypoplastic AML has been defined as AML with bone marrow cellularity less than 50% [10] or less than 40% [11]. Since an aspirate is usually hypocellular and there may be few circulating leukaemic cells, trephine biopsy can be essential for diagnosis (Figs 4.1 and 4.2). Careful examination of sections, supplemented by immunohistochemistry, permits a distinction from aplastic anaemia and hypocellular MDS.

Bone marrow fibrosis is most frequent in AML with megakaryocytic differentiation and in AML that follows chemotherapy or radiotherapy. It is a feature of the WHO-defined condition 'acute panmyelosis with fibrosis'. Fibrosis, either reticulin or collagen, generally prevents an adequate aspirate

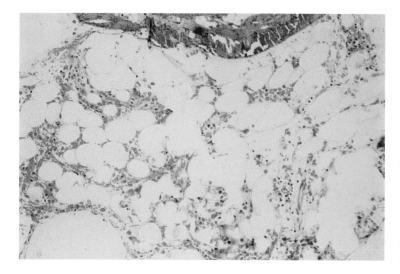

Fig. 4.1 Section of bone marrow (BM) trephine biopsy specimen, hypoplastic AML. The marrow is hypocellular with preservation of fat cells; however, normal haemopoietic cells are not seen. Resin-embedded, haematoxylin and eosin (H&E) ×10.

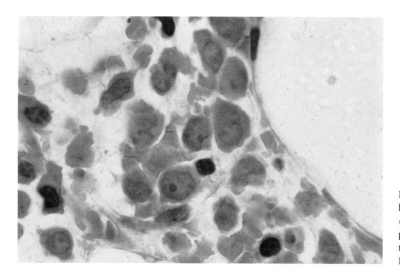

Fig. 4.2 Section of BM trephine biopsy specimen, hypoplastic AML (same patient as Fig. 4.1). High power examination reveals most of the cells present to be myeloblasts. Resin-embedded, H&E ×100.

and trephine biopsy histology is then essential for diagnosis.

Immunohistochemistry

Monoclonal and, to a much lesser extent, polyclonal antibodies that are useful in confirming a diagnosis of AML by immunohistochemistry are shown in Table 4.4 [12,13]. It is our practice to perform immunohistochemistry whenever there is diagnostic difficulty, for example when bone marrow aspi-

ration has failed and there are only low numbers of circulating blast cells. It is also possible to use immunohistochemistry to establish the baseline immunophenotype to permit comparison with follow-up samples.

Cytogenetic and molecular genetic analysis

The clinical and pathological features of AML are determined by the somatic mutation that occurred in the stem cell giving rise to the leukaemic clone.

Table 4.4 Monoclonal and polyclonal antibodies useful in immunohistochemistry for the diagnosis of acute myeloid leukaemia.

Specificity	Antibodies
Granulocytic and/or monocytic markers	Anti-myeloperoxidase, CD14, CD15, calprotectin (antibody Mac387), CD64, CD68, CD68R, anti-neutrophil elastase
Megakaryocyte/platelet markers	CD42b, CD61, anti-von Willebrand factor
Erythroid markers	Anti-glycophorin (A or C) – CD235a, CD236R , anti-spectrin, anti-haemoglobin A
Mast cell marker	Mast cell tryptase
Markers of immaturity	CD34, anti-terminal deoxynucleotidyl transferase

The resulting molecular genetic abnormality is therefore one of the most fundamental characteristics of any case of AML and it is appropriate that it be incorporated into classifications of this disease. The 2001 WHO classification included some genetic categories and more have been added in the 2008 revision. Genetic analysis includes cytogenetic and molecular genetic techniques. Cytogenetic studies include conventional cytogenetic analysis of cells in metaphase and fluorescence *in situ* hybridization (FISH) (a cytogenetic/molecular technique) of metaphase or interphase cells. The molecular technique most often employed, other than FISH, is the reverse transcriptase polymerase chain reaction (RT-PCR).

The FAB classification of acute myeloid leukaemia

Since the FAB classification is being gradually superseded by the WHO classification it will be discussed only briefly.

M0 AML

M0 AML is an acute leukaemia in which the blast cells show no cytological or cytochemical evidence of lineage commitment but immunophenotyping confirms myeloid differentiation (see Table 4.1). There are no Auer rods or granules and MPO, SBB, CAE and NSE are all negative, or are positive in less than 3% of blast cells. The presence of hypogranular neutrophils may provide a clue to the myeloid nature of the leukaemia.

M1 and M2 AML

The M1 and M2 FAB categories of AML show predominantly granulocytic differentiation, usually neutrophilic but sometimes to other granulocyte lineages (Fig. 4.3). In M1 AML differentiation is limited, whereas in M2 AML it is more extensive (Fig. 4.4) (see Table 4.1). Cells have granules that can be identified by MPO, SBB and CAE cytochemical stains. Auer rods may be present. The myeloid differentiation is obvious in M2 AML whereas cytochemical stains may be necessary for the recognition of M1 AML as myeloid. Similarly, in trephine biopsy sections, there is morphological evidence of maturation in M2 AML, whereas M1 AML may require immunohistochemistry for its recognition. When there is eosinophilic differentiation this is apparent in peripheral blood (Fig. 4.5) and bone marrow films and trephine biopsy sections which, in addition, may show Charcot–Leyden crystals (Figs 4.6–4.8).

M3 and M3 variant AML

This FAB category is identical to the WHO category of acute promyelocytic leukaemia with t(15;17) (q22;q12); *PML-RARA*, and is discussed on page 180.

M4 AML

M4 AML is characterized by differentiation to both granulocytic and monocytic lineages (Fig. 4.9; see Table 4.1). The granulocytic differentiation may be mainly neutrophilic or mainly eosinophilic. Occasionally differentiation is to the basophil lineage. The diagnosis can often be made from cytological features but is facilitated by a mixed esterase stain.

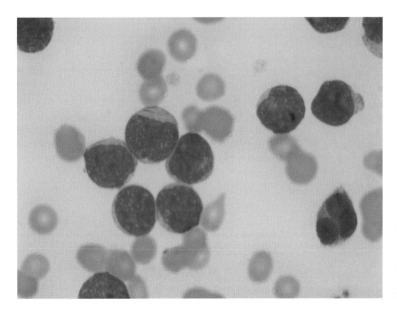

Fig. 4.3 BM aspirate from a patient with FAB M1 AML showing myeloblasts but no maturing cells. One blast cell contains an Auer rod. May-Grünwald-Giemsa (MGG) ×100.

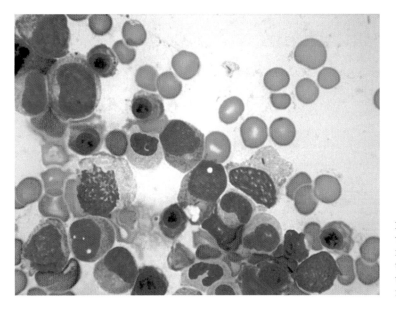

Fig. 4.4 BM aspirate from a patient with FAB M2 AML showing myeloblasts and maturing cells; there is granulocytic dysplasia and two cells in the centre contain Auer rods. MGG ×100.

M5 AML

M5 AML shows mainly monocytic differentiation. There may be very little maturation beyond the monoblast stage, designated M5a AML (Fig. 4.10), or substantial differentiation to monocytes, designated M5b (Fig. 4.11). A morphological diagnosis is generally straightforward in the case of M5b AML whereas M5a may show so little differentiation that it can be confused with large cell lymphoma. Cytochemistry or immunophenotyping is then needed for the diagnosis. Similarly, in trephine biopsy sections, M5b AML shows the irregu-

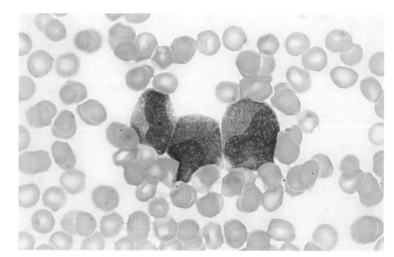

Fig. 4.5 Peripheral blood (PB) film from a patient with acute eosinophilic leukaemia (FAB M2Eo AML) showing eosinophil precursors with a mixture of primary and secondary granules. MGG ×100. (By courtesy of Dr A. Smith, Southampton.)

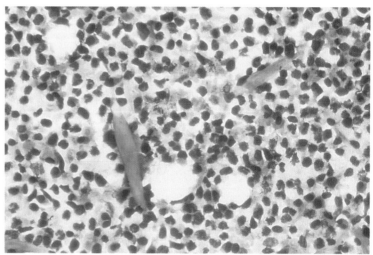

Fig. 4.6 BM aspirate from a patient with acute eosinophilic leukaemia (same patient as Fig. 4.5), showing eosinophils and their precursors and two Charcot–Leyden crystals. MGG ×40. (By courtesy of Dr A. Smith, Southampton.)

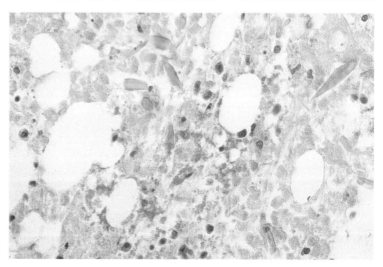

Fig. 4.7 Section of BM trephine biopsy specimen from a patient with acute eosinophilic leukaemia (same patient as Fig. 4.5), showing two Charcot–Leyden crystals in an area of necrotic bone marrow. Paraffin-embedded, H&E ×40.

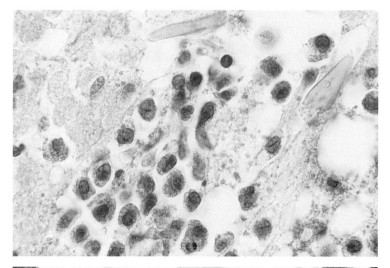

Fig. 4.8 Section of BM trephine biopsy specimen from a patient with acute eosinophilic leukaemia (same patient as Fig. 4.5), showing eosinophils and their precursors and two Charcot–Leyden crystals. Paraffin-embedded, H&E ×100.

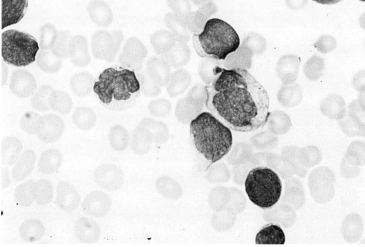

Fig. 4.9 BM aspirate film, FAB M4 AML, showing four myeloblasts, one monoblast and a monocyte. MGG ×100.

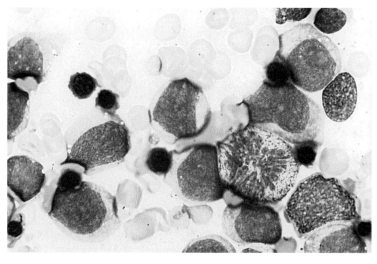

Fig. 4.10 BM aspirate film, FAB M5a AML, showing large blast cells with moderately abundant cytoplasm. MGG ×100.

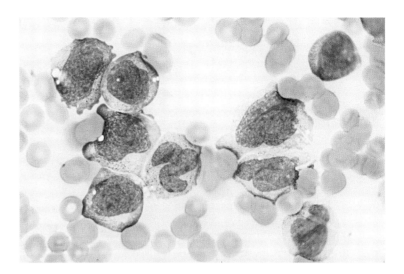

Fig. 4.11 BM aspirate film, FAB M5b AML, showing monoblasts, promonocytes and a monocyte. MGG ×100.

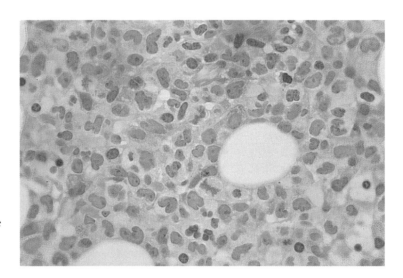

Fig. 4.12 BM trephine biopsy section, FAB M5b AML, showing replacement of haemopoietic marrow and fat spaces by a mixture of monoblasts, promonocytes and monocytes. Resin-embedded, H&E ×40.

lar nuclei of monocytes (Fig. 4.12) whereas in M5a AML there may be large cells with round nuclei and prominent nucleoli (Fig. 4.13) that require immunocytochemistry to make a distinction from large cell lymphoma.

M6 AML

M6 AML has a significant erythroid component, erythroblasts constituting at least 50% of bone marrow cells (Fig. 4.14). To make a diagnosis of M6 AML at least 30% of the non-erythroid cells must be blast cells. The diagnosis can only be made from

bone marrow examination, either from an aspirate or, with difficulty, by trephine biopsy (Figs 4.15 and 4.16).

M7 AML

M7 AML shows megakaryocytic differentiation. Sometimes megakaryoblasts and micromegakaryocytes have cytoplasmic blebs and cytoplasmic granules similar to those of platelets (Fig. 4.17) but often there are no distinguishing features and immunophenotyping is needed to establish their

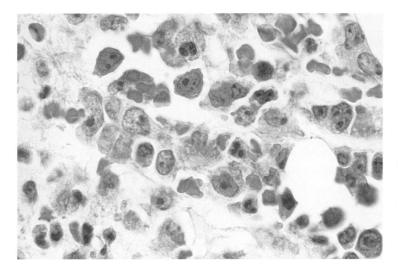

Fig. 4.13 BM trephine biopsy section, FAB M5a AML, showing monoblasts, which are large cells with plentiful cytoplasm and a prominent nucleolus. One blast (upper left) has phagocytosed red cells. Paraffin-embedded, H&E ×100. (By courtesy of Dr F. M. Wood, Vancouver.)

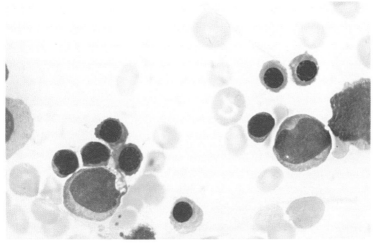

Fig. 4.14 BM aspirate film from a patient with M6 AML, showing two myeloblasts and numerous erythroblasts. MGG ×100.

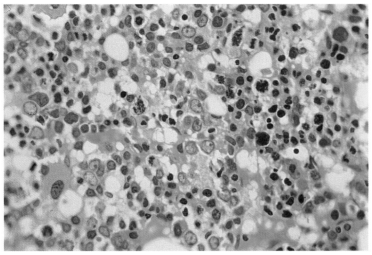

Fig. 4.15 Section of BM trephine biopsy specimen, M6 AML, showing a disorganized marrow containing large numbers of dysplastic erythroblasts and numerous myeloblasts. Paraffin-embedded, H&E ×40.

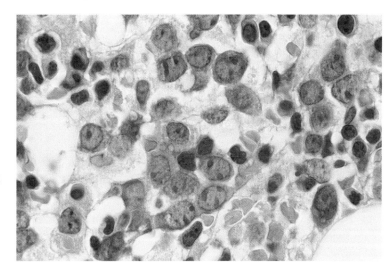

Fig. 4.16 Section of BM trephine biopsy specimen, M6 AML, showing disorganized architecture. There is an excess of immature erythroid cells, some of which have characteristic elongated nucleoli abutting on the nuclear membrane. Paraffin-embedded, H&E ×100.

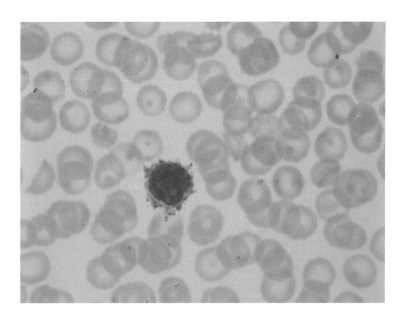

Fig. 4.17 PB film from a patient with M7 AML showing a micromegakaryocyte with cytoplasmic blebs and platelet-type granules. This patient had t(1;22) (p13;q13). MGG ×100.

lineage. Trephine biopsy sections show blast cells. There may also be micromegakaryocytes and fibrosis (reticulin with or without collagen) leading to the designation 'acute myelofibrosis' when there is a presentation with these bone marrow findings and few blast cells in the peripheral blood. In patients with fibrosis, aspiration may be difficult or impossible; histology and immunohistochemistry are then important in the diagnosis.

The WHO classification of acute myeloid leukaemia

Application of the 2008 WHO classification requires: (i) clinical history and physical examination (including recognition of Down's syndrome in neonates and infants and ascertainment of any history of exposure to irradiation or anti-cancer chemotherapy); (ii) full blood count (FBC), blood film and differential count; (iii) bone marrow aspirate and differential count; (iv) cytogenetic analysis; and (v) molecular analysis for *NPM1* and *CEBPA* mutations, particularly if cytogenetically normal. In addition, cytochemistry, immunophenotyping and trephine biopsy may be useful and genetic analysis for *FLT3* internal tandem duplication (*FLT3*-ITD) is advised. Cytochemistry, immunophenotyping or both are needed if it is not clear whether a case of acute leukaemia is AML or ALL. In addition, immunophenotyping is essential if it is intended to use this technique for monitoring for minimal residual disease (MRD). Trephine biopsy is useful if there is a poor aspirate, e.g. as a result of a hypocellular or fibrotic bone marrow.

Acute myeloid leukaemia with recurrent cytogenetic abnormalities

Acute myeloid leukaemia with t(8;21)(q22;q22); *RUNX1-RUNX1T1*
This subtype [14] constitutes about 5% of cases of AML. It is relatively more common in younger patients. Clinical features can include myeloid sarcomas. The majority of cases belong to the FAB M2 category, i.e. differentiation is mainly granulocytic rather than monocytic and maturation occurs. Granulocytic differentiation may be eosinophilic as well as neutrophilic. Prognosis is relatively good.

Peripheral blood
The peripheral blood may show large blasts with basophilic cytoplasm, a prominent Golgi zone and often a single, long, thin Auer rod, together with morphologically abnormal maturing cells (mainly neutrophilic lineage but sometimes including eosinophils). Occasional cases have giant granules.

Bone marrow cytology
A bone marrow aspirate shows a hypercellular marrow with an increase of blast cells although these are not necessarily more than 20% (Fig. 4.18). In addition to dysplastic maturing cells of neutrophil lineage, there are often increased eosinophils, which are usually cytologically normal.

Basophils and mast cells may be increased. Erythroid cells and megakaryocytes do not show dysplastic features.

Cytochemistry
Cytochemistry is not usually essential since granulocytic differentiation is obvious. However, it can be useful for the detection of Auer rods.

Bone marrow histology
There is usually a marked increase in cellularity with both increased blast cells and maturing cells of neutrophil and eosinophil lineages.

Immunophenotype
There is usually expression of CD34, human leukocyte antigen (HLA)-DR and CD13 and less strong expression of CD33. A subpopulation of maturing cells may express CD15 and CD65. CD56 may be expressed and expression correlates with worse prognosis. There may be aberrant expression of B-cell-associated antigens, CD19, PAX5 and CD79a; such aberrant expression can be useful in monitoring for MRD.

Cytogenetic and molecular genetic analysis
Cytogenetic analysis shows t(8;21)(q22;q22). The most frequent secondary cytogenetic abnormalities are –X in women, –Y in men and del(9q). Molecular analysis shows *RUNX1-RUNX1T1* fusion (previously known as *AML1-ETO*). The most frequent associated molecular abnormalities are mutation of *NRAS*, *KRAS* and *KIT*. *KIT* mutation correlates with a worse prognosis.

Acute myeloid leukaemia with inv(16)(p13.1q22) or t(16;16)(p13;q22); *CBFB-MYH11*
This subtype constitutes about 5–8% of cases of AML [14]. It is relatively more common in younger patients. Myeloid sarcomas can occur. The haematological features are usually those of acute myelomonocytic leukaemia with aberrant eosinophils and cases thus belong to the FAB M4 category; sometimes they are referred to as M4Eo. Prognosis is relatively good.

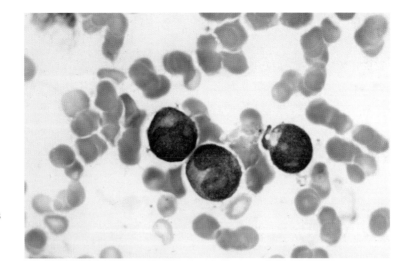

Fig. 4.18 Bone marrow aspirate from a patient with t(8;21) (q22;q22) showing three blast cells with prominent Golgi zone and peripheral cytoplasmic basophilia. MGG ×100

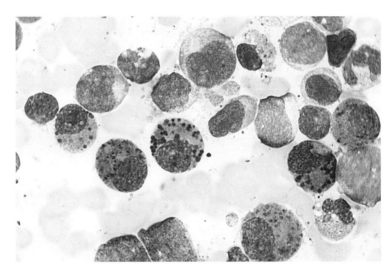

Fig. 4.19 BM aspirate from a patient with inv(16) (FAB M4 AML with eosinophilia), showing characteristic eosinophil myelocytes, eosinophils, a monocyte and blast cells. MGG ×100.

Peripheral blood

The peripheral blood usually shows blast cells and maturing cells of monocyte lineage. Eosinophils may be somewhat increased and are usually cytologically normal.

Bone marrow cytology

The bone marrow aspirate often shows a mixture of cells of monocyte and eosinophil lineages but cells of neutrophil lineage are relatively infrequent (Fig. 4.19). Some basophils may also be present.

Blast cells are increased but are not necessarily above 20%. The cells of eosinophil lineage are a mixture of myelocytes and mature eosinophils. In the great majority of cases the eosinophil myelocytes are morphologically abnormal with prominent pro-eosinophilic granules, which are basophilic in their staining characteristics, mixed with typical eosinophilic granules. The mature eosinophils may show cytological abnormalities such as nuclear hyperlobation or hypolobation or the presence of occasional pro-eosinophilic granules. Charcot–Leyden crystals may be present. Some cells of gran-

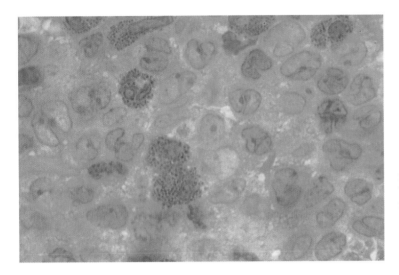

Fig. 4.20 Section of BM trephine biopsy specimen from a patient with inv(16) (FAB M4 AML with eosinophilia), showing monoblasts, myeloblasts, eosinophil myelocytes and eosinophils. Resin-embedded, H&E ×100.

ulocyte lineage, mainly immature cells, show Auer rods. There is usually retention of maturation in the monocyte lineage so that mature monocytes are present. Megakaryocytes and erythroid cells do not show dysplastic features.

Cytochemistry

Cytochemical stains are not essential. A double esterase stain, combining CAE and NSE, shows neutrophilic and monocytic differentiation. The eosinophils may show aberrant CAE positivity. SBB and MPO stains may show Auer rods in occasional eosinophils and their precursors as well as in neutrophil precursors.

Bone marrow histology

Trephine biopsy sections show a hypercellular marrow with the same abnormalities as described in the aspirate. Increased eosinophils and their precursors are apparent (Fig. 4.20) and Charcot–Leyden crystals may be present.

Immunophenotype

Flow cytometric immunophenotyping shows a mixed population of cells. There are immature cells (expressing CD34 and CD117), maturing cells of granulocyte lineages (expressing CD13, CD33, CD15, CD65 and MPO) and maturing cells of monocyte lineage (expressing CD4, CD11b, CD11c, CD14, CD36, CD64 and lysozyme). Aberrant

expression of CD2 occurs and can be useful for monitoring MRD.

Cytogenetic and molecular genetic analysis

Cytogenetic analysis shows either inv(16) (p13.1q22) or t(16;16)(p13;q22), the former considerably more often than the latter. The most frequent additional abnormalities are trisomy 8 and trisomy 22 (the latter fairly specific for this subtype). Trisomy 21 and del(7q) also occur. Molecular analysis shows *CBFB-MYH11* fusion. Molecular analysis is diagnostically important since the cytogenetic abnormality is subtle and can be missed. The most frequent associated genetic abnormality is a *KIT* mutation, correlating with a worse prognosis.

Acute myeloid leukaemia with t(15;17)(q22;q12); *PML-RARA*

This subtype of AML has the cytological features of acute hypergranular promyelocytic leukaemia or its variant (hypogranular/microgranular) form. In the FAB classification they are designated M3 and M3 variant AML. Patients are relatively young and typically present with haemorrhagic manifestations as a result of DIC. This subtype constitutes about 5–8% of cases of AML [14]. Rapid, correct diagnosis is of critical importance if specific targeted treatment is to be used and early death from haemorrhage avoided. The disease is very responsive to

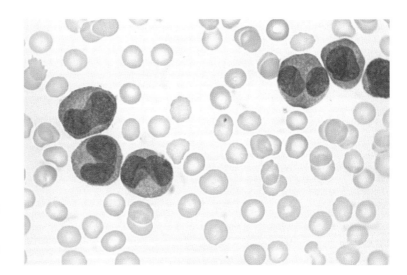

Fig. 4.21 PB film, hypogranular/microgranular variant of acute promyelocytic leukaemia, showing hypogranular promyelocytes with characteristic deeply lobulated nuclei. Several cells have very fine granules. MGG ×100.

all-*trans*-retinoic acid (ATRA) and arsenic trioxide and prognosis is now good.

Peripheral blood

The WBC is not usually greatly elevated and the number of circulating leukaemic cells tends to be low, sometimes very low. There is usually anaemia. The platelet count may be disproportionately low as a result of DIC. The abnormal promyelocytes are large cells, usually two to three times the diameter of an erythrocyte. Their cytoplasm is packed with granules which stain bright pink or reddish-purple. Some cells contain bundles of Auer rods ('faggot cells') or giant granules. No Golgi zone is apparent. The nucleus is usually round or oval but cytoplasmic granulation is so marked that the nuclear outline can be difficult to discern.

In the hypogranular variant, the WBC is usually elevated. Again, there is usually anaemia and marked thrombocytopenia. Abnormal promyelocytes are characteristically more frequent in the peripheral blood in the variant form than in cases with hypergranular promyelocytes. The variant promyelocytes may appear completely agranular or may have fine, dust-like reddish granules (Fig. 4.21). Some cells contain bundles of Auer rods or other crystalline inclusions. The nucleus is usually deeply lobed, often with two large lobes joined by a narrow bridge. The cytoplasm is usually weakly or moderately basophilic but some cases have promyelocytes with more marked basophilia and cyto-

plasmic protrusions or blebs. A careful search in cases of the variant form often discloses a minor population of more typical, hypergranular promyelocytes, occasionally with multiple Auer rods.

Bone marrow cytology

Bone marrow aspiration is often difficult since the hypercoagulable state leads to clotting of the specimen, even during aspiration. However, the bone marrow aspirate is important in diagnosis since there may be only infrequent leukaemic cells in the peripheral blood and, in the variant form, the bone marrow often contains a higher proportion of typical hypergranular cells than does the blood.

The bone marrow aspirate is usually intensely hypercellular. The number of blasts is relatively low, often less than 20%, since the predominant cell is an abnormal promyelocyte (Fig. 4.22). The predominant cells may be hypergranular promyelocytes or hypogranular bilobed promyelocytes with a variable admixture of hypergranular forms. In both morphological types there are usually some abnormal promyelocytes containing bundles of Auer rods. Hypergranular promyelocytes sometimes contain giant granules. There is a marked reduction in the number of normal maturing granulocytes. Erythroid cells and megakaryocytes are also considerably reduced in number but are cytologically normal. A few days after treatment with ATRA has commenced there is maturation

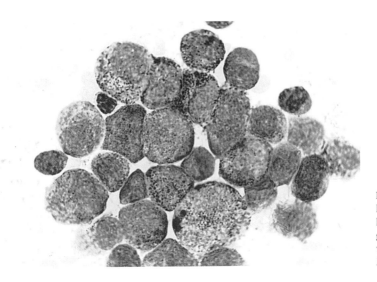

Fig. 4.22 BM aspirate film, hypergranular acute promyelocytic leukaemia, showing heavily granulated promyelocytes, one of which contains a giant granule. MGG ×100.

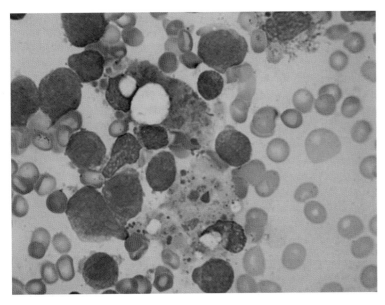

Fig. 4.23 BM aspirate from a patient with hypergranular acute promyelocytic leukaemia who had commenced ATRA therapy 4 days earlier, showing blast cells, promyelocytes and macrophages that have ingested giant granules. MGG ×100.

beyond the promyelocyte stage and giant granules and Auer rods may be seen in macrophages (Fig. 4.23).

Cytochemistry

Cytochemical stains are unnecessary in typical hypergranular acute promyelocytic leukaemia but are important in confirming a diagnosis of the variant form. Typically, there are strongly positive reactions with MPO, SBB and CAE stains and negative or weak reactions for NSE. In this subtype of

AML, Auer rods can be identified with MPO, SBB or CAE stains.

Bone marrow histology

There is usually marked hypercellularity with a homogeneous infiltrate of abnormal promyelocytes (Fig. 4.24). Occasional cases show little increase in cellularity, otherwise an unusual feature in *de novo* AML. The leukaemic cells have a characteristic appearance; they have prominent large granules that fill the cytoplasm and often obscure the

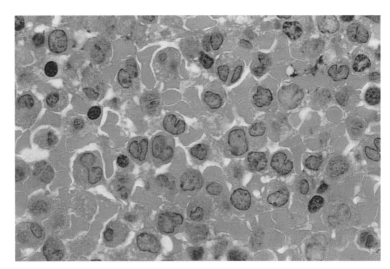

Fig. 4.24 Section of BM trephine biopsy specimen from a patient with hypergranular acute promyelocytic leukaemia showing abnormal promyelocytes with irregular, often bilobulated, nuclei containing prominent nucleoli and prominent cytoplasmic granules. Resin-embedded, H&E ×100.

nucleus. The nucleus may be oval or bilobed and has a single prominent nucleolus. Faggot cells may be detectable. In the variant form the granules are much smaller and may be inconspicuous; the nuclei are often bilobed.

Because of their hypergranularity, the leukaemic cells of typical cases can be readily recognized in haematoxylin and eosin (H&E)-stained sections of trephine biopsy specimens. A proportion of cases of the variant form can also be recognized from cytological features. Other variant cases, with very infrequent hypergranular cells, require confirmation by histochemistry (Leder's stain for CAE) or immunohistochemistry (e.g. demonstration of neutrophil elastase) if the diagnosis rests on the trephine biopsy specimen alone.

There is an accompanying reactive increase in small blood vessels in the bone marrow stroma [15]. Collagen fibrosis may be observed at presentation but this is quite uncommon [16]; it is greatly increased by treatment with ATRA [17]. ATRA therapy leads to maturation of the leukaemic clone with the bone marrow remaining hypercellular in contrast to the hypocellular marrow that is seen when chemotherapy is administered. Extensive bone marrow necrosis has been reported in association with hyperleucocytosis caused by ATRA [18].

Immunophenotype
The immunophenotype is very characteristic and diagnostically useful in the variant form. There is

usually no expression of CD34 or HLA-DR, strong expression of CD33 and heterogeneous expression of CD13; expression of MPO is strong. CD117 is usually expressed. CD34 positivity is more likely in the variant form. There may be aberrant expression of CD2 and CD56, the later correlating with a worse prognosis. In histological sections, demonstration of strong MPO and neutrophil elastase expression is helpful.

Cytogenetic and molecular genetic analysis
Both morphological subtypes are associated with t(15;17)(q22;q12) and a *PML-RARA* fusion gene. The most frequent additional cytogenetic abnormality is trisomy 8. Patients with a simple or complex variant translocation have an identical disease phenotype as long as a *PML-RARA* fusion gene is present, but this is not so for other translocations involving *RARA* that lead to different fusion genes. The most frequent additional molecular abnormalities are *FLT3*-ITD and tyrosine kinase domain mutations of *FLT3*. Molecular techniques are important for monitoring for MRD as well as for initial diagnosis.

Acute myeloid leukaemia with t(9;11)(p22;q23); *MLLT3-MLL*
The majority of cases of AML with t(9;11) have monocytic differentiation, most often falling into the FAB M5a category. This subtype of AML is much more common in children (9–12% or higher) than

adults (2%) [14]. Clinical presentation may include myeloid sarcomas and a pattern of tissue infiltration (gums and skin) typical of leukaemia with monocytic differentiation. Prognosis is intermediate.

Peripheral blood
The peripheral blood most often shows predominant monoblasts, with or without promonocytes. Monoblasts are large cells with a round or oval nucleus, a delicate chromatin pattern and plentiful cytoplasm. Promonocytes are similar cells except that the nucleus is irregular or lobated; in the WHO classification they are regarded as blast equivalents.

Bone marrow cytology
The bone marrow is typically infiltrated mainly by monoblasts.

Cytochemistry
Monocytic differentiation can be identified with an NSE stain. MPO may be negative.

Bone marrow histology
There is usually heavy infiltration by monoblasts with some maturing cells.

Immunophenotype
The immunophenotype may show features of monocytic differentiation such as expression of CD4, CD14 and HLA-DR. There may be lack of expression of CD34.

Cytogenetic and molecular genetic analysis
Cytogenetic analysis shows t(9;11)(p22;q23). Trisomy 8 is the most frequent additional abnormality. Molecular analysis shows *MLLT3-MLL*, previously known as *AF9-MLL*. Cases of acute leukaemia with other translocations involving the 11q23 breakpoint and the *MLL* gene have somewhat different clinical and haematological features from AML with t(9;11) and, in the 2008 WHO classification, these cases and those with t(9;11) no longer constitute a single category.

Acute myeloid leukaemia with t(6;9)(p23;q34); DEK-NUP214
This subtype constitutes less than 2% of cases of AML. The median age is low with many patients being children [14]. Cases usually fall into the FAB M2 or M4 categories. Prognosis is poor.

Peripheral blood
The peripheral film shows blast cells, dysplastic maturing cells of neutrophil lineage and sometimes increased basophils, which may be partly degranulated. Monocytes are sometimes increased.

Bone marrow cytology
The bone marrow aspirate shows increased blast cells and dysplastic maturing cells, often of basophil as well as neutrophil lineage. Blast cells may contain Auer rods. Trilineage dysplasia is usual (Fig. 4.25).

Cytochemistry
Some blast cells may contain SBB- and MPO-positive granules and Auer rods are likewise positive. Some blast cells may be of basophil lineage and others of neutrophil lineage. A toluidine blue stain shows metachromatic (pink) staining of granules in basophils and their precursors.

Bone marrow histology
There is a hypercellular marrow with both blast cells and maturing granulocytes. Basophils are not specifically identifiable in H&E-stained sections because of dissolution of their granules during aqueous fixation. Dysplastic features are present.

Immunophenotype
The immunophenotype shows expression of CD13, CD33, CD38 and HLA-DR whereas expression of CD34 and CD117 is variable [14]. Terminal deoxynucleotidyl transferase (TdT) expression is in seen in about half of patients [14].

Cytogenetic and molecular genetic analysis
Cytogenetic analysis shows t(6;9)(p23;q34), usually as the sole abnormality. Molecular analysis shows a *DEK-NUP214* fusion gene, previously known as *DEK-CAN*. An associated *FLT3*-ITD is very common.

Acute myeloid leukaemia with inv(3)(q21q26.2) or t(3;3)(q21;q26.2); RPN1-EVI1
This subtype represents about 1–2% of cases of AML [14]. The age range is wide. Cases can fall into any FAB category except acute promyelocytic leukaemia (FAB M3). Prognosis is poor.

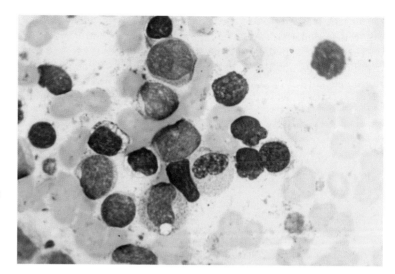

Fig. 4.25 BM aspirate film from a patient with t(6;9)(p23;q34) showing neutrophilic and basophilic differentiation; there is one heavily vacuolated basophil and, with toluidine blue, some of the blasts showed metachromatic staining. MGG ×100.

Peripheral blood

The peripheral blood shows blast cells and dysplastic features. In contrast to most subtypes of AML, the platelet count is often normal or even increased. Platelets may be large or hypogranular and 'bare' megakaryocyte nuclei can be seen.

Bone marrow cytology

A bone marrow aspirate shows increased blast cells and trilineage dysplasia with megakaryocyte dysplasia being particularly prominent (Fig. 4.26). In contrast to most cases of AML, megakaryocyte numbers are often normal or increased.

Cytochemistry

Cytochemical stains do not have any particular role.

Bone marrow histology

There is an increase of blast cells and usually prominent trilineage dysplasia. Some patients have a hypocellular marrow and some have fibrosis [14].

Immunophenotype

Blast cells usually express CD13, CD33, CD34, CD38 and HLA-DR [14]. In some cases CD7 is coexpressed. Some cases are of acute megakaryoblastic leukaemia and blast cells then express platelet glycoproteins (CD41, CD42b, CD61).

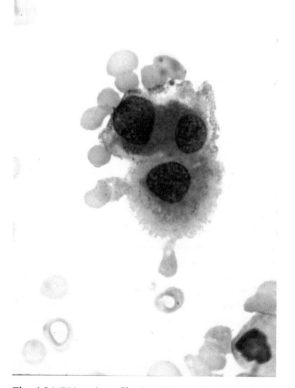

Fig. 4.26 BM aspirate film in AML associated with inv(3)(q21q26) showing three dysplastic megakaryocytes. MGG ×100.

Cytogenetic and molecular genetic analysis

Cytogenetic analysis most often shows inv(3)(q21q26.2) but sometimes t(3;3)(q21;q26.2). There is often also monosomy 7, del(7q) or a complex karyotype [14]. Molecular analysis shows *RPN1-EVI1* and *EVI1* is over-expressed.

Acute myeloid leukaemia with t(1;22)(p13;q13); *RBM15-MKL1*

The t(1;22)(p13;q13) translocation is associated with acute megakaryoblastic leukaemia (FAB M7) of infancy [14]. There may be hepatosplenomegaly so that the clinical presentation differs from 'acute myelofibrosis', which may be the presentation of other types of acute megakaryoblastic leukaemia in adults.

Peripheral blood

The peripheral blood shows blast cells, some with cytoplasmic pseudopods giving evidence of megakaryocytic differentiation; there may be micromegakaryocytes and giant platelets (Fig. 4.27).

Bone marrow cytology

A bone marrow aspirate shows increased blast cells but the number may not be very high, sometimes being less than 20%. There is megakaryocyte dysplasia including micromegakaryocytes.

Cytochemistry

MPO and SBB stains are negative.

Bone marrow histology

There is an increase in blast cells; increased reticulin deposition and collagen fibrosis are common [14].

Immunophenotype

Blast cells express platelet glycoproteins, CD41 and CD61 and, less often, CD42b; they may also express CD13, CD33 and CD36. CD34 and CD45 are often negative [14].

Cytogenetic and molecular genetic analysis

Usually t(1;22)(p13;q13) occurs as a single cytogenetic abnormality. Molecular analysis shows *RBM15-MKL1* (previously also known as *OTT-MAL*).

Acute myeloid leukaemia with *NPM1* mutation

This is a provisional entity in the 2008 WHO classification. The mutation is found in about a third of adults with AML, most often in association with a normal karyotype [14]. Cases usually fall into the FAB M4 or M5 categories. There may be a pattern of tissue infiltration consistent with monocytic dif-

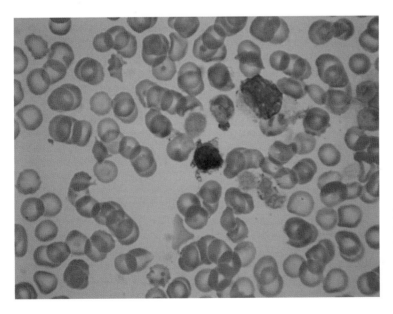

Fig. 4.27 PB film from a child with acute megakaryoblastic leukaemia associated with t(1;22) showing a megakaryoblast, a micromegakaryocyte and numerous giant platelets (same patient as Fig. 4.17). MGG ×100.

ferentiation. If there is no coexisting *FLT3*-ITD the prognosis is relatively good.

Peripheral blood
Blast cells are present. Cup-shaped nuclei have been noted in a proportion of cases but this finding is not specific [19].

Bone marrow cytology
The bone marrow aspirate shows increased blast cells. There is usually monocytic differentiation but granulocytic differentiation and erythroleukaemia are also seen. Some cases have multilineage dysplasia.

Cytochemistry
Cytochemistry shows the expected reactions but is not important in this diagnosis.

Bone marrow histology
There is a hypercellular marrow, most often with monocytic differentiation. Immunohistochemistry for NPM1 shows cytoplasmic expression of the protein, in addition to normal nuclear expression, which can be used as a surrogate marker for mutation of the gene.

Immunophenotype
Blast cells usually express CD13, CD33 and MPO and sometimes markers of monocytic differentiation, CD11b and CD14 [14]. There is usually no expression of CD34.

Cytogenetic and molecular genetic analysis
Cytogenetic analysis is usually normal but miscellaneous abnormalities are present in 5–15% of cases [14]. Molecular analysis has shown a number of different *NPM1* mutations, which are usually mono-allelic. A coexisting *FLT3*-ITD, present in about 40% of patients, is associated with a worse prognosis. Occasionally there is a coexisting *CEBPA* mutation.

Acute myeloid leukaemia with *CEBPA* mutation
This is a provisional entity in the 2008 WHO classification. A mutation of *CEBPA* is found in 6–15% of cases of AML, usually in association with a normal karyotype [14]. The AML can be of various FAB categories but is most often M1 or M2. *CEBPA* mutation is associated with a good prognosis.

Peripheral blood
The peripheral blood shows blast cells; usually these are myeloblasts but sometimes there is monocytic differentiation.

Bone marrow cytology
Bone marrow aspiration shows increased myeloblasts or, less often, monocytic differentiation.

Cytochemistry
Cytochemistry shows the expected reactions but is not important in this diagnosis.

Bone marrow histology
There is an increase of blast cells.

Immunophenotype
There is usually expression of CD13, CD33, CD34, CD11b, CD15 and HLA-DR [14]. CD7 expression is very frequent.

Cytogenetic and molecular genetic analysis
Cytogenetic analysis is normal in about three quarters of patients. *CEBPA* mutation is usually bi-allelic. *FLT3*-ITD coexists in up to a third of patients but its prognostic significance in this context is not yet clear.

Acute myeloid leukaemia with myelodysplasia-related changes
In the 2001 WHO classification a group of cases were designated AML with multilineage dysplasia. In the revised 2008 version of the WHO classification this category has been expanded and renamed. There are three qualifying criteria, which often overlap: the presence of dysplastic features in at least 50% of cells of at least two myeloid lineages; previous MDS or myelodysplastic syndrome/myeloproliferative neoplasm (MDS/MPN); and the presence of a myelodysplasia-related cytogenetic abnormality (see below) [20]. This subtype comprises a quarter to a third of cases of AML. It is mainly a disease of the elderly. Prognosis is poor, although the disease may be less rapidly progressive in those with prior MDS and a relatively low blast cell count.

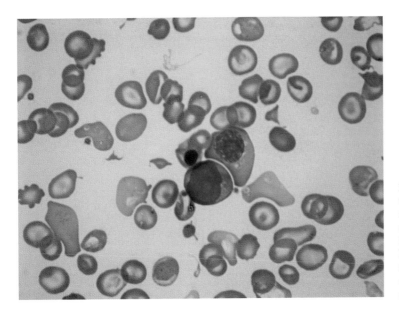

Fig. 4.28 PB film from a patient with AML with myelodysplasia-related changes showing gross anisocytosis and poikilocytosis including red cell fragments, basophilic stippling, a blast cell, a cytologically normal erythroblast and a dysplastic erythroblast (a macronormoblast). MGG ×100.

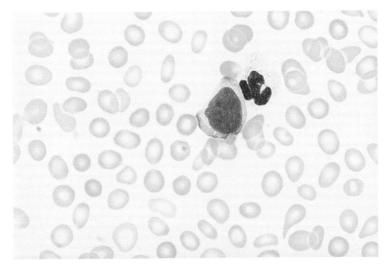

Fig. 4.29 PB film from a patient with AML with myelodysplasia-related changes (FAB M0 AML) showing anisocytosis, poikilocytosis, a blast cell and a hypogranular neutrophil. Assignment to this category was because of significant dysplasia and a previous history of MDS. MGG ×100.

Peripheral blood

There is often pancytopenia and sometimes macrocytosis. The blood film usually shows anisocytosis, poikilocytosis, basophilic stippling, dysplastic neutrophils (hypolobation and hypogranularity) and blast cells (Figs 4.28 and 4.29).

Bone marrow cytology

A bone marrow aspirate usually shows multilineage dysplasia (which may include ring sideroblasts) (Figs 4.30–4.32). Micromegakaryocytes are often present and there may also be multinucleated or other dysplastic megakaryocytes.

Cytochemistry

A periodic acid–Schiff (PAS) stain may show positivity of erythroblast cytoplasm, thus providing supporting evidence of erythroid dysplasia. MPO and SBB stains facilitate the detection of Auer rods.

Bone marrow histology

There is usually multilineage dysplasia. Megakaryocyte dysplasia may be more readily detected than in an aspirate film.

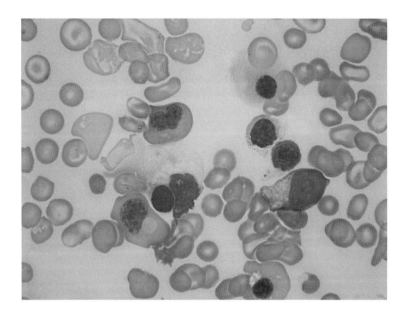

Fig. 4.30 BM film from a patient with AML with myelodysplasia-related changes (same patient as Fig. 4.28); cells present include a blast cell and two grossly dysplastic erythroblasts (both are megaloblastic). MGG ×100.

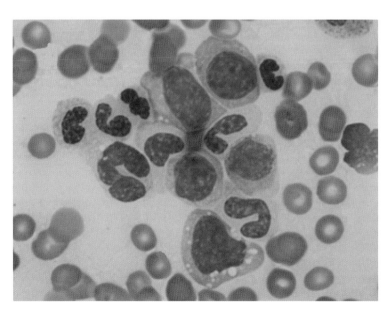

Fig. 4.31 BM film from a patient with AML with myelodysplasia-related changes showing severe dysplasia of cells of neutrophil lineage. MGG ×100.

Immunophenotype

The immunophenotype varies considerably between patients. However, aberrant expression of CD7 or CD56 by blast cells is common. Maturing cells may also show aberrant antigen expression.

Cytogenetic and molecular genetic analysis

The cytogenetic abnormalities shown in Table 4.8 (page 217), with the exception of inv(3) and t(6;9), lead to assignment to this category. In addition, cases are allocated to this category if they have any of the following recurrent cytogenetic abnormalities: t(3;5)(q25;q34), t(5;7)(q33;q11.2), t(5;10)(q33;q21), t(5;12)(q33;p12), t(5;17)(q33;p13) or a complex karyotype (greater than three unrelated abnormalities). The presence of an *NPM1* or *CEBPA* mutation does not exclude allocation to this category.

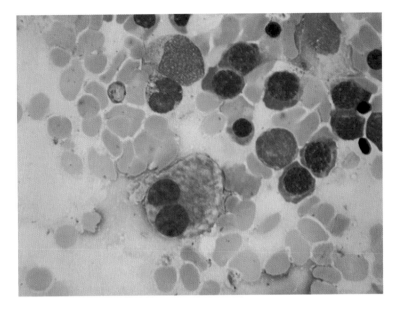

Fig. 4.32 BM aspirate from a patient with AML with myelodysplasia-related changes showing a dysplastic binucleated megakaryocyte. This patient's disease was assigned to this AML category both because of evolution from MDS (refractory cytopenia with multilineage dysplasia) and because of the presence of multilineage dysplasia. MGG ×100.

Therapy-related myeloid neoplasms

In the 2008 WHO classification therapy-related cases of AML, MDS and MDS/MPN have been grouped together in a single category [21]. The reason for this is that some cases of therapy-related MDS (t-MDS) have a prognosis as poor as that of therapy-related AML (t-AML). Cases are included in this category if the patients have been previously exposed to anti-cancer chemotherapy or irradiation. In contrast to the 2001 WHO classification, cases are no longer grouped according to whether exposure was to alkylating agents or topoisomerase-II-interactive drugs (although the clinical features and associated cytogenetic abnormalities differ and, to a lesser extent, so does the prognosis). Treatment with alkylating agents, nitrosoureas and irradiation can be followed in 5–10 years by t-MDS that progresses to t-AML. Therapy with topoisomerase-II-interactive drugs can be followed in 1–5 years by t-AML without there necessarily being a phase of t-MDS. The age range of patients with these disorders is wide. Some cases of therapy-related myeloid neoplasms follow autologous or allogeneic stem cell transplantation and some follow treatment of non-neoplastic disorders. The prognosis is generally poor, although it is considerably better in those patients who have a chromosomal rearrangement associated with a good prognosis in *de novo* AML. Patients with recurrent cytogenetic abnormalities are assigned to this AML category if they have been exposed to leukaemogenic drugs or irradiation.

Peripheral blood

There is often cytopenia together with features of multilineage dysplasia, particularly when t-MDS/t-AML follows the use of alkylating agents. In t-AML following topoisomerase-II-interactive drugs the features are similar to those of *de novo* AML with the same chromosomal abnormalities, although dysplastic features are sometimes present.

Bone marrow cytology

In cases related to alkylating agents, a bone marrow aspirate may be difficult to obtain because of hypocellularity or fibrosis. Trilineage dysplasia is usual with the blast cell count ranging from normal to counts diagnostic of AML. In cases following exposure to topoisomerase-II-interactive drugs the findings are usually of acute leukaemia, with the specific features depending on the chromosomal rearrangement; because of the frequent involvement of the *MLL* gene, myelomonocytic and monocytic differentiation is over-represented

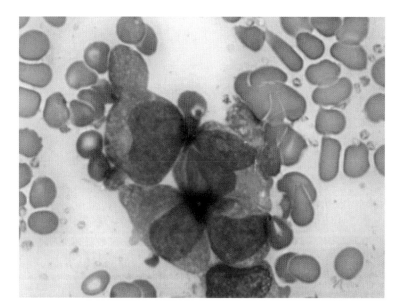

Fig. 4.33 BM aspirate from a patient with t-AML (FAB M5a AML) following exposure to doxorubicin for treatment of breast cancer. This patient had t(9;11) (p22;q23) but, in assigning the condition to a WHO category, the exposure to a genotoxic drug takes precedence over the recurrent cytogenetic abnormality. MGG ×100.

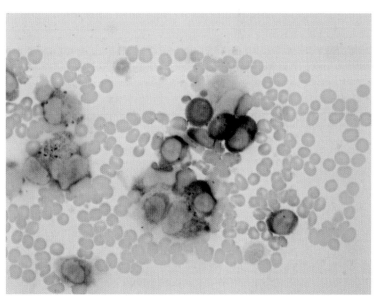

Fig. 4.34 BM aspirate from a patient with t-AML (same patient as Fig. 4.33) demonstrating that the blast cells are of monocyte lineage. ANAE ×50.

in comparison with *de novo* AML (Figs 4.33 and 4.34).

Cytochemistry
Cytochemistry is not usually very useful.

Bone marrow histology
Stromal changes, specifically reticulin or collagen fibrosis and hypocellularity, are common in alkylat-

ing agent-related cases. Trephine biopsy is therefore particularly useful.

Immunophenotype
The immunophenotype varies between cases. There may be aberrant expression of CD7 and CD56. CD34 is very useful for highlighting blast cells in trephine biopsy sections from patients with bone marrow fibrosis.

Cytogenetic and molecular genetic analysis

An abnormal karyotype is seen in about 90% of patients. The cytogenetic abnormalities that are seen following exposure to alkylating agents and related drugs are usually unbalanced and include abnormalities of chromosomes 5 and 7 and complex karyotypes. The abnormalities that follow use of topoisomerase-II-interactive drugs are usually balanced and include translocations with 11q23 (*MLL*) and 21q22 (*RUNX1*) breakpoints. The translocations that can follow treatment with topoisomerase-II-interactive drugs include some rearrangements that more often occur in *de novo* AML, such as t(8;21), t(15;17), inv(16) and t(16;16).

Acute myeloid leukaemia, not otherwise specified

Cases that cannot be assigned to the categories already discussed, are classified as 'acute myeloid leukaemia, not otherwise specified' (AML, NOS) and are divided further into morphological categories, most of which resemble those of the FAB classification [22]. However, these categories differ from those of the FAB classification because (i) all the subtypes of AML discussed above have been excluded, and (ii) the blast percentage for diagnosis differs from that of the FAB classification (20% rather than 30%). In addition, two new categories,

acute basophilic leukaemia and acute panmyelosis with fibrosis, have been recognized and the definition of erythroleukaemia has been expanded. Few data are available for the characteristics and outcome of AML, NOS so that extrapolations tend to be made from the similar FAB categories. Unless a patient has had successful cytogenetic analysis and has been investigated for *NPM1* and *CEBPA* mutation, assignment to AML, NOS is not strictly valid, but is all that is possible. (The cases used to illustrate this section have not been studied for these mutations.)

Acute myeloid leukaemia with minimal differentiation

This category resembles the FAB M0 category. There may be associated dysplasia, which can give a clue to the case being AML not ALL (Fig. 4.35). However, for all of these categories, the presence of multilineage dysplasia (as defined in the WHO classification) excludes the diagnosis of AML, NOS, cases being assigned instead to the category AML with myelodysplasia-associated features. Diagnosis requires flow cytometry immunophenotyping or immunohistochemistry since, by definition, cytochemical stains for MPO, SBB and NSE are positive in fewer than 3% of blast cells. Myeloid antigens are expressed and expression of CD7 and TdT may be more common than in AML in general. MPO

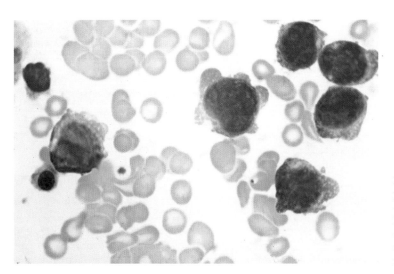

Fig. 4.35 BM aspirate from a patient with AML with minimal differentiation (FAB M0 AML). Blast cells were negative on all cytochemical stains and were identified as myeloid by immunophenotyping. MGG ×100.

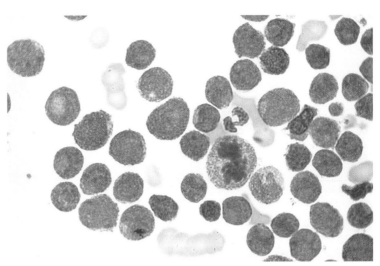

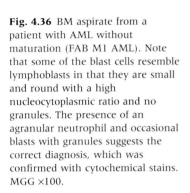

Fig. 4.36 BM aspirate from a patient with AML without maturation (FAB M1 AML). Note that some of the blast cells resemble lymphoblasts in that they are small and round with a high nucleocytoplasmic ratio and no granules. The presence of an agranular neutrophil and occasional blasts with granules suggests the correct diagnosis, which was confirmed with cytochemical stains. MGG ×100.

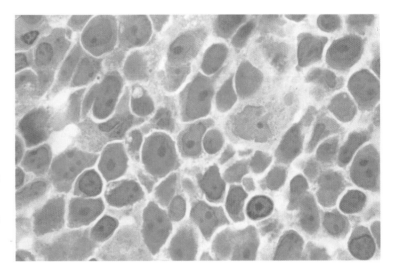

Fig. 4.37 Section of BM trephine biopsy specimen from a patient with AML without maturation (FAB M1 AML). There is a relatively uniform population of small blast cells with a high nucleocytoplasmic ratio and prominent nucleoli. Resin-embedded, H&E ×100.

protein is sometimes detected by immunophenotyping although cytochemical activity is absent. Cytologically and histologically, the findings are of small to medium-sized blast cells with no granules or Auer rods. There is a preferential association with abnormalities of chromosomes 5 and 7, trisomy 13 and translocations and deletions involving 12p [23]. *RUNX1* mutation and *FLT3*-ITD each occur in around a quarter of patients.

Acute myeloid leukaemia without maturation

This category resembles the FAB M1 category. Stains for SBB or MPO are positive in at least 3% of blast cells and granules or Auer rods may be present (Fig. 4.36). In trephine biopsy sections there may be little sign of maturation and immunohistochemistry may be necessary for diagnosis (Fig. 4.37). Flow cytometry shows expression of myeloid antigens.

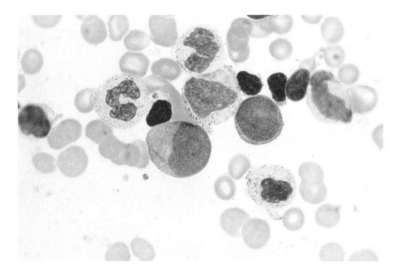

Fig. 4.38 BM aspirate from a patient with AML with maturation (FAB M2 AML), showing two myeloblasts, one of which contains a long slender Auer rod; there are abnormal maturing cells. MGG ×100.

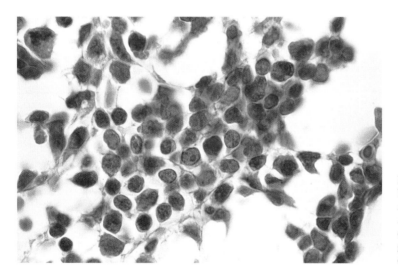

Fig. 4.39 Section of BM trephine biopsy specimen from a patient with AML with maturation (FAB M2 AML). There is a mixture of blast cells and maturing cells of the granulocytic series. Paraffin-embedded, H&E ×100.

Acute myeloid leukaemia with maturation

This category resembles the FAB M2 category. There is obvious granulocytic maturation (neutrophilic, eosinophilic or both but, by definition, not primarily basophilic) so that cytochemistry is unnecessary for diagnosis (Figs 4.38 and 4.39). There may be associated dysplasia and Auer rods may be present.

When there is eosinophilic differentiation, the eosinophil precursors often show nucleocytoplasmic asynchrony and immature granules with basophilic staining characteristics. The bone marrow shows an increase, often very marked, in eosinophils and their precursors. Occasionally Charcot–Leyden crystals are present, these being formed by crystallization of eosinophil granule contents. Bone marrow trephine biopsy sections show an increase of eosinophils and their precursors. These cells show strong peroxidase activity.

Flow cytometry shows expression of myeloid antigens but is not necessary for diagnosis.

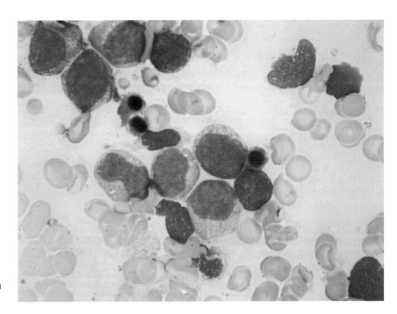

Fig. 4.40 BM aspirate in acute monoblastic leukaemia (FAB M5a category) showing monoblasts and a single promonocyte. MGG ×100.

Acute myelomonocytic leukaemia

This category resembles the FAB M4 category with there being both granulocytic and monocytic differentiation (see Fig. 4.9). A double esterase stain, combining CAE and NSE, can be used to confirm the diagnosis. Flow cytometry shows expression of myeloid antigens including expression of some that are typical of monocytic differentiation (see below).

Acute monoblastic and monocytic leukaemia

This category resembles the FAB M5 category, M5a (monoblastic) and M5b (monocytic), respectively. The dominant cell may be a monoblast (Fig. 4.40) or, alternatively, promonocytes and maturing monocytes may predominate (Fig. 4.41). In contrast to the FAB classification, promonocytes are regarded, in the WHO classification, as blast equivalents so that 20% monoblasts plus promonocytes in the peripheral blood or bone marrow is sufficient for the diagnosis of AML. In the case of acute monoblastic leukaemia, it is important to use either cytochemistry or immunophenotyping to confirm the diagnosis since cases can be confused morphologically with large cell lymphoma; some cases of

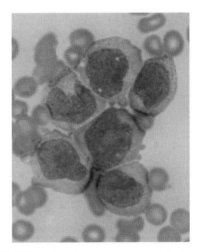

Fig. 4.41 BM aspirate in acute monocytic leukaemia (FAB M5b category) showing promonocytes with irregular and folded nuclei. MGG ×100.

acute monoblastic leukaemia do not exhibit NSE activity so that the diagnosis rests on morphology plus immunophenotyping. Acute monocytic leukaemia can usually be diagnosed reliably on the basis of morphology supplemented by cytochemistry. Flow cytometry shows variable expression of antigens characteristic of monocytic differentiation, such as CD4, CD11b, CD11c, CD14, CD64 and lysozyme. CD34 is expressed in only about a third of cases. Immunohistochemical demonstration of expression of CD68R and CD163 is useful. Some cases have prominent haemophagocytosis. This is particularly characteristic of cases associated with t(8;16)(p11.2;p13.3). This is not a specific WHO subtype and cases are therefore categorized as AML, NOS – acute monoblastic/monocytic leukaemia or acute myelomonocytic leukaemia, depending on the cytological features.

Acute erythroid leukaemia

The WHO classification recognizes two forms of AML with dominant erythroid differentiation. Erythroid/myeloid leukaemia resembles the FAB M6 category in having a significant population of myeloblasts, whereas pure erythroid leukaemia does not but instead has a neoplastic population that includes very immature erythroid cells (appearing undifferentiated or resembling proerythroblasts). The peripheral blood film may show myeloblasts or occasional dysplastic erythroid cells (Fig. 4.42). Relevant abnormalities are much more apparent in bone marrow aspirate and trephine biopsy specimens. The morphology of erythroid

cells varies between cases. In aspirates from some patients, erythroid cells show striking cytological abnormalities which may include nuclear lobulation, karyorrhexis, multinuclearity, gigantism or megaloblastic or sideroblastic erythropoiesis. In other patients, cytological abnormalities are quite minor. Coalescing empty cytoplasmic blocks and vacuoles are characteristic. Erythroblast cytoplasm may be PAS positive (blocks or diffuse) and focally NSE positive. In some patients there are numerous ring sideroblasts. In trephine biopsy sections the erythroid precursors are often markedly abnormal and may have bizarre appearances. They often show nuclear lobulation or fragmentation, marked variation in size or megaloblastic change. They are arranged in sheets without the formation of normal erythroblastic islands. Megakaryocytic dysplasia is often seen. Cytological features permit a distinction between erythroid cells and myeloblasts (Fig. 4.43).

Erythroid/myeloid leukaemia is usually readily diagnosed on morphological grounds but recognizing the lineage of the most immature cells of pure erythroid leukaemia may require immunophenotyping. Some cells express glycophorin, carbonic anhydrase or CD71 (transferrin receptor) but the most primitive cells may express only CD36 (which is not lineage-specific). In patients with a very high erythroid percentage, identification of blast cells among the non-erythroid component can be

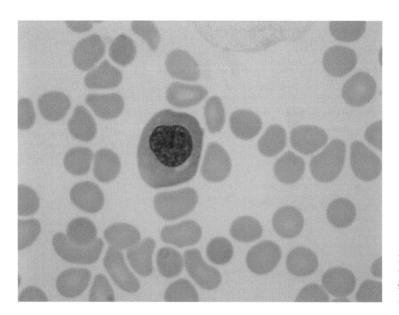

Fig. 4.42 PB film from a patient with acute erythroleukaemia showing a circulating megaloblast. MGG ×100.

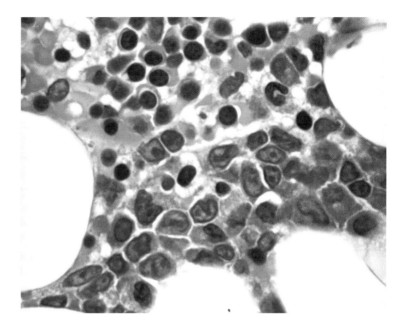

Fig. 4.43 Trephine biopsy section from a patient with erythroleukaemia. Erythroid cells are apparent at the top of the photograph; at the bottom are myeloblasts with irregular nuclei and prominent eosinophilic nucleoli. Paraffin-embedded, H&E ×60.

facilitated by immunohistochemistry for CD34. Many cases of FAB M6 AML are assigned to the WHO category of AML with myelodysplasia-related features on the basis of either multilineage dysplasia or relevant cytogenetic abnormalities so that cases categorized as 'acute erythroleukaemia' are quite uncommon.

Acute megakaryoblastic leukaemia

This WHO category resembles FAB M7 AML, but cases associated with t(1;22), t(3;3), inv(3), Down's syndrome or myelodysplasia-related features are excluded. Rare patients are young males with a mediastinal germ cell tumour and i(12p) in both megakaryoblasts and germ cell tumour cells. Assignment to this WHO category requires at least 20% blast cells, of which at least 50% are megakaryoblasts. Often the peripheral blood shows only pancytopenia with very infrequent or no circulating leukaemic blasts. Such patients usually lack organomegaly and have a fibrotic marrow; this condition has been described as 'acute myelofibrosis'. Other patients have features more typical of acute leukaemia, with hepatomegaly, splenomegaly and significant numbers of circulating blasts. Megakaryoblasts are similar in size to myeloblasts. They have a high nucleocytoplasmic ratio and

agranular, moderately basophilic cytoplasm. In some cases there are distinctive features that suggest their nature, such as the formation of peripheral cytoplasmic blebs or an association with circulating micromegakaryocytes, but in other cases there are no features to suggest lineage. There may be giant and hypogranular platelets. Bone marrow aspiration may be impossible or a poor aspirate containing scanty blasts may be obtained. In addition to megakaryoblasts, the aspirate may contain some micromegakaryocytes or other markedly dysplastic megakaryocytes. Blasts are negative with MPO, SBB and CAE stains. Acid phosphatase, PAS and α-naphthyl acetate esterase stains are negative in the more immature cells but may be positive in cells showing cytoplasmic maturation. Staining for α-naphthyl butyrate esterase is negative. The PAS stain sometimes shows a distinctive pattern with positivity being confined to cytoplasmic blebs. Flow cytometry shows expression of CD41 and CD61 and usually CD36. The marrow histology is very variable [24,25]. In those cases that present clinically as acute myelofibrosis, the marrow is largely replaced by fibrous tissue containing blasts and dysplastic megakaryocytes. In other cases the marrow is very hypercellular with an infiltrate of blasts, sometimes micromegakaryo-

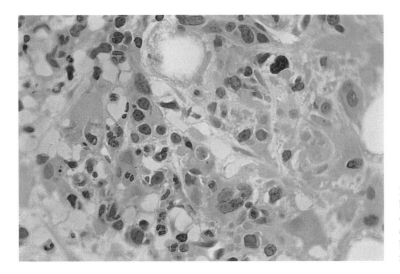

Fig. 4.44 Section of BM trephine biopsy specimen, M7 AML. There is collagen fibrosis and an infiltrate of dysplastic megakaryocytes and small blast cells. Resin-embedded, H&E ×40.

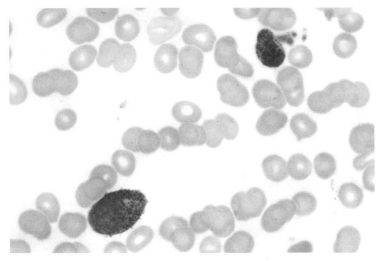

Fig. 4.45 PB film of a patient with acute basophilic leukaemia showing blasts with basophil-type granules. The granules are smaller than those of normal mature basophils. MGG ×100.

cytes and usually increased reticulin and scattered collagen fibres (Fig. 4.44). Dyserythropoiesis is common. Immunohistochemistry for CD42b, CD61 or von Willebrand antigen confirms the lineage.

Acute basophilic leukaemia

Acute basophilic leukaemia is a rare form of AML in which differentiation is primarily to basophils (Figs 4.45 and 4.46). Cases fall into the M1, M2 or M4 categories of the FAB classification. Cases that are *BCR-ABL1* positive or have t(6;9) are specifically excluded from this WHO category. There may be clinical features of hyperhistaminaemia. The blood film shows blast cells and some maturing basophils.

The blast cells may have occasional basophilic granules. Maturing basophils may be hypogranular and vacuolated. Granules stain metachromatically with toluidine blue. MPO, SBB and CAE stains are negative. A PAS stain may show blocks and lakes of positive material. On flow cytometric immunophenotyping, blast cells are seen to express CD13, CD33 or both and also CD11c, CD123, CD203c and usually CD9 [22]. The bone marrow aspirate shows 20% or more blast cells, usually with maturation to dysplastic basophils. Trephine biopsy sections show increased blast cells. Basophilic differentiation can be identified by immunohistochemistry but not in H&E-stained sections.

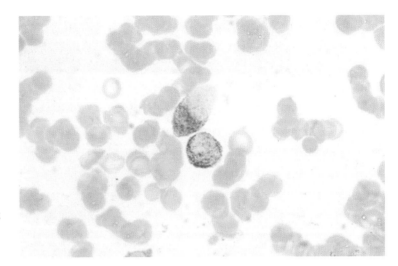

Fig. 4.46 PB film of a patient with acute basophilic leukaemia showing that the granules stain metachromatically with toluidine blue. Toluidine blue ×100.

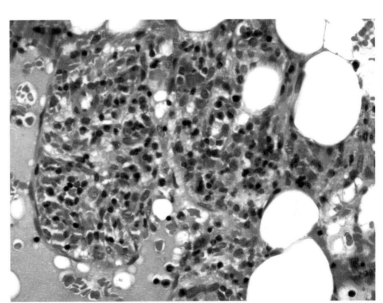

Fig. 4.47 BM trephine biopsy section from a patient with acute panmyelosis with myelofibrosis showing disorderly haemopoiesis and increased immature cells. Paraffin-embedded, H&E ×40.

Acute panmyelosis with myelofibrosis

This rare entity presents acutely and is characterized pathologically by trilineage differentiation associated with bone marrow reticulin fibrosis. It has some features in common with those cases of acute megakaryocytic leukaemia that are associated with the clinicopathological features of 'acute myelofibrosis'. It has to be distinguished from AML with myelodysplasia-related features and refractory anaemia with excess of blasts (RAEB) with fibrosis. There is pancytopenia. The blood film may show small numbers of blast cells, neutrophil dysplasia or macrocytosis. The bone marrow aspirate is often inadequate for diagnosis because of the associated reticulin fibrosis. Increased blasts cells and multilineage dysplasia may be apparent. Bone marrow histology is critical in making the diagnosis, with immunohistochemistry being important in showing trilineage differentiation. Immature cells of granulocytic, erythroid and megakaryocyte lineages are increased; micromegakaryocytes and other dysplastic features may be prominent (Figs 4.47–

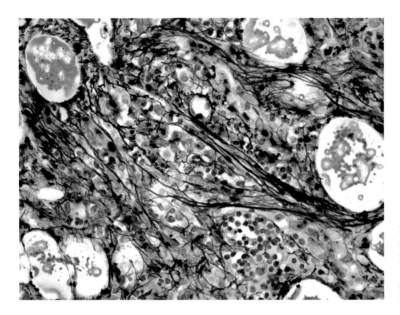

Fig. 4.48 BM trephine biopsy section from a patient with acute panmyelosis with myelofibrosis (same patient as Fig. 4.47) showing grade 4 fibrosis. Paraffin-embedded, reticulin stain ×40.

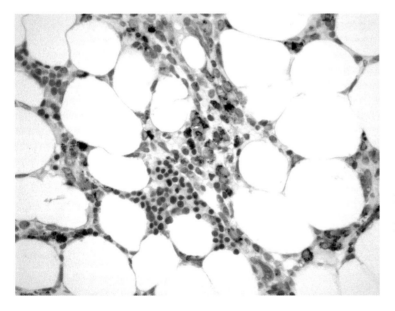

Fig. 4.49 BM trephine biopsy section from a patient with acute panmyelosis with myelofibrosis (same patient as Fig. 4.47) showing immature haemopoietic cells that are expressing CD34. Paraffin-embedded, immunohistochemistry for CD34 ×40.

4.52). The blast cell count is not very high, often around 20–25%, Reticulin is increased and occasionally there is collagen deposition.

Myeloid proliferations related to Down's syndrome

Down's syndrome is associated with two distinct leukaemic processes: transient abnormal myelopoi-esis (which is a spontaneously remitting leukaemia of neonates) and acute megakaryoblastic leukaemia occurring in older infants.

Transient abnormal myelopoiesis

This condition is specific to the fetus or neonate with Down's syndrome, including mosaic Down's

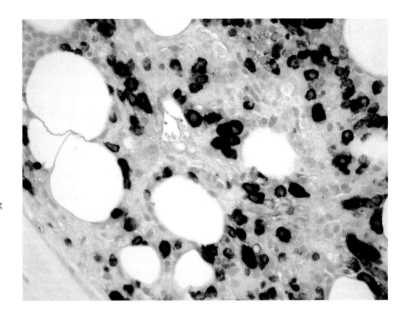

Fig. 4.50 BM trephine biopsy section from a patient with acute panmyelosis with myelofibrosis (same patient as Fig. 4.47) showing low numbers of dispersed myeloperoxidase-positive cells – a mixture of myeloblasts, promyelocytes and myelocytes. Paraffin-embedded, immunohistochemistry for MPO ×40.

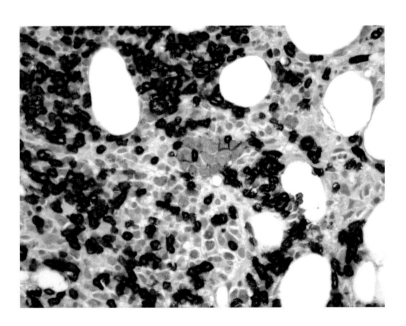

Fig. 4.51 BM trephine biopsy section from a patient with acute panmyelosis with myelofibrosis (same patient as Fig. 4.47) showing strongly glycophorin-positive maturing erythroblasts and erythrocytes and a cluster of more weakly positive proerythroblasts, which are forming a 'pseudo-ALIP'. Paraffin-embedded, immunohistochemistry for glycophorin A (CD235A) ×40.

syndrome. In addition to a constitutional trisomy 21 or related lesion, there is a somatic *GATA1* mutation and occasionally also an acquired clonal chromosomal rearrangement. Differentiation is predominantly to the megakaryocyte lineage but in some cases there is an increase of myeloblasts and proerythroblasts (Fig. 4.53). There may be circulating micromegakaryocytes. The peripheral blood may show a higher percentage of blast cells than the bone marrow. Remission usually occurs in 4–6 weeks, but around a quarter of infants develop a non-transient AML several years later.

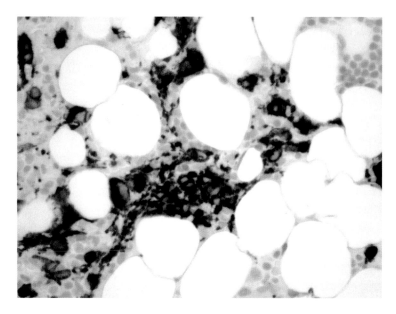

Fig. 4.52 BM trephine biopsy section from a patient with acute panmyelosis with myelofibrosis (same patient as Fig. 4.47) showing megakaryoblasts and several small dysplastic megakaryocytes. Paraffin-embedded, immunohistochemistry for CD61 ×40.

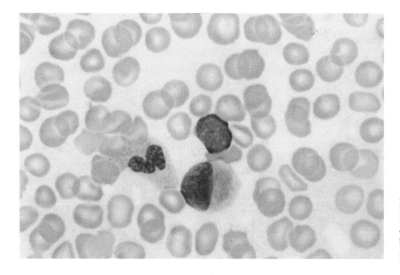

Fig. 4.53 PB film of a baby with Down's syndrome and transient abnormal myelopoiesis showing a blast cell, a neutrophil and a micromegakaryocyte. MGG ×100.

Myeloid leukaemia associated with Down's syndrome

There is a specific association of Down's syndrome with acute megakaryoblastic leukaemia occurring during the first 5 years of life (Fig. 4.54). There may be preceding MDS and in some children prior transient abnormal myelopoiesis is documented. A *GATA1* mutation is consistently present. The prognosis is considerably better than that of other AML in children.

Blastic plasmacytoid dendritic cell neoplasm

Plasmacytoid dendritic cell neoplasm is a rare neoplasm now thought to be of dendritic cell lineage and distinct from CD56-positive AML [26–29]. In the 2001 WHO classification it was designated blastic natural killer (NK) cell lymphoma and it is also known as CD4-positive CD56-positive haematodermic neoplasm. The disease often involves multiple sites with a predilection for the skin,

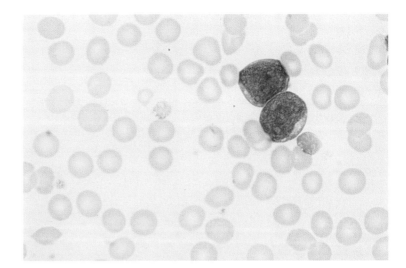

Fig. 4.54 BM aspirate of a patient with Down's syndrome and acute megakaryoblastic leukaemia (FAB M7 category) showing two megakaryoblasts and two giant platelets. MGG ×100.

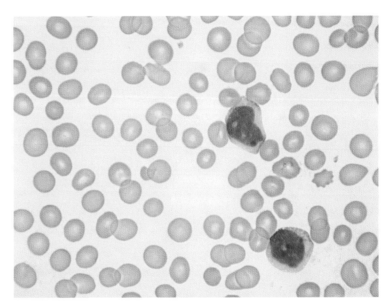

Fig. 4.55 PB film from a patient with blastic plasmacytoid dendritic cell neoplasm showing two blast cells with small nucleoli and agranular cytoplasm containing a few small vacuoles. MGG ×100.

peripheral blood and bone marrow. The condition may be better defined immunologically than morphologically, being a neoplasm of CD4-positive CD56-positive cells with no expression of B, T or myeloid immunophenotypic markers [30]. About 20% of patients develop chronic myelomonocytic leukaemia or AML [29]. The prognosis is poor.

Peripheral blood
Neoplastic cells with blastic morphology may be present in the peripheral blood (Fig. 4.55).

Anaemia, neutropenia and thrombocytopenia are common. In a minority of patients, myeloid cells show dysplastic features.

Bone marrow cytology
There may be bone marrow infiltration by blasts with a variable nucleocytoplasmic ratio and weakly basophilic, agranular, often vacuolated cytoplasm which may show pseudopodia-like extensions [30,31] (Fig. 4.56). Neoplastic cells tend to be

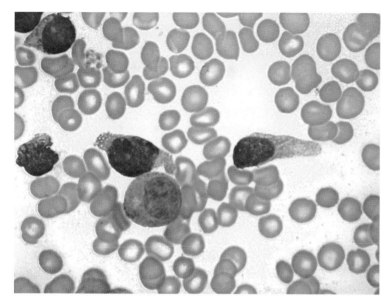

Fig. 4.56 BM aspirate film from a patient with blastic plasmacytoid dendritic cell neoplasm (same patient as Fig. 4.55) showing two neoplastic cells with cytoplasmic tails; one cell has fine cytoplasmic vacuoles. In this patient cytoplasmic tails were quite prominent in the BM aspirate and trephine biopsy sections but were not a feature of circulating neoplastic cells. MGG ×100.

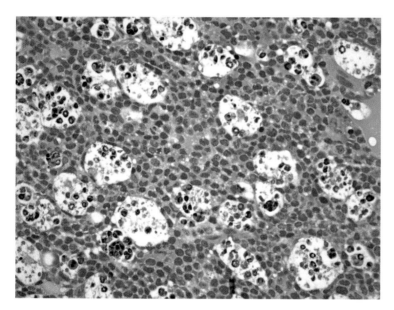

Fig. 4.57 Trephine biopsy section from a patient with blastic plasmacytoid dendritic cell neoplasm. There is almost total replacement of normal haemopoietic cells by an infiltrate of somewhat pleomorphic, medium-sized blast cells. The patient also had several skin nodules with a similar infiltrate. In the bone marrow (but not in the skin) massive apoptosis was apparent, with prominent macrophages throughout the infiltrate having cytoplasm expanded by apoptotic cell fragments (leading to a 'starry sky' appearance). Paraffin-embedded, H&E ×40.

cytologically uniform in a single patient but vary from small/medium to medium/large between patients. Nuclei may be regular or irregular and nucleoli may be present. In a minority of patients, myeloid cells show dysplastic features [30].

Cytochemistry
The MPO stain is negative.

Flow cytometric immunophenotyping
Flow cytometry shows that the tumour cells express CD4 and do not express CD3, CD8, CD16 or CD57. There is variable expression of CD2, CD7 and TdT and expression of CD123.

Bone marrow histology and immunohistochemistry
Bone marrow infiltration, when present, varies

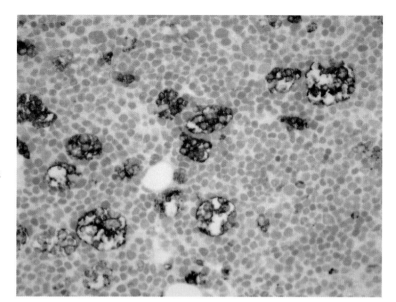

Fig. 4.58 Trephine biopsy section from a patient with blastic plasmacytoid dendritic cell neoplasm (same patient as Fig. 4.57). The macrophages containing apoptotic neoplastic cell fragments have been accentuated by immunohistochemistry. In this patient only occasional neoplastic cells are positive for CD68. Paraffin-embedded, immunoperoxidase for CD68 ×40.

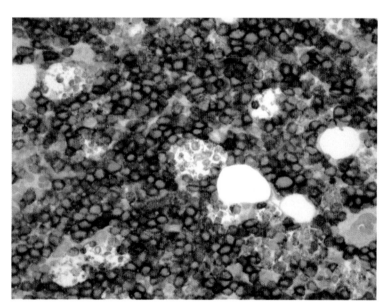

Fig. 4.59 Trephine biopsy section from a patient with blastic plasmacytoid dendritic cell neoplasm (same patient as Fig. 4.57) showing strong expression of CD123. Paraffin-embedded, immunoperoxidase for CD123 ×40.

from interstitial to a packed marrow pattern. Infiltrating cells are medium-sized cells resembling lymphoblasts or myeloblasts; sometimes cells and nuclei are elongated. There may be a high rate of apoptosis and a 'starry sky' appearance (Fig. 4.57). Neoplastic cells show expression of CD4, CD43, CD45RA, CD56 and more specific plasmacytoid dendritic cell markers, CD123 and BDCA2 (blood dendritic cell antigen 2)/CD303

and TCL1 (Figs. 4.58–4.60). CD56 (which is not expressed by mature plasmacytoid dendritic cells) is occasionally negative. About half of cases express CD68 [29]. There is variable expression of cytoplasmic CD3ε, CD7 and CD33. CD8 is not expressed. Cytotoxic granule-associated molecules are usually negative. TdT is expressed in about a third of cases in a variable proportion of cells [29] (Fig. 4.61).

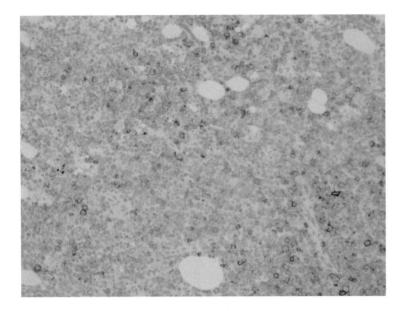

Fig. 4.60 Trephine biopsy section from a patient with blastic plasmacytoid dendritic cell neoplasm (same patient as Fig. 4.57) showing expression of CD56. Paraffin-embedded, immunoperoxidase for CD56 ×20.

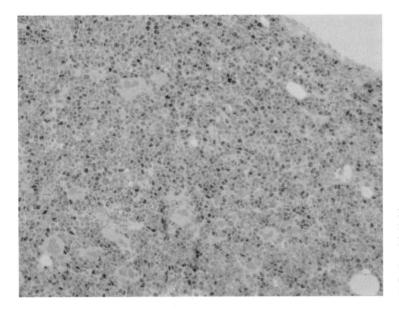

Fig. 4.61 Trephine biopsy section from a patient with blastic plasmacytoid dendritic cell neoplasm (same patient as Fig. 4.57) showing nuclear expression of TdT. Paraffin-embedded, immunoperoxidase for CD56 ×20.

Cytogenetic and molecular genetic analysis

TCR and *IGH* genes are germline. Complex cytogenetic abnormalities are common, including del(5q), del(6q) and del(12p) and deletions of 4q23, 9p13-p11 and 9q12-q34 [28].

Problems and pitfalls in the diagnosis of AML

Because of the extended use of genetic data in the 2008 WHO classification, difficulties will occur in the classification of those cases for which cytogenetic or molecular genetic information cannot be obtained.

It is sometimes difficult to distinguish cases of FAB M0 and M1 AML from ALL on the basis of examination of H&E-stained sections. Some histological features are useful. ALL is usually associated with effacement of the bone marrow whereas, in AML, there may be residual myeloid cells showing dysplastic features. In comparison with the blast cells of AML, ALL blasts tend to have less cytoplasm and their chromatin is more condensed. If difficulty is experienced in making the distinction and if diagnosis depends on the trephine biopsy sections, immunohistochemistry should be used. Antibodies reactive with CD68, CD117, lysozyme, neutrophil elastase and MPO are useful in distinguishing AML from ALL in trephine biopsy sections; these should be used in conjunction with antibodies reactive with lymphoid cell-associated antigens. The antigen (calprotectin) detected by the MAC387 antibody is also myeloid-associated, being expressed by cells of the monocyte lineage and by mature cells of the granulocyte lineage. To distinguish AML with erythroid or megakaryocytic differentiation from ALL it is necessary to use antibodies reactive with antigens such as glycophorin and spectrin or CD42b, CD61 and von Willebrand factor. However, it should be noted that immunohistochemistry for MPO and other myeloid antigens is less sensitive for the detection of myeloid differentiation than cytochemistry and immunophenotyping by flow cytometry. For this reason there are some cases of FAB M0 and M1 AML that cannot be distinguished from ALL histologically, even with the help of immunohistochemistry.

Other diagnostic problems relate mainly to FAB M6 and M7 categories and to hypoplastic AML. M6 AML and megaloblastic anaemia can be confused with each other in trephine biopsy sections or, less often, in a bone marrow aspirate. This is a very serious error which must be avoided. It arises mainly because the diagnosis of AML is not considered or because a case of M6 has megaloblastic erythropoiesis. Diagnostic error can be avoided by careful attention to cytological details supplemented, when necessary, by assays of vitamin B_{12} and folic acid. A therapeutic trial of haematinic agents is useful when there is diagnostic uncertainty.

FAB M7 AML and acute panmyelosis with myelofibrosis, when accompanied by dense fibrosis, can be confused with primary myelofibrosis (chronic idiopathic myelofibrosis). Clinical and haematological features of these two conditions differ. Marked splenomegaly is usual in primary myelofibrosis but not in FAB M7 AML or acute panmyelosis with fibrosis. A leucoerythroblastic anaemia with marked poikilocytosis is likewise usual in primary myelofibrosis but not in M7 AML or acute panmyelosis. Bone marrow aspiration

usually fails or yields inadequate material for diagnosis in all these conditions. However, histology shows increased blast cells in M7 AML and acute panmyelosis and not in primary myelofibrosis. AMLs with myelofibrosis can also be confused with bone marrow infiltration by a non-haemopoietic tumour with secondary myelofibrosis. Dysplastic megakaryocytes and metastatic tumour cells can be distinguished by immunohistochemistry.

Hypoplastic AML must be distinguished from aplastic anaemia and from hypoplastic MDS. In contrast to cases of typical AML, pancytopenia is usual and peripheral blood blast cells are often absent or infrequent. The bone marrow aspirate is often hypocellular and may therefore not be optimal for diagnosis. In hypoplastic MDS there may also be some circulating blast cells and an inadequate bone marrow aspirate, whereas there is no increase in blast cells in aplastic anaemia. Accurate differential diagnosis of these three conditions requires good quality sections of trephine biopsy specimens. Increased reticulin deposition and dysplastic megakaryocytes suggest a diagnosis of AML or MDS rather than aplastic anaemia. Sections need to be examined carefully with high power magnification so that the proportion of blast cells can be estimated. If there are at least 20% blast cells the diagnosis is AML and, if blasts are increased but less than 20%, the diagnosis is MDS. Immunohistochemical staining for CD34 is helpful in highlighting blast cells.

Acute myeloid leukaemia of the FAB M5a subtype can sometimes be confused with large cell non-Hodgkin lymphoma. If monocytes are very immature they may lack peroxidase and NSE activity. Flow cytometry immunophenotyping or immunohistochemistry is then very important in making the correct diagnosis.

Leukaemoid reactions can simulate AML very closely. For example, a patient has been reported with a hypocellular bone marrow containing 34% blast cells that expressed CD34 and CD117; the appearances were found to be the result of alcohol abuse and infection [32].

Acute leukaemia of ambiguous lineage

The 2008 WHO classification includes a group of acute leukaemias regarded as 'of ambiguous

208   CHAPTER 4

Table 4.5 Acute leukaemias of ambiguous lineage including mixed phenotype acute leukaemia (MPAL)[33].

Designation	Usual lineages
Acute undifferentiated leukaemia	Does not express myeloperoxidase, esterase, cCD3, cCD22, cCD79a or strong CD19
MPAL with t(9;22) (q34;q11.2) and *BCR-ABL1* fusion	B, myeloid; less often T, myeloid or B, T, myeloid
MPAL with t(v;11) (v;q23) and *MLL* rearrangement	B, myeloid (usually B, monoblastic)
MPAL, B/myeloid, NOS	B, myeloid
MPAL, T/myeloid, NOS	T, myeloid
MPAL, NOS – rare types	T, B or T, B, myeloid
NK cell lymphoblastic leukaemia/lymphoma	Expresses CD56 and CD7 or CD2 or, occasionally, cCD3

c, cytoplasmic; NK, natural killer; NOS, not otherwise specified.

lineage', which includes conditions previously designated 'biphenotypic' and 'bilineage' acute leukaemia. New diagnostic criteria have been proposed [33]. These rare conditions are summarized in Table 4.5 [33].

The myelodysplastic syndromes

As discussed at the beginning of this chapter, the myelodysplastic syndromes are diseases resulting from a clonal haemopoietic disorder characterized by dysplastic, ineffective haemopoiesis. There is thus often a discrepancy between a hypercellular bone marrow and peripheral cytopenia. In any one patient, different haemopoietic lineages are not necessarily affected to the same degree and there may be defective production of cells of one lineage while in another lineage normal numbers of cells are produced. There may even be increased production of cells of one or more lineages – for

example, neutrophils, monocytes or platelets – despite other features typical of MDS. In some instances this is sufficient to lead to classification as a myelodysplastic/myeloproliferative neoplasm.

The MDS are predominantly diseases of the elderly with an incidence of the order of 3–12 per 100000 per year. They are more frequent in men than in women and more frequent in white Americans than black or Asian Americans [34].

Clinical features of MDS result from the various cytopenias; there may be haemorrhage, susceptibility to infections and symptoms of anaemia. Some patients have hepatomegaly and splenomegaly. MDS show a tendency to evolve into higher grade MDS and AML. Most cases of MDS are apparently primary but a minority are secondary to exposure of the bone marrow to known mutagens, such as alkylating agents. There are some differences in laboratory and clinical features between primary MDS and t-MDS.

Diagnosis of MDS requires consideration of clinical, peripheral blood, bone marrow and cytogenetic features. Peripheral blood and bone marrow aspirate findings are most important and, in a straightforward case, may be all that is required for diagnosis. Bone marrow trephine biopsy in general offers only supplementary information; however, sometimes it is necessary for confirmation of the diagnosis, for example, when an excess of blasts or an abnormal localization of blasts is detected in a patient who has other features suggestive but not diagnostic of MDS. Bone marrow trephine biopsy is particularly important in patients with a hypocellular marrow including some patients with t-MDS, in whom a hypocellular bone marrow with increased fibrosis often leads to a non-diagnostic aspirate. In some patients, a firm diagnosis cannot be made on cytological and histological features alone but diagnosis is possible when these are supplemented by cytogenetic analysis or other tests giving information about clonality. An iron stain should be performed in all patients with suspected MDS; this demonstrates any ring sideroblasts as well as permitting an assessment of iron stores. An MPO or SBB stain should be performed at least in all patients with any increase in blasts and preferably in all patients; this will facilitate the detection of Auer rods, which are of importance both in diagnosis and in classification.

The MDS are a heterogeneous group of disorders with very variable prognoses. They can be divided into various disease categories which have more uniform clinicopathological characteristics. For several decades the most widely used categorization was that proposed by the FAB group [1,2,5,35] (Table 4.6) but this has now been supplanted by the WHO classification [36,37] (Table 4.7). The most important difference between the FAB and WHO classifications is that the latter uses 20% (rather than 30%) blast cells in the peripheral blood or bone marrow as the general criterion for a diagnosis of AML rather than MDS. In addition, the RAEB-T category (refractory anaemia with excess of blasts in transformation) has been abolished and chronic myelomonocytic leukaemia (CMML) (see page 280) has been assigned to a new group of disorders designated MDS/MPN rather than to MDS. There are a considerable number of other, more minor, changes.

Some morphological abnormalities are characteristic of MDS, without being specific for this diag-

nosis, while others show sufficient specificity to be useful in confirming the diagnosis. Although the MDS are heterogeneous they also have many features in common. We shall therefore describe these syndromes as a group before discussing specific WHO categories.

Peripheral blood

Anaemia is seen in the great majority of patients. Red cells are usually normochromic and either normocytic or macrocytic. In patients with sideroblastic erythropoiesis there is commonly a dimorphic blood film with a mixture of a minority population of hypochromic microcytes and a majority population of normochromic cells which are either normocytic or, more often, macrocytic. Pappenheimer bodies, the nature of which can be confirmed with an iron stain, may be present. Microcytosis is seen in certain rare variants including acquired haemoglobin H disease. Some patients have occasional circulating erythroblasts, which may include dys-

Table 4.6 The FAB classification of the myelodysplastic syndromes [1,2,5,35].

Category	Peripheral blood			Bone marrow
Refractory anaemia (RA) or cytopenia	Anaemia* Blasts ≤1% Monocytes ≤1 × 10⁹/l		*and*	Blasts <5%, ringed refractory sideroblasts ≤15% of erythroblasts
Refractory anaemia with ringed sideroblasts (RARS)	Anaemia Blasts ≤1% Monocytes ≤1 × 10⁹/l		*and*	Blasts <5%, ringed sideroblasts >15% of erythroblasts
Refractory anaemia with excess of blasts (RAEB)	Anaemia Blasts >1% Blasts <5% Monocytes ≤1 × 10⁹/l		*or* *and*	Blasts ≥5% Blasts ≤20%
Chronic myelomonocytic leukaemia (CMML)	Blasts <5% Monocytes >1 × 10⁹/l Granulocytes often increased		*and*	Blasts ≤20%, promonocytes often increased
Refractory anaemia with excess of blasts in transformation (RAEB-T)	Blasts ≥5%	*or*	Auer rods in blasts in *or* blood or marrow	Blasts >20% *but* <30%

*Or in the case of refractory cytopenia, either neutropenia or thrombocytopenia.

plastic forms such as megaloblasts and, in patients with sideroblastic erythropoiesis, ring sideroblasts.

Neutropenia is common, particularly in RAEB. Neutrophils often show dysplastic features including reduced granulation and the acquired or pseudo-Pelger–Huët anomaly. Hypogranular and

Table 4.7 The WHO classification of *de novo* myelodysplastic syndromes [36,37].

Refractory cytopenia with unilineage dysplasia (RCUD)
Refractory anaemia (RA)
Refractory neutropenia (RN)
Refractory thrombocytopenia (RT)
Refractory anaemia with ring sideroblasts (RARS)
Refractory cytopenia with multilineage dysplasia (RCMD)*
Refractory anaemia with excess blasts 1 (RAEB-1)
Refractory anaemia with excess blasts 2 (RAEB-2)
Myelodysplastic syndrome, unclassified (MDS-U)
Myelodysplastic syndrome with isolated del(5q)
Provisional entity: refractory cytopenia of childhood (RCC)†

*With or without ring sideroblasts.
†Includes cases meeting criteria for RCMD but not cases that in adults would be classified as RAEB.

agranular neutrophils (Fig. 4.62) indicate defective formation of secondary granules; agranular neutrophils are highly specific for MDS [38]. The acquired Pelger–Huët anomaly refers to hypolobulation of nuclei associated with dense chromatin clumping (Fig. 4.62); nuclei of mature neutrophils may be completely non-lobed, dumb-bell or peanut-shaped, or bilobed with their shape resembling a pair of spectacles. This abnormality resembles the inherited Pelger–Huët anomaly, hence its name. The acquired anomaly is highly characteristic of MDS and almost pathognomonic [38]. Eosinophil and basophil counts are commonly reduced but, in a small minority of patients, are increased; dysplastic forms with abnormalities of either nuclear shape or cytoplasmic granulation can occur. Monocytosis is sometimes present and monocytes may show cytological abnormalities such as increased cytoplasmic basophilia or nuclei of unusual shape. Blast cells may be present in the peripheral blood in all categories of MDS but particularly in RAEB. They usually have the cytological features of myeloblasts with scanty cytoplasm and few granules. Auer rods are sometimes present. Other granulocyte precursors are quite uncommon in the peripheral blood.

The platelet count is usually either normal or reduced, although in a minority of patients it is increased. Dysplastic features that may be noted in platelets include hypogranular and agranular forms ('grey' platelets) and giant platelets.

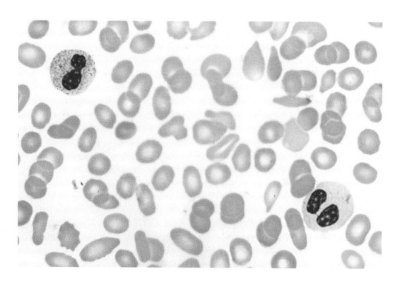

Fig. 4.62 PB film from a patient with MDS, showing anisocytosis, poikilocytosis and two pseudo-Pelger–Huët neutrophils, one of which is also hypogranular. MGG ×100.

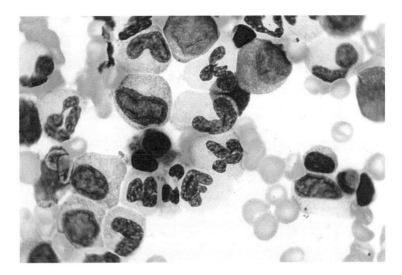

Fig. 4.63 BM aspirate, FAB RA category (WHO RCMD category), showing a binucleate micromegakaryocyte which is budding platelets. MGG ×100.

Patients with MDS have an increased incidence of autoimmune thrombocytopenia [39].

Bone marrow cytology

The bone marrow is hypercellular in the majority of patients but is sometimes normocellular and in about 10% of patients is hypocellular. Hypercellularity may be due to increased erythroid or granulocytic precursors or both. Hypocellularity is more frequent in t-MDS and in MDS following benzene [40].

Erythropoiesis may be normoblastic, macronormoblastic or megaloblastic. In patients with sideroblastic erythropoiesis there are some erythroblasts with poorly haemoglobinized or vacuolated cytoplasm. Other dysplastic features may include binuclearity and multinuclearity, internuclear bridges, nuclear lobulation, irregularity or fragmentation of nuclei, gigantism, increased pyknosis and basophilic stippling. The bone marrow erythroid component (calculated from cellularity and the percentage of erythroblasts) has been found predictive of response to therapy with erythropoietin plus granulocyte–macrophage colony-stimulating factor (GM-CSF) [41].

Granulopoiesis is usually increased. Granulocyte precursors may be increased in relation to mature cells. Defects of granulation may be apparent from the promyelocyte stage onwards and defects of nuclear lobulation may also be present.

Megakaryocyte numbers are usually normal or increased but sometimes decreased. One of the features most specific for MDS is the presence of micromegakaryocytes [38], cells of about the size of a myeloblast with one or two small round nuclei (Fig. 4.63). Megakaryocytes may also be of normal size but have a large non-lobated nucleus (Fig. 4.64); this abnormality is less specific for MDS but is characteristic of cases with 5q– as an acquired chromosomal abnormality [42]. Other megakaryocyte abnormalities include bizarre nuclear shapes and the presence of multiple separate nuclei. Poor granulation of megakaryocyte cytoplasm is also common in the MDS and has been found to be highly specific [43].

The bone marrow aspirate may show non-specific abnormalities such as increased numbers of macrophages, sea-blue histiocytes, lymphocytes, plasma cells or mast cells.

Cytochemistry

The cytochemical stain of most value is an iron stain. This should be performed in all cases of suspected MDS, in order to quantify iron stores and to detect and enumerate ring sideroblasts and other abnormal sideroblasts. Ring sideroblasts have iron-positive granules in a circle close to the nuclear membrane (Fig. 4.65). In the WHO classification the defining criteria for a ring sideroblast are that there are at least five granules around at least a

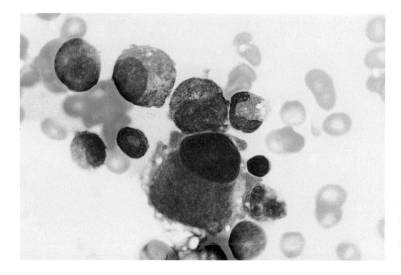

Fig. 4.64 BM aspirate, FAB RA category (WHO MDS with isolated del(5q) category), 5q– syndrome, showing a megakaryocyte of normal size with a hypolobated nucleus. MGG ×100.

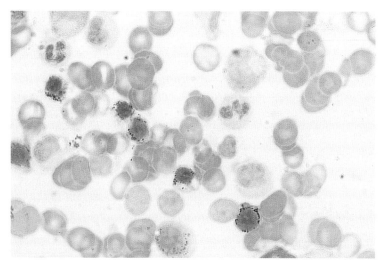

Fig. 4.65 BM aspirate, FAB RARS category (WHO RARS category), showing numerous ring sideroblasts, several of which can be seen to have defectively haemoglobinized cytoplasm. Perls' stain ×100.

third of the nuclear circumference [44]. Other abnormal sideroblasts have scattered iron-positive granules which are both larger and more numerous than those of normal sideroblasts. Ring sideroblasts are highly suggestive of MDS if the other known causes of sideroblastic erythropoiesis (see page 462) can be eliminated. Abnormal sideroblasts other than ring sideroblasts are common both in MDS and in other disorders of erythropoiesis and so are not useful in the differential diagnosis of suspected MDS. Other cytochemical stains are of use in identifying abnormal cells of megakaryocyte lineages and in characterizing blasts. MPO and SBB stains will identify myeloblasts and facilitate the detection of Auer rods and may also show cells of the neutrophil lineage to have defective primary granules. Non-specific esterase stains are useful for identifying monoblasts and promonocytes; NSE and PAS stains can be useful for identifying abnormal megakaryocytes.

Bone marrow histology

In the majority of cases the marrow is hypercellular (Fig. 4.66), but in a significant minority it is hypocellular [45,46]. There may be considerable variation of the cellularity between adjacent

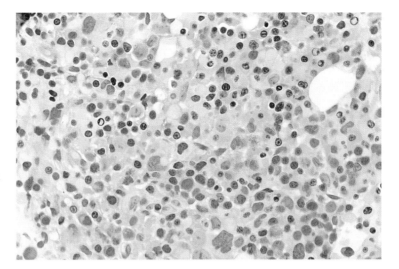

Fig. 4.66 BM trephine biopsy section, FAB RA category (WHO RCMD category), showing marked hypercellularity with disorganization of haemopoiesis and marked dyserythropoiesis. Note the apoptotic erythroblasts with peripheral condensation of their nuclear chromatin. Resin-embedded, H&E ×40.

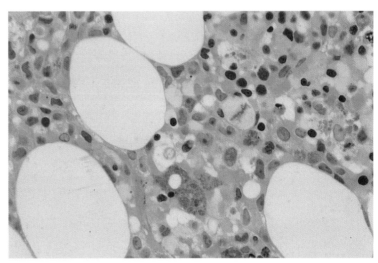

Fig. 4.67 BM trephine biopsy section, FAB RAEB-T category (WHO AML), showing increased numbers of blasts forming a small cluster (centre) (an abnormal localization of immature precursors or ALIP). Resin-embedded, H&E ×100.

intertrabecular spaces [47]. In addition to cytological evidence of dysplasia, there is derangement of normal architecture. In histological sections, dysplasia is most obvious in the erythroid precursors and megakaryocytes; however, the acquired Pelger–Huët anomaly can be detected in good quality sections of paraffin-embedded material and, in good resin-embedded material, Auer rods may also be identified. Disturbance of normal architecture results in groups of granulocytic precursors being found in the central parts of intertrabecular spaces (Fig. 4.67), referred to as 'abnormal localization of immature precursors' (ALIP), and erythroid precursors and megakaryocytes being in the para-

trabecular regions. Erythroblastic islands may be poorly formed or very large. The cells within clusters sometimes appear abnormally uniform, as if arrested in maturation, and there may be discrepancy between adjacent clusters showing maturation apparently synchronized at different stages. Erythroid precursors may be multinucleated or show nuclear budding or fragmentation, megaloblastic change or cytoplasmic vacuolation (Fig. 4.68). Megakaryocytic dysplasia is present in the vast majority of cases and is usually more apparent in histological sections than in marrow films. Megakaryocytes are usually increased in number and clustering is often seen (Fig. 4.69). Typically

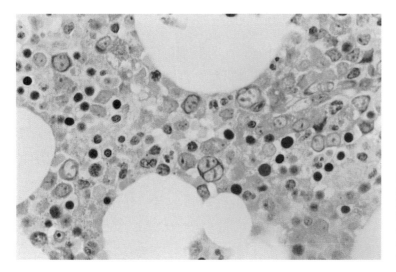

Fig. 4.68 BM trephine biopsy section in MDS showing numerous immature erythroid cells including a binucleate form; the erythroblasts are not grouped into a compact erythroid island. Paraffin-embedded, Giemsa ×100.

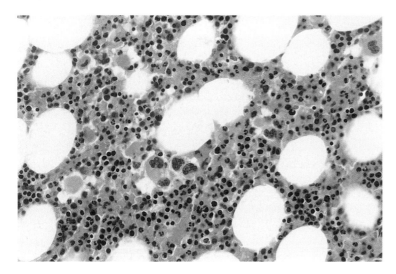

Fig. 4.69 BM trephine biopsy section, FAB RA category (WHO RCMD category), showing an aggregate of dysplastic megakaryocytes. Paraffin-embedded, H&E ×20.

they have hypolobated nuclei, which are often hyperchromatic. Small dysplastic megakaryocytes, including micromegakaryocytes, can be detected [46,48] but they are seen more readily in aspirate films than in H&E-stained trephine biopsy sections. Increased emperipolesis may be apparent [49]. Some patients have multinucleated megakaryocytes (Fig. 4.70). Immunohistochemical staining for CD42b and CD61 may be used to accentuate abnormal megakaryocytes [50] (Fig. 4.71) and is particularly useful for the detection of micromegakaryocytes. Increased numbers of apoptotic erythroid and granulocytic precursors, reflecting ineffective haemopoiesis, are often seen [51] (see

Fig. 4.66). In a minority of cases, haemopoietic cells, particularly megakaryocytes, are present within sinusoids [49]. Reticulin fibrosis has been reported in a fifth [52] to almost a half [46] of cases of MDS, as defined by the FAB group. It is more common in CMML (now designated MDS/MPN) than in other FAB subtypes [46,52]. The presence of reticulin fibrosis correlates with megakaryocyte numbers and atypia [52]. Severe collagen fibrosis is rare in all subtypes [46,52]; it is seen most often in t-MDS. Reticulin fibrosis correlates with unfavourable cytogenetic abnormalities and is indicative of a worse prognosis. Other non-specific reactions are commonly seen including oedema,

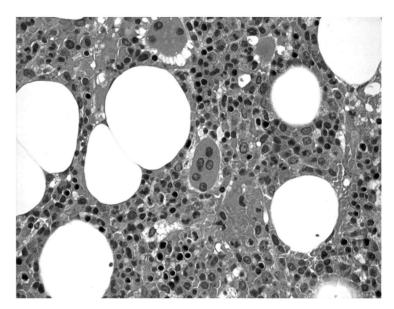

Fig. 4.70 BM trephine biopsy section, MDS (WHO RCMD category) showing a hypercellular marrow with two multinucleated megakaryocytes. Paraffin-embedded, H&E ×20.

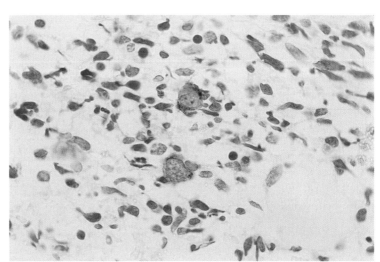

Fig. 4.71 BM trephine biopsy section, therapy-related MDS, showing small dysplastic megakaryocytes. Paraffin-embedded, immunoperoxidase for CD61 ×100.

ectasia of sinusoids, increased numbers of plasma cells and increased numbers of lymphoid follicles. Haemosiderin-laden macrophages are a frequent finding, particularly in patients who have received transfusions.

One feature that has been the subject of much debate is the significance of ALIP, the presence of small groups of immature granulocytic precursors (promyelocytes and myeloblasts) in a central position within intertrabecular spaces (see Fig. 4.67). Some studies have found this phenomenon to be an independent predictor of prognosis and to be associated with an increased incidence of leukaemic transformation [53]. Although ALIP is more frequent in the subtypes of myelodysplasia with increased numbers of blasts in the marrow, several studies have failed to confirm any independent influence on prognosis [46,47,54]. Others, however, have confirmed prognostic significance independent of the blast percentage in an aspirate [49] or in histological sections [55]. It should be noted that it can be difficult, particularly in paraffin-embedded sections, to distinguish between small groups of immature erythroid precursors and the clusters of immature cells of granulocytic lineage that constitute ALIP. Immunohistochemistry can be useful. Other histological features found to be of poor prognostic significance, in a study using multivariate analysis, were an elevated blast percentage, increased haemosiderin, megakaryocyte atypia and reduced erythropoiesis, while increased mast cells were of good prognostic significance [55].

Trephine biopsy is particularly important in the diagnosis of hypoplastic MDS and MDS with fibrosis, in both of which an aspirate can be misleading. The former diagnosis is clinically important since there may be a response to anti-thymocyte globulin.

Flow cytometric immunophenotyping

In higher grade MDS there may be an increase in precursor cells that are positive for CD34, CD117 or both; these immature cells are usually also positive for CD38. In general there is a correlation between the percentage of blast cells and the percentage of cells expressing CD34. Immunophenotyping can be used to confirm the lineage of any blast cells. If a large panel of monoclonal antibodies is used, and if the laboratory is familiar with normal patterns and the changes that occur in reactive conditions, flow cytometry can also provide evidence of dysplasia; underexpression or over-expression of antigens or aberrant antigen expression on cells of granulocyte, monocyte or erythroid lineage may be detected.

Immunohistochemistry

The value of immunohistochemistry in MDS can be summarized as follows:

1 Abnormal topography can be highlighted, e.g. the presence of ALIP or the presence of erythroid cells or megakaryocytes in a paratrabecular position.

2 Immature granulocyte lineage cells that constitute ALIP can be distinguished from clusters of immature erythroid cells (Fig. 4.72), using antibodies such as CD68, anti-MPO and anti-neutrophil elastase antibodies, to identify immature granulocytic cells, and antibodies reactive with glycophorin or spectrin to identify early erythroid cells.

3 Abnormally large erythroid islands can be identified very easily and the altered maturation of cells within and between islands is highlighted.

4 Micromegakaryocytes can be identified and the presence of megakaryocyte clustering or dysplasia highlighted by immunohistochemistry for CD42b and CD61 (see Fig. 4.71).

5 Diagnostic and prognostic information can be gained by the use of CD34 antibodies (Fig. 4.73): the presence of more than 5% CD34-positive cells may be useful in distinguishing patients with and without MDS [56]; the presence of more than 1% CD34-positive cells indicates a worse prognosis in

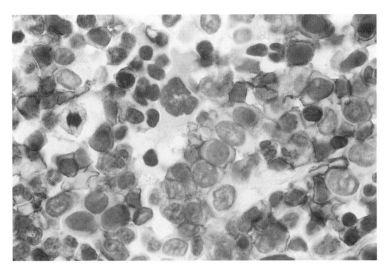

Fig. 4.72 Trephine biopsy section from a patient with FAB RARS category (WHO RARS category) of MDS showing a clump of early erythroid cells that can be distinguished from an ALIP by their weak but definite reaction with anti-glycophorin. Paraffin-embedded, immunoperoxidase anti-glycophorin ×100.

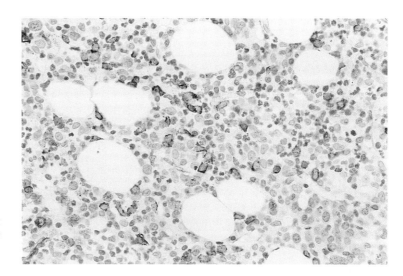

Fig. 4.73 Trephine biopsy section from a patient with RAEB showing numerous CD34-positive immature cells. Paraffin-embedded, immunoperoxidase CD34 ×40.

MDS as a whole and within the RAEB category [57]; clusters of CD34-positive cells are predictive of progression in refractory anaemia [56] and of leukaemic transformation [57]; and CD34 is important in identifying blast cells in MDS with fibrosis.
6 The distinction from reactive conditions can be facilitated with anti-MPL antibodies, which may show reduced expression in MDS [58]; however, such antibodies have not become generally available for diagnostic use.
7 The distinction between hypocellular MDS and aplastic anaemia can be facilitated (see below).

Cytogenetic and molecular genetic analysis
The cytogenetic abnormalities associated with MDS are heterogeneous. The most characteristic abnormalities are monosomies, deletions and unbalanced translocations. Abnormalities often observed include monosomy 5, monosomy 7, trisomy 8, del(5q), del(7q), del(9q) and del(20q). In MDS related to alkylating agents, monosomies and deletions of chromosomes 5 and 7 are common, whereas MDS related to topoisomerase-II-interactive drugs is characterized by balanced translocations with 3q26, 11q23 and 21q22 breakpoints.

Clonal cytogenetic abnormalities can confirm the diagnosis of MDS when cytological abnormalities are not definitive. The abnormalities that are accepted in the WHO classification as providing presumptive evidence of MDS are shown in Table 4.8 [36]. The type of abnormality found is also of

Table 4.8 Cytogenetic abnormalities that provide presumptive evidence of myelodysplastic syndrome (MDS) if detected in a patient with refractory cytopenia[36].*

Unbalanced (in order of frequency)	Balanced
–7 or del(7q)	t(11;16)(q23;p13.3)†
–5 or del(5q)	t(3;21)(q26.2;q22.1)†
i(17q) or t(17p)	t(1;3)(p36.3;q21.2)
–13 or del(13q)	t(2;11)(p21;q23)
del(11q)	inv(3)(q21.6q26.2)
del(12p) or t(12p)	t(6;9)(p23;q34)
del(9q)	
idic(X)(q13)	

*−Y, +8 and del(20q) are not accepted as presumptive evidence of MDS in the WHO classification.
†Mainly associated with therapy-related MDS, in which diagnostic difficulty is not likely to occur.

prognostic significance. Isolated del(5q) is prognostically good whereas complex karyotypes and 17p– (which correlates with granulocyte dysplasia and *TP53* loss) are prognostically adverse.

MDS is typically associated with multiple oncogenic events, the formation of fusion genes, mutations of oncogenes and both mutation and loss of cancer-suppressing genes. Genes that may be mutated include *NRAS*, *TP53*, *IRF1*, *BCL2*, *CDKN2B* (*p15^{INK4b}*), *EVI1* and *MLL*.

Table 4.9 International Prognostic Scoring System (IPSS) of the International Myelodysplastic Syndrome Working Group (updated to exclude a score for 20–30% blast cells since such cases are no longer regarded as MDS) [59].* (Reprinted by permission of *Blood*, **89**, 2079–2088, 1997.)

	Score			
Prognostic variables	0	0.5	1.0	1.5
Blasts (%)	<5%	5–10	–	11–19
Karyotype†	Good	Intermediate	Poor	
Cytopenias‡	0–1	2–3		

*Individual scores are summed and cases are then assigned to four risk groups, indicative of an increasingly bad prognosis. A score of 0 is indicative of low risk; a score of 1 is indicative of intermediate risk 1; a score of 1.5–2.0 is indicative of intermediate risk 2; a score of ≥2.5 is indicative of high risk.
†Good prognosis karyotype: normal, −Y, del(5q), del(20q). Poor prognosis karyotype: complex (≥3 abnormalities) or chromosome 7 abnormalities. Intermediate prognosis karyotype: other abnormalities.
‡Cytopenias: Hb <100 g/l, neutrophil count <1.5 × 10⁹/l, platelet count <100 × 10⁹/l.

*Cytopenias: Hb $<100\,g/l$, neutrophil count $<1.5 \times 10^9/l$, platelet count $<100 \times 10^9/l$.

Determining prognosis

Since MDS is an extremely heterogeneous disorder, establishing a diagnosis is just the first step in the clinical management of patients. It is important also to make an assessment of prognosis. The most widely accepted scheme is that of the International Myelodysplastic Syndrome Working Group [59] (Table 4.9).

The WHO classification of the myelodysplastic syndromes

The WHO classification requires examination of peripheral blood and bone marrow aspirate films, a 200-cell peripheral blood differential count, a 500-cell differential count of the bone marrow (on an aspirate film or a trephine biopsy imprint) and a Perls' stain of a bone marrow film [36]. To assess the presence or absence of dysplasia it is advised that cytological features of at least 200 neutrophils and precursors, 200 erythroid precursors and 30 megakaryocytes (in films or sections) be assessed. Cytogenetic analysis is also necessary in order to recognize 'myelodysplastic syndrome with isolated del(5q)' and to assign cases with t(8;21), inv(16), t(16;16) and t(15;17) to the diagnostic category of AML rather than MDS. A diagnosis of MDS is made when cases fit the criteria for the individual WHO subtypes and when the patient has not been exposed to cytotoxic chemotherapy or

BOX 4.1

Diagnostic criteria for refractory cytopenia with unilineage dysplasia

- Unicytopenia (anaemia, neutropenia or thrombocytopenia) or bicytopenia
- Dysplasia in at least 10% of cells of one myeloid lineage (not necessarily the lineage that is cytopenic)
- No blasts or rare blasts (<1%) in the blood
- Bone marrow blasts <5%
- Bone marrow ring sideroblasts <15%

irradiation. Patients who meet the criteria for MDS but have been exposed to such genotoxic agents are categorized as therapy-related MDS and are grouped with therapy-related AML.

Refractory cytopenia with unilineage dysplasia

Refractory cytopenia with unilineage dysplasia (RCUD) constitutes 10–20% of cases of MDS. Patients are usually middle aged or elderly. Prognosis is relatively good with a median survival of more than 5 years and a low rate of transformation to AML [60]. Diagnostic criteria are shown in Box 4.1. Refractory anaemia (RA) is the most common form of RCUD but a minority of patients

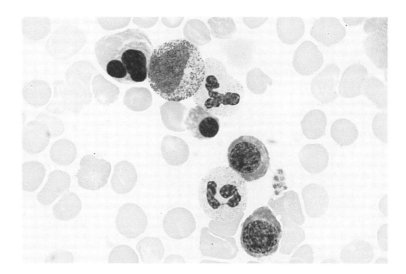

Fig. 4.74 BM aspirate, WHO RA category, showing erythroid hyperplasia and hypogranular neutrophils; note a dysplastic binucleated erythroblast. MGG ×100.

have refractory neutropenia or refractory thrombocytopenia. If there is no clonal cytogenetic abnormality, it is important to exclude other diseases and deficiency states that could cause secondary dysplasia with associated cytopenia. If there is doubt as to the diagnosis the patient should be regarded as having 'idiopathic cytopenia of undetermined significance' rather than MDS.

Peripheral blood

Often morphological and numerical abnormalities are confined to the erythroid series but some patients have bicytopenia. Red cells are usually normochromic and either normocytic or macrocytic with variable anisocytosis and poikilocytosis. Dysplasia is confined to a single myeloid lineage, which is usually but not necessarily the same lineage that manifests cytopenia. A minority of patients have thrombocytosis but the count is less than 450×10^9/l. In patients with refractory neutropenia there may be dysplastic features such as hypolobation and hypogranularity.

Bone marrow cytology

The bone marrow is usually hypercellular as a result of increased erythropoiesis (Fig. 4.74). A minority of patients show marked erythroid hypoplasia, sometimes with an apparent arrest of erythropoiesis at the proerythroblast stage. Erythropoiesis usually shows dysplastic features. Ring sideroblasts

may be present but constitute less than 15% of erythroblasts.

In RA the granulocyte series and megakaryocytes may be apparently normal or may be quantitatively increased or dysplastic (as long as only one myeloid lineage is dysplastic). In refractory neutropenia there is usually dysgranulopoiesis and in refractory thrombocytopenia dysplastic megakaryocytes (hypolobated, binucleated or multinucleated).

Bone marrow histology

There are often no histological features of diagnostic importance in trephine biopsy specimens of patients with RCUD. The marrow is usually hypercellular but hypocellular forms do occur. Increased erythropoiesis and dyserythropoiesis are usually present and are easily seen in tissue sections (see Fig. 4.66). The granulocytic series may appear relatively normal. Dysplastic megakaryocytes may be present but if these are more than 10% and erythropoiesis is also dysplastic the diagnosis become refractory cytopenia with multilineage dysplasia. The number of CD34-positive cells is normal.

Cytogenetic analysis

Clonal cytogenetic abnormalities may be present and may include del(20q), trisomy 8 and abnormalities of chromosome 5, chromosome 7 or both. Abnormalities of chromosome 5 can include del(5q) but not as an isolated anomaly.

Refractory anaemia with ring sideroblasts

Refractory anaemia with ring sideroblasts (RARS) has also been referred to as primary acquired sideroblastic anaemia. It constitutes about 10% of cases of MDS. Diagnostic criteria are shown in Box 4.2. Patients are mainly middle aged or elderly. Prognosis is relatively good with a low rate of leukaemic transformation [44]. Refractory anaemia with ring sideroblasts is usually either an incidental diagnosis in the elderly or is diagnosed because of symptoms of anaemia. It is important to exclude drug toxicity, lead poisoning and copper deficiency when considering a diagnosis of RARS. This subtype of MDS is very rare in children and if it is suspected an alternative diagnosis, e.g. a mitochondrial cytopathy or congenital sideroblastic anaemia, should be considered.

Peripheral blood

There is anaemia which is sometimes normocytic but more often macrocytic. The film is dimorphic,

---

BOX 4.2

Diagnostic criteria for refractory anaemia with ring sideroblasts

- Anaemia or bicytopenia
- No blasts in the blood
- Bone marrow blasts <5%
- Bone marrow ring sideroblasts at least 15% and other dyserythropoietic features may be present

---

consequent on the presence of a minor population of hypochromic and microcytic red cells. Occasional cells contain Pappenheimer bodies. There may be a small number of circulating erythroblasts, among which may be some ring sideroblasts. Abnormalities of neutrophils and platelets can occur but are uncommon and, if present, are seen in fewer than 10% of cells. A significant minority of patients have thrombocytosis but by definition the platelet count is less than 450×10^9/l.

Bone marrow cytology

The bone marrow is usually hypercellular and shows increased erythropoiesis. Erythropoiesis is usually normoblastic or macronormoblastic. A proportion of erythroblasts, which correspond to the ring sideroblasts, are micronormoblasts or show defective haemoglobinization or cytoplasmic vacuolation (Fig. 4.75). Basophilic stippling may be present. Other dysplastic features in red cells may be present. Abnormalities can occur in other lineages but they are uncommon and by definition are present in less than 10% of cells.

An iron stain shows that at least 15% of erythroblasts are ring sideroblasts (see Fig. 4.65). These cells are defined as erythroblasts in which there are at least five iron-containing granules surrounding at least a third of the nuclear circumference. Up to 70% or 80% of erythroblasts may be ring sideroblasts and they may be associated with other abnormal sideroblasts. Iron stores are commonly increased.

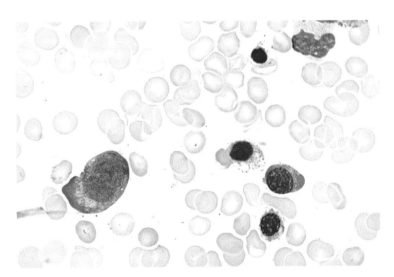

Fig. 4.75 BM aspirate, WHO RARS category, showing five erythroblasts, two of which show defectively haemoglobinized, heavily granulated cytoplasm. MGG ×100.

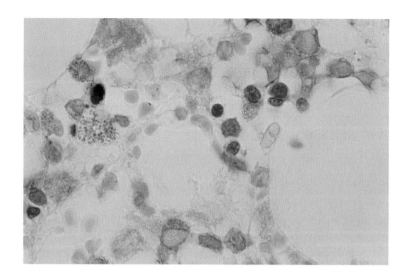

Fig. 4.76 BM clot section, WHO RARS category, showing two ring sideroblasts with blue iron-containing granules arranged around the nucleus. Paraffin-embedded, Perls' stain ×100.

Bone marrow histology

Trephine biopsy is not usually very useful in the diagnosis of RARS. Bone marrow histology may be relatively normal with the only abnormality being increased erythropoiesis with large, poorly formed erythroid islands. There is often an increase in stainable iron within macrophages. Ring sideroblasts can be seen in resin-embedded sections of trephine biopsies and occasionally in paraffin-embedded sections of marrow clot sections (Fig. 4.76); they are not visible in sections of paraffin-embedded or other decalcified trephine biopsy specimens. The granulocytic series is usually normal. Dysplastic megakaryocytes are present in a minority of cases but by definition are below 10%. The number of CD34-positive cells is normal.

Cytogenetic analysis

Clonal cytogenetic abnormalities are present in a minority of patients. They are usually single aberrations.

Refractory cytopenia with multilineage dysplasia

Refractory cytopenia with multilineage dysplasia (RCMD) constitutes around 30% of MDS. Diagnostic criteria are shown in Box 4.3. Patients are most often elderly. Median survival is about 30 months, with about 10% of patients showing transformation to AML by 30 months [61].

BOX 4.3

Diagnostic criteria for refractory cytopenia with multilineage dysplasia

- Cytopenia
- No blasts or rare blasts (<1%) in the blood
- Bone marrow blasts <5%
- No Auer rods
- Dysplasia in at least 10% of cells of at least two myeloid lineages
- Ring sideroblasts may be 15% or more of bone marrow erythroblasts, or not

---

Peripheral blood

There is a normocytic or macrocytic anaemia. Anisocytosis and poikilocytosis may be marked. Granulocytic dysplasia is common, usually some combination of hypogranularity, hypolobation (acquired Pelger–Huët anomaly) and abnormal chromatin clumping.

Bone marrow cytology

The bone marrow is usually hypercellular with bilineage or trilineage dysplasia. Some patients have 15% or more ring sideroblasts.

Bone marrow histology

Trephine biopsy sections show bilineage or trilineage dysplasia. The content of CD34-positive early haemopoietic cells is normal.

Cytogenetic analysis

Clonal cytogenetic abnormalities are common. These may include del(20q), trisomy 8, abnormalities of chromosomes 5 or 7 or both and complex cytogenetic abnormalities. Abnormalities of chromosome 5 can include del(5q) but not as an isolated anomaly. Patients with a complex karyotype have a worse prognosis than other patients.

Refractory anaemia with excess of blasts

Refractory anaemia with excess of blasts (RAEB) comprises about 40% of cases of MDS [62] and is divided into RAEB-1 and RAEB-2 on the basis of the number of blasts cells and the presence or absence of Auer rods. *De novo* MDS with fibrosis (MDS-F) is usually a variant of RAEB. Diagnostic criteria are shown in Boxes 4.4 and 4.5. Patients are usually middle aged or elderly. Diagnosis usually follows the development of symptoms of anaemia or the occurrence of bruising, bleeding or infection. Some patients have splenomegaly. Prognosis is poor, due either to bone marrow failure or transformation to AML (estimated to occur in a quarter of RAEB-1 patients and a third with RAEB-2). The worst prognosis is seen in those RAEB-2 patients who have 11–19% bone marrow blast cells; they have a median survival of about 3 months, in comparison with about 12 months in patients in whom a diagnosis of RAEB-2 is based on other criteria [62].

Peripheral blood

The peripheral blood shows normocytic or macrocytic anaemia, sometimes with a minor population of hypochromic microcytes. Anisocytosis and poikilocytosis are often marked. Neutropenia and thrombocytopenia are common. Monocytes may be increased but by definition are less than 1×10^9/l. Some blast cells are usually present. Dysplastic features in neutrophils, neutrophil precursors and platelets are commonly present. Dysplastic changes in the neutrophil lineage may include hypogranularity of neutrophils or precursors, hypolobation of neutrophils, increased chromatin clumping of neutrophils or precursors, abnormally long filaments between nuclear lobes and pseudo-Chédiak–Higashi granules or Auer rods in blast cells. Platelet changes include platelet anisocytosis and large and hypogranular platelets.

Bone marrow cytology

The bone marrow is usually hypercellular. Any or all lineages may be increased and trilineage dysplasia is common. The percentage of blasts is usually increased, although a case may qualify to be categorized as RAEB on the basis of increased peripheral blood blasts or Auer rods without an increase in bone marrow blasts. Erythropoiesis may be sideroblastic but, because of the excess of blasts, the case is nevertheless categorized as RAEB rather than as RARS.

BOX 4.4

Diagnostic criteria for refractory anaemia with excess of blasts 1

- Cytopenia
- Monocyte count <1 × 10⁹/l
- No Auer rods
- Dysplasia in at least 10% of cells of one or more myeloid lineages *and*

  either

  Peripheral blood blast cells 2–4% and bone marrow blast cells <5%

  or

  Bone marrow blast cells 5–9%

BOX 4.5

Diagnostic criteria for refractory anaemia with excess of blasts 2

- Cytopenia
- Monocyte count <1 × 10⁹/l
- Dysplasia in at least 10% of cells of one or more myeloid lineages *and*

  either

  Peripheral blood blast cells 5–19%

  or

  Bone marrow blast cells 10–19%

  or

  Auer rods present

An iron stain may show ring sideroblasts, other abnormal sideroblasts and increased iron stores. Either an MPO or a SBB stain should be performed routinely both to confirm the lineage of the blasts and to facilitate detection of Auer rods.

In MDS with fibrosis the bone marrow aspirate is usually inadequate for diagnosis.

Bone marrow histology

Bone marrow biopsy is not usually essential for diagnosis but can give useful supplementary information. Histology is usually markedly abnormal. The majority of cases have increased or normal cellularity with only a small number of cases having a hypocellular marrow. Dyserythropoiesis and megakaryocytic dysplasia are seen in almost all cases (Fig. 4.77). Blasts are generally increased in number but it is not uncommon for the percentage of blasts seen in the biopsy sections to be less than that observed in marrow aspirates taken at the same time [46]. With immunohistochemistry, increased numbers of CD34-positive cells are usually readily demonstrable, with counts in the region of 10% or more; ALIP is seen in most cases. Megakaryocytes may be abnormally situated, against the trabeculum.

Myelodysplastic syndrome with fibrosis is diagnosed when there is accompanying coarse reticulin fibrosis with or without collagen fibrosis. Megakaryocytes are often increased and conspicuously dysplastic. Since the bone marrow aspirate is often inadequate, a trephine biopsy is important in the diagnosis of MDS-F. Immunohistochemistry for CD34 is particularly useful in this variant to identify the increased numbers of immature cells.

Cytogenetic analysis

Clonal cytogenetic abnormalities similar to those observed in RCMD are common.

Myelodysplastic syndrome with isolated del(5q) (the '5q– syndrome')

Myelodysplastic syndrome with isolated del(5q) (often referred to as the 5q– syndrome) is a subtype of MDS characterized by refractory anaemia, hypolobated megakaryocytes and an isolated interstitial deletion of part of the long arm of chromosome 5. Diagnostic criteria are shown in Box 4.6. Patients

---

BOX 4.6

Diagnostic criteria for myelodysplastic syndrome with isolated del(5q)

- Anaemia
- No or rare blast cells in peripheral blood (<1%)
- Blast cells <5% in bone marrow
- No Auer rods
- Isolated del(5q)

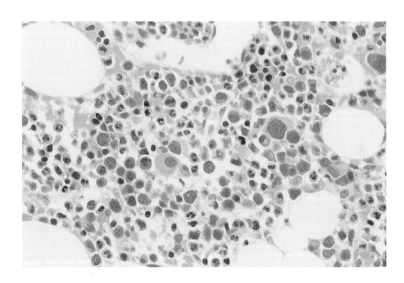

Fig. 4.77 BM trephine biopsy section, WHO RAEB category, showing dysplastic megakaryocytes including micromegakaryocytes. Resin-embedded, H&E ×40.

tend to be middle aged or elderly with a female predominance and a relatively good prognosis.

Peripheral blood

The peripheral blood shows anaemia, which is often macrocytic. There may be a minor population of hypochromic microcytes. There may be cytopenia but usually the white cell count is normal and the platelet count is usually normal or increased.

Bone marrow cytology

The bone marrow is typically hypercellular. Some patients have ring sideroblasts and these may be 15% or more. There are characteristic megakaryocytes; these are more than 30 µm in diameter but have non-lobulated nuclei (see Fig. 4.64).

Bone marrow histology

The bone marrow is usually hypercellular with increased numbers of characteristic hypolobated megakaryocytes. The content of CD34-positive early haemopoietic cells is normal.

Cytogenetic and molecular genetic analysis

The length of the interstitial deletion is variable but there is a common deleted segment. FISH studies show that, although morphological abnormalities may be confined to one or two lineages, this is a trilineage disorder [63]. The essential molecular lesion may be haploinsufficiency of *RPS14* [64].

Myelodysplastic syndrome, unclassified

The criteria for a diagnosis of MDS, unclassified are shown in Box 4.7.

Refractory cytopenia of childhood

Because MDS in childhood has characteristics that differ from MDS in adults the 2008 WHO classification has introduced a provisional entity, refractory cytopenia of childhood (RCC), that constitutes about half of childhood MDS [37]. The WHO criteria are shown in Box 4.8. There appears to be some overlap between RCC and cases that other groups would regard as aplastic anaemia. Furthermore, the presence of congenital abnormalities in some children raises the possibility of a missed diagnosis of a constitutional haematological

abnormality in cases included in this WHO category. Childhood RCMD is incorporated in RCC but cases that meet the criteria of RAEB are categorized as RAEB-1 or RAEB-2.

BOX 4.7

Diagnostic criteria for myelodysplastic syndrome, unclassified (MDS-U)

- Pancytopenia in a patient who would otherwise fit the criteria for RCUD

  or

  Peripheral blood blasts 1% on two occasions in a patient who would otherwise meet the criteria for RCUD or RCMD

  or

  Unequivocal dysplasia is not present in 10% of cells in any lineage but a clonal cytogenetic abnormality giving presumptive evidence of MDS is present (see Table 4.8, page 217)

  and

- Peripheral blood blast cells are not greater than 1%
- Bone marrow blast cells <5%

BOX 4.8

Diagnostic criteria for refractory cytopenia of childhood (refractory cytopenia with multilineage dysplasia included)*

- *History and examination*: inherited bone marrow disorders, Down's syndrome and prior genotoxic therapy are excluded
- *Peripheral blood*: dysplastic changes in at least 10% of neutrophils (unless severe neutropenia), blast cells less than 2%
- *Bone marrow aspirate*: dysplastic changes in at least 10% of cells of at least two myeloid lineages, blast cells less than 5%
- *Trephine biopsy*: erythroid islands with at least 20 cells, maturation arrest with excess of proerythroblasts, increased mitoses in erythroid cells, micromegakaryocytes (on immunohistochemistry) and other dysplastic megakaryocytes (unless megakaryocytes are absent)

*Criteria for RAEB not met and chromosomal rearrangements diagnostic of AML not present.

Peripheral blood

The peripheral blood shows anaemia, which is often macrocytic, and either neutrophil dysplasia or severe neutropenia.

Bone marrow cytology

The bone marrow is hypocellular in about three quarters of patients and shows the features described in Box 4.8.

Bone marrow histology

The bone marrow is hypocellular in about three quarters of patients. Erythropoiesis is dysplastic. Megakaryocytes are either absent or dysplastic.

Cytogenetic analysis

Cytogenetic analysis is usually normal. Some patients have trisomy 8 (associated with a good prognosis). Others have monosomy 7 (the most frequent abnormality) or a complex karyotypic abnormality (both associated with a poor prognosis).

Problems and pitfalls in the diagnosis of myelodysplastic syndromes

Diagnostic errors can result from a failure to assess clinical features, peripheral blood and bone marrow cytology, bone marrow histology and the results of cytogenetic analysis in all cases. Cytology and histology are complementary in the investigation of MDS since sometimes one will give information that could not be gained from the other. For example, ring sideroblasts and neutrophil dysplasia are best detected in an aspirate, whereas ALIP is detected only by means of trephine biopsy. Similarly, it is sometimes cytogenetic analysis that permits an unequivocal diagnosis when other features have been suggestive of MDS but not pathognomonic. If patients have unexplained cytopenia but the criteria for MDS are not met, categorization as idiopathic cytopenia of undetermined significance is appropriate.

Some cases of MDS have pathological features that are strongly suggestive of the diagnosis. In other patients the diagnosis of MDS is a presumptive one, based on the presence of features that are characteristic but not diagnostic. In the latter group

the exclusion of other diagnoses is particularly important. A careful clinical assessment is essential, in order to exclude relevant systemic illness and exposure to drugs, alcohol, heavy metals and growth factors. Some of the non-neoplastic causes of bone marrow dysplasia are discussed on page 500. Important pitfalls are relevant drug exposure that has not been disclosed to the pathologist and unexpected HIV positivity.

If dysplastic features are confined to the erythroid lineages it is important to consider alternative causes of dyserythropoiesis such as the congenital dyserythropoietic anaemias and various thalassaemic conditions. Unstable haemoglobins are also sometimes associated with quite marked dyserythropoiesis.

It can sometimes be difficult to distinguish megaloblastic erythropoiesis as a feature of MDS from that attributable either to a deficiency of vitamin B_{12} or folic acid or to the administration of drugs that interfere with DNA synthesis (Fig. 4.78). A useful feature is the lack of associated white cell changes – giant metamyelocytes and hypersegmented neutrophils – when megaloblastosis is a feature of MDS. However, it should be noted that white cell abnormalities may be lacking in megaloblastic erythropoiesis caused by drug exposure. Occasionally cohesive clumps or sheets of erythroid cells, all at a similar stage of maturation, can be confused with infiltration by carcinoma cells (Fig. 4.79).

The differential diagnosis of RARS includes sideroblastic erythropoiesis secondary to drugs or heavy metals (see page 501), copper deficiency (see page 521), the mitochondrial cytopathies (see page 522) and thiamine-responsive anaemia with diabetes mellitus and sensorineural deafness. The latter condition may show granulocytic and megakaryocytic dysplasia in addition to ring sideroblasts [65]. Ring sideroblasts are also present in significant numbers in some patients with erythropoietic protoporphyria [66].

The differential diagnosis of hypoplastic AML and hypoplastic MDS (Fig. 4.80) has been discussed on page 207. Immunohistochemistry can be of some value in making a distinction between hypoplastic MDS and aplastic anaemia [67,68]. Cases of hypocellular MDS have been found to have higher numbers of CD34-positive cells and cells expressing proliferating cell nuclear antigen [67].

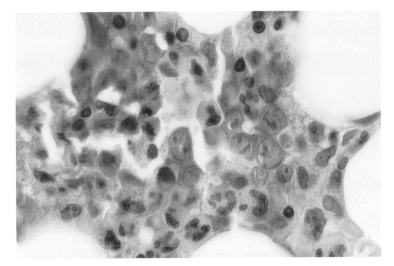

Fig. 4.78 BM trephine biopsy section from an HIV-positive patient taking a high dose of zidovudine. The patient had megaloblastic erythropoiesis and a cluster of early megaloblasts was confused with ALIP; the linear nucleoli of the megaloblasts is a clue to their true nature. Paraffin-embedded, H&E ×100.

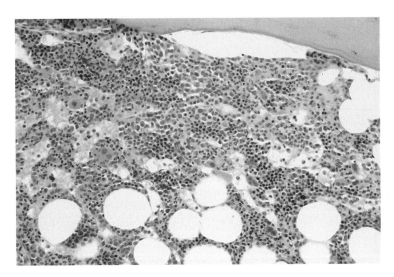

Fig. 4.79 BM trephine biopsy section from a patient with RARS showing large sheets of dysplastic erythroid cells separated by dilated sinusoids; the growth pattern appears so cohesive that the appearance could be confused with infiltration by carcinoma cells. Paraffin-embedded, H&E ×10.

Abnormal localization of immature precursors should not be confused with clusters of immature erythroid cells. Immunohistochemistry may help but it should be noted that not all blast cells express CD34 and, in addition, CD34 is not totally specific for myeloblasts since it can also be expressed by early erythroid cells (e.g. in megaloblastic anaemia or congenital dyserythropoietic anaemia) and by dysplastic megakaryocytes.

Lymphoid aggregates are sometimes present in MDS, giving rise to a differential diagnosis with non-Hodgkin lymphoma, particularly T-cell lymphoma, with associated dysplastic features. It should also be remembered that some patients with lymphomatous infiltration of the bone marrow have secondary dysplastic changes resembling those of MDS (Fig. 4.81).

In the rare patients with MDS who present with isolated thrombocytopenia it is sometimes difficult to make a distinction from autoimmune thrombocytopenic purpura. Dysplastic features may be very minor.

It should be noted that, even with a careful assessment of clinical features and use of all available diagnostic methods, it may still not be possible to make a firm diagnosis of MDS. In such patients

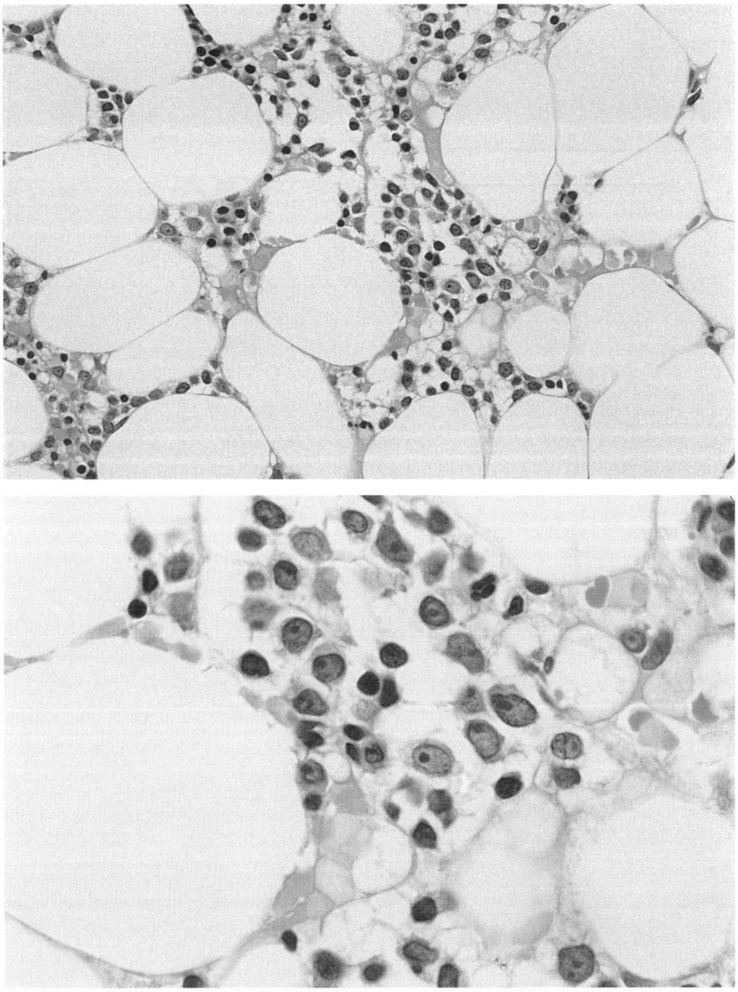

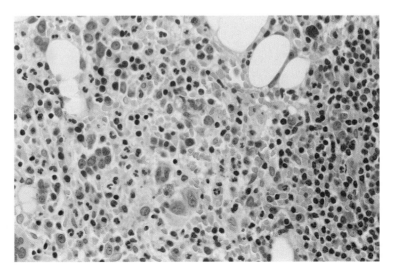

(a)

(b)

Fig. 4.80 BM trephine biopsy sections from a patient with hypoplastic MDS (RAEB) showing a disorganized marrow of low cellularity. (a) Paraffin-embedded, H&E ×40. (b) At higher power it is apparent that blast cells are increased. Paraffin-embedded, H&E ×100.

Fig. 4.81 BM trephine biopsy section from a patient with low grade T-cell lymphoma with secondary myelodysplasia; small hypolobated megakaryocytes are apparent. Paraffin-embedded, H&E ×40.

follow-up with regular review of the diagnosis is necessary.

Histiocytic neoplasms

Malignant histiocytosis

Malignant histiocytosis is a disease caused by the proliferation in tissues of a neoplastic clone of cells of monocyte/macrophage lineage; the abnormal cells show variable phagocytic activity. This disease may be regarded as the tissue counterpart of acute monocytic leukaemia. It differs from myeloid sarcoma with monocytic differentiation in that the cells of the neoplastic clone are widely distributed in peripheral tissues rather than forming localized tumours. In the 2008 WHO classification, malignant histiocytosis is regarded as histiocytic sarcoma with involvement of multiple sites.

It appears clear that, in the past, a significant proportion of cases reported as malignant histiocytosis [69,70] or as histiocytic medullary reticulosis [71] (usually regarded as a form of the same disease) were actually other conditions [72–76]. The majority of cases interpreted as malignant histiocytosis were either reactive histiocytosis consequent on viral or other infections or reactive histiocytosis occurring as a response to large cell anaplastic lymphoma and other T-lineage lymphomas. A less common cause of confusion is a T-cell lymphoma in which the lymphoma cells are themselves phagocytic [77]. It is important that the term malignant histiocytosis be restricted to cases in which neoplastic cells are of monocyte lineage. The term histiocytic medullary reticulosis has now been abandoned since the availability of immunophenotyping and other techniques has led to the recognition that, in the great majority of cases, the histiocytic proliferation and florid haemophagocytosis were secondary to a T-cell lymphoma [75,76] or a viral infection [74]. The reactive haemophagocytic syndromes are discussed on pages 138–144.

The diagnosis of malignant histiocytosis rests on clinical, histological, cytochemical and immunophenotypic grounds. Neoplastic cells are primitive and although phagocytosis occurs it is not prominent [72]. Neoplastic cells can be demonstrated, by cytochemical staining or immunophenotyping, to belong to the monocyte lineage and not to the T-lymphocyte lineage whereas, in haemophagocytic syndromes secondary to a T-cell lymphoma, there is an admixture of reactive, mainly mature, phagocytic histiocytes and immature neoplastic cells of lymphoid lineage [75].

Common clinical features of malignant histiocytosis are hepatomegaly, splenomegaly, lymphadenopathy, skin infiltration and systemic symptoms such as malaise, fever and weight loss.

Peripheral blood

Pancytopenia is common. Small numbers of immature cells of monocyte/macrophage lineage may be present in the blood (Fig. 4.82).

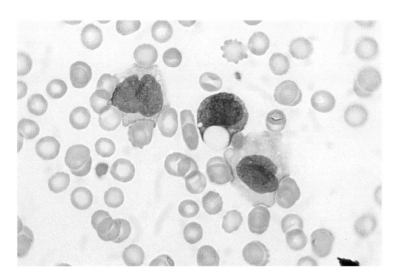

Fig. 4.82 PB film from a patient with malignant histiocytosis showing anaemia, thrombocytopenia and three abnormal cells of monocyte lineage, one of which has a phagocytic vacuole. MGG ×100.

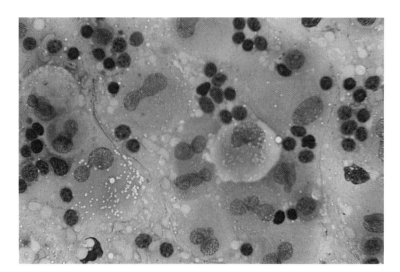

Fig. 4.83 BM aspirate from a patient with malignant histiocytosis associated with t(9;11)(p22;q23). MGG ×40. (By courtesy of Dr R. Brunning, Minneapolis.)

Bone marrow cytology

At the onset of disease, the bone marrow may show minimal or no infiltration by neoplastic cells. With more advanced disease there may be heavy infiltration (Fig. 4.83). The majority of neoplastic cells have the morphological features of monoblasts. Cells are large and usually have a round nucleus with nucleoli and a diffuse chromatin pattern. Cytoplasm is plentiful and moderately basophilic. A variable number of maturing cells with kidney-shaped nuclei and more abundant cytoplasm are also present [72]. Some cells are phagocytic and are seen to have ingested granulocytes and their precursors, erythroblasts and platelets; however, phagocytosis is much less marked than in reactive haemophagocytosis.

Bone marrow histology

Bone marrow infiltration has been reported to be more commonly detected by trephine biopsy than by bone marrow aspiration [78]. The bone marrow may appear normal at the time of diagnosis or may show a focal infiltrate of neoplastic cells (Fig. 4.84). In the later stages of the disease diffuse replacement of haemopoietic tissue commonly occurs [70,79,80] (Fig. 4.85). The infiltrate is largely composed of immature cells with large pleomorphic nuclei which may be lobulated and contain prominent nucleoli; there are moderate amounts of basophilic cytoplasm. Mitoses are usually numerous. A variable component of more mature cells of monocytic lineage may be present.

Cytogenetic and molecular genetic analysis

Some cases of malignant histiocytosis have been associated with translocations that are also associated with AML with monocytic differentiation, such as t(9;11)(p22;q23) [80] and t(8;16)(p11;p13).

Problems and pitfalls

The diagnosis of malignant histiocytosis is fraught with pitfalls and should be made with great circumspection. A minor degree of haemophagocytosis may be seen but marked haemophagocytosis suggests an alternative diagnosis. In children, familial or sporadic lymphohistiocytosis is likely and investigation for herpesvirus infection is indicated. In adults, reactive haemophagocytosis is often caused by mycobacterial or herpesvirus infection or by a T-cell lymphoma. Molecular analysis to demonstrate T-cell receptor gene rearrangement can be useful. Cytogenetic analysis is indicated if malignant histiocytosis appears likely, since it may confirm the diagnosis.

Histiocytic sarcoma

Histiocytic sarcoma [81] (previously referred to as 'true histiocytic lymphoma') initially presenting at

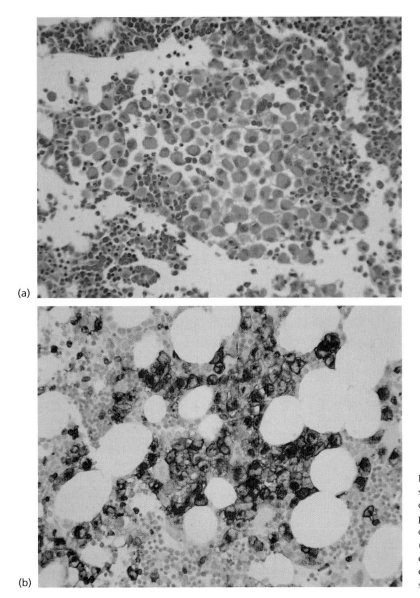

(a)

(b)

Fig. 4.84 BM trephine biopsy sections showing nodular collections of abnormal histiocytes as a prodromal stage in the development of acute monoblastic leukaemia (FAB M5b category). (a) Paraffin-embedded, H&E ×20. (b) Paraffin-embedded, immunohistochemical staining for CD14 ×20.

extramedullary sites may subsequently infiltrate the bone marrow. The patterns of infiltration reported are interstitial, patchy focal and diffuse [82]. Rarely, the initial site of disease may be the bone marrow; in one reported patient, presentation was with bone pain and diffuse sheets of atypical histiocytes replaced haemopoietic cells [83].

Langerhans cell histiocytosis

Langerhans cell histiocytosis, previously known as histiocytosis X, is a heterogeneous disease or group of diseases characterized by proliferation of Langerhans cells [84,85]. The proliferation is clonal and neoplastic [86]. Localized and disseminated forms occur. Haematological involvement occurs in the disseminated forms of the disease, which in the

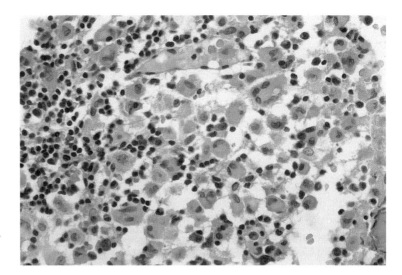

Fig. 4.85 BM trephine biopsy section, malignant histiocytosis (same patient as Fig. 4.82) Paraffin-embedded, H&E ×20. (By courtesy of Dr R. Brunning, Minneapolis.)

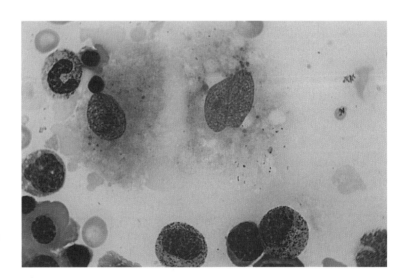

Fig. 4.86 BM aspirate film in Langerhans cell histiocytosis. MGG ×100. (By courtesy of Dr R. Brunning, Minneapolis.)

past have been referred to by the eponymous terms Letterer–Siwe disease of infants and Hand–Schüller–Christian disease. Bone marrow infiltration is seen mainly in infants and children.

Peripheral blood

The peripheral blood may be normal or there may be pancytopenia as a consequence either of hypersplenism or of bone marrow infiltration. Rarely a leukaemia of Langerhans cells occurs.

Bone marrow cytology

The bone marrow aspirate may show Langerhans cells together with a mixed population including eosinophils, monocytes, lipid-laden macrophages, lymphocytes and plasma cells [87,88]. Haemophagocytosis may occur. Langerhans cells are large and slightly irregular in shape. The nucleus is usually oval, somewhat irregular and sometimes grooved with delicately clumped chromatin and inconspicuous nucleoli (Fig. 4.86). The cytoplasm

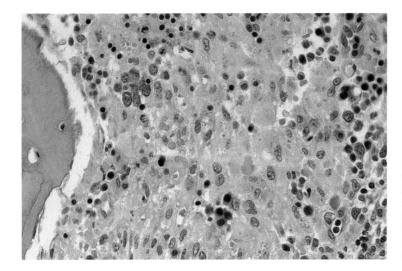

Fig. 4.87 BM trephine biopsy section in Langerhans cell histiocytosis showing an admixture of Langerhans cells and normal haemopoietic cells (same patient as Fig. 4.86). Paraffin-embedded, H&E ×20. (By courtesy of Dr R. Brunning, Minneapolis.)

is weakly basophilic with occasional azurophilic granules. Ultrastructural examination demonstrates Birbeck granules.

Cytochemistry

Langerhans cells have been variously reported as expressing [89] or not expressing [90,91] tartrate-resistant acid phosphatase and similarly as expressing [90] or not expressing [91] non-specific esterase.

Bone marrow histology

In those cases with marrow involvement, the bone marrow contains clusters or sheets of Langerhans cells together with eosinophils, neutrophils, lymphocytes, plasma cells, monocytes, phagocytic macrophages, lipid-laden macrophages and giant cells (Fig. 4.87). Xanthomatous transformation (accumulation of sheets of large, pale, lipid-filled macrophages) and fibrosis may occur [87,88]. Langerhans cells have a characteristic appearance [85]. The nuclei are usually convoluted or twisted and longitudinal grooves may be present; chromatin is delicate and nucleoli are inconspicuous; their cytoplasm is plentiful and slightly eosinophilic.

Immunophenotype

Langerhans cells are positive for CD1a, CD4 and HLA-DR. Lysozyme and CD68 are variably expressed [85].

Immunohistochemistry

Immunohistochemical staining shows Langerhans cells to express S100 protein in the nucleus and cytoplasm, although only a small proportion of cells may stain positively in some cases. Langerhans cells are also positive for vimentin, CD1a, CD4 and CD207 (langerin). Positivity for CD1a and CD207 are the most reliable immunophenotypic markers; expression of CD68 and CD68R is weak or absent and cells are negative for CD14, calprotectin (monoclonal antibody Mac387) and factor XIIIA (the A subunit of factor XIII).

Cytogenetic and molecular genetic analysis

A familial tendency to the development of Langerhans cell histiocytosis has been described [92]. A clonal cytogenetic abnormality, t(7;12)(q11.2;p13) has been reported in a single case of eosinophilic granuloma [93].

Problems and pitfalls

It should be noted that Langerhans cell histiocytosis often causes focal lesions, even when widespread throughout the skeleton, and a targeted biopsy of a radiologically suspicious lesion may be more informative than a standard iliac crest trephine biopsy.

Langerhans cell histiocytosis has been confused with systemic mastocytosis, hairy cell leukaemia and malignant melanoma. Careful assessment of

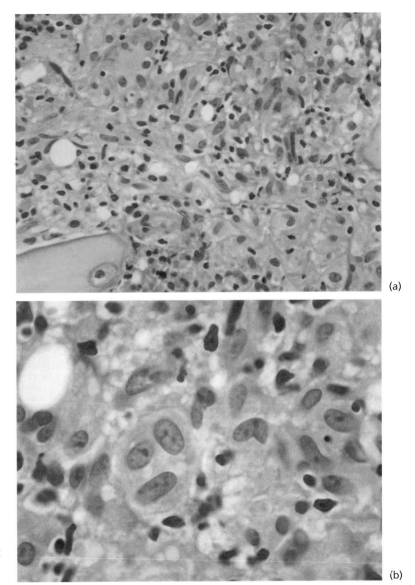

(a)

(b)

Fig. 4.88 BM trephine biopsy sections from a patient with non-Langerhans cell histiocytosis. Most of the histiocytes are epithelioid cells, with occasional multinucleated variants and cells with more irregular nuclei resembling Langerhans cells. Langerhans cells would express CD68R only weakly. Histiocytes in this patient's bone marrow were also negative for CD1a and S100 protein. (a) Paraffin-embedded H&E ×40. (b) Paraffin-embedded, H&E ×100.

continued

cytological features, supplemented by immunohistochemistry, will resolve these difficulties.

Rare histiocytoses of non-Langerhans cell type also occur and may involve bone marrow, sometimes presenting at this site (Fig. 4.88). They may resemble Langerhans cell histiocytosis morphologi-cally but are clinically and pathologically heterogeneous. They are thought to originate from cells either resembling those of Rosai–Dorfman disease, which are strongly S100 positive, or from cells related to dermal dendrocytes, which express factor XIIIA.

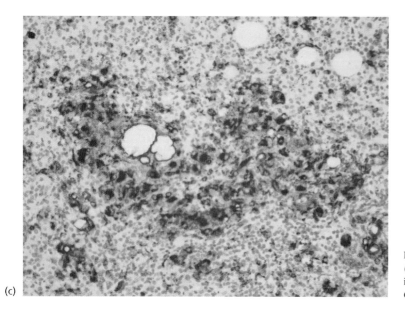

(c)

Fig. 4.88 (continued) (c) Paraffin-embedded, immunohistochemical staining for CD68R ×10.

Interdigitating dendritic cell sarcoma

A small number of patients with disseminated interdigitating dendritic cell sarcoma have had bone marrow infiltration, and another patient had bone marrow necrosis followed by fibrosis [94,95].

Disseminated juvenile xanthogranuloma

This somewhat ill-defined, possibly clonal, condition and its adult form, Erdheim–Chester disease, is characterized by an accumulation of lipid-laden macrophages [85,96]. Bone marrow aspirates may show foamy macrophages. Trephine biopsy sections may demonstrate infiltration by lipid-laden and other macrophages, multinucleated giant cells and lymphocytes.

References

1 Bennett JM, Catovsky D, Daniel MT, Flandrin G, Galton DAG, Gralnick HR and Sultan C (1976) Proposals for the classification of the acute leukaemias (FAB cooperative group). *Br J Haematol*, **33**, 451–458.

2 Bennett JM, Catovsky D, Daniel MT, Flandrin G, Galton DAG, Gralnick HR and Sultan C (1985) Proposed revised criteria for the classification of acute myeloid leukemia. *Ann Intern Med*, **103**, 626–629.

3 Vardiman JW, Brunning RD, Arber DA, Le Beau MM, Porwit A, Tefferi A, Bloomfield CD and Thiele J (2008) Introduction and overview of the classification of the myeloid neoplasms. In: Swerdlow SH, Campo E, Harris NL, Jaffe ES, Pileri SA, Stein H, Thiele J and Vardiman JW (eds) *World Health Organization Classification of Tumours of Haematopoietic and Lymphoid Tissues*. IARC Press, Lyon, pp. 19–30.

4 Hayhoe FGJ and Quaglino D (1988) *Haematological Cytochemistry*, 2nd edn. Churchill Livingstone, Edinburgh.

5 Bain BJ (2010) *Leukaemia Diagnosis*, 3rd edn. Wiley–Blackwell, Oxford.

6 Islam A, Frisch B and Henderson ES (1989) Plastic embedded core biopsy: a complementary approach to bone marrow aspiration for diagnosing acute myeloid leukaemia. *J Clin Pathol*, **42**, 300–306.

7 Islam A, Catovsky D, Goldman JM and Galton DAG (1985) Bone marrow biopsy changes in acute leukaemia. I: Observations before chemotherapy. *Histopathology*, **9**, 939–957.

8 Islam A, Catovsky D, Goldman J and Galton DAG (1984) Bone marrow fibre content in acute myeloid leukaemia before and after treatment. *J Clin Pathol*, **37**, 1259–1263.

9 Wilkins BS, Bostanci AG, Ryan MF and Jones DB (1993) Haemopoietic regrowth after chemotherapy: an immunohistochemical study of bone marrow trephine biopsy specimens. *J Clin Pathol*, **46**, 915–921.

10 Needleman SW, Burns P, Dick FR and Armitage JO (1981) Hypoplastic acute leukemia. *Cancer*, **48**, 1410–1414.

11 Howe RB, Bloomfield CD and McKenna RW (1982) Hypocellular acute leukemia. *Am J Med*, **72**, 391–395.

12 Horny H-P, Wehrmann M, Steinke B and Kaiserling E (1994) Assessment of the value of immunohisto-chemistry in the subtyping of acute leukemia on routinely processed bone marrow biopsy specimens with particular reference to macrophage-associated antibodies. *Hum Pathol*, **25**, 810–814.

13 Manaloor EJ, Neiman RS, Heilman DK, Albitar M, Casey T, Vatuone T *et al.* (2000) Immunohistochemistry can be used to subtype acute myeloid leukemia in routinely processed bone marrow biopsy specimens: comparison with flow cytometry. *Am J Clin Pathol*, **113**, 814–822.

14 Arber DA, Brunning RD, Le Beau MM, Falini B, Vardiman JW, Porwit A, Thiele J and Bloomfield C (2008) Acute myeloid leukaemia with recurrent genetic abnormalities. In: Swerdlow SH, Campo E, Harris NL, Jaffe ES, Pileri SA, Stein H, Thiele J and Vardiman JW (eds) *World Health Organization Classification of Tumours of Haematopoietic and Lymphoid Tissues*. IARC Press, Lyon, pp. 110–133.

15 Padró T, Ruiz S, Bieker R, Bürger H, Steins M, Kienast J *et al.* (2000) Increased angiogenesis in the bone marrow of patients with acute myeloid leukemia. *Blood*, **95**, 2637–2644.

16 Mori A, Wada H, Okada M, Takatsuka H, Tamura A, Fujimori Y *et al.* (2000) Acute promyelocytic leukemia with marrow fibrosis at initial presentation: possible involvement of transforming growth factor-β_1. *Acta Haematol*, **103**, 220–223.

17 Hatake K, Ohtsuki T, Uwai M, Takahashi H, Izumi T, Yoshida M *et al.* (1996) Tretinoin induces bone marrow collagenous fibrosis in acute promyelocytic leukaemia: new adverse but reversible effect. *Br J Haematol*, **93**, 646–649.

18 Lopez P and Hayme O (1992) Case report: all-*trans* retinoic acid, hyperleucocytosis and marrow infarction. *Am J Hematol*, **41**, 305–306.

19 Kroschinsky FP, Schäkel U, Fischer R, Mohr B, Oelschlaegel U, Repp R *et al.* on behalf of the DSIL (Deutsche Studieninitiative Leukämie) Study Group (2008) Cup-like acute myeloid leukemia: new disease or artificial phenomenon? *Haematologica*, **93**, 283–286.

20 Arber DA, Brunning RD, Orazi A, Bain BJ, Porwit A, Vardiman JW, Le Beau MM and Greenberg PL (2008) Acute myeloid leukaemia with myelodysplasia-related changes. In: Swerdlow SH, Campo E, Harris NL, Jaffe ES, Pileri SA, Stein H, Thiele J and Vardiman JW (eds) *World Health Organization Classification of Tumours of Haematopoietic and Lymphoid Tissues*. IARC Press, Lyon, pp. 124–126.

21 Vardiman JW, Arber DA, Brunning RD, Larson RA, Matutes E, Baumann I and Thiele J (2008) Therapy-related myeloid neoplasms. In: Swerdlow SH, Campo E, Harris NL, Jaffe ES, Pileri SA, Stein H, Thiele J and Vardiman JW (eds) *World Health Organization Classification of Tumours of Haematopoietic and Lymphoid Tissues*. IARC Press, Lyon, pp. 127–128.

22 Arber DA, Brunning RD, Orazi A, Porwit A, Peterson L, Thiele J and Le Beau MM. Acute myeloid leukaemia, not otherwise specified. In: Swerdlow SH, Campo E, Harris NL, Jaffe ES, Pileri SA, Stein H, Thiele J and Vardiman JW (eds) *World Health Organization Classification of Tumours of Haematopoietic and Lymphoid Tissues*. IARC Press, Lyon, pp 130–139.

23 Stasi R and Amadori S (1999) AML-M9: a review of laboratory features and proposal of new diagnostic criteria. *Blood Cell Mol Dis*, **25**, 120–129.

24 Lorand-Metz I, Vassallo J, Aoki RY and de Souza CA (1991) Acute megakaryoblastic leukaemia: importance of bone marrow biopsy in diagnosis. *Leuk Lymphoma*, **4**, 74–75.

25 Penchansky L, Taylor SR and Krause JR (1989) Three infants with acute megakaryoblastic leukaemia simulating metastatic tumour. *Cancer*, **64**, 1366–1371.

26 Chan JK, Sin VC, Wong KF, Ng CS, Tsang WY, Chan CH *et al.* (1997) Nonnasal lymphoma expressing the natural killer cell marker CD56: a clinicopathologic study of 49 cases of an uncommon aggressive neoplasm. *Blood*, **89**, 4501–4513.

27 Chaperot L, Bendriss N, Manches O, Gressin R, Maynadié M, Trimoreau F *et al.* (2004) Identification of a leukaemic counterpart of the plasmacytoid dendritic cells. *Blood*, **99**, 3210–3217.

28 Dijkman R, van Doom R, Szuhai K, Willemze R, Vermeer MH and Tensen CP (2007) Gene-expression profiling and array-based CGH classify CD4+CD56+ hematodermic neoplasm and cutaneous myelomonocytic leukemia as distinct disease entities. *Blood*, **109**, 1720–1727.

29 Facchetti F, Jones DM and Petrella T (2008) Blastic plasmacytoid dendritic cell neoplasm. In: Swerdlow SH, Campo E, Harris NL, Jaffe ES, Pileri SA, Stein H, Thiele J and Vardiman JW (eds) *World Health Organization Classification of Tumours of Haematopoietic and Lymphoid Tissues*. IARC Press, Lyon, pp. 145–147.

30 Feuillard J, Jacob M-C, Valensi F, Maynadié M, Gressin R, Chaperot L *et al.* (2002) Clinical and biological features of CD4$^+$CD56$^+$ malignancies. *Blood*, **99**, 1556–1563.

31 Kassam S, Rice A, Morilla R and Bain BJ (2007) Case 35: an unusual haematological neoplasm characterized by cells with cytoplasmic tails. *Leuk Lymphoma*, **48**, 1208–1210.

32 Bianco M, Turner J and Rosenthal N (2005) Increased blasts mimicking acute leukemia in a patient with polysubstance abuse. *Arch Path Lab Med*, **129**, e35–e38.

33 Borowitz MJ, Béné M-C, Harris NL, Porwit A and Matutes E (2008) Acute of ambiguous lineage. In:

Swerdlow SH, Campo E, Harris NL, Jaffe ES, Pileri SA, Stein H, Thiele J and Vardiman JW (eds) *World Health Organization Classification of Tumours of Haematopoietic and Lymphoid Tissues*. IARC Press, Lyon, pp. 150–155.

34 Rollison DE, Howlader N, Smith MT, Strom SS, Merritt WD, Ries LA *et al.* (2008) Epidemiology of myelodysplastic syndromes and chronic myeloproliferative disorders in the United States, 2001–2004, using data from the NAACCR and SEER programs. *Blood*, **112**, 45–52.

35 Bennett JM, Catovsky D, Daniel MT, Flandrin G, Galton DAG, Gralnick HR and Sultan C (1982) Proposals for the classification of the myelodysplastic syndromes. *Br J Haematol*, **51**, 189–199.

36 Brunning RD, Orazi A, Germing U, Le Beau MM, Porwit A, Baumann I, Vardiman JW and Hellstrom-Lindberg E (2008) Myelodysplastic syndromes/neoplasms, overview. In: Swerdlow SH, Campo E, Harris NL, Jaffe ES, Pileri SA, Stein H, Thiele J and Vardiman JW (eds) *World Health Organization Classification of Tumours of Haematopoietic and Lymphoid Tissues*. IARC Press, Lyon, pp. 88–93.

37 Baumann I, Niemeyer CM, Bennett JM and Shannon K (2008) Childhood myelodysplastic syndrome. In: Swerdlow SH, Campo E, Harris NL, Jaffe ES, Pileri SA, Stein H, Thiele J and Vardiman JW (eds) *World Health Organization Classification of Tumours of Haematopoietic and Lymphoid Tissues*. IARC Press, Lyon, pp. 105–107.

38 Kuriyama K, Tomonaga M, Matsuo T, Ginnai I and Ichimaru M (1986) Diagnostic significance of detecting pseudo-Pelger–Huët anomalies and micromegakaryocytes in myelodysplastic syndrome. *Br J Haematol*, **63**, 665–669.

39 Fernández-Lago C and Romero E (1998) Myelodysplastic syndromes associated with immune thrombocytopenia. *Br J Haematol*, **102**, 342–345.

40 Natelson EA (2007) Benzene-induced acute myeloid leukemia: a clinician's perspective. *Am J Hematol*, **82**, 826–830.

41 Stasi R, Pagano A, Terzoli E and Amadori S (1999) Recombinant human granulocyte-macrophage colony-stimulating factor plus erythropoietin for the treatment of cytopenias in patients with myelodysplastic syndromes. *Br J Haematol*, **105**, 141–148.

42 Thiede T, Engquist L and Billstrom R (1988) Application of megakaryocytic morphology in diagnosing 5q– syndrome. *Eur J Haematol*, **41**, 434–437.

43 Wong KF and Chan JKC (1991) Are 'dysplastic' and hypogranular megakaryocytes specific markers for myelodysplastic syndrome? *Br J Haematol*, **77**, 509–514.

44 Hasserjian RP, Gatterman N, Bennett JM, Brunning RD and Thiele J (2008) Refractory anaemia with ring sideroblasts. In: Swerdlow SH, Campo E, Harris NL, Jaffe ES, Pileri SA, Stein H, Thiele J and Vardiman JW (eds) *World Health Organization Classification of Tumours of Haematopoietic and Lymphoid Tissues*. IARC Press, Lyon, pp. 96–97.

45 Yoshida Y, Oguma S, Uchjino H and Maekawa T (1988) Refractory myelodysplastic syndromes with hypocellular bone marrow. *J Clin Pathol*, **41**, 763–767.

46 Rios A, Cañizo C, Sanz MA, Vallespi T, Sanz G, Torrabadella M *et al.* (1990) Bone marrow biopsy in myelodysplastic syndromes: morphological characteristics and contribution to the study of prognostic factors. *Br J Haematol*, **75**, 26–33.

47 Frisch B and Bartl R (1986) Bone marrow histology in myelodysplastic syndromes. *Scand J Haematol*, **36** (Suppl. 45), 21–37.

48 Thiele J and Fischer R (1991) Megakaryocytopoiesis in haematological disorders: diagnostic feature of bone marrow biopsies. *Virchows Archiv (A)*, **418**, 87–97.

49 Mangi MH and Mufti GJ (1992) Primary myelodysplastic syndromes: diagnostic and prognostic significance of immunohistochemical assessment of bone marrow biopsies. *Blood*, **79**, 198–205.

50 Fox SB, Lorenzen J, Heryet A, Jones M, Gatter KC and Mason DY (1990) Megakaryocytes in myelodysplasia: an immunohistochemical study on bone marrow trephines. *Histopathology*, **17**, 69–74.

51 Clark DM and Lampert IA (1990) Apoptosis is a common histopathological finding in myelodysplasia: the correlate of ineffective haematopoiesis. *Leuk Lymphoma*, **2**, 415–418.

52 Maschek H, Georgii A, Kaloutsi V, Werner M, Bandecar K, Kressel M-G *et al.* (1992) Myelofibrosis in primary myelodysplastic syndromes: a retrospective study of 352 patients. *Eur J Haematol*, **48**, 208–214.

53 Tricot G, de Wolf Peeters C, Hendrickx B and Verwilghen RL (1984) Bone marrow histology in myelodysplastic syndromes. *Br J Haematol*, **56**, 423–430.

54 Delacrétaz F, Schmidt P-M, Piguet D, Bachmann F and Costa J (1987) Histopathology of myelodysplastic syndromes: the FAB classification. *Am J Clin Pathol*, **87**, 180–186.

55 Maschek H, Gutzmer R, Choritz H and Georgii A (1994) Life expectancy in primary myelodysplastic syndromes: a prognostic score based upon histopathology from bone marrow biopsies of 569 patients. *Eur J Haematol*, **53**, 280–287.

56 Baur AS, Meugé-Moraw C, Schmidt P-M, Parlier V, Jotterand M and Delacrétaz F (2000) CD34/QBEND10 immunostaining in bone marrow biopsies: an additional parameter for the diagnosis and classification of myelodysplastic syndromes. *Eur J Haematol*, **64**, 71–79.

57 Soligo DA, Oriani A, Annaloro C, Cortelezzi A, Calori R, Pozzoli E *et al.* (1994) CD34 immunohistochemistry of bone marrow biopsies: prognostic significance in

primary myelodysplastic syndromes. *Am J Hematol*, **46**, 9–17.

58 Yoon S-Y, Li C-Y and Tefferi A (2000) Megakaryocyte c-Mpl expression in chronic myeloproliferative disorders and the myelodysplastic syndrome: immunoperoxidase staining patterns and clinical correlates. *Eur J Haematol*, **65**, 170–174.

59 Greenberg P, Cox C, Le Beau MM, Fenaux P, Morel P, Sanz G *et al.* (1997) International Scoring System for evaluating prognosis in myelodysplastic syndromes. *Blood*, **89**, 2079–2088.

60 Brunning RD, Hasserjian RP, Porwit A, Bennett JM, Thiele J and Hellstrom-Lindberg E (2008) Refractory cytopenia with unilineage dysplasia. In: Swerdlow SH, Campo E, Harris NL, Jaffe ES, Pileri SA, Stein H, Thiele J and Vardiman JW (eds) *World Health Organization Classification of Tumours of Haematopoietic and Lymphoid Tissues.* IARC Press, Lyon, pp. 94–95.

61 Brunning RD, Bennett JM, Matutes E, Orazi A, Vardiman JW and Thiele J (2008) Refractory cytopenia with multilineage dysplasia. In: Swerdlow SH, Campo E, Harris NL, Jaffe ES, Pileri SA, Stein H, Thiele J and Vardiman JW (eds) *World Health Organization Classification of Tumours of Haematopoietic and Lymphoid Tissues.* IARC Press, Lyon, pp. 98–99.

62 Orazi A, Brunning RD, Hasserjian RP, Germing U and Thiele J (2008) Refractory anaemia with excess of blasts. In: Swerdlow SH, Campo E, Harris NL, Jaffe ES, Pileri SA, Stein H, Thiele J and Vardiman JW (eds) *World Health Organization Classification of Tumours of Haematopoietic and Lymphoid Tissues.* IARC Press, Lyon, pp. 100–101.

63 Bigoni R, Cuneo A, Milani R, Cavazzini P, Bardi A, Roberti MG *et al.* (2001) Multilineage involvement in the 5q– syndrome: a fluorescent *in situ* hybridization study on bone marrow smears. *Haematologica*, **86**, 375–381.

64 Ebert BL, Pretz J, Bosco J, Chang CY, Tamayo P, Galili N *et al.* (2008) Identification of RPS14 as a 5q– syndrome gene by RNA interference screen. *Nature*, **451**, 335–339.

65 Bazarbachi A, Haidar J, Salem Z, Solh H and Ayas M (1997) Thiamine-responsive myelodysplasia. *Blood*, **90** (Suppl. 1), 264b.

66 Rademakers LHRM, Koningsberger JC, Sorber CWJ, Faile HBDL, Hattum JV and Mars JJM (1993) Accumulation of iron in erythroblasts of patients with erythropoietic protoporphyria. *Eur J Clin Invest*, **23**, 130–138.

67 Orazi A, Albitar M, Heerema NA, Haskins S and Neiman RS (1997) Hypoplastic myelodysplastic syndromes can be distinguished from acquired aplastic anemia by CD34 and PRNA immunostaining of bone marrow biopsy specimens. *Am J Clin Pathol*, **107**, 268–274.

68 Horny H-P, Wehrmann M, Schlicker HUH, Eichstaedt A, Clemens MR and Kaiserling E (1995) QBENDIO for the diagnosis of myelodysplastic syndromes in routinely processed bone marrow biopsy specimens. *J Clin Pathol*, **48**, 291–294.

69 Warnke RA, Kim H and Dorfman RF (1975) Malignant histiocytosis (histiocytic medullary reticulosis). I. Clinicopathological study of 29 cases. *Cancer*, **35**, 215–230.

70 Lampert IA, Catovsky D and Bergier N (1978) Malignant histiocytosis: a clinicopathological study of 12 cases. *Br J Haematol*, **40**, 65–77.

71 Scott RB and Robb-Smith AHT (1939) Histiocytic medullary reticulosis. *Lancet*, **ii**, 194–198.

72 Manoharan A and Catovsky D (1981) Histiocytic medullary reticulosis revisited. In: Schmalz IF, Huhn D and Schaefer HE (eds) *Haematology and Blood Transfusion*, vol. **27**, *Disorders of the Monocyte Macrophage System.* Springer Verlag, Berlin.

73 Wilson MS, Weiss LM, Gatter KC, Mason DY, Dorfman RF and Warnke RA (1990) Malignant histiocytosis: a reassessment of cases previously reported in 1975 based on paraffin section immunophenotyping studies. *Cancer*, **66**, 530–536.

74 Su I-J, Lin D-T, Hsieh H-C, Lee SH, Chen J, Chen RL, Lee CY and Chen JY (1990) Fatal primary Epstein Barr virus infection masquerading as histiocytic medullary reticulosis in young children in Taiwan. *Hematol Pathol*, **4**, 189–195.

75 Falini B, Pileri S, de Solas I, Martelli MF, Mason DY, Delsol G, Gatter KC and Fagioli M (1990) Peripheral T-cell lymphoma associated with hemophagocytic syndrome. *Blood*, **75**, 434–444.

76 Robb-Smith AHT (1990) Before our time: half a century of histiocytic medullary reticulosis: a T-cell teaser. *Histopathology*, **17**, 279–293.

77 Kadin ME, Kamoun M and Lamberg J (1981) Erythrophagocytic T-γ lymphoma: a clinicopathological entity resembling malignant histiocytosis. *N Engl J Med*, **304**, 648–653.

78 Sonneveld P, van Lom K, Kappers-Klunne M, Prins MER and Abels J (1990) Clinico-pathological diagnosis and treatment of malignant histiocytosis. *Br J Haematol*, **75**, 511–516.

79 Ralfkiaer E, Delsol G, O'Connor NTJ, Brandtzaeg P, Brousset P, Vejlsgaard GL and Mason DY (1990) Malignant lymphomas of true histiocytic origin. A clinical, histological, immunophenotypic and genotypic study. *J Pathol*, **160**, 9–17.

80 Brunning RD (1999) Malignant histiocytosis. *Br J Haematol*, **107**, 679.

81 Grogan TM, Pileri SA, Chan JKC, Weiss LM and Fletcher CDM (2008) Histiocytic sarcoma. In: Swerdlow SH, Campo E, Harris NL, Jaffe ES, Pileri SA, Stein H, Thiele J and Vardiman JW (eds) *World Health Organization Classification of Tumours of Haematopoietic*

and Lymphoid Tissues. IARC Press, Lyon, pp. 356–357.

82 Lauritzen AF, Delsol G, Hansen NE, Horn T, Ersbøll J, Hou-Jensen K and Ralfkiaer E (1994) Histiocytic sarcomas and monoblastic leukemias: a clinical, histologic and immunophenotypical study. *Am J Clin Pathol*, **102**, 45–54.

83 Copie-Bergman C, Wotherspoon AC, Norton AJ, Diss TC and Isaacson PG (1998) True histiocytic lymphoma: a morphologic, immunochemical, and molecular genetic study of 13 cases. *Am J Surg Pathol*, **22**, 1386–1392.

84 Malone M (1991) The histiocytoses of childhood. *Histopathology*, **19**, 105–119.

85 Jaffe R, Weiss LM and Facchetti F (2008) Langerhans cell histiocytosis. In: Swerdlow SH, Campo E, Harris NL, Jaffe ES, Pileri SA, Stein H, Thiele J and Vardiman JW (eds) *World Health Organization Classification of Tumours of Haematopoietic and Lymphoid Tissues.* IARC Press, Lyon, pp. 358–360.

86 Willman CL, Busque L, Griffith BB, Favara BE, McClain KL, Duncan MH and Gilliland DG (1994) Langerhans'-cell histiocytosis (histiocytosis X) – a clonal proliferative disease. *N Engl J Med*, **331**, 154–160.

87 Frisch B, Lewis SM, Burkhardt R and Bartl R (1985) *Biopsy Pathology of the Bone Marrow.* Chapman & Hall, London.

88 Favara BE and Jaffe R (1987) Pathology of Langerhans' cell histiocytosis. *Hematol Oncol Clin North Am*, **1**, 75–97.

89 Mufti GJ, Flandrin G, Schaefer H-E, Sandberg AA and Kanfer EJ (1996) *An Atlas of Malignant Haematology.* Martin Dunitz, London.

90 Weiss LM, Grogan TM, Müller-Hermelink H-K, Stein H, Dura T, Favara B, Paulli M and Feller AC (2001) Langerhans cell histiocytosis. In: Jaffe ES, Harris NL, Stein H and Vardiman JW (eds) *World Health Organization Classification of Tumours: Pathology and genetics of tumours of haematopoietic and lymphoid tissues.* IARC Press, Lyon, pp. 280–282.

91 Lauritzen AF and Ralfkiaer E (1995) Histiocytic lymphoma *Leuk Lymphoma*, **18**, 73–80.

92 Arico M, Nichols K, Whitlock JA, Arceci R, Haupt R, Mittler U *et al.* (1999) Familial clustering of Langerhans cell histiocytosis. *Br J Haematol*, **107**, 883–888.

93 Betts DR, Leibundgut KE, Feldges A, Pluss HJ and Niggli EK (1998) Cytogenetic abnormalities in Langerhans cell histiocytosis. *Br J Cancer*, **77**, 552–555.

94 Kawachi K, Nakatani Y, Inavama Y, Kawano N, Toda N and Misugi K (2002) Interdigitating dendritic cell sarcoma of the spleen: report of a case with a review of the literature. *Am J Surg Pathol*, **26**, 530–537.

95 Pillay K, Solomon R, Daubenton JD and Sinclair-Smith CC (2004) Interdigitating dendritic cell sarcoma: a report of four paediatric cases and review of the literature. *Histology*, **44**, 283–291.

96 Al-Quran S, Reith J, Bradley J and Rimsza L (2002) Erdheim–Chester disease: case report, PCR-based analysis of clonality, and review of literature. *Mod Pathol*, **15**, 666–672.

FIVE

MYELOPROLIFERATIVE AND MYELODYSPLASTIC/ MYELOPROLIFERATIVE NEOPLASMS AND RELATED CONDITIONS

The myeloproliferative neoplasms are a group of diseases, which have in common that they result from proliferation of a clone of neoplastic myeloid cells derived from a mutated haemopoietic stem cell. In the 2008 revision of the World Health Organization (WHO) classification of tumours of haematopoietic and lymphoid tissues the designation of this group of conditions is 'myeloproliferative neoplasms' (MPN) rather than 'myeloproliferative disorders' or 'myeloproliferative diseases' [1,2]. Evidence suggests that, even when differentiation is predominantly to cells of a single lineage, the disorder has arisen in a multipotent myeloid stem cell or, at least in some cases, in a pluripotent stem cell capable of giving rise to cells of both myeloid and lymphoid lineages. For an increasing number of these disorders mutations in tyrosine kinase genes, thought to be important in pathogenesis, have been discovered. In MPN, maturation of neoplastic cells is relatively normal and cells retain some responsiveness to normal physiological controls; for this reason they may be regarded as relatively benign neoplasms. However, this group of conditions shows a greater or lesser propensity to evolve into a malignant neoplasm, resembling acute leukaemia, which rapidly leads to death. In the case of chronic granulocytic leukaemia, prior to the introduction of therapy with tyrosine kinase inhibitors, acute transformation was very frequent and occurred at a median interval of

only 2–3 years. Polycythaemia vera, primary myelofibrosis and systemic mastocytosis undergo acute transformation less often and usually after a longer chronic phase. An acute transformation is least frequent in essential thrombocythaemia.

The MPN differ from the myelodysplastic syndromes (MDS) in that, early in the course of the disease, haemopoiesis is effective with overproduction of cells of at least one lineage. Dysplastic features are either absent or not prominent. However, with disease progression haemopoiesis may become ineffective and dysplastic features may appear. Some patients cannot be readily assigned to one or other category of disease because of the presence of both myeloproliferative and myelodysplastic features; such cases fall into the group of disorders now designated myelodysplastic/myeloproliferative neoplasms (MDS/MPN) in the WHO classification.

Bone marrow reticulin or collagen fibrosis can be a prominent feature of MPN and MDS/MPN. It should be noted that the 2008 WHO classification incorporates a proposed scale for grading fibrosis in these conditions [3] (Table 5.1).

The correct diagnosis and classification of MPN is dependent on a structured approach in which clinical features and peripheral blood, bone marrow cytological, histological, cytogenetic and molecular characteristics are all assessed. For the chronic myeloid leukaemias, careful examination of a blood film is often more important than examination of a bone marrow aspirate.

The 2008 WHO classification of MPN and MDS/ MPN, which is followed in this chapter, is shown in Table 5.2.

Bone Marrow Pathology. By Barbara Bain, David Clark and Bridget Wilkins. © 2010, Blackwell Publishing.

Table 5.1 Semiquantitative grading of reticulin and collagen deposition in MPN and MDS/MPN [3].*

Grade	Description
0	Scattered linear reticulin with no intersections (cross-overs), corresponding to normal bone marrow
1	Loose network of reticulin with many intersections, especially in perivascular areas
2	Diffuse and dense increase in reticulin with extensive intersections, occasionally with focal bundles of collagen and/or focal osteosclerosis
3	Diffuse and dense increase in reticulin with extensive intersections and coarse bundles of collagen, often associated with osteosclerosis

*Fibre density is assessed only in haemopoietic areas.

Myeloproliferative neoplasms

Chronic myelogenous leukaemia, BCR-ABL1+ (chronic granulocytic leukaemia)

Chronic myelogenous leukaemia, *BCR-ABL1* positive, also known as chronic granulocytic leukaemia and chronic myeloid leukaemia, is a distinct, easily recognizable disease [4]. For brevity and clarity we shall use the designation 'chronic granulocytic leukaemia' (CGL); the now more commonly employed 'chronic myeloid leukaemia' (CML) is open to misinterpretation since it is sometimes used as a generic term, encompassing also *BCR-ABL1*-negative conditions. CGL is an uncommon condition resulting from the neoplastic proliferation of an early haemopoietic precursor cell that can differentiate into cells of granulocyte, monocyte, erythroid, megakaryocyte and, under certain circumstances, lymphoid lineages. Approaching 95% of patients with CGL have an acquired chromosomal abnormality in the leukaemic clone consisting of a reciprocal translocation between the long arms of chromosomes 9 and 22, t(9;22)(q34;q11.2). The abnormal chromosome 22 (22q–) is known as the Philadelphia (Ph) chromosome. As a result of this translocation, a hybrid gene is formed on 22q–, by fusion of part of

Table 5.2 The WHO classification of the myeloproliferative and myelodysplastic/ myeloproliferative neoplasms [2].

Myeloproliferative neoplasms
Chronic myelogenous leukaemia, Philadelphia chromosome positive (t(9;22)(q34;q11.2), *BCR-ABL1* positive)
Chronic neutrophilic leukaemia
Chronic eosinophilic leukaemia, not otherwise specified
Primary myelofibrosis
Polycythaemia vera
Essential thrombocythaemia
Mastocytosis
Myeloproliferative neoplasm, unclassifiable

Myelodysplastic/myeloproliferative neoplasms
Chronic myelomonocytic leukaemia
Atypical chronic myeloid leukaemia, *BCR-ABL1* negative
Juvenile myelomonocytic leukaemia
Other myelodysplastic/myeloproliferative disorder, unclassifiable

the *ABL1* (Abelson) oncogene from the long arm of chromosome 9 with part of a chromosome 22 gene known as *BCR* (breakpoint cluster region). This fusion gene encodes an abnormal tyrosine kinase. Patients whose cells lack the t(9;22) and the resultant Ph chromosome, but in whom the disease is identical to Ph-positive disease in all other respects, have a *BCR-ABL1* fusion gene demonstrable by molecular techniques [5]. This is not the case with atypical chronic myeloid leukaemia, which is a *BCR-ABL1*-negative condition (see below).

Chronic granulocytic leukaemia is very largely a disease of adult life but cases occur from childhood onwards. The overall incidence is 1–2 per 100000 per year with a slow increase occurring with increasing age. The disease is more common in men than in women with a male : female ratio of about 1.5 : 1. Patients may present with symptoms of anaemia, abdominal fullness, splenic discomfort or pain or, rarely, features of leucostasis due to a very high white blood cell count (WBC). However, because of the insidious onset of the disease, many patients have only minor symptoms at the time of diagnosis. Sometimes the disease is diagnosed from a routine blood count in an asymptomatic patient.

Physical examination usually reveals splenomegaly although this is not marked until the WBC exceeds 100×10^9/l. Hepatomegaly is also common.

Initially the disease pursues a chronic course, in which patients are often maintained in reasonably good health. However, the prognosis, in the absence of stem cell transplantation or treatment with imatinib or other tyrosine kinase inhibitors, is ultimately very poor because of almost invariable transformation to an acute leukaemia that is refractory to treatment. Acute transformation is often preceded by an accelerated phase in which the disease becomes resistant to therapy. The median survival in CGL, in the absence of treatment, is about 2.5 years. Median survival in the absence of allogeneic stem cell transplantation or tyrosine kinase inhibitor therapy is of the order of 5 years. With the use of imatinib, the 5-year survival is now around 90%.

Assessment of peripheral blood features is of major importance in the diagnosis of CGL; bone marrow cytological and histological features are of lesser value. Diagnostic criteria are summarized in Fig. 5.1.

Peripheral blood

The WBC is elevated, usually to between 20 and 500×10^9/l. The predominant cell types in the peripheral blood are neutrophils and myelocytes (Fig. 5.2); immature granulocytic cells are also present with blasts and promyelocytes usually being less than 10–15% of cells [6]. Basophils are almost invariably increased and the absolute eosinophil count is increased in the great majority of patients; eosinophil and basophil myelocytes are usually present. Granulocytes show normal maturation. A normocytic normochromic anaemia is usual. There may be circulating erythroblasts; the presence of

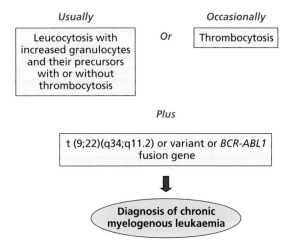

Fig. 5.1 WHO 2008 criteria for a diagnosis of chronic myelogenous leukaemia, *BCR-ABL1* positive (also known as chronic granulocytic leukaemia and chronic myeloid leukaemia).

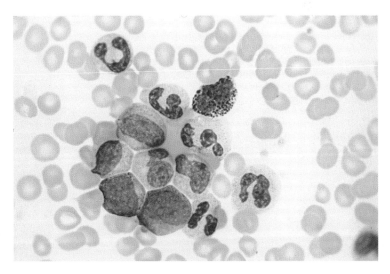

Fig. 5.2 Peripheral blood (PB) from a patient with CGL showing neutrophils and their precursors and one basophil. May-Grünwald-Giemsa (MGG) ×100.

2% or more nucleated red blood cells has been associated with a worse prognosis (pre-imatinib era) [7]. The platelet count is usually normal or elevated but does not often exceed $1000 \times 10^9/l$. Rare patients with Ph-positive *BCR-ABL1*-positive disease have thrombocytosis without leucocytosis; this condition is now recognized as a variant of CGL. Occasional patients have thrombocytopenia. Some giant platelets are usually present and occasional 'bare' megakaryocyte nuclei are seen.

During successful chronic phase treatment, the peripheral blood count and film usually become almost normal although a degree of basophilia and occasional immature granulocytes may persist. Patients presenting with or developing extensive bone marrow fibrosis have marked anisocytosis and poikilocytosis with prominent teardrop poikilocytes. The accelerated phase may be marked by increasing basophilia, persistent leucocytosis or the reappearance of anaemia. Acute transformation may follow an accelerated phase or the appearance of features of bone marrow fibrosis or be heralded by the appearance of dysplastic features (such as the acquired Pelger–Huët anomaly of neutrophils or the presence of circulating micromegakaryocytes) or there may be the abrupt appearance of increasing numbers of circulating blasts in a previously stable patient.

Acute transformation is myeloid in about two thirds of cases and lymphoblastic or mixed in the remainder. Myeloblasts may show neutrophilic or basophilic differentiation. Megakaryoblastic trans-

formation is not uncommon. Rarely, transformation is monoblastic, eosinophilic, hypergranular promyelocytic or erythroblastic. Alternatively, there may be hybrid cells with both basophil and mast cell features. Often a single patient has blasts of diverse types, usually a mixture of megakaryoblasts and myeloblasts, but occasionally a mixture of lymphoblasts and blasts of one or more myeloid lineages. As the number of blast cells in the blood increases there is a gradual disappearance of mature cells and anaemia and thrombocytopenia develop. The presence of more than 20% circulating blasts is an acceptable criterion for a diagnosis of acute transformation.

The neutrophil alkaline phosphatase score can be useful in confirming a diagnosis of chronic granulocytic leukaemia since it is low in about 95% of cases. However, cytochemistry is redundant when cytogenetic and molecular genetic techniques are available.

Treatment with hydroxycarbamide (previously known as hydroxyurea), interferon-α or the tyrosine kinase inhibitor, imatinib (previously known as STI571 or imatinib mesylate), usually leads to the loss of most of the peripheral blood features of CGL.

Bone marrow cytology

In the chronic phase of CGL, the bone marrow is intensely hypercellular with an increase in granulocytes and their precursors and often also megakaryocytes (Fig. 5.3). The myeloid : erythroid ratio is greater than 10 : 1, usually of the order of 25 : 1

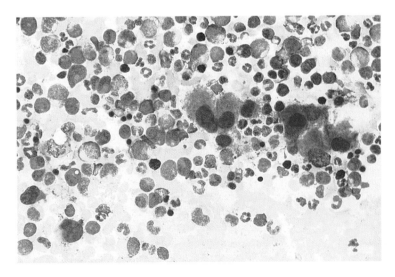

Fig. 5.3 Bone marrow (BM) aspirate film from a patient with CGL showing an increase of all granulocytic lineages and a clump of megakaryocytes with hypolobulated nuclei. MGG ×40.

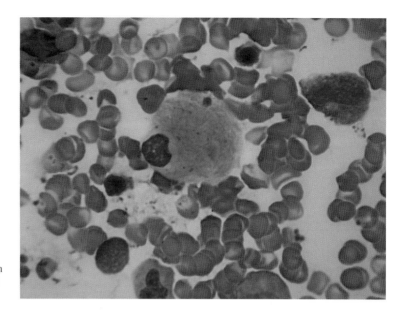

Fig. 5.4 BM aspirate film, CGL, showing a storage cell with characteristics intermediate between those of a pseudo-Gaucher cell and a sea-blue histiocyte. MGG ×100.

[2]. Precursors of neutrophils, eosinophils and basophils are all increased. Cellular maturation is normal. Erythropoiesis is reduced but morphologically normal. The average size and lobulation of megakaryocytes is reduced but micromegakaryocytes with one or two small round nuclei, as seen in MDS, are not usually a feature of the chronic phase of CGL. As a consequence of the increased cell turnover, macrophages and various storage cells are often prominent (see below).

Treatment of CGL with hydroxycarbamide or interferon is associated with a reduction in granulopoiesis and megakaryocyte numbers and an increase in erythropoiesis. If a cytogenetic response occurs, megakaryocyte size returns towards normal. Treatment with imatinib is associated with a complete morphological response, even in the absence of a cytogenetic response, indicating that the effect of *BCR-ABL1* is being blocked [8]. During imatinib treatment storage cells may be prominent, including cells with features intermediate between sea-blue histiocytes and pseudo-Gaucher cells (Fig. 5.4).

During the accelerated phase, the bone marrow may show increasing basophilia, some increase of blast cells or the appearance of dysplastic features. Bone marrow aspiration may become difficult or impossible because of increasing bone marrow fibrosis.

With the onset of acute transformation, the bone marrow is steadily replaced by blasts showing the usual cytological features of the lineage involved. Acute transformation can be diagnosed if bone marrow blasts exceed 20%.

Bone marrow histology [9–13]

The marrow is hypercellular with a loss of fat cells (Figs 5.5 and 5.6). In most cases more than 95% of the marrow cavity is occupied by haemopoietic cells. There is a marked increase in granulocytic precursors with a variable degree of left shift. The normal topographic relationship of haemopoiesis is retained, with granulopoiesis occurring predominantly in the paratrabecular, peri-arterial and pericapillary areas, although the more mature granulocytic precursors extend into the central areas of intertrabecular marrow. The increased numbers of basophils are not detected in haematoxylin and eosin (H&E)-stained histological sections because of dissolution of their granules during processing. Eosinophil precursors are increased in the majority of cases. A feature that may be helpful in distinguishing CGL from a leukaemoid reaction with granulocytic hyperplasia is that in CGL there is a loss of fat cells from the very earliest stages of the disease; the loss of paratrabecular fat cells is marked, whereas it has been reported that these are often preserved in a leukaemoid reaction [13].

Megakaryopoiesis and, to a lesser extent, erythropoiesis occurs in the perisinusoidal areas. There

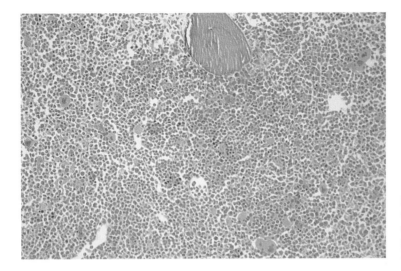

Fig. 5.5 BM trephine biopsy section, CGL, showing a packed marrow with a marked increase in granulocytic cells. Resin-embedded, H&E ×10.

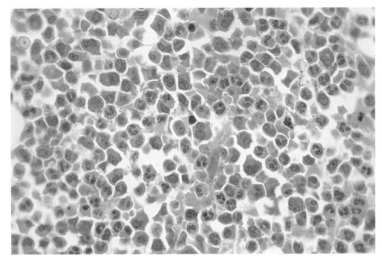

Fig. 5.6 BM trephine biopsy section, CGL, showing a marked increase in granulocytic cells with left shift. Resin-embedded, H&E ×40.

may be some megakaryocytes within sinusoids and also some near bony trabeculae [14]. Megakaryocytes are usually increased in number, often forming small clusters of cells; in some cases this is a striking feature. The average size and nuclear lobe count of megakaryocytes is decreased (Figs 5.7 and 5.8). The megakaryocytic morphology is variable, with most patients having both relatively normal forms and smaller cells with small, hypolobated nuclei.

Increased numbers of mast cells and plasma cells are commonly seen, usually in a perivascular position. Pseudo-Gaucher cells may be present (see Fig. 9.38): these are macrophages that contain phagocytosed glycolipids and also haemosiderin,

formed as a consequence of increased cell turnover. Pseudo-Gaucher cells have been reported in as many as 30% of cases [15]. Sea-blue histiocytes may also be found. There may be some attenuation of bone trabeculae [16]. Bone marrow vascularity is increased [17]. Marrow necrosis is uncommon and, when present, is usually a sign of impending blast transformation.

Reticulin is often increased and occasionally the fibrosis is severe enough to cause confusion with primary myelofibrosis [18]. In one series of patients, increased reticulin, with or without collagen deposition, was seen in a quarter of patients [15]. Fibrosis is more common in cases with

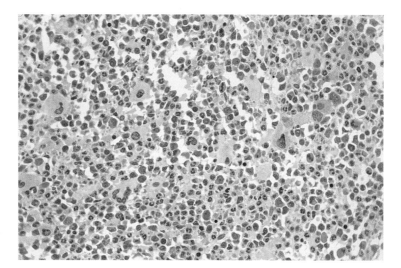

Fig. 5.7 BM trephine biopsy section, CGL with prominent megakaryocytic component, showing increased numbers of megakaryocytes with hypolobulated nuclei and increased granulocytes. Resin-embedded, H&E ×20.

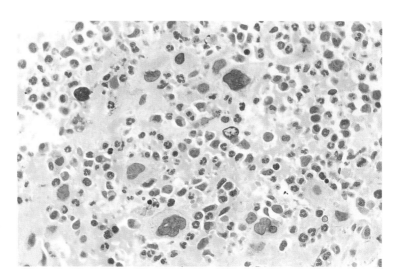

Fig. 5.8 BM trephine biopsy section, CGL, with prominent megakaryocytic component, showing increased granulocytes and numerous megakaryocytes with hyperchromatic, hypolobulated nuclei. Resin-embedded, H&E ×40.

marked megakaryocytic proliferation [11] (Fig. 5.9), correlating with the number of megakaryocytes and their precursors [15]. Identification of small dysplastic megakaryocytes is aided by immunohistochemistry (CD42b or CD61). In multivariate analysis, increased reticulin correlates with a worse prognosis (pre-imatinib era) [15]. Increased reticulin deposition may be present at the time of diagnosis although it is seen more often in the accelerated phase and in some cases in blast transformation. Depending on the therapeutic agent used, there may be progressive reticulin deposition during therapy (see below).

Heavy deposition may predict impending blast transformation. Severe fibrosis may be accompanied by osteosclerosis.

If a cytogenetic response occurs as a result of therapy, there is normalization of histological features. For example, cellularity generally decreases and small hypolobated megakaryocytes are replaced by cytologically normal forms. Increasing reticulin deposition is often seen during interferon therapy and to a lesser extent during busulphan therapy [19]. During hydroxycarbamide treatment reticulin fibrosis may regress [20]. Lymphoid aggregates are increased, particularly during interferon therapy

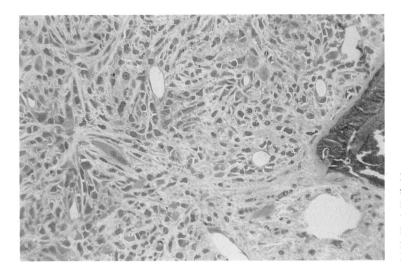

Fig. 5.9 BM trephine biopsy section, CGL with fibrosis, showing marked collagen fibrosis and 'streaming' of haemopoietic cells including numerous hypolobulated megakaryocytes. Resin-embedded, H&E ×20.

[21]. Bone marrow aplasia is a rare complication of interferon therapy [22].

When patients still in the chronic phase are treated with imatinib there is generally a morphological response, even in the absence of a cytogenetic response [8]. Granulocytic excess usually resolves by 2 months, often with a period of granulocytic hypoplasia [8]. The increase in megakaryocytes resolves by 5 months [8]. Erythropoiesis recovers towards normal [8]. Sea-blue histiocytes often persist in the first few months and then gradually disappear [8]. Gelatinous transformation has been reported in occasional patients [23]. In one study, bone marrow vascularity slowly decreased to normal without any clear correlation with cytogenetic response [17], whereas in another study reduction in microvessels was associated with cytogenetic response [24]. Reticulin fibrosis resolves over time [24,25]. Reactive lymphoid aggregates, containing a mixture of T and B lymphocytes, are common [8,21]. Imatinib therapy has been associated with increased bone formation [26].

Prognostic features demonstrated in chronic phase CGL pre-imatinib included the number of megakaryocytes [15,27], the degree of reticulin and collagen fibrosis (indicative of worse prognosis) [15,27] and the proportion of erythroid precursors (indicative of a better prognosis) [27].

Accumulation of immature granulocytic precursors (myeloblasts and promyelocytes) in the paratrabecular (Fig. 5.10) and perivascular regions are often seen in the accelerated phase, preceding the blast phase [28]. There may also be intrasinusoidal haemopoiesis in this phase of the disease.

Blast transformation [29–32] may involve part or all of a trephine biopsy specimen. Areas of involvement contain sheets of blasts, which usually have a single prominent nucleolus and often show considerable pleomorphism. In megakaryoblastic transformation there are usually large numbers of dysplastic megakaryocytes, often with bizarre morphology, in addition to numerous megakaryoblasts. Otherwise it is often not possible to determine the lineage of blasts from H&E-stained sections. Moderate or severe myelofibrosis is seen in approximately 40% of cases of both myeloid and lymphoid transformation and is an almost universal finding in megakaryoblastic transformation. Myelofibrosis may make marrow aspiration impossible so that a biopsy is necessary to establish the diagnosis of blast transformation. Acute transformation can be diagnosed if trephine biopsy sections show extensive focal infiltration by blast cells, even if peripheral blood and bone marrow aspirate blast cells are less than 20%.

Immunohistochemistry is of limited value during the chronic phase of the disease but can be useful in the accelerated phase and in blast transformation. Increased numbers of CD34-positive cells are observed in the accelerated phase and transformation [33] and generally correlate with an increase of blast cells. Immunohistochemistry can be useful

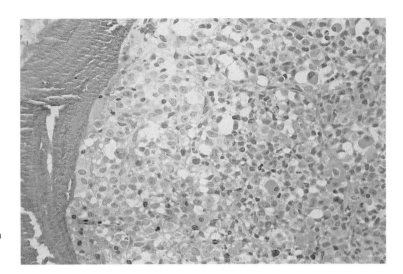

Fig. 5.10 BM trephine biopsy section, CGL in accelerated phase, showing accumulation of blasts in a broad paratrabecular band. Resin-embedded, H&E ×20.

to distinguish between myeloid and lymphoid transformation and, using CD42b or CD61, to confirm megakaryoblastic transformation. CD79a is more reliable than CD20 for the identification of B-lineage blast crisis. Basophils can be identified using BB1 or 2D7 monoclonal antibodies [34] but this is not usually necessary. Immature basophils may also express mast cell tryptase [34].

Cytogenetic and molecular genetic analysis

Chronic granulocytic leukaemia is typically associated with t(9;22)(q34;q11.2) and with the formation of a *BCR-ABL1* fusion gene. *BCR-ABL1* fusion can also result from variant and complex translocations and from cryptic chromosomal rearrangements. The diagnosis of CGL cannot be sustained if *BCR-ABL1* is lacking. The *BCR-ABL1* fusion gene usually encodes a 210 kD protein with tyrosine kinase activity, which has an important role in the pathogenesis of the disease. In uncommon molecular variants there is either a p190 protein (sometimes associated with prominent monocytosis) or a p230 protein (associated with predominantly neutrophilic differentiation or marked thrombocytosis). The diagnosis of CGL can be confirmed by conventional cytogenetic analysis, fluorescence *in situ* hybridization (FISH) or a reverse transcriptase polymerase chain reaction (RT-PCR).

A significant minority of patients with CGL have, in addition to t(9;22), a fairly large deletion of chromosome 9 sequences centromeric to the *ABL1*

gene [35]. This has been found to correlate with a worse prognosis in patients treated with hydroxycarbamide or interferon but only if the deletion spans the breakpoint [36]; the inferior outcome is abrogated by imatinib treatment [37].

The accelerated phase and blast transformation are often associated with cytogenetic evolution. Extra cytogenetic abnormalities often include i(17q) and further copies of the Ph chromosome.

Problems and pitfalls

The chronic phase of CGL is so characteristic that, as long as peripheral blood as well as bone marrow features are considered, misdiagnosis is unlikely. Leukaemoid reactions very rarely simulate CGL, basophilia and the characteristic different count being absent. Because of their sensitivity to imatinib, it is important to identify not only haematologically typical cases of CGL but also Ph-positive *BCR-ABL1*-positive cases presenting with thrombocytosis and to distinguish these from essential thrombocythaemia; they have different bone marrow histological features (Fig. 5.11) and a different disease course from essential thrombocythaemia, showing a marked propensity to develop typical CGL or myelofibrosis [38] or to transform into acute leukaemia [38,39]. The presence of more than 3–5% of basophils in a patient presenting with thrombocytosis is predictive of Ph positivity [39,40].

In patients who present already in accelerated phase (Fig. 5.12) or acute transformation, diagnosis

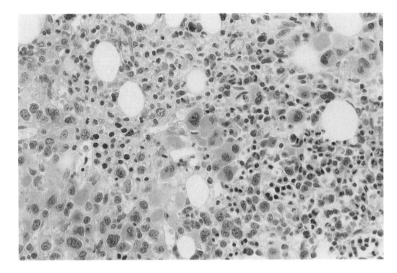

Fig. 5.11 BM trephine biopsy section in CGL presenting with isolated thrombocytosis showing a marked increase in megakaryocytes. The average size of megakaryocytes is reduced and there is a tendency to hypolobation; the increase in granulopoiesis was minimal. Paraffin-embedded, H&E ×20. (By courtesy of Dr R. Cuthbert.)

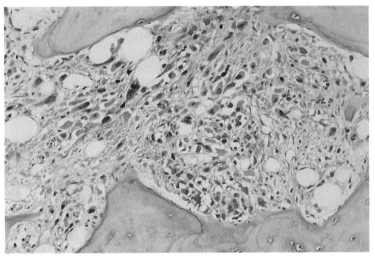

Fig. 5.12 Section of BM trephine biopsy specimen from a patient presenting in an accelerated phase of CGL showing granulocytic dysplasia, increased numbers of megakaryocytes (most of which are dysplastic) and osteomyelofibrosis. The correct diagnosis was revealed by cytogenetic analysis which showed normal metaphases, a clonal population with t(9;22) as the sole abnormality and a sideline showing cytogenetic evolution. Paraffin-embedded, H&E ×20.

is more difficult. These cases can be confused with atypical chronic myeloid leukaemia (aCML) or with acute myeloid leukaemia (AML). Genetic analysis is needed for diagnosis.

In an appropriate haematological context, the *BCR-ABL1* fusion gene is a defining feature of CGL. Because of the responsiveness to imatinib therapy, cytogenetic/molecular analysis in patients presenting with apparent aCML or AML has become of considerable importance.

Chronic neutrophilic leukaemia

Chronic neutrophilic leukaemia is a rare condition, occurring mainly in the elderly. The incidence in

the USA has been estimated at 0.01 per 100 000 per year [41]. Familial cases have been reported [42]. Splenomegaly and hepatomegaly are often present. In the WHO classification, a WBC at least 25×10^9/l is a prerequisite for the diagnosis [43]. Diagnostic criteria of the 2008 WHO classification are summarized in Fig. 5.13.

Peripheral blood

The peripheral blood shows an increase in mature neutrophils and band forms (Fig. 5.14) without any eosinophilia or basophilia and with very few neutrophil precursors (almost always less than 5%). Some cases have shown heavy neutrophil granula-

WBC at least 25×10^9/l

Plus

Neutrophils and band forms more than 80% of peripheral blood cells and no dysplasia

Plus

Promyelocytes, myelocytes and metamyelocytes <10% of peripheral blood cells

Plus

Blast cells <5% in blood and <20% in bone marrow

Plus

No evidences of another MPN or MDS (monocytes <1 x 10^9/l) or rearrangement of *PDGFRA*, *PDGFRB* or *FGFR1*

Plus

Hepatosplenomegaly

Plus

Clonality demonstrated if a cause of reactive neutrophilia or a paraprotein present

Diagnosis of chronic neutrophilic leukaemia

Fig. 5.13 The 2008 WHO criteria for a diagnosis of chronic neutrophilic leukaemia. MDS, myelodysplastic syndrome; MPN, myeloproliferative neoplasm; WBC, white blood cell count.

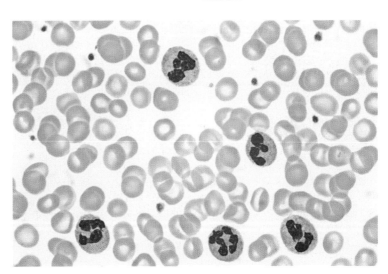

Fig. 5.14 PB film in chronic neutrophilic leukaemia showing an increase of mature neutrophils. MGG ×100.

tion. Cases with dysplastic features have been reported but the WHO classification excludes these from the designation 'chronic neutrophilic leukaemia' [43].

Bone marrow cytology

The bone marrow is hypercellular with an increase in neutrophils and their precursors (Fig. 5.15), with no disproportionate increase in immature cells.

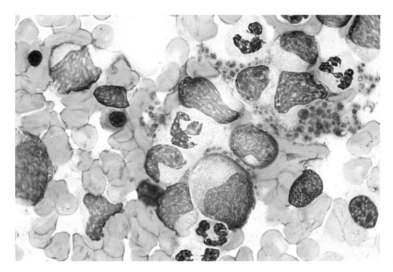

Fig. 5.15 BM aspirate film in chronic neutrophilic leukaemia showing an increase of neutrophils and precursors; neutrophils appear hypogranular and have nuclear projections. MGG ×100.

Bone marrow histology

The bone marrow is hypercellular with an increase in neutrophils and their precursors. Abnormal localization of immature neutrophil precursors is sometimes seen and megakaryocytes may be atypical with some clustering [44]. An increase of reticulin is uncommon [43].

Cytogenetic and molecular genetic analysis

No specific cytogenetic or molecular genetic abnormality has been recognized. Clonal abnormalities described have included trisomy 8, trisomy 9, trisomy 21, del(11q), del(20q) and del(12p). The *JAK2* V617F mutation is present in occasional patients [45] and has sometimes been homozygous.

Problems and pitfalls

A distinction should be drawn between chronic neutrophilic leukaemia, which is Ph negative and *BCR-ABL1* negative, and the neutrophilic variant of chronic granulocytic leukaemia, which is Ph positive and *BCR-ABL1* positive but is associated with a p230 rather than p210 BCR-ABL1 protein. The distinction is based on cytogenetic and molecular genetic features rather than on cytology. The neutrophil alkaline phosphatase score is normal or high in chronic neutrophilic leukaemia and low in CGL but this test is redundant if genetic analysis is available.

A neutrophilic leukaemoid reaction can occur in association with multiple myeloma (Fig. 5.16) and monoclonal gammopathy of undetermined significance [46]. It is essential to investigate patients with apparent neutrophilic leukaemia for the presence of a paraprotein to avoid misdiagnosis of this leukaemoid reaction as neutrophilic leukaemia.

Polycythaemia vera

Polycythaemia vera (PV; preferred WHO terminology), also known as polycythaemia rubra vera or primary proliferative polycythaemia, is an MPN in which the dominant feature is excessive production of erythrocytes by the marrow with a resultant increase in the circulating red cell mass and the venous haematocrit. Frequently there is also an increase in cells of other haemopoietic cell lineages, both in the marrow and in the peripheral blood, reflecting the origin of the neoplastic clone from a multipotent myeloid stem cell.

Most patients present between the ages of 40 and 70 years but there are rare instances of well-documented cases in young adults, adolescents and even young children [47]. The reported incidence varies from 0.35 to 2.6 per 100 000 per year [48]. Many of the disease features are related to hyperviscosity of the blood and to the arterial or venous thromboses that occur; these include headache, a feeling of fullness of the head, dizziness, tinnitus, dyspnoea, visual disturbance, Raynaud's phenomenon, erythromelalgia, claudication and gangrene. Pruritus may occur, probably consequent on histamine secretion by basophils. Up to 70% of cases

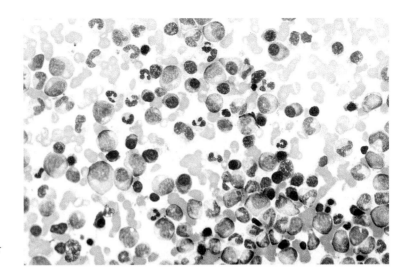

Fig. 5.16 BM aspirate film from a patient with a neutrophilic leukaemoid reaction to multiple myeloma showing granulocytic hyperplasia and increased plasma cells. MGG ×40. (By courtesy of Dr G. Lucas, Manchester.)

have been found to have splenomegaly and 40% hepatomegaly.

Polycythaemia vera must be distinguished from secondary polycythaemia which is usually a consequence of either chronic generalized tissue hypoxia (for example, due to high altitude, chronic hypoxic pulmonary disease or cyanotic congenital heart disease) or of inappropriate erythropoietin production (usually a result of chronic renal hypoxia or ectopic production of erythropoietin by a renal or other tumour). In many patients with secondary polycythaemia, the cause is readily apparent but sometimes there is diagnostic difficulty and the differential diagnosis then depends on consideration of clinical, peripheral blood and bone marrow features. Hepatomegaly and splenomegaly are not features of secondary polycythaemia.

Polycythaemia vera and secondary polycythaemia must also be distinguished from pseudo- or relative polycythaemia, which is a consequence of a decreased plasma volume rather than an increased red cell mass.

Polycythaemia vera may enter a 'burnt out' or 'spent' phase in which there is initially a reduction of red cell production followed by the development of splenomegaly and bone marrow fibrosis; with disease progression, there is development of all the clinical and pathological features usually associated with primary myelofibrosis. The designation 'spent phase of polycythaemia' has been suggested for the phase of the disease when there is a stable haem-

atocrit and marked splenomegaly with minimal fibrosis and the designation 'transitional state polycythaemia vera' when there is persisting erythrocytosis with progressive myelofibrosis [49]. The final stage of this progression is designated post-polycythaemic myelofibrosis A small proportion of patients, particularly those who have been treated with alkylating agents or ^{32}P, develop AML. The incidence of acute leukaemia is much increased in those in whom myelofibrosis has developed, but acute transformation can also occur without any warning signs or, occasionally, following the appearance of myelodysplastic features.

Historically, untreated PV had a median survival of about 1.5 years but with currently available treatment the median survival is about 12 years.

Although not specific for the disease, diagnosis of PV has been facilitated by the discovery of its very frequent association with a gain-of-function mutation in exon 14 of the *JAK2* gene, most often *JAK2* V617F (see below). JAK2 is a tyrosine kinase in the signalling pathway of many haemopoietic growth factors.

A pre-polycythaemic stage of PV is now recognized in which there is borderline or mild erythrocytosis with a variable combination of other features such as thrombocytosis, the *JAK2* V617F mutation, low serum erythropoietin, consistent bone marrow histology and growth of endogenous erythroid colonies from the blood [50]. Rarely, patients who present with unexplained portal or hepatic vein

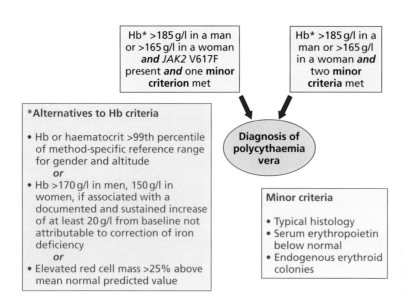

| Hb* >185 g/l in a man or >165 g/l in a woman *and* JAK2 V617F present *and* one **minor criterion** met | Hb* >185 g/l in a man or >165 g/l in a woman *and* two **minor criteria** met |

*Alternatives to Hb criteria

- Hb or haematocrit >99th percentile of method-specific reference range for gender and altitude
  or
- Hb >170 g/l in men, 150 g/l in women, if associated with a documented and sustained increase of at least 20 g/l from baseline not attributable to correction of iron deficiency
  or
- Elevated red cell mass >25% above mean normal predicted value

Diagnosis of polycythaemia vera

Minor criteria

- Typical histology
- Serum erythropoietin below normal
- Endogenous erythroid colonies

Fig. 5.17 The 2008 WHO criteria for a diagnosis of polycythaemia vera. Hb, haemoglobin concentration.

thrombosis and a normal blood count subsequently develop PV [51]. Patients presenting with such thrombosis should be investigated for an MPN with serum erythropoietin assay, *JAK2* V617F analysis and trephine biopsy [51].

The diagnostic criteria of the 2008 WHO classification are summarized in Fig. 5.17 [50].

Peripheral blood

The blood count shows an elevation of the red cell count, haemoglobin concentration (Hb) and haematocrit. As a consequence of the increased blood viscosity, the blood film shows crowding together of the red cells, an appearance described as a 'packed film'. In some patients, iron stores have been exhausted and there is also microcytosis and hypochromia. The WBC is commonly elevated due to an increase in the neutrophil count; occasionally neutrophilia is marked. Absolute basophilia is often present. Small numbers of immature granulocytes or erythroblasts may be present. Many patients have a moderately elevated platelet count. An elevated WBC (above $15 \times 10^9/l$) is associated with a higher risk of myocardial infarction [52] and correlates with subsequent development of post-polycythaemic myelofibrosis [53]. The minority of patients with an exon 12 *JAK* mutation rather than the usual *JAK2* V617F mutation generally present with isolated erythrocytosis [54].

Bone marrow cytology

The bone marrow usually shows a marked increase in erythroid precursors and often some increase of granulocytes, granulocyte precursors and megakaryocytes (Fig. 5.18). Cells of eosinophil and basophil lineages, as well as those of neutrophil lineage, may be increased. The average size and nuclear lobation of megakaryocytes is increased. Iron stores are usually absent and the features of superimposed iron deficiency may be present.

Bone marrow histology [9,55–59]

There is usually marked hypercellularity relative to the patient's age, with haemopoietic cells often filling more than 90% of the marrow space. There is commonly an increase in cells of all three haemopoietic lineages (but particularly erythroid lineage and megakaryocytes). Erythropoiesis is morphologically normal (Fig. 5.19). Megakaryocyte morphology is often abnormal with a spectrum from small hypolobated to large hyperlobated forms; the average size of megakaryocytes is considerably increased, as is their nuclear lobation. Often there is clustering of megakaryocytes (Fig. 5.19). There may be an increase in emperipolesis and in mitotic figures in megakaryocytes [14]. Neutrophil granulopoiesis is increased and sometimes also eosinophil production. Many cases

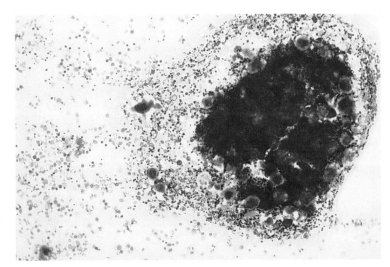

Fig. 5.18 BM aspirate film, polycythaemia vera, showing a markedly hypercellular bone marrow fragment showing increased erythroid and granulocyte precursors and increased megakaryocytes. MGG ×10.

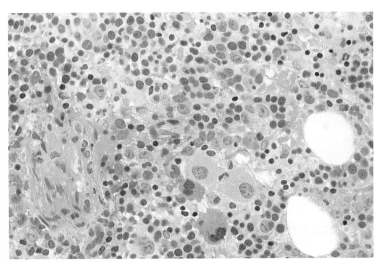

Fig. 5.19 BM trephine biopsy section, polycythaemia vera, showing hypercellularity, increased erythroid precursors and a cluster of immature megakaryocytes. Resin-embedded, H&E ×40.

show a mild increase in reticulin, with about 10% of patients showing a moderate or marked increase [57]. Around a third of patients show an increase in small vessels [58]. Sinusoids are usually increased in number and may be dilated. Marrow iron stores are decreased or absent (but it should be noted that assessment of decalcified trephine biopsy specimens is unreliable; the bone marrow aspirate is more reliable). Lymphoid nodules have been reported in up to 20% of patients in some series. There may be osteoporosis with attenuation of trabeculae [16]. The minority of patients with an exon 12 *JAK2* mutation rather than the usual *JAK2* V617F mutation have increased erythroid precursors without morpho-

logical abnormalities of megakaryocytes or of the granulocyte series [54].

Up to 30% of patients with PV develop severe marrow fibrosis, which is morphologically indistinguishable from primary myelofibrosis (see page 260); this is more common in cases with marked megakaryocytic proliferation.

Cytogenetic and molecular genetic analysis

A minority of patients have clonal cytogenetic abnormalities at diagnosis, of which del(20q) is the most characteristic. Other recurrent abnormalities include trisomy 8, trisomy 9, trisomy 1q, del(13q), del(1p) and del(9p). Detection is enhanced by the use of FISH with probes for 9p21, 20q12 and the centromere of chromosome 8. Loss of heterozygosity for 9p is frequently observed [60].

Molecular genetic analysis is of more importance than cytogenetic analysis. A gain-of-function point mutation, *JAK2* V617F, is present in about 95% of patients [45,61,62]; it is likely to be a second event, contributing to disease progression; it is homozygous in over a quarter of patients [63] (those with loss of heterozygosity of 9p as a result of mitotic recombination leading to acquired isodisomy, sometimes referred to as uniparental disomy). The mutation is present in cells of all myeloid lineages and, in some patients, also in B, T or natural killer (NK) lymphocytes [64]. When AML supervenes in PV, the leukaemic blasts cells may lack the *JAK2* mutation that was initially present [65] supporting the view that this mutation is not the primary pathogenetic event. The discovery of this *JAK2* mutation means that the molecular response to treatment can now be studied; it has been shown that the molecular response to imatinib and interferon-α is minor [66].

A minority of patients, who have a somewhat different phenotype, have a *JAK2* mutation (point mutation, small deletion or deletion/insertion) in exon 12 rather than in exon 14 [54]. The *JAK2* V617F (exon 14) mutation can be detected in peripheral blood granulocytes whereas detection of exon 12 mutations usually requires analysis of bone marrow cells [54]. Rare patients have both *JAK2* V617F and a *JAK2* exon 12 mutation [67].

Problems and pitfalls

The diagnosis of PV previously required isotopic dilution studies to demonstrate a true polycythaemia and exclude relative polycythaemia (elevation of the Hb because of reduction of plasma volume). Following the discovery that the great majority of patients with PV have a detectable acquired *JAK2* mutation, providing evidence of a clonal bone marrow disorder, the importance of estimating the red cell mass has greatly declined. The 2008 WHO classification permits the diagnosis of PV without a study of red cell mass if the Hb is greater than 185 g/l in a man or greater than 165 g/l in a woman and if certain other criteria are met [50] (Fig. 5.17). Bone marrow examination is not indicated in patients with relative polycythaemia but, if done, is normal. Serum erythropoietin is usually normal

in relative polycythaemia but is occasionally reduced [68,69].

Polycythaemia vera also needs to be distinguished from secondary polycythaemia. This distinction has become easier with the discovery of the *JAK2* mutation. Testing for the mutation can be done on peripheral blood granulocytes at an early stage in the investigation of a patient and investigations can then be targeted either at PV or at other causes of a high Hb. Peripheral blood basophilia is not seen in secondary polycythaemia and neutrophilia and thrombocytosis are unusual. In contrast to PV, superimposed iron deficiency is uncommon in secondary cases and trephine biopsy sections show only moderate hypercellularity. There is increased erythropoiesis but the other haemopoietic cell lineages are normal. In particular, the megakaryocytic abnormalities seen in PV are not present, reticulin is normal and sinusoids are not increased [55,56]. Lymphoid nodules are more prevalent in PV than in healthy subjects but may also be increased in some reactive conditions associated with secondary polycythaemia. Increased plasma cells and increased cellular debris within macrophages, seen in some cases of secondary polycythaemia, are said not to be features of PV [59]. Typical cases of PV can be distinguished readily from secondary polycythaemia on histological grounds. However, not all cases can be recognized and some patients in whom a diagnosis of PV can be made on the basis of clinical or clinical and cytogenetic features do not have diagnostic histopathological features [55,57]. Cases of PV associated with exon 12 mutation and early *JAK2* V617F-associated cases are not always distinguishable histologically from reactive polycythaemia. Immunohistochemistry using a monoclonal antibody directed at the thrombopoietin receptor, MPL, has been reported to be useful in distinguishing PV from secondary erythrocytosis; in secondary erythrocytosis there is uniform, moderate to strong staining of megakaryocytes whereas in PV staining is either weak or heterogeneous [70]. Unfortunately the antibody clone used in this study has not survived and there are currently no commercially available antibodies reactive with paraffin-embedded tissues.

Some patients in whom no underlying cause of secondary polycythaemia can be found do not have any clinical, haematological or histopathological features that permit a diagnosis of PV. If such patients lack a detectable *JAK2* mutation (exon 12, exon 14 or other) the appropriate diagnosis is 'idiopathic erythrocytosis'. In the past, with prolonged follow-up, some, but not all, of this group of patients developed features such as splenomegaly, neutrophilia or basophilia, indicating in retrospect that the correct diagnosis was PV. It is probable that this sequence of events will be much less frequent now that molecular investigation is likely to be done early.

Essential thrombocythaemia

Essential thrombocythaemia (ET), in common with other MPN, is a disease resulting from the clonal proliferation of a multipotent myeloid stem cell but with the predominant disease features resulting from increased platelet production. The disease is seen at all ages but is predominately one of middle and old age. The reported incidence varies from 0.1 to 2.53 per 100 000 per year with the higher figures appearing more probable [48]. In several series of patients there has been a marked female predominance [48]. ET is characterized by a marked thrombocytosis (usually 1000–4000 $\times$ 10^9/l) often resulting in haemorrhagic or thrombotic episodes or both. At least 20% of patients are asymptomatic and are diagnosed incidentally from routine blood counts. With the widespread use of automated blood counters the proportion of patients in whom the diagnosis is made incidentally, before the occurrence of symptoms, is steadily increasing. About two thirds of symptomatic patients suffer venous or arterial thrombosis or symptoms attributable to small vessel obstruction, such as headache, dizziness, visual disturbance, paraesthesiae and peripheral vascular insufficiency. About a third of symptomatic patients have abnormal bleeding, for example into the gastro-intestinal tract or subcutaneous tissues.

Moderate splenomegaly was reported in up to 40% of cases in early series of patients and hepatomegaly in up to 20% [39], but if the 2008 WHO diagnostic criteria are used the prevalence is much lower. Occasional patients suffer repeated splenic infarcts, resulting in splenic atrophy and hyposplenism. Pruritus occurs in a minority of patients.

Although ET may terminate in MDS, AML or myelofibrosis, the chronic phase of the disease is usually very long. Transformation to AML occurs in about 1% of patients. No accurate data are available on prognosis in the absence of treatment since, before the general availability of automated blood cell counters, only the more severe cases were recognized. With currently available treatment, life expectancy shows little reduction from normal.

In the 2008 WHO classification, a sustained platelet count of at least 450×10^9/l is required to establish the diagnosis [71,72]. Previously, a count of at least 600×10^9/l was required but a lower cut-off point is important for recognition of a larger group of patients who may have thrombotic complications, splenomegaly and typical histological features before reaching the previous threshold. Diagnostic criteria of the 2008 WHO classification are summarized in Fig. 5.20 [72].

Peripheral blood

The blood film shows an increased number of platelets with the average platelet size being increased. There are usually some giant platelets and agranular and hypogranular platelets; platelet aggregates may also be present. Occasional 'bare' megakaryocyte nuclei are seen. Mild leucocytosis, neutrophilia and occasional immature granulocytes may be present but the WBC does not usually exceed 20×10^9/l. A WBC above 11×10^9/l (but, curiously, not an increased platelet count) correlates with an increased risk of thrombosis [73]. Absolute basophilia is sometimes present but basophils are usually only 1–2% [31,48]. Rarely, in patients who have suffered splenic infarction, features of hyposplenism are found (Howell–Jolly bodies, acanthocytes, target cells and occasional spherocytes). Patients who have suffered haemorrhagic episodes may show features of iron deficiency.

Bone marrow cytology

The bone marrow aspirate shows an increase in megakaryocytes, which are generally large and hyperlobated (Fig. 5.21). On flow cytometric analysis, megakaryocytes can be shown to be increased in number, diameter, volume and ploidy [74]. In some cases there is a mild to moderate overall increase in cellularity. There is no more

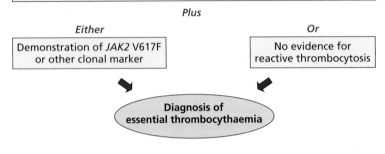

| Sustained platelet count ≥450 × 10⁹/l |

Plus

Bone marrow biopsy specimen showing proliferation mainly of the megakaryocytic lineage with increased numbers of enlarged, mature megakaryocytes

Plus

Criteria for other myeloid neoplasms not met, e.g. not PV (ferritin normal or Hb does not rise with iron), not PMF, not CML (*BCR-ABL1* negative), not MDS (fewer than 15% ring sideroblasts, not 5q– syndrome)

Plus

Either
Demonstration of *JAK2* V617F or other clonal marker

Or
No evidence for reactive thrombocytosis

Diagnosis of essential thrombocythaemia

Fig. 5.20 The 2008 WHO criteria for a diagnosis of essential thrombocythaemia. CML, chronic myeloid leukaemia; Hb, haemoglobin concentration; MDS, myelodysplastic syndrome; PMF, primary myelofibrosis; PV, polycythaemia vera.

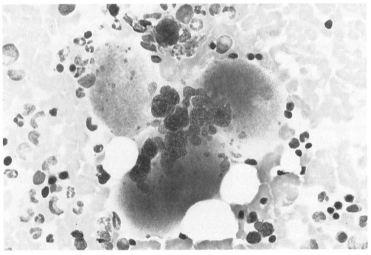

Fig. 5.21 BM aspirate, essential thrombocythaemia, showing four megakaryocytes, one of which is small while three are very large with hyperlobulated nuclei. MGG ×40.

than a minor increase in granulopoiesis and erythropoiesis.

In patients who are treated with anagrelide, a reduction in megakaryocyte number, diameter, size and ploidy is demonstrable [74,75].

Bone marrow histology [10,14,76]
Trephine biopsy findings are extremely variable and in some cases there may be no specific diagnostic features [76]. The marrow is usually somewhat hypercellular, relative to the patient's age,

although this is not as marked as in the other MPN. Cellularity is higher in those with a *JAK2* mutation than in those with a *MPL* mutation (in whom cellularity is usually normal or decreased) or those with neither mutation [77]. There may be an increase in granulocytic and erythroid precursors but this is not usual in those with an *MPL* mutation [77]. Sometimes the bone marrow is normocellular or even hypocellular. Megakaryocytes are increased in number in all cases but the degree of increase is very variable and does not correlate closely with

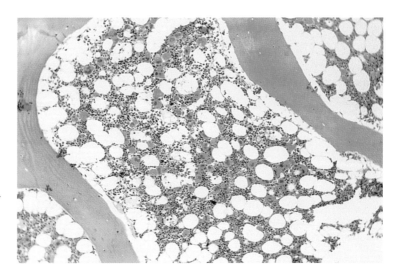

Fig. 5.22 BM trephine biopsy section, essential thrombocythaemia, showing mild hypercellularity with a marked increase in megakaryocytes, which are forming large clusters. Resin-embedded, H&E ×10.

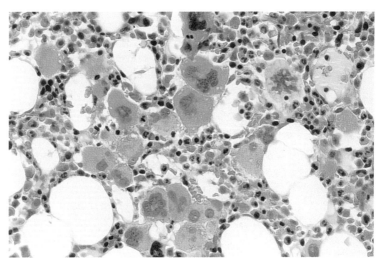

Fig. 5.23 BM trephine biopsy section, essential thrombocythaemia, showing clustering of megakaryocytes. The megakaryocytes are mainly large and hyperlobated, although some small forms are present. Resin-embedded, H&E ×40.

the platelet count. Loose clusters of megakaryocytes are commonly seen but tight clustering is uncommon and involves only a small number of cells (Fig. 5.22). The average size of megakaryocytes is increased, as is the lobation of their nuclei; these appearances have been referred to as staghorn-like (Fig. 5.23). The nuclear chromatin pattern is normal, in contrast to the hyperchromatic nuclei that may be seen in primary myelofibrosis [10]. In comparison with PV and cellular stages of primary myelofibrosis, megakaryocytes in ET are less pleomorphic and small megakaryocytes are not increased. Some megakaryocytes may be sited abnormally, close to the endosteum of trabec-

ulae, and emperipolesis and mitotic figures may be increased [14]. A mild focal increase in reticulin sometimes occurs but, if there is marked reticulin fibrosis, a diagnosis of primary myelofibrosis with thrombocytosis is more likely. Dilated sinusoids with intrasinusoidal megakaryocytes or other haemopoietic cells are likewise not a feature of ET.

Small blood vessels may be increased; in one study, this was found in 12% of patients [58]. Increased angiogenesis correlates with increased reticulin deposition [58]. Immunohistochemistry for MPL expression has been reported as clinically useful [78–81] but no antibody reactive in fixed, paraffin-embedded tissues is currently available.

In patients with ET who are treated with anagrelide, reduction in megakaryocyte size has been noted [75]. Increased fibrosis was observed in some ET patients receiving anagrelide in a large randomized controlled trial [82].

Cytogenetic and molecular genetic analysis

A small minority of patients with ET have a clonal cytogenetic abnormality detectable by standard cytogenetic analysis, most often trisomy 8, del(13q), trisomy 9, del(20q) or an abnormality of 9q. Other recurrent abnormalities include dup(1q), del(5q), del(7q) and del(17q) [83]. FISH analysis detects a much larger proportion of patients with abnormalities, 15% in a study that used probes to detect +8, +9, del(13)(q14) and del(20)(q12) [84]. By definition, there is no t(9;22)(q34;q11.2) or *BCR-ABL1*, such cases being classified as CGL.

JAK2 V617F is detectable in granulocytic and erythroid cells in about 50% of patients [45,61–63]; as in PV and primary myelofibrosis, it is likely to be a second event since, when evolution to AML occurs, the blast cells may lack the *JAK2* mutation [85]. Its presence correlates with the presence of del(20q) and trisomy 9 [65]. The mutation is homozygous due to mitotic recombination (acquired isodisomy) in about 3% of patients [63]. The presence of *JAK2* V617F correlates with an increased risk of thrombosis [73]. An *MPL* gain-of-function mutation (e.g. *MPL* W515L, *MPL* W515K, *MPL* W515S or *MPL* S505N) is found in 4–5% of patients and may coexist with *JAK2* V617F [77,86,87].

Some patients in whom a diagnosis of ET is made appear, on analysis of X-linked polymorphisms, to have polyclonal haemopoiesis [80,88,89]; this unexpected observation is likely to reflect insensitivity of the techniques used since some patients with apparently polyclonal haemopoiesis on X-liked polymorphism analysis have a clonal *JAK2* mutation [90]. Conversely, granulocyte monoclonality can be detected by X-linked polymorphism analysis in some patients who lack a *JAK2* mutation [91].

Problems and pitfalls

It is necessary to distinguish ET from reactive thrombocytosis. Peripheral blood features can be useful. In ET there are often giant platelets, some agranular platelets and occasionally circulating megakaryocyte nuclei. In contrast, the platelets in reactive thrombocytosis are small and normally granulated and circulating megakaryocyte nuclei are not seen. In reactive thrombocytosis, basophilia is not seen and neutrophilia is usually absent. In reactive thrombocytosis, the bone marrow aspirate and trephine biopsy sections often show an increase in megakaryocyte number and size and an increase in emperipolesis but megakaryocytes are cytologically normal; they do not occur in large clusters or close to the endosteum [14]. The bone marrow reticulin is also normal.

Since marked thrombocytosis can occur not only in ET but also in PV, CGL and primary myelofibrosis, the diagnosis is, in part, one of exclusion. Making a distinction from CGL (see above) is important because of the therapeutic implications and with cytogenetic/molecular genetic analysis is quite straightforward. The distinction from PV, particularly with coexisting iron deficiency or the prepolycythaemic phase of PV, and from the prefibrotic stage of primary myelofibrosis is both more difficult and less important. Peripheral blood features are not usually helpful since giant platelets, agranular platelets, megakaryocyte fragments, neutrophilia and basophilia can be seen in any MPN. The bone marrow aspirate and trephine biopsy are more useful but it should be noted that even experienced haematopathologists show poor concordance in distinguishing between ET and prefibrotic primary myelofibrosis [92]. Features that may be useful in making a distinction between various MPN that may cause thrombocytosis are summarized in Table 5.3. In prefibrotic early stage primary myelofibrosis, megakaryocytes are usually markedly abnormal, whereas in ET they are cytologically less atypical. Although megakaryocytic dysplasia also tends to be more marked in PV than in ET, distinguishing between these two conditions on histological grounds can be difficult. Some authors have considered that the lack of atypia of megakaryocytes in ET permits this distinction to be made [14], whereas others have suggested that, in the majority of instances, the two conditions cannot be distinguished on this basis [39]. The serum erythropoietin is of some value but it should be noted that low or even undetectable values are sometimes seen in ET as well as in PV [69,93]. If clinical, hae-

Table 5.3 Bone marrow histological features that may be of use in distinguishing essential thrombocythaemia from other myeloproliferative neoplasms.

	Polycythaemia vera	Essential thrombocythaemia	Primary myelofibrosis, prefibrotic	Primary myelofibrosis, fibrotic
Cellularity	Increased: erythropoiesis increased, often trilineage increase	Usually normal or moderately increased, occasionally reduced: megakaryocytes increased; granulopoiesis and erythropoiesis no more than mildly increased	Increased: increased megakaryocytes and granulopoiesis	Focally increased, normal or hypocellular: megakaryocytes often still increased
Megakaryocyte size, cytological features and distribution	Loose clusters; may be adjacent to endosteum; vary in size from smaller than normal to larger than normal, but with average size increased; nuclear lobation varies from hypolobated to hyperlobated with an overall increase	Loose clusters or dispersed; may be adjacent to endosteum; mainly large to giant with deeply lobated staghorn-like nuclei; less pleomorphic than those of polycythaemia vera and early primary myelofibrosis	Dense clusters; some adjacent to endosteum or within sinusoids; markedly atypical including 'cloud-like', 'balloon-like' or hyperchromatic nuclei; increased 'bare' megakaryocyte nuclei	Large clusters or sheets of atypical megakaryocytes may persist; increased proportion of small megakaryocytes; may be elongated; hyperchromatic nuclei are prominent
Reticulin	Normal or slightly increased	Normal or slightly increased	Normal or slightly increased	Markedly increased
Collagen	Usually absent	Absent	Absent	Usually present
Osteosclerosis	Absent	Absent	Absent	May be present

matological and histopathological features are all considered then genuine diagnostic difficulty occurs only in cases with complicating iron deficiency and in pre-polycythaemic PV. The presence of a *JAK2* V617F mutation does not help but the absence of both this mutation and exon 12 mutations makes PV highly improbable. Generally the Hb and red cell mass are increased in PV and are normal in ET. A therapeutic trial of iron therapy permits the distinction to be made but may not be justifiable since making a precise diagnosis does not as yet influence therapy.

It is desirable for cytogenetic and molecular genetic (*JAK2* and *BCR-ABL1*) analysis to be performed in all patients in whom a diagnosis of ET appears likely. However, if such analysis is not done as a routine it should at least be performed whenever there are any features suggesting the possibility of Ph positivity or pre-polycythaemic or iron-deficient PV. The neutrophil alkaline phosphatase score has been found to be unhelpful in identifying Ph-positive cases, which should be classified as a variant of CGL, whereas a marked increase in the basophil count or the presence of sheets of atypical megakaryocytes (see Fig. 5.11) have been found predictive of Ph positivity and indicate the need for genetic analysis. However, because of the therapeutic implications, it is prudent to exclude Ph positivity in all patients with apparent ET who do not have a *JAK2* V617F mutation.

Occasional cases of systemic mastocytosis present with thrombocytosis as their predominant haematological manifestation. Careful examination of trephine biopsy sections should permit their distinction from ET. However, it should be noted that ET and systemic mastocytosis may coexist.

The presence of significant numbers of ringed sideroblasts in a bone marrow aspirate is likely to indicate a diagnosis of refractory anaemia with ring sideroblasts and thrombocytosis rather than ET (see page 287).

Primary myelofibrosis

'Primary' or 'chronic idiopathic' myelofibrosis has also been known as myelofibrosis with myeloid metaplasia, agnogenic myeloid metaplasia and chronic megakaryocytic granulocytic myelosis. The WHO expert group now favours the designation 'primary myelofibrosis' but it should be noted that the terms 'primary', 'idiopathic' and 'agnogenic' are equally inappropriate since this condition is known to be an MPN in which the fibrosis is a response to the myeloid neoplasm. 'Myelofibrosis with myeloid metaplasia' is also inaccurate since the presence of haemopoietic cells in the liver and spleen represents clonal extramedullary haemopoiesis rather than true metaplasia.

Primary myelofibrosis (PMF) is an MPN characterized by splenomegaly, a leucoerythroblastic anaemia and marrow fibrosis; hepatomegaly is observed less often than splenomegaly. The reported incidence is 0.3–1.5 per 100 000 per year with a median age of onset of 65–75 years [48,49]. There is extramedullary haemopoiesis, particularly in the spleen but also in the liver and sometimes in other organs such as kidney, lymph nodes, adrenals, lung, gastro-intestinal tract, skin, dura and pleural and peritoneal cavities. The disease is due to proliferation of a clone of neoplastic cells arising from a multipotent myeloid stem cell or possibly sometimes from a pluripotent lymphoid–myeloid stem cell. Proliferation of bone marrow fibroblasts with deposition of reticulin and collagen is reactive to the myeloid proliferation.

Myelofibrosis, indistinguishable from PMF, may also develop following PV and, less often, ET. CGL may likewise evolve into myelofibrosis or, less often, patients whose myeloid cells are Ph positive may present with a condition that is otherwise indistinguishable from PMF. Cases with preceding PV or with an increased red cell mass are classified as post-polycythaemic myelofibrosis. Cases with previous ET are classified as post-essential thrombocythaemia myelofibrosis. Cases with Ph or BCR-ABL1 positivity represent evolution of CGL, usually accelerated phase or blast transformation.

Primary myelofibrosis is a chronic disorder in which patients may remain relatively asymptomatic until the later stages. It is not uncommon for the diagnosis to be incidental. Except in the prefibrotic–early stage of the disease, some degree of splenomegaly is almost invariable and splenomegaly is often very marked. Slight or moderate hepatomegaly is also common. Not surprisingly, survival is longest in those patients who are asymptomatic at the time of diagnosis. Overall, approximately 50% of patients will be alive 5 years after diagnosis. Reported median survival is 3–6 years from diagnosis [49]. Myelofibrosis sometimes terminates in a condition resembling CML with very striking myeloid proliferation and increasing hepatomegaly and splenomegaly. In 10–20% of cases, PMF terminates by transformation to acute leukaemia; this is usually a megakaryocytic/megakaryoblastic or myeloblastic transformation but, rarely, it is lymphoblastic, suggesting that the disease may have arisen in a pluripotent rather than a multipotent stem cell. Leukaemic transformation should be suspected when there is a rapid increase in splenic size or the sudden development of anaemia or thrombocytopenia. Other causes of death include infection, haemorrhage and heart failure.

Various diagnostic criteria have been proposed in the past [39,94], but these are now superseded by the WHO 2008 classification [3] (Fig. 5.24).

Peripheral blood

The most characteristic peripheral blood findings of PMF are pancytopenia, a leucoerythroblastic blood film and striking poikilocytosis including teardrop poikilocytes (Fig. 5.25). There is sometimes a mild basophil leucocytosis. Granulocytes and platelets may show dysplastic features such as hypolobation of neutrophil nuclei, reduced granulation of eosinophils or large or hypogranular platelets. Occasional circulating micromegakaryocytes can be seen. In the early stages of the disease, when the bone marrow is hypercellular, there is often thrombocytosis and sometimes leucocytosis rather than

Major criteria

- Megakaryocytes increased with characteristic atypia *and* either reticulin or collagen deposition *or* hypercellularity with increased granulopoiesis
- Does not meet criteria for another MPN
- *Either* *JAK2* V617F or other clonal marker *or* no evidence that fibrosis could be secondary

Minor criteria

- Leucoerythroblastosis
- Increased LDH
- Anaemia
- Splenomegaly

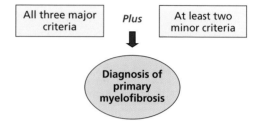

All three major criteria

Plus

At least two minor criteria

Diagnosis of primary myelofibrosis

Fig. 5.24 The 2008 WHO criteria for a diagnosis of primary myelofibrosis. LDH, lactate dehydrogenase.

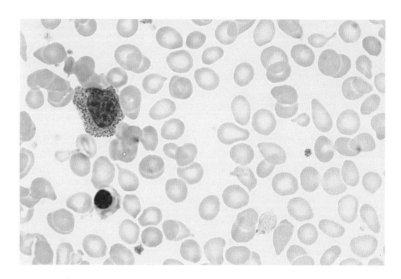

Fig. 5.25 PB film, primary myelofibrosis, showing anisocytosis, poikilocytosis (including teardrop poikilocytes), a myelocyte and an erythroblast. MGG ×100.

cytopenia. Leucoerythroblastic features and teardrop poikilocytes may also be absent [95]. With disease progression, leucopenia, neutropenia and thrombocytopenia supervene and a leucoerythroblastic blood film with prominent teardrop poikilocytes is then consistently present.

Peripheral blood features at presentation may be of prognostic significance. A worse prognosis has been associated with an Hb of less than 100 g/l, 1% or more circulating blasts, more than 10% immature granulocytes and a WBC of less than 4 or more

than $30 \times 10^9/l$ [96]. A study using multivariate analysis found an Hb of less than 100 g/l, a WBC of $20 \times 10^9/l$ or more and a platelet count of $300 \times 10^9/l$ or less to be associated with a worse prognosis [97].

In the final phase of PMF, a progressive rise of the WBC can be seen with counts up to 100–200 $\times 10^9/l$ and the appearance in the peripheral blood of increasing numbers of blasts, promyelocytes and myelocytes. Eosinophilia and basophilia may also occur in this phase and, apart from the red cell changes, the blood film can be

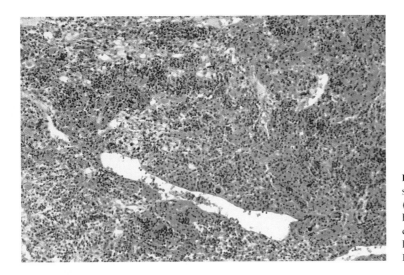

Fig. 5.26 BM trephine biopsy section, primary myelofibrosis (cellular phase), showing marked hypercellularity, with an increase in cells of all three haemopoietic cell lineages, and ectatic sinusoids. Paraffin-embedded, H&E ×10.

indistinguishable from that of chronic myeloid leukaemia. In other patients in whom an acute transformation occurs there is a rapid rise in the blast count with worsening anaemia, neutropenia and thrombocytopenia.

Peripheral blood immunophenotyping can be used to demonstrate an increase of CD34-positive cells. Primary myelofibrosis appears to be the only MPN in which this increase occurs [3].

Bone marrow cytology

As a consequence of the fibrosis, aspiration of bone marrow is often difficult. In the earlier disease stages, however, an aspirate is sometimes obtained and shows very hypercellular fragments with an increase in cells of all lineages; maturation is fairly normal although there may be some dysplastic features. In the later stages of the disease, there is often failure to obtain an aspirate (a 'dry tap') or attempted aspiration yields only blood (a 'blood tap'). Diagnosis then rests on the peripheral blood findings and trephine biopsy histology.

Bone marrow histology

In the early stages, the marrow may be diffusely hypercellular with an increase in all haemopoietic cell lineages with relatively normal maturation [95,98] (Figs 5.26 and 5.27). However, megakaryocytes often predominate and immature and dysplastic forms are usually present. Megakaryocytic morphology is extremely variable; the nuclei may

be small and hypolobated or hyperchromatic and hyperlobated. Micromegakaryocytes and 'bare' megakaryocyte nuclei are increased. Some megakaryocytes have bulky, lightly staining nuclei with rounded lobes. Mitotic figures are increased. Megakaryocytes may be clustered (Fig. 5.27) or sited abnormally, close to the endosteum [14] or within sinusoids. Reduced megakaryocyte expression of MPL has been reported [81]. Granulocyte precursors may show an abnormal clustering centrally in the intertrabecular spaces [99]. In hypercellular marrows there is usually only a mild to moderate increase in reticulin (Fig. 5.28). In some series as many as 20–30% of patients in the hypercellular phase show no reticulin fibrosis, representing the prefibrotic stage of PMF [12]. Later there is a more marked increase in reticulin with coarse fibres running in parallel bundles. Streaming of haemopoietic cells may be noted when reticulin is increased (Fig. 5.29). Marrow sinusoids are increased in number, distended and contain foci of haemopoietic cells (Fig. 5.26); in the early stages this feature may be more easily detected in sections stained for reticulin. A greater degree of angiogenesis correlates with increasing spleen size [58] and worse prognosis [30]. The interstitium may be oedematous and show an increase of lymphocytes, plasma cells, mast cells and macrophages. The prevalence of reactive lymphoid nodules is increased. The interstitium may also contain platelets that have been released inappropriately within the

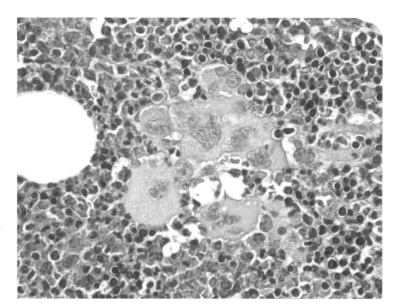

Fig. 5.27 BM trephine biopsy section, primary myelofibrosis (cellular phase), showing a cluster of megakaryocytes with varied size and other morphogical features; most nuclei are poorly or irregularly lobated (including some with cloud-like features and occasional staghorn forms). The background cellularity is markedly increased. Paraffin-embedded, H&E ×20.

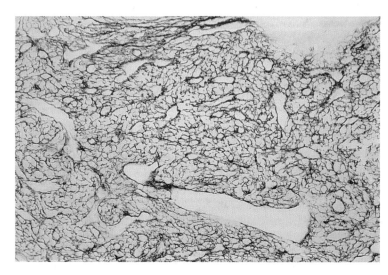

Fig. 5.28 BM trephine biopsy section, primary myelofibrosis (cellular phase), showing grade 3 reticulin deposition with numerous ectatic sinusoids outlined (same patient as in Fig. 5.26). Paraffin-embedded, Gordon and Sweet stain ×10.

marrow rather than into sinusoids; these can be visualized by immunohistochemistry (CD42b or CD61).

As the degree of fibrosis increases, granulocytic and erythroid precursors in the marrow decrease and morphological abnormalities in the megakaryocytic series become more pronounced. In severely fibrotic marrows there is fibroblast proliferation and collagen deposition (Figs 5.30 and 5.31). Sinusoids may be obliterated by progressive fibrosis but capillaries are very numerous [100]. Fibrotic changes are often focal with marked variability within a single biopsy specimen; one intertrabecular space may show hypercellular marrow while an adjacent one shows dense fibrosis. In severely fibrotic marrows there may also be an increase of osteoblasts with new bone formation resulting in osteosclerosis (Fig. 5.31); the thickening of bone trabeculae is often marked. Bone deposition may be both by appositional osteoid deposition and by metaplastic bone formation in the marrow cavity [99]. Newly deposited bone is of woven type. In

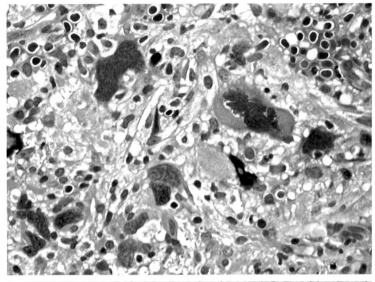

Fig. 5.29 BM trephine biopsy section, primary myelofibrosis (fibrotic phase), showing residual haemopoietic cells, which include numerous dysplastic megakaryocytes, and collagen fibrosis. Megakaryocytes have bizarre hyperchromatic nuclei. Paraffin-embedded. H&E ×40.

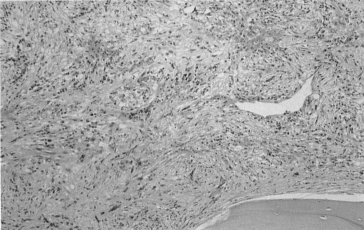

Fig. 5.30 BM trephine biopsy section, primary myelofibrosis (fibrotic phase), showing marked collagen fibrosis, with reduction in all haemopoietic cell lineages. Paraffin-embedded, H&E ×10.

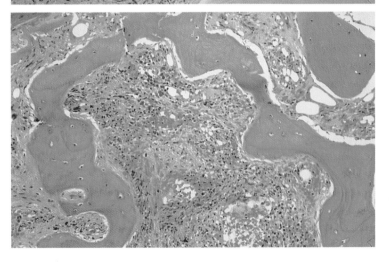

Fig. 5.31 BM trephine biopsy section, osteomyelosclerosis, showing irregular thickening of bone trabeculae and marked collagen fibrosis of the intervening marrow. Paraffin-embedded, H&E ×10.

the osteosclerotic phase there may also be an increased proportion of unmineralized osteoid (osteomalacia) [16]. Osteomyelosclerosis has been associated with delayed engraftment and an increased incidence of acute graft-versus-host disease in patients treated by bone marrow transplantation [101].

It is generally considered that PMF progresses from a hypercellular phase to a hypocellular fibrotic phase and this sequence of events may be seen by serial biopsy [98,102,103]. However, the rate of progression is very variable between patients and progressive changes have not always been observed [76]. In some patients, sequential biopsies show a decrease rather than an increase in fibrosis; to what extent this is due to variation in the degree of fibrosis from one part of the bone marrow to another cannot be readily determined. Some patients develop osteosclerosis disproportionate to the accompanying degree of fibrosis. Increasing age and an increased number of megakaryocytes have been found to predict progression from the prefibrotic to the fibrotic phase [104].

Patients who present in a hypercellular phase of myelofibrosis have longer survivals than those who present with fully developed osteomyelosclerosis [97].

Therapy with anagrelide is associated with an increased number of megakaryocytes despite a fall in the platelet count [105]. The megakaryocytes appear left shifted suggesting that the drug interferes with megakaryocyte maturation rather than proliferation. This suggestion is supported by the observation that megakaryocyte numbers are also increased in healthy volunteers given this drug. Thalidomide therapy has led to increased megakaryocyte numbers and platelet count in some patients and a reduction in bone marrow vascularity in a minority [106]. Lenalidomide therapy also leads to a haematological response in a significant minority of patients and in a small minority there is a reduction of reticulin fibrosis and angiogenesis [107].

Amyloidosis occasionally develops in patients with PMF [108] and amyloid deposition in the bone marrow has been observed [109].

When acute transformation supervenes in PMF, increasing numbers of blasts are seen in biopsy sections.

Cytogenetic and molecular genetic analysis

Clonal cytogenetic abnormalities are present in about a third of patients. The most common are del(13q), del(20q), trisomy 8, trisomy 9, del(12p), i(17q) and partial trisomy of 1q. Detection is enhanced by the use of FISH with probes for 9p21, 13q14, 20q12 and the centromere of chromosome 8. The der(6)t(1;6)(q21-23;p21.3) rearrangement may be specific for PMF [110]. The detection of del(13)(q11-13q14-22) is also strongly suggestive. Using comparative genomic hybridization, abnormalities are found in about 80% of cases; the most frequently observed is gain of 9p with gains of 2q, 3p, 12q and 13q also being common [111]. Worse prognosis has been associated with trisomy 8, 12p–, −7 and 7q– [112].

The gain-of-function *JAK2* V617F mutation is present in about 50% of patients [45,61–63,65]; it is likely to be a second event, contributing to disease progression. *JAK2* V617F is homozygous, as a result of mitotic recombination, in about a third of patients with this mutation. It can sometimes be detected also in B cells, T cells and NK cells, in addition to myeloid cells [113]. The presence of this mutation correlates with a higher WBC and neutrophil count and less likelihood of needing blood transfusion but significantly worse survival [114]. An *MPL* gain-of-function mutation, either *MPL* W515L or *MPL* W515K is found in 5–8% of patients and may coexist with a *JAK2* V617F mutation [86,115]; its presence correlates with worse anaemia [115]. A further 11% of patients have a different MPL mutation, either *MPL* W515S or *MPL* S505N, sometimes with a coexisting *JAK2* mutation [87].

Problems and pitfalls

Primary myelofibrosis needs to be distinguished from acute myelofibrosis, from myelofibrosis following other MPN, and from myelofibrosis secondary to non-haemopoietic disorders.

Acute myelofibrosis is a clinicopathological syndrome sometimes associated with AML, either acute megakaryoblastic leukaemia or acute panmyelosis with myelofibrosis. Prominent megakaryoblastic proliferation is usual. Clinical features differ from those of PMF in that splenomegaly is not usually present. The peripheral blood film lacks the teardrop poikilocytes and leucoerythroblastic

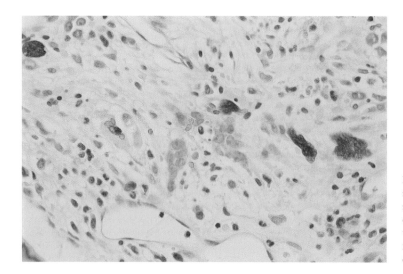

Fig. 5.32 BM trephine biopsy section in osteomyelosclerosis showing entrapped, dysplastic erythroid cells and megakaryocytes which might be mistaken for metastatic malignant cells. Paraffin-embedded, H&E ×40.

features that are typical of PMF. There is usually pancytopenia and there may be circulating blast cells. Bone marrow aspiration is often impossible. Trephine biopsy sections usually show numerous megakaryocytes but, in addition, there are increased blast cells, a feature that is not seen in PMF.

Distinction between primary myelofibrosis and that following other MPN is not possible on histological grounds alone (see Fig. 5.9). The identification of Ph-positive cases is important in view of the generally worse prognosis and the possibility of successful tyrosine kinase inhibitor therapy. This can be achieved by molecular analysis for *BCR-ABL1* performed on peripheral blood cells. Otherwise making a distinction between primary myelofibrosis and that following another MPN is not of clinical significance.

Making a correct diagnosis of myelofibrosis secondary to infiltration by carcinoma or lymphoma is, however, of considerable clinical significance. The blood film in patients with secondary myelofibrosis (for example, that due to bone marrow metastases) may be virtually indistinguishable from that of PMF, there being pancytopenia, a leucoerythroblastic blood film and striking poikilocytosis. However, an increased basophil count, circulating micromegakaryocytes and dysplastic features do not occur. Bone marrow aspiration is usually difficult whether the patient has primary or secondary myelofibrosis. However, sometimes non-haemopoietic malignant cells can be aspirated,

thus providing a diagnosis. Often a trephine biopsy is necessary to make this distinction. When there is dense fibrosis it is necessary to look carefully for malignant cells embedded in the fibrous tissue. Sometimes it is difficult to distinguish metastatic carcinoma cells from small dysplastic megakaryocytes or dysplastic erythroblasts (Fig. 5.32). When necessary, immunohistochemistry to identify megakaryocytes, erythroid cells or cells of epithelial origin (see Tables 2.6 and 10.1) can be used to confirm the nature of abnormal cells. Infiltration by lymphoma, particularly by Hodgkin lymphoma, can also lead to dense bone marrow fibrosis. Immunohistochemistry can again be useful to distinguish Reed–Sternberg cells and mononuclear Hodgkin cells from carcinoma cells or dysplastic megakaryocytes. Primary myelofibrosis also needs to be distinguished from fibrosis associated with bone disease (see pages 589–593).

The prefibrotic and early fibrotic stages of PMF can be difficult to distinguish from other MPN, particularly from ET. Bone marrow histology is crucial.

Chronic eosinophilic leukaemia, not otherwise specified

Chronic eosinophilic leukaemia is a subtype of CML in which differentiation is entirely or predominantly to eosinophils. In the 2008 WHO classification, cases that result from rearrangement of the *PDGFRA*, *PDGFRB* or *FGFR1* genes fall into a

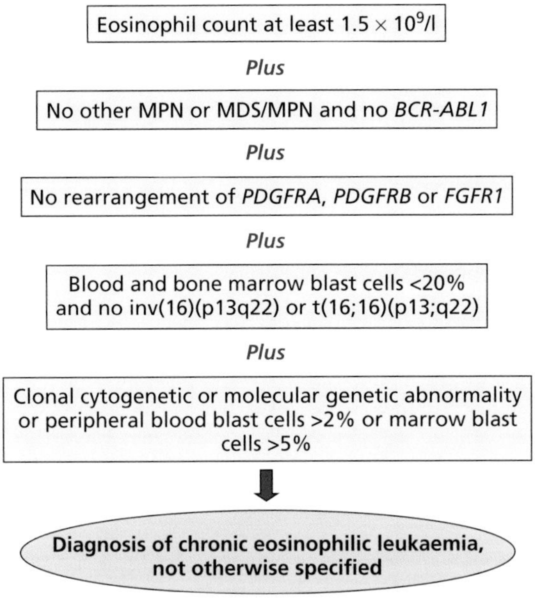

| Eosinophil count at least 1.5 × 10⁹/l |

Plus

| No other MPN or MDS/MPN and no *BCR-ABL1* |

Plus

| No rearrangement of *PDGFRA*, *PDGFRB* or *FGFR1* |

Plus

| Blood and bone marrow blast cells <20% and no inv(16)(p13q22) or t(16;16)(p13;q22) |

Plus

| Clonal cytogenetic or molecular genetic abnormality or peripheral blood blast cells >2% or marrow blast cells >5% |

Diagnosis of chronic eosinophilic leukaemia, not otherwise specified

Fig. 5.33 The 2008 WHO criteria for a diagnosis of chronic eosinophilic leukaemia, not otherwise specified. MDS, myelodysplastic syndrome; MPN, myeloproliferative neoplasm.

distinct category (see page 288) leaving cases that lack these specific genetic abnormalities in the category designated 'chronic eosinophilic leukaemia, not otherwise specified (CEL, NOS)' [116]. In the WHO classification, an eosinophil count of at least 1.5 × 10⁹/l is a prerequisite for the diagnosis. Diagnostic criteria are summarized in Fig. 5.33. The leukaemic clone usually arises from a multipotent haemopoietic stem cell. Eosinophilic leukaemia must be distinguished from reactive eosinophilia, which is secondary to another disorder, such as allergy, a parasitic infection or a non-haemopoietic neoplasm. Clinical features of eosinophilic leukaemia may include hepatosplenomegaly and anaemia but, in addition, there may be tissue damage as a consequence of release of eosinophil granule contents. Such tissue damage often includes damage to the myocardium and endocardium with consequent heart failure.

Peripheral blood

The blood film shows increased eosinophils and sometimes increased neutrophils or monocytes. In some patients there are circulating blast cells but,

by definition, these are less than 20% or the case is regarded as AML. A blast cell count of 2% or more is accepted in the WHO classification as evidence that the eosinophilia represents eosinophilic leukaemia. The eosinophils may be cytologically normal or may show abnormalities such as degranulation, cytoplasmic vacuolation, hypolobation or hyperlobation. It should be noted, however, that striking cytological abnormalities in eosinophils do not provide reliable evidence that a disorder is leukaemic in nature since they can also be seen in patients with reactive eosinophilia.

Bone marrow cytology

The bone marrow aspirate shows an increase of eosinophils and their precursors (Fig. 5.34). Blast cells may be increased and a count of 5% or more provides evidence of the leukaemic nature of the condition. By definition, blasts are less than 20%. The eosinophil myelocytes may contain some pro-eosinophilic granules, which have basophilic staining characteristics. Eosinophils may have granules showing aberrant positivity for naphthol AS-D chloroacetate esterase (CAE) and the cytoplasm may be periodic acid–Schiff (PAS) positive [44]. Charcot–Leyden crystals may be present.

Bone marrow histology

The trephine biopsy sections show increased eosinophils and eosinophil precursors, with or without an increase in blast cells (Fig. 5.35). Charcot–Leyden crystals may be present [117].

Cytogenetic and molecular genetic analysis

Miscellaneous clonal cytogenetic abnormalities may be present, e.g. trisomy 8, i(17q) and del(20q) [116,118]. A rare translocation, t(8;9)(p22;p24), leading to *PCM1-JAK2* fusion is more specifically associated with CEL and aCML with eosinophilic differentiation [119]. By definition, t(9;22), *BCR-ABL1*, rearrangement of *PDGFRA*, *PDGFRB* and *FGFR1* and inv(16) with *CBFB-MYH11* are specifically excluded. The *JAK2* V617F mutation is found in occasional patients with otherwise unexplained hypereosinophilia, permitting a diagnosis of CEL [45]. The techniques of molecular genetics can also be used to establish clonality in patients with suspected CEL, NOS, e.g. by analysis for X-linked polymorphisms in female patients.

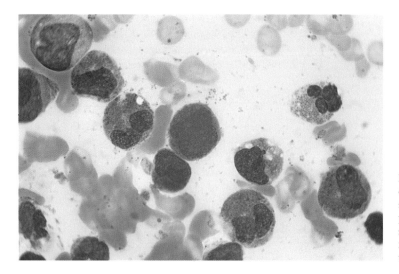

Fig. 5.34 BM aspirate film, chronic eosinophilic leukaemia NOS, showing increased eosinophils and precursors and several blast cells; some eosinophils have abnormal nuclear shapes and cytoplasmic vacuolation. MGG ×100.

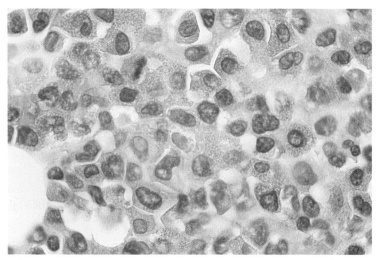

Fig. 5.35 BM trephine biopsy section, chronic eosinophilic leukaemia NOS, showing that normal haemopoietic cells have been largely replaced by eosinophils and their precursors (same patient as Fig. 5.34). Paraffin-embedded, H&E ×100.

Problems and pitfalls

Making a distinction between chronic eosinophilic leukaemias and the idiopathic hypereosinophilic syndrome (see page 488) is problematical. The latter diagnosis is one of exclusion, being made when there is no firm evidence of leukaemia and when no potential cause of reactive eosinophilia has been identified. Although the nature of this condition in an individual patient is, by definition, uncertain, on prolonged follow-up some patients develop AML, thus providing strong circumstantial evidence that the initial disorder was CEL with subsequent acute transformation having occurred. Others develop a clonal cytogenetic abnormality,

suggesting that the disorder was clonal from the beginning with a further mutation having occurred in a clone that was initially cytogenetically normal. However, not all cases of initially unexplained hypereosinophilic syndrome are actually leukaemic. Immunophenotypic and molecular investigation has shown that some such patients have cytokine-driven hypereosinophilia consequent on the presence of a clone of T lymphocytes [120,121]. An initially occult lymphoproliferative disorder subsequently becomes overt in some patients [120]. For this reason cases of the idiopathic hypereosinophilic syndrome should not be assumed to have eosinophilic leukaemia. We recommend that such

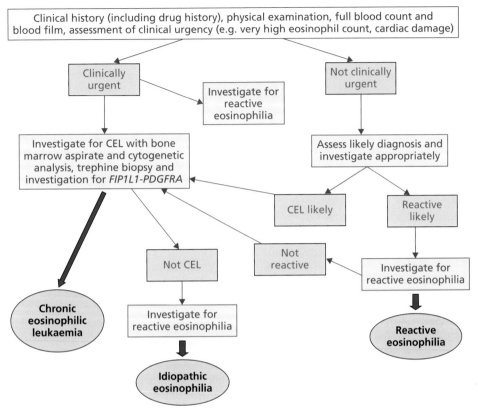

Fig. 5.36 A flow chart showing the diagnostic pathway for investigation of unexplained eosinophilia including suspected chronic eosinophilic leukaemia (CEL).

patients be investigated for underlying causes of eosinophilia, such as parasitic infection, and should have cytogenetic and molecular genetic analysis performed. It is essential that they are investigated for a *FIP1L1-PDGFRA* fusion gene (see page 288). When facilities permit, consideration should be given to investigation for aberrant T lymphocyte populations. If there is no specific evidence supporting a diagnosis of leukaemia and if no other cause of hypereosinophilia is found the case should be classified as 'idiopathic'. Some such patients will subsequently be recognized, in retrospect, as having had CEL. Figure 5.36 summarizes the diagnostic process in unexplained eosinophilia including suspected eosinophilic leukaemia.

Systemic mastocytosis

Mast cell proliferation may be confined to the skin or may be generalized, the latter condition being designated systemic mastocytosis. Systemic mastocytosis is a rare condition resulting from a neoplastic proliferation of mast cells. Mast cells are derived from a multipotent myeloid stem cell (or, at least in some cases, a pluripotent lymphoid–myeloid stem cell [122]) and the mast cell proliferation is often associated with increased proliferation of other myeloid lineages. Systemic mastocytosis is classified as an MPN in the 2008 WHO classification and has been divided into indolent systemic mastocytosis, systemic mastocytosis with associated clonal haematological non-mast cell lineage disease (SM-AHNMD) and aggressive systemic mastocytosis [123] (Table 5.4). The diagnostic criteria are summarized in Fig. 5.37. The WHO expert group have also included acute mast cell leukaemia in the group of conditions designated 'mastocytosis' within the broad grouping of MPN (although classification as AML might seem more appropriate).

Table 5.4 The WHO classification of mastocytosis [123].

Cutaneous mastocytosis
Indolent systemic mastocytosis
Systemic mastocytosis with associated clonal,
    haematological non-mast cell lineage disease
Aggressive systemic mastocytosis
Mast cell leukaemia
Mast cell sarcoma
Extracutaneous mastocytoma

Various organs may be involved in systemic mastocytosis, including the bone marrow, liver, spleen, lymph nodes and skin; the most typical skin lesions are those of urticaria pigmentosa. Patients often have symptoms related to the release of secretory products by the neoplastic mast cells; these include abdominal pain, nausea and vomiting, diarrhoea, flushing and bronchospasm [124–126]. Serum tryptase is elevated and a level above 20 ng/ml can be included in the diagnostic criteria for this disease.

Systemic mastocytosis may pursue either an indolent or an aggressive clinical course. Although patients can be divided into two or three groups with varying prognosis on the basis of clinical and haematological features [127,128], there is actually a continuous spectrum of disease characteristics.

Major criterion

• Multifocal, dense infiltrates of mast cells (≥15 mast cells in aggregates) in sections of BM and/or other extracutaneous tissues

Minor criteria

• In biopsy sections >25% of the mast cells are spindle shaped or have atypical morphology or in BM aspirate >25% are immature or atypical
• Activating point mutation at codon 816 of *KIT* in extracutaneous tissue
• Mast cells express CD2 and/or CD25
• Serum tryptase persistently >20ng/ml (unless there is another myeloid neoplasm)

Major criterion +
1 minor criterion
or
3 of 4 minor criteria

Diagnosis of systemic mastocytosis

Fig. 5.37 The 2008 WHO criteria for a diagnosis of systemic mastocytosis. BM, bone marrow.

Patients whose disease has an aggressive course are less likely to have skin involvement and more likely to have hepatomegaly, splenomegaly, leucocytosis, anaemia and thrombocytopenia [127,128]. In multivariate analysis, a higher percentage of mast cells in bone marrow films, the presence of an associated clonal non-mast cell haematological disorder and the absence of urticaria pigmentosa were found to be indicative of worse prognosis [129]. The explanation of the poor prognostic significance of the absence of urticaria pigmentosa is likely to relate to the greater degree of mast cell abnormality in patients lacking skin manifestations [129]. Prognosis is worst in the minority of patients with overt mast cell leukaemia.

Patients with systemic mastocytosis may develop MDS, all five French–American–British (FAB) categories of MDS having been observed [130]. Systemic mastocytosis may also terminate in AML, this sometimes appearing abruptly and sometimes following a period of myelodysplasia. The leukaemia is occasionally mast cell leukaemia (see page 278) but more often is another category of AML. Commonest are acute myeloblastic or acute myelomonocytic leukaemia but occasional cases of erythroleukaemia or megakaryoblastic leukaemia have also been reported [130].

Peripheral blood [126,128,131,132]
In patients with an indolent clinical course the peripheral blood is most often normal but a minority of patients show evidence of abnormal proliferation of cells of one or more myeloid lineages (neutrophilia, eosinophilia, basophilia, monocytosis, thrombocytosis). Circulating mast cells are usually not noted.

In patients in whom the clinical course is aggressive, peripheral blood evidence of a myeloid disorder is more prominent. The majority of patients have neutrophilia, many have eosinophilia, basophilia or monocytosis, and a minority have thrombocytosis. Cytopenias are also common, particularly anaemia and thrombocytopenia but sometimes leucopenia and neutropenia. Hypogranular and hypersegmented eosinophils may be present [132]. In some patients the peripheral blood features closely resemble those of CGL. Some patients have myelodysplastic features such as the acquired Pelger–Huët anomaly of neutrophils. Occasional patients have circulating mast cells, usually in small

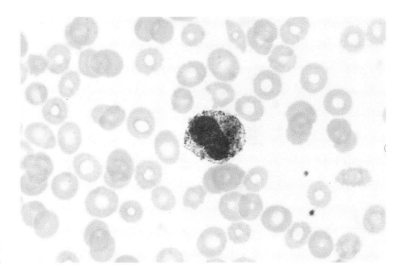

Fig. 5.38 PB film, systemic mastocytosis, showing an abnormal hypogranular mast cell. MGG ×100.

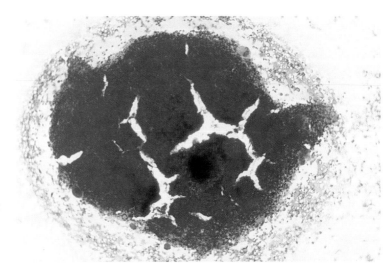

Fig. 5.39 BM aspirate film, systemic mastocytosis, showing an intensely hypercellular fragment due mainly to an increase of granulocytes and their precursors. MGG ×10.

numbers (Fig. 5.38). In the few patients in whom mast cell leukaemia supervenes there are larger numbers of circulating mast cells, usually with atypical cytological features such as hypogranularity or nuclear lobation.

Bone marrow cytology

The bone marrow aspirate is normo- or hypercellular and contains increased numbers of mast cells (Fig. 5.39). These may be under-represented in an aspirate in comparison with a trephine biopsy section because of the fibrosis provoked by mast cell proliferation. They may also remain in the fragments so that fragments as well as cell trails should

be examined carefully. Clusters of mast cells may be present [131]. When mast cells are cytologically normal they are easily identifiable as oval or elongated cells with a central non-lobated nucleus and with the cytoplasm packed with purple granules; when they are cytologically atypical they may sometimes be confused with basophils. Atypical features include nuclear lobation (Fig. 5.40), smaller granules than normal, hypogranularity (Fig. 5.40) and a primitive chromatin pattern. Most often neoplastic mast cells are spindle shaped and hypogranular. Mast cells in systemic mastocytosis have been classified, according to their cytological features in bone marrow films as follows:

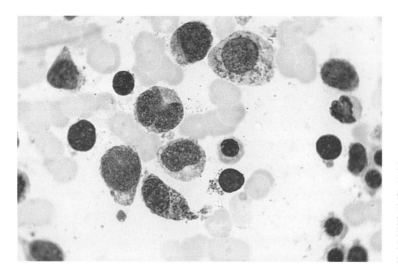

Fig. 5.40 BM aspirate film, systemic mastocytosis, showing two abnormal mast cells and three cells that are probably mast cell precursors. One mast cell is hypogranular and both have a higher nucleocytoplasmic ratio than normal mast cells. MGG ×100.

(i) cytologically normal; (ii) atypical I (with cytoplasmic elongations, eccentric oval nuclei and hypogranularity); (iii) atypical II (with bilobed or multilobed nuclei, analogous to promastocytes when mast cells are cultured *in vitro*); and (iv) atypical III (blast cells with metachromatically-staining granules) [129]. In a comparison of cytological features in systemic mastocytosis and reactive mastocytosis, fusiform cells and cells with reduced and irregularly distributed granules were found to be much more common in systemic mastocytosis, while irregular lobated nuclei were seen only in systemic mastocytosis [133]. However, in an uncommon variant of systemic mastocytosis that is seen particularly in children, designated well-differentiated systemic mastocytosis, the mast cells are cytologically much more normal [134]. In patients whose disease pursues an indolent clinical course, the bone marrow is usually normocellular and contains a relatively small number of cytologically fairly normal mast cells. Those patients whose disease is aggressive are more likely to show a hypercellular marrow with increased granulopoiesis and larger numbers of mast cells, which are cytologically atypical. Sperr *et al.* [129] found that having more than 5% of mast cells in bone marrow films or having 10% or more of atypical, type II or type III, mast cells correlated with worse survival; the percentage of mast cells in films remained significant in multivariate analysis [129]. The mast cell percentage in films was prognostically significant despite the fact that less than 5% of mast cells in films did not preclude heavy mast cell infiltration demonstrated histologically [129].

Increased granulopoiesis may involve neutrophil, eosinophil and basophil lineages. In some patients there are increased numbers of megakaryocytes. The bone marrow appearances may be confused with those of CGL if the presence of large numbers of mast cells is not appreciated. In some cases there are myelodysplastic features such as ring sideroblasts or hypolobated megakaryocytes. Many patients whose disease does not meet the criteria for any of the MDS nevertheless have dysplastic features in myeloid cells [133].

Mast cell granules stain with Alcian blue as well as with Romanowsky stains (such as Giemsa and May–Grüwald–Giemsa (MGG)) and stain metachromatically with toluidine blue; they are myeloperoxidase (MPO) and Sudan black B (SBB) negative and PAS and CAE positive. By immunocytochemistry or immunofluorescence, mast cells react positively with monoclonal antibodies (McAb) of CD9, CD33, CD45, CD68 and CD117 clusters and with McAb directed against mast cell tryptase and, sometimes, chymotryptase. Flow cytometry can be applied to bone marrow aspirates and is a sensitive technique for the detection of neoplastic mast cells [135]. Mast cells are identified by light-scattering characteristics and expression of CD117; neoplastic mast cells generally show aberrant expression of CD2 and CD25 and increased expression of CD63

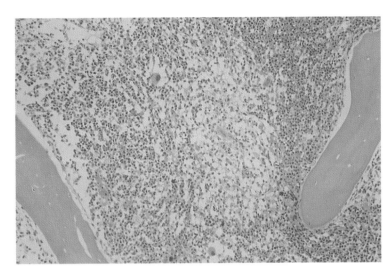

Fig. 5.41 BM trephine biopsy section, systemic mastocytosis, showing marked hypercellularity with a loose focal aggregate of mast cells (centre). Paraffin-embedded, H&E ×10.

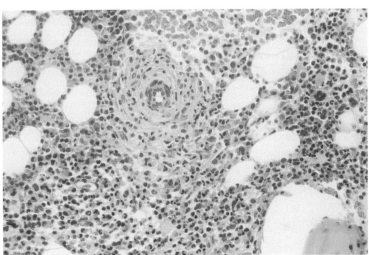

Fig. 5.42 BM trephine biopsy section, systemic mastocytosis, showing concentric mast cells encircling a vessel. Paraffin-embedded, H&E ×25. (By courtesy of Dr B. I. Dalal, Vancouver.)

and CD69 [135]. However, CD2 and CD25 may not be expressed in cases with better differentiated mast cells [122] and, conversely, they may be expressed also in the mast cells of CEL with *PDGFRA* or *PDGFRB* rearrangement.

Bone marrow histology

The marrow biopsy histology is abnormal in the great majority of cases [124,125,136] (Fig. 5.41), but in one study only one of two bilateral biopsies was found to be positive in 15–20% of patients [137]. The most common finding is focal infiltration by mast cells, often in paratrabecular and perivascular areas or as intertrabecular nodules. There may be an accompanying interstitial infiltrate [138]. Perivascular lesions may be associated with prominent medial and adventitial hypertrophy and collagen fibrosis. There may be layers of mast cells encircling vessels (Fig. 5.42). Eosinophils are present in variable numbers, often concentrated at the periphery of the infiltrated areas (Figs 5.43 and 5.44). Lymphocytes, plasma cells, macrophages and fibroblasts are also frequently seen in the areas of infiltration. Occasionally lymphocytes are aggregated either at the centre or at the periphery of a focal lesion [125,139]; immunocytochemical analysis has shown the lymphocytes to be a mixture of B and T cells [140]. B cells have been

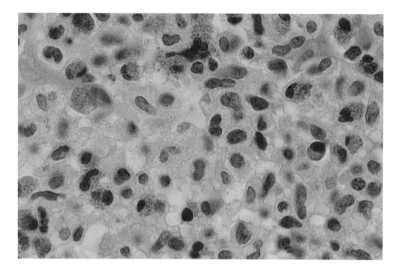

Fig. 5.43 BM trephine biopsy section, systemic mastocytosis (same patient as Fig. 5.41), showing numerous abnormal mast cells – with marked variation in nuclear shape and moderate amounts of pale-staining cytoplasm – eosinophils and small numbers of lymphocytes. Paraffin-embedded, H&E ×100.

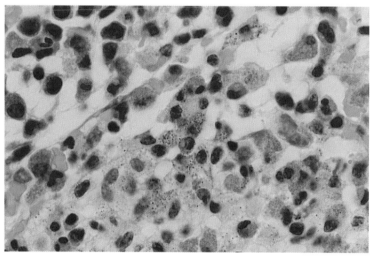

Fig. 5.44 BM trephine biopsy section, systemic mastocytosis (same patient as Fig. 5.41), showing basophilic granules in the cytoplasm of mast cells. Paraffin-embedded, Giemsa ×100.

reported to be more numerous than [141] or equal in number to [142] T cells. They do not show any immunophenotypic abnormality and are polyclonal [142]. There is usually a dense network of reticulin fibres associated with areas of infiltration and sometimes there is collagen deposition. There may be osteosclerosis, osteoporosis or evidence of increased bone turnover with osteoclasts, osteoblasts and the amount of osteoid all being increased [139]; paratrabecular fibrosis, which is sometimes present, may be related to increased bone turnover.

The morphology of the mast cells is variable and this may cause difficulty in their recognition, espe-

cially in H&E-stained sections. They may be either spindle shaped, thus resembling fibroblasts (Fig. 5.45), or have abundant pale pink cytoplasm and irregularly shaped nuclei, leading to confusion with macrophages. A Giemsa stain shows purple cytoplasmic granules (Fig. 5.44), although these are often quite scanty. With a toluidine blue stain the granules are deep pink or purple (Fig. 5.46). Decalcification of specimens can lead to loss of metachromatic staining with toluidine blue. Zenker's and B5 fixatives may interfere with both Giemsa and toluidine blue reactivity. Mast cells have CAE activity, which may be demonstrated in both paraffin- and resin-embedded sections using

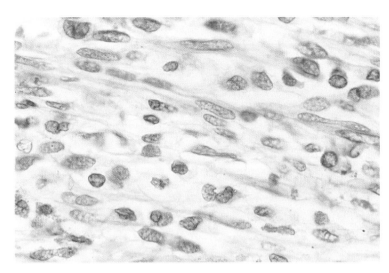

Fig. 5.45 BM trephine biopsy section, systemic mastocytosis, showing spindle-shaped mast cells. Paraffin-embedded, H&E ×100. (By courtesy of Dr Wendy Erber and Dr L. Matz.)

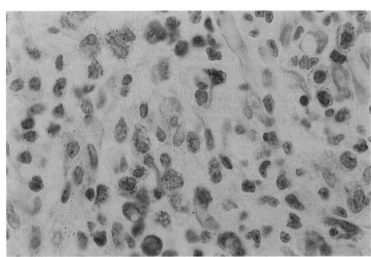

Fig. 5.46 BM trephine biopsy section, systemic mastocytosis (same patient as Fig. 5.41), showing purple metachromatic granules in the cytoplasm of mast cells. Paraffin-embedded, toluidine blue ×100.

Leder's stain; however, this stain does not work well in acid-decalcified paraffin-embedded specimens and it should be noted that neutrophil myelocytes will also stain strongly. In resin-embedded specimens, ε-aminocaproate activity, which is specific for mast cells, can be demonstrated. In paraffin-embedded sections, mast cell tryptase is the preferred immunohistochemical stain since it has a high degree of specificity and sensitivity (Fig. 5.47). Mast cells also express mast cell chymase, vimentin, CD45, CD68, CD117, lysozyme, S100, α_1-anti-trypsin and α_1-anti-chymotrypsin [143]. Although CD68 (Fig. 5.48) is expressed by mast cells it is not specific. CD68 broad-specificity monoclonal antibodies, such as KP1, stain normal, reactive and neoplastic mast cells whereas antibodies with more restricted specificity (CD68R), such as PG-M1, do not stain normal or reactive mast cells but may stain neoplastic mast cells in patients with aggressive systemic mastocytosis [138]. In systemic mastocytosis (and also in MDS) there is an increase in tryptase-positive mast cells but generally no increase in chymase-positive mast cells [144]. There is usually aberrant expression of CD2, CD25 or both, which can be diagnostically useful and is a minor criterion for diagnosis in the WHO classification. In well-differentiated systemic mastocytosis, however, the mast cells may fail to express

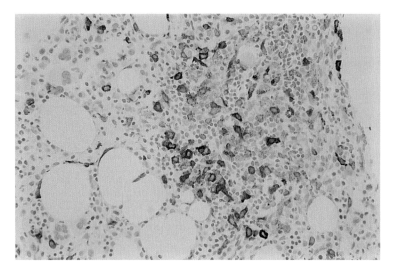

Fig. 5.47 BM trephine biopsy section, systemic mastocytosis, showing increased mast cells, some of which are spindle shaped. Paraffin-embedded, immunohistochemistry for mast cell tryptase ×20.

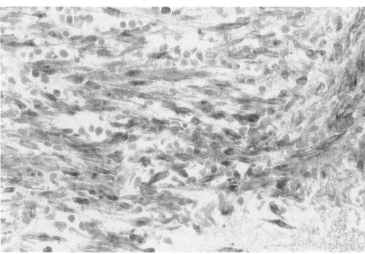

Fig. 5.48 BM trephine biopsy section, systemic mastocytosis, (same patient as Fig. 5.45) immunohistochemistry (alkaline phosphatase–anti-alkaline phosphatase (APAAP) technique) with a CD68 McAb. Paraffin-embedded ×40. (By courtesy of Dr Wendy Erber, Perth.)

these antigens [134]. About two thirds of cases of systemic mastocytosis give positive reactions with a monoclonal antibody to tartrate-resistant acid phosphatase [145]. CD117 (KIT) is expressed by normal and neoplastic mast cells. It is also expressed, but more weakly, by CD34-positive haemopoietic precursors, by a minority of other early haemopoietic cells (which are cytologically probably pro-erythroblasts and promyelocytes) and by occasional small lymphocytes (probably a subset of NK cells [146]). Stem cell factor (the ligand of KIT) can be detected in mast cells with both a membrane-bound and granular pattern of staining [141]. Neoplastic mast cells show aberrant nuclear expres-

sion of phosphorylated STAT5, a downstream target of mutated KIT; this is not seen in normal or reactive mast cells but was detected in a patient with eosinophilic leukaemia with a *FIP1L1-PDGFRA* fusion gene [147].

Diffuse replacement of the marrow by neoplastic mast cells occurs infrequently. In these cases the infiltrate is much more monomorphic than when lesions are focal. The mast cells are usually spindle shaped and may show nuclear atypia. There is marked reticulin fibrosis and osteosclerosis is often present. Often there are atypical mast cells in the peripheral blood allowing a diagnosis of mast cell leukaemia to be made [136].

Lennert and Parwaresch [127] used the marrow biopsy findings to divide patients into prognostic groups. They described three main patterns of involvement: type I, in which there is focal infiltration, but the intervening haemopoietic marrow is normal; type II, in which there are focal lesions and a marked increase in granulopoiesis with loss of fat spaces; and type III in which there is diffuse replacement of the haemopoietic marrow. Type I corresponds to indolent systemic mastocytosis, type II to aggressive systemic mastocytosis and type III to mast cell leukaemia. Others have found a hypercellular bone marrow to have an adverse prognostic significance [126].

Cytogenetic and molecular genetic analysis

Clonal cytogenetic abnormalities have been demonstrated in a number of cases of systemic mastocytosis [148]. Abnormalities detected have included trisomy 8, trisomy 9, trisomy 11, del(5q), del(7q), monosomy 7 and del(20q).

A *KIT* mutation, most often D816V, is found in more than 90% of patients with both indolent and aggressive systemic mastocytosis if sensitive techniques are used [122]. In one study the mutation was identified in cells of other lineages in a significant proportion of patients: CD34-positive haemopoietic stem cells (34%), eosinophils (31%), monocytes (21%), neutrophils (21%) and lymphocytes (10%) [122]. Well-differentiated systemic mastocytosis shows a wider spectrum of *KIT* mutations, I817V, N819Y and F522C having been described, in addition to D816V [134]. The most frequently observed mutations are in the tyrosine kinase domain but, exceptionally, there is a mutation in the transmembrane domain [149]; in this patient there were unusual round, well-granulated mast cells, but whether this is a consistent association remains to be established.

Problems and pitfalls

Because infiltrates are typically focal and resistant to aspiration, bone marrow infiltration by neoplastic mast cells cannot be excluded by a normal aspirate. We have observed a normal aspirate despite quite heavy infiltration of a trephine biopsy specimen. It is also important to realize that mast cell infiltration detected in a trephine biopsy specimen may be quite minor despite the patient having major systemic symptoms. Immunohistochemistry for mast cell tryptase is invaluable in the detection of infiltration since neoplastic mast cells may be cytologically atypical and may have reduced metachromatic staining with Giemsa or toluidine blue stains. However, the application of appropriate immunohistochemical stains will occur only if the correct diagnosis is suspected.

Misdiagnosis of systemic mast cell disease is not uncommon, largely because the mast cells are misidentified as fibroblasts or macrophages (including epithelioid cells). Focal marrow lesions may be misinterpreted as granulomas or focal infiltrates of lymphoma, such as angioimmunoblastic T-cell lymphoma or lymphoplasmacytic lymphoma. Confusion with primary myelofibrosis has occurred; however, when marrow fibrosis occurs as a response to systemic mastocytosis, mast cells are recognizable in the fibrous tissue, permitting a distinction from other causes of myelofibrosis. In patients with a heavy mast cell infiltrate, misdiagnosis as hairy cell leukaemia is possible because of the even spacing of nuclei, a feature which is also typical of hairy cell leukaemia. The two crucial elements in reaching a correct diagnosis are that Giemsa-stained sections are routinely examined and that the cell types in any apparent granulomas or infiltrates are determined. The 'pseudo-granulomas' of systemic mast cell disease commonly have eosinophils and lymphocytes associated with them and sometimes lymphoid nodules and plasma cells; the mast cells may show atypical features. Mast cells are also often associated with focal marrow infiltrates of lymphoplasmacytic lymphoma (see page 327). However, these reactive mast cells are morphologically normal and are a minority population in the areas of infiltration. In angioimmunoblastic T-cell lymphoma there may be focal or diffuse infiltration by a heterogeneous population of cells that often includes plasma cells, lymphocytes and many eosinophils (see page 376). However, immunoblasts, which are not a feature of systemic mastocytosis, are present and often prominent.

By definition, cutaneous mastocytosis is confined to the skin. However, bone marrow infiltration occasionally develops in patients who initially had mast cell infiltration apparently involving only the skin. In a study of paediatric cases of apparent cutaneous mastocytosis, 10 out of 15 trephine

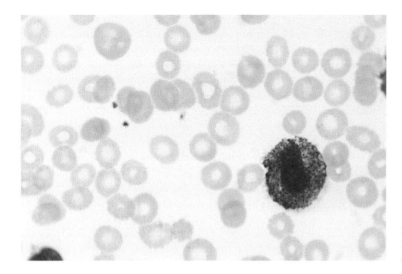

Fig. 5.49 PB film in acute mast cell leukaemia showing circulating abnormal mast cell. MGG ×100.

biopsies showed focal perivascular and peritrabecular aggregates of mast cells, eosinophils and early myeloid cells [131,150]. Similarly, of a series of 30 adults presenting with urticaria pigmentosa, there were 18 with bone marrow infiltration [151]. In addition, a clonal cytogenetic abnormality has been reported in the bone marrow of a patient with urticaria pigmentosa suggesting occult infiltration by neoplastic cells [148]. Immunohistochemistry for mast cell tryptase, to demonstrate the presence of focal aggregates of mast cells, is recommended if a trephine biopsy is performed in the investigation of patients with cutaneous mastocytosis.

The abnormal infiltrates reported in association with drug hypersensitivity, designated 'eosinophilic fibrohistiocytic lesions' [152], are now known to represent proliferation of eosinophils and neoplastic mast cells, mainly in patients with indolent systemic mastocytosis.

Many patients with systemic mastocytosis have evidence of involvement of other myeloid lineages. In some patients, the platelet count, WBC or Hb is so greatly elevated that a diagnosis of ET, CGL or PV is made. It is likely that such cases represent an MPN with differentiation to several lineages, rather than the coexistence of two separate diseases. Similarly, the emergence of MDS or AML in patients with systemic mastocytosis is likely to represent evolution of the neoplastic clone. In the 2008 WHO classification both these groups of cases are categorized as 'systemic mastocytosis with associated clonal haematological non-mast cell lineage disease' rather than as 'myeloproliferative neoplasm, unclassifiable' or 'myelodysplastic/myeloproliferative neoplasm, unclassifiable'.

Acute mast cell leukaemia

Acute mast cell leukaemia is a rare condition which can occur *de novo* or as a transformation of systemic mastocytosis.

Peripheral blood

The blood film shows immature mast cells which have round, oval or lobulated nuclei and a variable number of granules of mast cell type (Fig. 5.49). The presence of more than 10% mast cells in the blood has been found to correlate with more than 20% in bone marrow films and is therefore likely to indicate mast cell leukaemia, as defined in the WHO classification [123,129].

Bone marrow cytology

The bone marrow aspirate shows immature cells of mast cell lineage. Immunocytochemistry for mast cell tryptase can be used to demonstrate mast cell differentiation if this is not certain from cytological features. In the WHO classification, 20% of mast cells in an aspirate is a criterion for a diagnosis of mast cell leukaemia [123].

Cytochemistry

Mast cells stain metachromatically with toluidine blue. They are CAE positive.

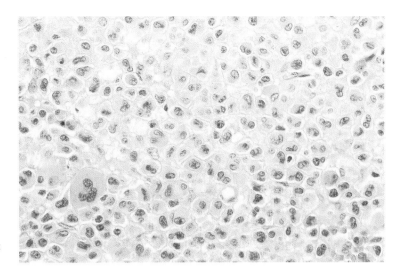

Fig. 5.50 BM trephine biopsy section from a patient with acute mast cell leukaemia showing replacement of the marrow by mast cells. Paraffin-embedded, H&E ×40.

Bone marrow histology

Trephine biopsy sections show effacement of the bone marrow by immature mast cells. These have more voluminous cytoplasm than most other myeloid blast cells so that, in an H&E-stained section, the round, oval or lobulated nuclei appear spaced apart (Fig. 5.50). With Giemsa staining, granules may be apparent. Immunohistochemistry for mast cell tryptase confirms the lineage.

Myeloproliferative neoplasm, unclassifiable

Occasional patients are seen who clearly have an MPN but whose disease either cannot be readily classified or, alternatively, has characteristics of two, usually distinct, MPN. This is acknowledged by the inclusion in the WHO classification of a category for unclassifiable cases [153]. Diagnostic criteria are shown in Fig. 5.51. Others have already drawn attention to this group of patients [103,148,154,155].

Pettit *et al.* [154] reported a group of patients with a condition intermediate between PV and PMF which they designated 'transitional myeloproliferative disorder'. In these patients the criteria for PV were generally met but, in addition, there was moderate or marked splenomegaly, a leucoerythroblastic blood film, extramedullary haemopoiesis and a hypercellular marrow with increased reticulin. In the majority of patients the condition had stable characteristics for a number of years and thus did not appear to represent a transient

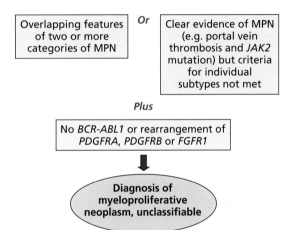

Fig. 5.51 The 2008 WHO criteria for a diagnosis of myeloproliferative neoplasm, unclassifiable. MPN, myeloproliferative neoplasm.

phase between PV and post-polycythaemic myelofibrosis.

The Polycythaemia Vera Study Group [103] used the designation 'undifferentiated chronic myeloproliferative disorder' for another group of patients with splenomegaly and a leucoerythroblastic blood film without an increased red cell mass, Ph chromosome or significant marrow fibrosis.

Patients have also been described with features of both systemic mastocytosis and a variety of MPN, including CGL, PV, ET and PMF [148]. Such cases might be better categorized as 'myeloproliferative disease, unclassifiable' although in the WHO classification they are designated 'systemic mastocytosis with associated clonal haematological non-mast cell lineage disease'.

The existence of patients with characteristics of two MPN, or with features of MPN without specific features allowing assignation to a defined disease category, is not surprising. This is because, firstly, all MPN are the result of mutation of a multipotent or pluripotent stem cell with the potential for proliferation and differentiation into cells of various lineages and, secondly, reticulin and collagen deposition are a common secondary change in various subtypes of MPN.

Myelodysplastic/myeloproliferative neoplasms

The 2001 WHO classification adopted the concept of a group of haematological neoplasms with features of both the myelodysplastic syndromes and the myeloproliferative neoplasms. This concept has been retained in the 2008 classification. There are four defined entities within this group together with a more heterogeneous group of unclassifiable cases.

Chronic myelomonocytic leukaemia

Chronic myelomonocytic leukaemia (CMML) was assigned by the FAB group to the MDS. Subsequently it was suggested that cases should be divided into MDS type and myeloproliferative disorder type. The WHO group, recognizing the presence of both dysplasia and proliferative features, assigns CMML to MDS/MPN. As defined by the FAB group [156], the peripheral blood monocyte count in CMML is greater than 1×10^9/l but peripheral blood blasts are less than 5% and bone marrow blasts not greater than 20%. The WHO definition is similar: an MDS/MPN with a monocyte count of greater than 1×10^9/l, no Ph chromosome or $BCR-ABL1$ fusion gene, and fewer than 20% blasts plus promonocytes in the blood and marrow [157]. In addition, in cases that do not have significant dysplasia in two or more myeloid lineages there must be a clonal cytogenetic abnormality or unexplained monocytosis must persist for at least 3 months. Diagnostic criteria are summarized in Fig. 5.52.

CMML needs to be distinguished from aCML with which it shares some features. It has been recommended that cases in which more than 15% of circulating white cells are granulocyte precursors should be categorized as aCML and cases with fewer as CMML [5]. Although a bone marrow examination is essential for the diagnosis of CMML, careful consideration of the peripheral blood features is equally important in the differential diagnosis. A trephine biopsy offers only supplementary information.

The incidence in the USA has been estimated at 0.37 per 100 000 per year [41]. Clinically, CMML is characterized by features of anaemia and, often, by hepatomegaly and splenomegaly. In a minority of patients there is tissue infiltration by monocytic cells resulting in lymphadenopathy, skin infiltration and serous effusions. Diagnosis is usually either incidental or occurs when the patient develops symptoms of anaemia or when organomegaly is noted.

In the WHO classification, CMML is divided into two grades of disease: CMML-1 (blasts plus promonocytes <5% in peripheral blood and <10% in bone marrow); and CMML-2 (blasts plus promono-

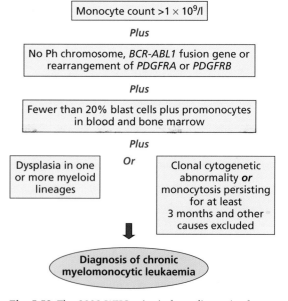

Fig. 5.52 The 2008 WHO criteria for a diagnosis of chronic myelomonocytic leukaemia.

cytes 5–19% in blood or 10–19% in bone marrow or Auer rods present) [157].

Peripheral blood

There is usually anaemia, most often normocytic but sometimes macrocytic or with a dimorphic blood film. There is monocytosis. The monocytes may be morphologically normal or may show atypical features such as nuclei of bizarre shapes or increased cytoplasmic basophilia or granulation. The neutrophil count is often elevated but this is not necessary for the diagnosis. The neutrophils may be morphologically normal or a varying proportion may show dysplastic features. Granulocyte precursors are infrequent, usually less than 5%. Blasts (plus promonocytes) may be present, their number being of prognostic significance (less than 5% versus 5–19%) [157]. The platelet count may be normal or low.

Bone marrow cytology

The bone marrow is hypercellular. There is an increase of granulocyte precursors (Fig. 5.53). An increase of monocytes and their precursors is often evident but this is not always so, probably because monocyte precursors can be difficult to distinguish from promyelocytes and because mature monocytes leave the marrow early. The blast (plus promonocyte) count in the marrow may be increased up to a level of 19%. Whether these cells are less than 10% or 10–19% is of prognostic significance [157].

An iron stain may show abnormal sideroblasts, increased iron stores or both. Some patients have dysplastic erythroblasts and megakaryocytes but this is not necessarily so. An MPO or SBB stain should be performed in all cases with an increase of blast cells, both to confirm the lineage and to exclude the presence of Auer rods. A non-specific esterase stain such as α-naphthyl acetate esterase is useful in identifying monocyte precursors and is most useful when combined with a CAE stain to show cells of neutrophil lineage.

Bone marrow histology

The diagnosis of CMML is usually established from peripheral blood and bone marrow aspirate features; trephine biopsy does not have a major role in diagnosis. Almost all cases have a hypercellular marrow and increased granulopoiesis. Some also show an increase in cells of monocytic lineage (Fig. 5.54). There may be nodules of plasmacytoid dendritic cells, these being part of the neoplastic clone [158–160]. Similar nodules are seen in some cases of MDS. These cells show variable CD68 and CD68R positivity, low proliferative activity and no expression of lysozyme and CD163; in half or more of patients they express CD123. Their presence appears to correlate with resistance to intensive chemotherapy [159]. Some, but not all, cases of CMML show erythroid and megakaryocytic dysplasia. Abnormal localization of immature precursors (see page 215) is sometimes present and there may

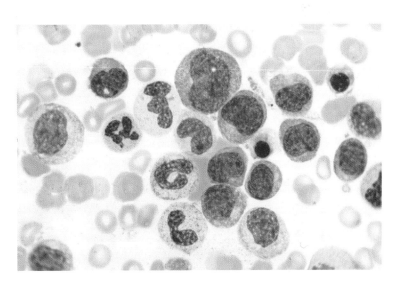

Fig. 5.53 BM aspirate, CMML, showing increased granulocytes and precursors. MGG ×100.

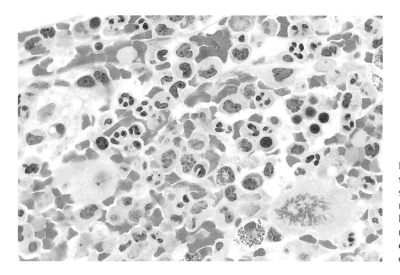

Fig. 5.54 BM trephine biopsy section from a patient with CMML showing increased neutrophils, monocytes and precursor cells, a hypolobated megakaryocyte and a megakaryocyte in mitosis. Paraffin-embedded, H&E ×40. (By courtesy of Dr D. Swirsky, Leeds.)

be an absolute increase in blasts. CD34 immuno-histochemistry is of little use since monoblasts and promonocytes are usually CD34 negative. Reticulin deposition is often diffusely increased.

Atypical chronic myeloid leukaemia, *BCR-ABL1* negative

Atypical chronic myeloid leukaemia (aCML) [5,161–163] is a rare Ph-negative, *BCR-ABL1*-negative condition with a higher median age of onset and a worse prognosis than CGL. Diagnostic criteria are summarized in Fig. 5.55. Common clinical features are anaemia and splenomegaly. The disorder appears to arise in a multipotent myeloid stem cell or possibly, since occasional lymphoblastic transformations have been observed, in a pluri-potent stem cell.

Assessment of peripheral blood features is of major importance in the diagnosis. Bone marrow cytology and histology are of less importance.

Peripheral blood

The WBC is elevated with an increase of neutrophils and their precursors (Fig. 5.56). Monocytosis is more marked than in CGL, while eosinophilia and basophilia are less marked and may be absent. The WBC at presentation is, on average, not as high as in CGL while the anaemia is more severe. The platelet count is not often elevated but is commonly reduced. Maturation of cells is less normal than in CGL and clear dysplastic features may be

Leucocytosis with dysplastic neutrophils and precursors; precursors (promyelocytes to metamyelocytes) at least 10% of leucocytes, basophils usually less than 2%

Plus

Fewer than 10% monocytes in blood

Plus

Fewer than 20% blast cells in blood and bone marrow

Plus

Hypercellular bone marrow with dysplasia at least in granulocyte lineage

Plus

No Ph chromosome, *BCR-ABL1* fusion gene or rearrangement of *PDGFRA* or *PDGFRB*

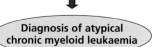

Diagnosis of atypical chronic myeloid leukaemia

Fig. 5.55 The 2008 WHO criteria for a diagnosis of atypical chronic myeloid leukaemia, *BCR-ABL1* negative.

present. Some cases show marked clumping of nuclear chromatin in neutrophils and precursors. Distinction from CMML is largely on the basis of the sum of promyelocytes, myelocytes and meta-myelocytes being 15% or higher in aCML but usually less than 5% in CMML [2].

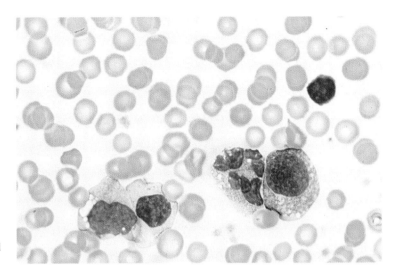

Fig. 5.56 PB film, aCML, *BCR-ABL1* negative, showing a myelocyte, a bizarre macropolycyte, an abnormal monocyte, an unidentifiable cell and a lymphocyte. MGG ×100.

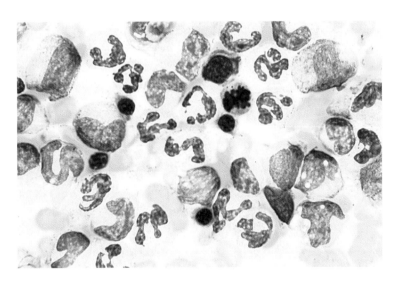

Fig. 5.57 BM aspirate film, aCML, *BCR-ABL1* negative (same patient as Fig. 5.56), showing increased granulocytes, monocytes and precursor cells. MGG ×100.

Bone marrow cytology

The bone marrow is hypercellular. Both granulocytic and monocytic precursors are increased (Fig. 5.57) although the cellularity is not increased to the extent that is seen in CGL and the myeloid:erythroid ratio is generally less than 10:1. Blasts may be increased but are less than 20%. Megakaryocytes are decreased in about a third of cases.

Bone marrow histology

The marrow histology in aCML may resemble that of CGL, particularly when examined at low power. However, the marrow is much more disorderly with disruption of normal architecture. There is marked hypercellularity with predominance of the granulocytic series. Erythroblasts are distributed as single cells or small groups throughout the marrow with well-formed erythroblastic islands being difficult to identify. Megakaryocytes may be increased in number and sometimes appear abnormal; they are more pleomorphic than in CGL. When monocytes are increased (Fig. 5.58) this is the morphological feature that most readily distinguishes aCML from CGL. The monocytes are recognized by their irregular nuclei with chromatin being less condensed than in neutrophil nuclei and moderate

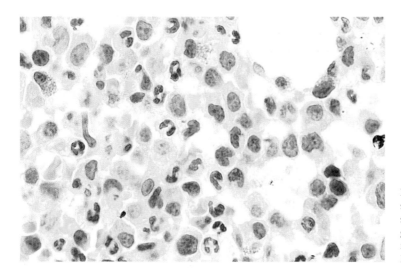

Fig. 5.58 BM trephine biopsy section, aCML, *BCR-ABL1*-negative, showing increased granulocytes and granulocyte precursors and numerous abnormal monocytes. Paraffin-embedded, H&E ×100.

amounts of cytoplasm, which stains pink with H&E. Atypical CML shows a variable degree of reticulin and collagen fibrosis and osteosclerosis can occur.

Cytogenetic and molecular genetic analysis
There is no specific cytogenetic or molecular genetic abnormality associated with aCML. Some cases are cytogenetically normal while others show clonal cytogenetic abnormalities such as trisomy 8. Mutations of *NRAS* or *KRAS* are present in about a third of patients.

Problems and pitfalls
Leukaemoid reactions can sometimes simulate aCML. Consideration of the clinical features and, if necessary, re-examination of blood and bone marrow after a period of follow-up, permits the correct diagnosis to be made.

Making the distinction between aCML and CGL is not always possible on histological grounds alone. Cytogenetic and molecular genetic analysis are necessary to distinguish aCML from CGL presenting in accelerated phase. Likewise, CMML and aCML often cannot be distinguished histologically; consideration of the blood count and film is necessary.

Juvenile myelomonocytic leukaemia
Juvenile myelomonocytic leukaemia (JMML) is a Ph-negative *BCR-ABL1*-negative condition that occurs mainly in children less than 5 years of age.

This term encompasses not only the condition previously designated 'juvenile chronic myeloid leukaemia' but also the infantile monosomy 7 syndrome and other myelodysplastic/myeloproliferative neoplasms of childhood [1,164,165]. There is an increased incidence in children with neurofibromatosis type 1 and Noonan's syndrome. Three quarters of affected children are under the age of 3 years, with the incidence in boys being twice that in girls. Clinical features often include anaemia, hepatomegaly, splenomegaly, lymphadenopathy and rash. Erythropoiesis may show reversion to features of fetal erythropoiesis (high haemoglobin F and red cell carbonic anhydrase and low haemoglobin A_2). There is often hypergammaglobulinaemia and there is an increased prevalence of autoantibodies. Diagnostic criteria are shown in Fig. 5.59.

Peripheral blood
The blood film shows neutrophilia, prominent monocytosis and sometimes granulocyte precursors or nucleated red blood cells (Fig. 5.60). Anaemia and thrombocytopenia are usual. In cases in which haemoglobin F is increased, a Kleihauer test shows a population of haemoglobin F-containing cells (Fig. 5.61).

Bone marrow cytology
The bone marrow shows increased cells of granulocyte and sometimes monocyte lineages. There may be dysplastic features (Fig. 5.62).

Bone marrow histology

Features are similar to those of CMML in adults. The monocytic component may be inconspicuous.

Cytogenetic and molecular genetic analysis

The Ph chromosome and the *BCR-ABL1* fusion gene are absent. Many cases are cytogenetically normal

Monocytes >1 × 10⁹/l

Plus

Fewer than 20% blast cells (plus promonocytes) in blood and bone marrow

Plus

No Ph chromosome or *BCR-ABL1* fusion gene

Plus

Two or more of the following criteria:
• Haemoglobin F increased for age
• Immature granulocytes in the peripheral blood
• WBC >10 × 10⁹/l
• Clonal chromosomal abnormality (monosomy 7 not excluded)
• Myeloid progenitors hypersensitive to GM-CSF *in vitro*

Diagnosis of juvenile myelomonocytic leukaemia

Fig. 5.59 The 2008 WHO criteria for a diagnosis of juvenile myelomonocytic leukaemia. GM-CSF, granulocyte–macrophage colony-stimulating factor; WBC, white blood cell count.

at presentation but develop clonal abnormalities during the course of the disease. Overall, 40–67% have been reported to be cytogenetically normal, 25–33% have been found to have monosomy 7, and 10–25% to have had other chromosomal abnormalities including trisomy 8 and other abnormalities of chromosome 7 [164].

About 15% of children with JMML have clinical features of neurofibromatosis, such as *café-au-lait* spots. These children have a constitutional abnormality of one *NF1* gene and often a somatic deletion of the normal allele, which can be the result of acquired isodisomy. In addition to children with clinical features of neurofibromatosis, a similar number of patients with JMML have been found to have mutations of the *NF1* gene without clinical features of the disease [164]. Mutations in *RAS* oncogenes (*NRAS* and *KRAS2*) are also common, being observed in 15–30% of patients. Another group of children have a mutation in *PTPN11*, the gene that is mutated in Noonan's syndrome. Since *PTPN11* encodes a protein in the RAS pathway and the *NF1* gene product is a negative regulator of *RAS*, the mechanisms of leukaemogenesis are likely to be related in these three groups of mutations (which are largely mutually exclusive) [164,165].

Problems and pitfalls

Leukaemoid reactions resulting from herpesvirus infections can simulate JMML; such reactions have been observed following Epstein–Barr virus infec-

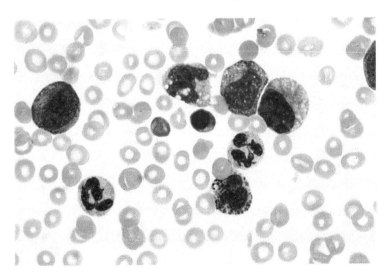

Fig. 5.60 PB, juvenile chronic myeloid leukaemia, showing a monocyte, a basophil, dysplastic neutrophils, neutrophil precursors and thrombocytopenia. MGG ×100.

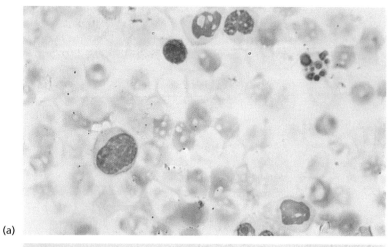

(a)

(b)

Fig. 5.61 Kleihauer test on PB of a patient with juvenile myelomonocytic leukaemia (same patient as Fig. 5.60) showing numerous haemoglobin F-containing cells which stain pink: (a) patient; (b) negative control. Kleihauer test ×100.

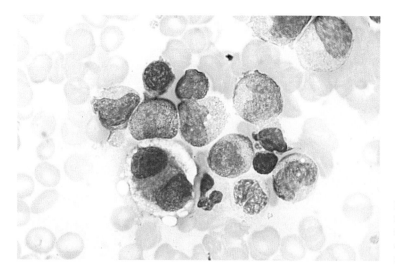

Fig. 5.62 BM aspirate film, juvenile myelomonocytic leukaemia, showing granulocyte precursors and a dysplastic binucleated micromegakaryocyte. MGG ×100.

tion, cytomegalovirus infection and human herpes-virus 6 infection. Reversion to features of fetal erythropoiesis, which occurs in JMML, is not seen in leukaemoid reactions. Investigation of these features plus cytogenetic and molecular genetic analysis and appropriate viral studies is useful when there is diagnostic difficulty.

It should be noted that children with Noonan's syndrome, in addition to having an increased incidence of JMML, can also develop a similar syndrome that resolves without treatment [166].

Myelodysplastic/myeloproliferative neoplasms, unclassifiable

In addition to those patients who conform to the three specific categories of MDS/MPN of the WHO classification there are other patients with features of both myelodysplasia and myeloproliferation [167,168]; the diagnostic criteria are shown in Fig. 5.63. For example, coexistence of sideroblastic erythropoiesis and thrombocytosis is relatively common [155] and is often designated refractory anaemia with ring sideroblasts and thrombocytosis (RARS-T) (Fig. 5.64). In the 2008 WHO classification this is recognized as a provisional entity; the diagnostic criteria are coexistence of anaemia with more than 15% ring sideroblasts with a platelet count of at least 450×10^9/l [168]. Such patients

often have splenomegaly, an increased WBC and increased reticulin deposition in the bone marrow. The karyotype is usually normal. There is quite often a *JAK2* V617F mutation, which is homozygous

| Meets criteria for one of the categories of MDS | *And* | Prominent myeloproliferative features, e.g. platelet count at least 450×10^9/l or WBC at least 13×10^9/l |

Plus

No preceding history of MDS or MPN and cannot be assigned to a more specific category of MDS/MPN

And

No *BCR-ABL1* or rearrangement of *PDGFRA*, *PDGFRB* or *FGFR1*
No isolated del(5q), t(3;3)(q21;q26.2) or inv(3)(q21q26.2)

Diagnosis of myelodysplastic/ myeloproliferative neoplasm, unclassifiable

Fig. 5.63 The 2008 WHO criteria for a diagnosis of myelodysplastic/myeloproliferative neoplasm (MDS/MPN), unclassifiable. WBC, white blood cell count.

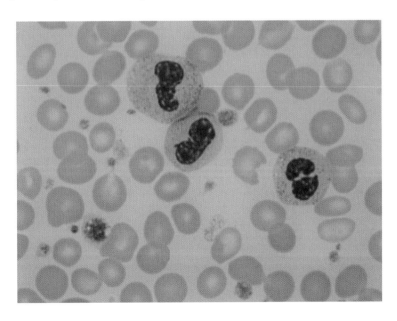

Fig. 5.64 PB film from a patient with refractory anaemia with ring sideroblasts and thrombocytosis showing mild anisopoikilocytosis, dysplastic neutrophils, thrombocytosis and giant platelets; there is one hypochromic erythrocyte. MGG ×100.

in about half of patients [169,170]. The disease may evolve into myelofibrosis.

A number of patients have been described with coexistence of systemic mastocytosis and a myelo-dysplastic/myeloproliferative neoplasm [148]. In the WHO classification these are included in the group 'systemic mast cell disease with associated haematological neoplasm' rather MDS/MPN, unclassified.

Myeloid and lymphoid neoplasms with rearrangement of *PDGFRA*, *PDGFRB* or *FGFR1*

The 2008 WHO classification recognizes a group of haematological neoplasms best characterized by their genetic abnormalities – rearrangement of one of three specific genes that encode aberrant tyrosine kinases [171,172]. The three groups of neoplasms have some characteristics in common, particularly the usual presentation as a chronic myeloid neoplasm and the frequent occurrence of eosinophilic differentiation, but they also have characteristics that differ. A lymphoid component is recognized in the case of disorders with a rearrangement of *PDGFRA* and *FGFR1*. The therapeutic implications of these diagnoses illustrate the importance of moving, when possible, to a molecular classification of haemopoietic neoplasms. Neoplasms associated with rearrangement of *PDGFRA* and *PDGFRB* are responsive to imatinib therapy. *FGFR1*-related neoplasms also lead to expression of a constitutively activated tyrosine kinase, rendering possible the development of an effective inhibitor of the gene product and meanwhile being an indication for consideration of stem cell transplantation.

Myeloid and lymphoid neoplasms with rearrangement of *PDGFRA*

The most common among this group of neoplasms is CEL associated with a *FIP1L1-PDGFRA* fusion gene that results from a cryptic deletion at 4q12 [173]. Less often there are translocations leading to this fusion gene or a variant. Most patients present in chronic phase with eosinophilic leukaemia. They usually have splenomegaly and may have cardiac and other tissue damage as a result of release of

eosinophil granule contents. A minority of patients present with either AML with eosinophilia or T-lymphoblastic lymphoma with eosinophilia. Acute transformation can occur when the initial presentation was CEL. There is a remarkable male predominance in this neoplasm. Most patients are young to middle aged. The condition is very sensitive to imatinib therapy.

In the cytogenetic/molecular variant associated with t(4;22)(q12;q11) and *BCR-PDGFRA* fusion, the haematological features appear to be intermediate between those of CEL associated with *FIP1L1-PDGFRA* fusion and those of CGL. Acute lymphoblastic transformation (T or B lineage) can occur in these cases also.

Peripheral blood
There is usually, perhaps invariably, hypereosinophilia. Eosinophils may be cytologically normal or abnormal (hypogranular, vacuolated and with nuclear abnormalities) (Fig. 5.65). Neutrophils are sometimes increased and there may be anaemia and thrombocytopenia. Blast cells are not usually increased.

Bone marrow cytology
The bone marrow shows an increase of eosinophils and their precursors (Fig. 5.66).

Bone marrow histology
Bone marrow trephine biopsy sections show an increase of eosinophils and their precursors. In the majority of patients there is also an increase of mast cells, which may be cytologically abnormal (Fig. 5.67); usually these are less frequent that in systemic mastocytosis but sometimes the mast cell infiltration is quite marked and there are cohesive clusters. Often the mast cells show aberrant expression of CD25 but usually not of CD2 (whereas in systemic mastocytosis expression of both CD2 and CD25 is usual). In one patient the mast cells resembled those of systemic mastocytosis in showing over-expression of phosphorylated nuclear STAT5, likely to be induced by the aberrant tyrosine kinase activity [147].

Cytogenetic and molecular genetic analysis
Cytogenetic analysis is usually normal. Molecular analysis for the *FIP1L1-PDGFRA* fusion gene is nec-

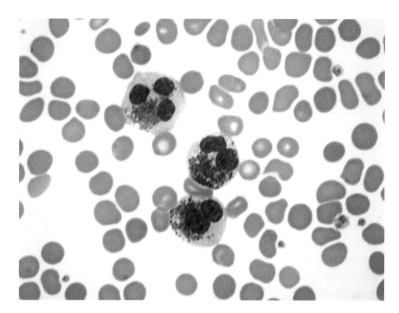

Fig. 5.65 PB film from a patient with a myeloproliferative neoplasm associated with *FIP1L1-PDGFRA* showing three partially degranulated eosinophils. MGG ×100.

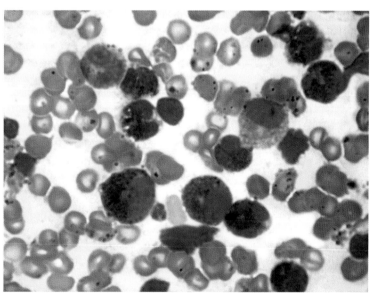

Fig. 5.66 BM film from a patient with a myeloproliferative neoplasm associated with *FIP1L1-PDGFRA* (same patient as Fig. 5.65) showing an increase of eosinophils and precursors. MGG ×100.

essary. PCR (preferably nested PCR) and FISH can be used.

Problems and pitfalls
The differential diagnosis includes other causes of hypereosinophilia. A diagnosis of 'idiopathic hyper-eosinophilic syndrome' should never be made without exclusion of CEL associated with *PDGFRA*

rearrangement. If this molecular lesion is found, the diagnosis is not idiopathic hypereosinophilic syndrome.

Systemic mastocytosis is an important differential diagnosis. Despite the increase in mast cells in both conditions, this is a quite different disease from systemic mastocytosis with a different molecular lesion and different therapeutic and prognostic implications.

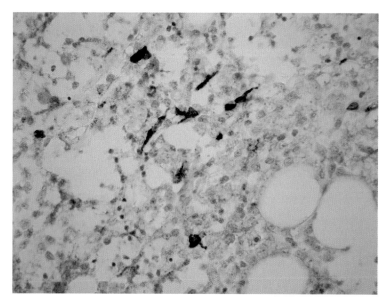

Fig. 5.67 BM trephine biopsy section from a patient with a myeloproliferative neoplasm associated with *FIP1L1-PDGFRA* showing an increase of mast cells, most of which are spindle shaped. Paraffin-embedded, immunoperoxidase for mast cell tryptase ×40.

Myeloid neoplasms with rearrangement of *PDGFRB*

The most common among this group of neoplasms is an MPN or MDS/MPN associated with a t(5;12) (q31~33;p12) and an *ETV6-PDGFRB* fusion gene. The most frequent haematological manifestation is CMML with eosinophilia but some patients have CEL or aCML. Acute transformation can occur. This condition is about twice as common in men as in woman with peak incidence being in early middle age. Splenomegaly is common. Myeloid neoplasms associated with *PDGFRB* rearrangement are sensitive to imatinib and when this treatment is available the previously poor prognosis is likely to be ameliorated.

Peripheral blood
There is usually eosinophilia and sometimes monocytosis or neutrophilia. Neutrophil precursors may be present. There may be anaemia or thrombocytopenia.

Bone marrow cytology
The bone marrow aspirate shows a hypercellular marrow (Fig. 5.68), usually with increased eosinophils and precursors and a variable increase in cells of monocyte and neutrophil lineage.

Bone marrow histology
Bone marrow trephine biopsy sections show a hypercellular marrow with a variable increase of cells of eosinophil, neutrophil and monocyte lineage. Increased mast cells may be observed and these may be spindle shaped. The mast cells often show aberrant expression of CD2 and CD25.

Cytogenetic and molecular genetic analysis
In addition to the most often observed translocation, t(5;12)(q31~33;p12) leading to *ETV6-PDGFRA*, there are at least 14 variant translocations, all involving *PDGFRB*. Molecular analysis (e.g. FISH) can be used to confirm *PDGFRB* rearrangement, but FISH does not always detect an abnormality that is present and if it is negative or not available a trial of imatinib may be justified in patients with a 5q31~33 breakpoint.

Problems and pitfalls
This condition should not be confused with systemic mastocytosis. Because of the therapeutic implications, its correct identification is important.

Myeloid and lymphoid neoplasms with rearrangement of *FGFR1*
This is a cytogenetically and molecularly heterogeneous group of conditions. Nevertheless there are

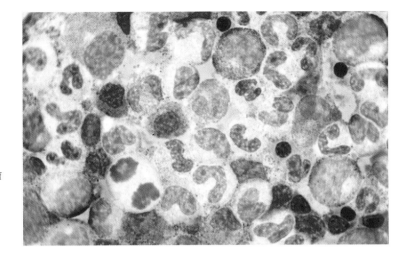

Fig. 5.68 BM aspirate film from a patient with chronic eosinophilic leukaemia associated with t(5;12) (p33;p12) showing a hypercellular marrow with an increase in cells of neutrophil and eosinophil lineage. MGG ×100. (By courtesy of Dr E. Granjo, Porto [174]; reprinted by permission of *Hematol J*, **1** (Suppl. 1), 74, 2000.)

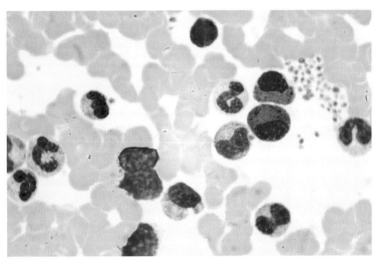

Fig. 5.69 BM aspirate film from a patient with chronic myelomonocytic leukaemia with eosinophilia associated with t(8;13) (p11;q12) showing neutrophil, and two eosinophil, precursors; the two eosinophil myelocytes have some granules with basophilic staining characteristics, a non-specific feature seen in both reactive and neoplastic conditions. MGG ×100. (Courtesy of Dr Donald Macdonald, London.)

clinical and haematological features in common between the different genetic subgroups associated with *FGFR1* rearrangement. Most patients present with CEL with early transformation to AML or lymphoblastic lymphoma/leukaemia. The lymphoid neoplasm is most often of T lineage but sometimes B lineage. Usual clinical features are hepatosplenomegaly, lymphadenopathy and systemic symptoms. Most patients are young adults. There is only a modest male predominance. Prognosis is currently poor.

Peripheral blood
Eosinophilia and neutrophilia are usual and some patients have monocytosis.

Bone marrow cytology and histology
The bone marrow is hypercellular with patients who present in chronic phase showing a variable increase of cells of neutrophil, eosinophil and monocyte lineages (Fig. 5.69). Some patients have bone marrow infiltration by myeloblasts or lymphoblasts.

Cytogenetic and molecular genetic analysis
The four most frequently observed cytogenetic/molecular genetic abnormalities are shown in Table 5.5 [172]. In addition, there have been small numbers of reports of other similar cases with other translocations leading to *FGFR1* rearrangement. Trisomy 21 is the most common secondary abnormality.

Table 5.5 The more common of the myeloid and lymphoid neoplasms associated with a rearrangement of *PDGFRA*, *PDGFRB* or *FGFR1* (abbreviated from reference [171]).

Gene rearranged	Fusion gene	Cytogenetic abnormality
PDGFRA	*FIP1L1-PDGFRA*	Usually none (cryptic deletion), sometimes a translocation with a 4q12 breakpoint
	BCR-PDGFRA	t(4;22)(q12;q11)
PDGFRB	*ETV6-PDGFRB*	t(5;12)(q31-33;p12)
	HIP1-PDGFRB	t(5;7)(q33;q11.2)
	CCDC6-PDGFRB	t(5;10)(q33)(q21)
FGFR1	*FGFR1OP1-FGFR1*	t(6;8)(q27;p11-12)
	CEP110-FGFR1	t(8;9)(p11;q32-34)
	ZNF198-FGFR1	t(8;13)(p11;q12)
	BCR-FGFR1	t(8;22)(p11;q11)

References

1 Jaffe ES, Harris NL, Stein H and Vardiman JW (eds) (2001) *World Health Organization Classification of Tumours: Pathology and genetics of tumours of haematopoietic and lymphoid tissues.* IARC Press, Lyon.

2 Vardiman J, Brunning RD, Arber DA, Le Beau MM, Porwit A, Tefferi A, Bloomfield CD and Thiele J (2008) Introduction and overview of the classification of myeloid neoplasms. In: Swerdlow SH, Campo E, Harris NL, Jaffe ES, Pileri SA, Stein H, Thiele J and Vardiman JW (eds) *World Health Organization Classification of Tumours of Haematopoietic and Lymphoid Tissue*, 4th edn. IARC Press, Lyon, pp. 18–30.

3 Thiele J, Kvasnicka HM, Tefferi A, Barosi G and Orazi A (2008) Primary myelofibrosis. In: Swerdlow SH, Campo E, Harris NL, Jaffe ES, Pileri SA, Stein H, Thiele J and Vardiman JW (eds) *World Health Organization Classification of Tumours of Haematopoietic and Lymphoid Tissue*, 4th edn. IARC Press, Lyon, pp. 44–50.

4 Vardiman J, Melo J, Baccarani M and Thiele J (2008) Chronic myelogenous leukaemia, BCR-ABL1-positive. In: Swerdlow SH, Campo E, Harris NL, Jaffe ES, Pileri SA, Stein H, Thiele J and Vardiman JW (eds) *World Health Organization Classification of Tumours of Haematopoietic and Lymphoid Tissue*, 4th edn. IARC Press, Lyon, pp. 32–37.

5 Shepherd PC, Ganesan TS and Galton DA (1987) Haematological classification of the chronic myeloid leukaemias. *Bailliere's Clin Haematol*, **1**, 887–906.

6 Spiers AS, Bain BJ and Turner JE (1977) The peripheral blood in chronic granulocytic leukaemia. Study of 50 untreated Philadelphia-positive cases. *Scand J Haematol*, **18**, 25–38.

7 Thiele J, Kvasnicka HM, Zirbes TK, Flucke U, Niederle N, Leder LD *et al.* (1998) Impact of clinical and morphological variables in classification and regression tree-based survival (CART) analysis of CML with special emphasis on dynamic features. *Eur J Haematol*, **60**, 35–46.

8 Braziel RM, Launder TM, Druker BJ, Olson SB, Magenis RE, Mauro MJ *et al.* (2002) Hematopathologic and cytogenetic findings in imatinib mesylate-treated chronic myelogenous leukemia patients: 14 months experience. *Blood*, **100**, 435–441.

9 Burkhardt R, Frisch B and Bartl R (1982) Bone biopsy in haematological disorders. *J Clin Pathol*, **35**, 257–284.

10 Burkhardt R, Bartl R, Jager K, Frisch B, Kettner G, Mahl G and Sund M (1986) Working classification of chronic myeloproliferative disorders based on histological, haematological, and clinical findings. *J Clin Pathol* **39**, 237–252.

11 Lazzarino M, Morra E, Castello A, Inverardi D, Coci A, Pagnucco G *et al.* (1986) Myelofibrosis in chronic granulocytic leukaemia: clinicopathologic correlations and prognostic significance. *Br J Haematol*, **64**, 227–240.

12 Rozman C, Cervantes F. and Feliu E (1989) Is the histological classification of chronic granulocytic leukaemia justified from the clinical point of view? *Eur J Haematol*, **42**, 150–154.

13 Schmid C, Frisch B, Beham A, Jager K and Kettner G (1990) Comparison of bone marrow histology in early chronic granulocytic leukemia and in leukemoid reaction. *Eur J Haematol*, **44**, 154–158.

14 Thiele J and Fischer R (1991) Megakaryocytopoiesis in haematological disorders: diagnostic features of bone marrow biopsies. An overview. *Virchows Arch A Pathol Anat Histopathol*, **418**, 87–97.

15 Thiele J, Kvasnicka HM, Schmitt-Graeff A, Zirbes TK, Birnbaum F, Kressmann C et al. (2000) Bone marrow features and clinical findings in chronic myeloid leukemia – a comparative, multicenter, immunohistochemical and morphometric study of 614 patients. *Leuk Lymphoma*, **36**, 295–308.

16 Frisch B and Bartl R (1999) *Biopsy Interpretation of Bone and Bone Marrow: Histology and immunohistology in paraffin and plastic*, 2nd edn. Arnold, London.

17 Rumpel M, Friedrich T and Deininger MWN (2003) Imatinib normalizes bone marrow vascularity in patients with chronic myeloid leukemia in first chronic phase. *Blood*, **101**, 4641–4642.

18 Clough V, Geary CG, Hashmi K, Davson J and Knowlson T (1979) Myelofibrosis in chronic granulocytic leukaemia. *Br J Haematol*, **42**, 515–526.

19 Thiele J, Kvasnicka HM, Fischer R and Diehl V (1997) Clinicopathological impact of the interaction between megakaryocytes and myeloid stroma in chronic myeloproliferative disorders: a concise update. *Leuk Lymphoma*, **24**, 463–481.

20 Thiele J, Kvasnicka HM, Schmitt-Graeff A, Spohr M, Diehl V, Zancovich R et al. (2000) Effects of interferon and hydroxyurea therapy on bone marrow fibrosis in chronic myelogenous leukaemia: a comparative retrospective multicentric histological and clinical study. *Br J Haematol*, **108**, 64–71.

21 Roberts MM, Ross DM, Hughes TP and To LB (2005) Lymphoid foci in the bone marrow of patients with chronic myeloid leukaemia treated with imatinib. *Blood*, **106**, 568a.

22 Chiusolo P, Sica S, Laurenti L, Piccirillo N, Giordano G and Leone G (2000) Fatal bone marrow aplasia during interferon-α treatment in chronic myelogenous leukemia. *Haematologica*, **85**, 212.

23 Ram R, Gafter-Gvili A, Okon E, Pazgal I, Shpilberg O and Raanani P (2008) Gelatinous transformation of bone marrow in chronic myeloid leukemia during treatment with imatinib mesylate: a disease or a drug effect? *Acta Haematol*, **119**, 104–107.

24 Kvasnicka HM, Thiele J, Staib P, Schmitt-Graff A, Griesshammer M, Klose J et al. (2004) Reversal of bone marrow angiogenesis in chronic myeloid leukemia following imatinib mesylate (STI571) therapy. *Blood*, **103**, 3549–3551.

25 Beham-Schmid C, Apfelbeck U, Sill H, Tsybrovsky O, Hofler G, Haas OA and Linkesch W (2002) Treatment of chronic myelogenous leukemia with the tyrosine kinase inhibitor STI571 results in marked regression of bone marrow fibrosis. *Blood*, **99**, 381–383.

26 Fitter S, Dewar AL, Kostakis P, To LB, Hughes TP, Roberts MM et al. (2008) Long-term imatinib therapy promotes bone formation in CML patients. *Blood*, **111**, 2538–2547.

27 Thiele J, Kvasnicka HM, Niederle N, Kloke O, Schmidt M, Lienhard H et al. (1995) Clinical and histological features retain their prognostic impact under interferon therapy of CML: a pilot study. *Am J Hematol*, **50**, 30–39.

28 Islam A (1988) Prediction of impending blast cell transformation in chronic granulocytic leukaemia. *Histopathology*, **12**, 633–639.

29 Peterson LC, Bloomfield CD and Brunning RD (1976) Blast crisis as an initial or terminal manifestation of chronic myeloid leukemia. A study of 28 patients. *Am J Med*, **60**, 209–220.

30 Islam A, Catovsky D, Goldman J and Galton DAG (1980) Histological study of chronic granulocytic leukaemia in blast transformation. *Br J Haematol*, **46**, 326.

31 Williams WC and Weiss GB (1982) Megakaryoblastic transformation of chronic myelogenous leukemia. *Cancer*, **49**, 921–926.

32 Muehleck SD, McKenna RW, Arthur DC, Parkin JL and Brunning RD (1984) Transformation of chronic myelogenous leukemia: clinical, morphologic, and cytogenetic features. *Am J Clin Pathol*, **82**, 1–14.

33 Orazi A, Neiman RS, Cualing H, Heerema NA and John K (1994) CD34 immunostaining of bone marrow biopsy specimens is a reliable way to classify the phases of chronic myeloid leukemia. *Am J Clin Pathol*, **101**, 426–428.

34 Valent P, Agis H, Sperr W, Sillaber C and Horny H-P (2008) Diagnostic and prognostic value of new biochemical and immunohistochemical parameters in chronic myeloid leukemia. *Leuk Lymphoma*, **49**, 635–638.

35 Sinclair PB, Nacheva EP, Leversha M, Telford N, Chang J, Reid A et al. (2000) Large deletions at the t(9;22) breakpoint are common and may identify a poor-prognosis subgroup of patients with chronic myeloid leukemia. *Blood*, **95**, 738–743.

36 Kreil S, Pfirrmann M, Haferlach C, Waghorn K, Chase A, Hehlmann R et al. (2007) Heterogeneous prognostic impact of derivative chromosome 9 deletions in chronic myelogenous leukemia. *Blood*, **110**, 1283–1290.

37 Kim DH, Popradi G, Sriharsha L, Kamel-Reid S, Chang H, Messner HA and Lipton JH (2008) No significance of derivative chromosome 9 deletion on the clearance of BCR/ABL fusion transcripts, cytogenetic or molecular response, loss of response, or treatment failure to imatinib mesylate therapy for chronic myeloid leukemia. *Cancer*, **113**, 772–781.

38 Michiels JJ, Berneman Z, Schroyens W, Kutti J, Swolin B, Ridell B et al. (2004) Philadelphia (Ph) chromosome-positive thrombocythemia without features of chronic myeloid leukemia in peripheral blood: natural history and diagnostic differentiation from Ph-negative essential thrombocythaemia. *Annals Hematol*, **83**, 504–512.

39 Murphy S, Iland H, Rosenthal D and Laszlo J (1986) Essential thrombocythemia: an interim report from the Polycythemia Vera Study Group. *Semin Hematol*, **23**, 177–182.

40 Stoll DB, Peterson P, Exten R, Laszlo J, Pisciotta AV, Ellis JT *et al.* (1988) Clinical presentation and natural history of patients with essential thrombocythemia and the Philadelphia chromosome. *Am J Hematol*, **27**, 77–83.

41 Rollison DE, Howlader N, Smith MT, Strom SS, Merritt WD, Ries LA *et al.* (2008) Epidemiology of myelodysplastic syndromes and chronic myeloproliferative disorders in the United States, 2001–2004, using data from the NAACCR and SEER programs. *Blood*, **112**, 45–52.

42 Kojima K, Yasukawa M, Hara M, Nawa Y, Kimura Y, Narumi H and Fujita S (1999) Familial occurrence of chronic neutrophilic leukaemia *Br J Haematol*, **105**, 428–430.

43 Bain BJ, Brunning RD, Vardiman JW and Thiele J (2008) Chronic neutrophilic leukaemia. In: Swerdlow SH, Campo E, Harris NL, Jaffe ES, Pileri SA, Stein H, Thiele J and Vardiman JW (eds) *World Health Organization Classification of Tumours of Haematopoietic and Lymphoid Tissue*, 4th edn. IARC Press, Lyon, pp. 38–39.

44 Foucar K (2001) *Bone Marrow Pathology*, 2nd edn. ASCP Press, Chicago.

45 Jones AV, Kreil S, Zoi K, Waghorn K, Curtis C, Zhang L, Score J *et al.* (2005) Widespread occurrence of the *JAK2* V617F mutation in chronic myeloproliferative disorders. *Blood*, **106**, 2162–2168.

46 Standen GR, Steers FJ and Jones L (1993) Clonality of chronic neutrophilic leukaemia associated with myeloma: analysis using the X-linked probe M27β. *J Clin Pathol*, **46**, 297–298.

47 Cario H, Schwarz K, Herter JM, Komrska V, McMullin MF, Minkov M *et al.* (2008) Clinical and molecular characterisation of a prospectively collected cohort of children and adolescents with polycythaemia vera. *Br J Haematol*, **142**, 622–626.

48 Ridell B, Carneskog J, Wedel H, Vilén L, Dufva IH, Mellqvist U-H *et al.* (2000) Incidence of chronic myeloproliferative disorders in the city of Göteborg, Sweden 1983–1992. *Eur J Haematol*, **65**, 267–271.

49 Tefferi A (2000) Myelofibrosis with myeloid metaplasia. *N Engl J Med*, **342**, 1255–1265.

50 Thiele J, Kvasnicka HM, Orazi A, Tefferi A and Birgegard G (2008) Polycythaemia vera. In: Swerdlow SH, Campo E, Harris NL, Jaffe ES, Pileri SA, Stein H, Thiele J and Vardiman JW (eds) *World Health Organization Classification of Tumours of Haematopoietic and Lymphoid Tissue*, 4th edn. IARC Press, Lyon, pp. 40–43.

51 McNamara C, Juneja S, Wolf M and Grigg A (2002) Portal or hepatic vein thrombosis as the first presentation of a myeloproliferative disorder in patients with normal peripheral blood counts. *Clin Lab Haematol*, **24**, 239–242.

52 Landolfi R, Di Gennaro L, Barbui T, De Stefano V, Finazzi G, Marfisi R *et al.* (2007) Leukocytosis as a major thrombotic risk factor in patients with polycythemia vera. *Blood*, **109**, 2446–2453.

53 Passamonti F, Rumi E, Caramella M, Elena C, Arcaini L, Boveri E *et al.* (2008) A dynamic prognostic model to predict survival in post-polycythemia vera myelofibrosis. *Blood*, **111**, 3383–3387.

54 Scott LM, Tong W, Levine RL, Scott MA, Beer PA, Stratton MR *et al.* (2007) JAK2 exon 12 mutations in polycythemia vera and idiopathic erythrocytosis. *N Engl J Med*, **356**, 459–468.

55 Vykoupil KF, Thiele J, Stangel W, Krmpotic E and Georgii A (1980) Polycythemia vera. I. Histopathology, ultrastructure and cytogenetics of the bone marrow in comparison with secondary polycythemia. *Virchows Arch A Pathol Anat Histopathol*, **389**, 307–324.

56 Lucie NP and Young GA (1983) Marrow cellularity in the diagnosis of polycythaemia. *J Clin Pathol*, **36**, 180–183.

57 Ellis JT, Peterson P, Geller SA and Rappaport H (1986) Studies of the bone marrow in polycythemia vera and the evolution of myelofibrosis and second hematologic malignancies. *Semin Hematol*, **23**, 144–155.

58 Mesa RA, Hanson CA, Rajkumar SV, Schroeder G and Tefferi A (2000) Evaluation and clinical correlations of bone marrow angiogenesis in myelofibrosis with myeloid metaplasia. *Blood*, **96**, 3374–3380.

59 Thiele J, Kvasnicka HM, Zankovich R and Diehl V (2001) The value of bone marrow histology in differentiating between early stage polycythemia vera and secondary (reactive) polycythemias. *Haematologica*, **86**, 368–374.

60 Kralovics R, Buser AS, Teo S-S, Coers J, Tichelli A, van der Maas PC and Skoda RC (2003) Comparison of molecular markers in a cohort of patients with chronic myeloproliferative disorders. *Blood*, **102**, 1869–1871.

61 Baxter EJ, Scott LM, Campbell PJ, East C, Fourouclas N, Swanton S *et al.* (2005) Acquired mutation of the tyrosine kinase *JAK2* in human myeloproliferative disorders. *Lancet*, **365**, 1054–1061.

62 Kralovics R, Passamonti F, Buser AS, Teo SS, Tiedt R, Passweg JR *et al.* (2005) A gain-of-function mutation of JAK2 in myeloproliferative disorders. *N Engl J Med*, **352**,1779–1790.

63 Khwaja A (2006) The role of Janus kinases in haemopoiesis and haematological malignancy. *Br J Haematol*, **134**, 366–384.

64 Ishii T, Bruno E, Hoffman R and Xu M (2006) Involvement of various hematopoietic-cell lineages

by the JAK2V^{617F} mutation in polycythemia vera. *Blood*, **108**, 3128–3134.

65 Campbell PJ, Baxter EJ, Beer PA, Scott LM, Bench AJ, Huntly BJ *et al.* (2006) Mutation of JAK2 in the myeloproliferative disorders: timing, clonality studies, cytogenetic associations, and role in leukemic transformation. *Blood*, **108**, 3548–3555.

66 Jones AV, Silver RT, Waghorn K, Curtis C, Kreil S, Zoi K *et al.* (2006) Minimal molecular response in polycythemia vera patients treated with imatinib or interferon alpha. *Blood*, **107**, 3339–3341.

67 Li S, Kralovics R, de Libero G, Theocharides A, Gisslinger H and Skoda RC (2008) Clonal heterogeneity in polycythemia vera patients with *JAK2* exon12 and JAK2-V617F mutations. *Blood*, **111**, 3863–3866.

68 Carneskog J, Safai-Kutti S, Suurküla M, Wadenvik H, Bake B, Lindstedt G and Kutti J (1998a) The red cell mass, plasma erythropoietin and spleen size in apparent polycythaemia. *Eur J Haematol*, **62**, 43–48.

69 Messinezy M, Westwood NB, El-Hemaidi I, Marsden JT, Sherwood RS and Pearson TC (2002) Serum erythropoietin values in erythrocytoses and in primary thrombocythaemia *Br J Haematol*, **117**, 47–53.

70 Tefferi A, Yoon S-Y and Li C-Y (2000) Immunohistochemical staining for megakaryocyte c-mpl may complement morphologic distinction between polycythemia vera and secondary erythrocytosis. *Blood*, **96**, 771–772.

71 Lengfelder E, Hochhaus A, Kronawitter U, Höche D, Queisser W, Jahn-Eder M *et al.* (1998) Should a platelet limit of 600 × 10^9/l be used as a diagnostic criterion in essential thrombocythaemia? An analysis of the natural course including early stages. *Br J Haematol*, **100**, 15–23.

72 Thiele J, Kvasnicka HM, Orazi A, Tefferi A and Gisslinger H (2008) Essential thrombocythaemia. In: Swerdlow SH, Campo E, Harris NL, Jaffe ES, Pileri SA, Stein H, Thiele J and Vardiman JW (eds) *World Health Organization Classification of Tumours of Haematopoietic and Lymphoid Tissue*, 4th edn. IARC Press, Lyon, pp. 48–50.

73 Carobbio A, Finazzi G, Antonioli E, Guglielmelli P, Vannucchi AM, Delaini F *et al.* (2008) Thrombocytosis and leukocytosis interaction in vascular complications of essential thrombocythemia. *Blood*, **112**, 3135–3137.

74 Torner A (2002) Effects of anagrelide on in vivo megakaryocyte proliferation and maturation in essential thrombocythemia. *Blood*, **99**, 1602–1609.

75 Solberg LA, Tefferi A, Oles KJ, Tarach JS, Petitt RM, Forstrom LA and Silverstein MN (1997) The effects of anagrelide on human megakaryocytopoiesis. *Br J Haematol*, **99**, 174–180.

76 Wolf BC and Neiman RS (1988) The bone marrow in myeloproliferative and dysmyelopoietic syndromes. *Hematol Oncol Clin North Am*, **2**, 669–694.

77 Beer PA, Campbell PJ, Scott LM, Bench AJ, Erber WN, Bareford D *et al.* (2008) MPL mutations in myeloproliferative disorders: analysis of the PT-1 cohort. *Blood*, **112**, 141–149.

78 Mesa RA, Hanson CA, Li C-Y, Yoon S-Y, Rajkumar SV, Schroeder G and Tefferi A (2002) Diagnostic and prognostic value of bone marrow angiogenesis and megakaryocyte c-Mpl expression is essential thrombocythaemia. *Blood*, **99**, 4131–4137.

79 Teofili L, Pierconti F, Di Febo A, Maggiano N, Vianelli N, Ascani S *et al.* (2002) The expression pattern of c-*mpl* in megakaryocytes correlates with thrombotic risk in essential thrombocythemia. *Blood*, **100**, 714–717.

80 Harrison CN, Gale RE, Pezella F, Mire-Sluis A, Machin SJ and Linch DC (1999) Platelet c-mpl is dysregulated in patients with essential thrombocythaemia but this is not of diagnostic value. *Br J Haematol*, **107**, 139–147.

81 Yoon S-Y, Li C-Y and Tefferi A (2000) Megakaryocyte c-Mpl expression in chronic myeloproliferative disorders and the myelodysplastic syndrome: immunoperoxidase staining patterns and clinical correlates. *Eur J Haematol*, **65**, 170–174.

82 Harrison CN, Campbell PJ, Buck G, Wheatley K, East CL, Bareford D *et al.* (2005) Hydroxyurea compared with anagrelide in high-risk essential thrombocythemia. *N Engl J Med*, **353**, 33-45.

83 Steensma DP and Tefferi A (2002) Cytogenetic and molecular genetic aspects of essential thrombocythemia. *Acta Haematol*, **108**, 55–65.

84 Zamora L, Espinet B, Florensa L, Besses C, Salido M and Sole F (2003) Incidence of trisomy 8 and 9, deletion of D13S319 and D20S108 loci and BCR/ABL translocation in non-treated essential thrombocythemia patients: an analysis of bone marrow cells using interphase fluorescence in situ hybridization. *Haematologica*, **88**, 110–111.

85 Rossi D, Deambrogi C, Capello D, Cerri M, Lunghi M, Parvis G *et al.* (2006) *JAK2*^{V617F} mutation in leukaemic transformation of philadelphia-negative chronic myeloproliferative disorders. *Br J Haematol*, **135**, 267–268.

86 Pardanani AD, Levine RL, Lasho T, Pikman Y, Mesa RA, Wadleigh M *et al.* (2006) MPL515 mutations in myeloproliferative and other myeloid disorders: a study of 1182 patients. *Blood*, **108**, 3472–3476.

87 Tefferi A (2008) JAK and MPL mutations in myeloid malignancies. *Leuk Lymphoma*, **49**, 388–397.

88 Harrison CN, Gale RE, Machin SJ and Linch DC (2002) A large proportion of patient with a diagnosis of essential thrombocythaemia do not have a clonal disorder and may be at lower risk of thrombotic complications. *Blood*, **93**, 417–424.

89 Harrison CN (2005) Essential thrombocythaemia: challenges and evidence-based management. *Br J Haematol*, **130**, 153–165.

90 Gale RE, Allen AJR and Linch DC (2006) Lack of correlation of clonality status with the level of Val17Phe JAK2 mutant in essential thrombocythaemia (ET) indicates that the JAK2 mutation, when present, is not the primary pathogenic event. *Br J Haematol*, **133** (Suppl. 1), 12.

91 Levine RL, Belisle C, Wadleigh M, Zahrieh D, Lee S, Chagnon P *et al.* (2006) X-inactivation-based clonality analysis and quantitative JAK2V617F assessment reveal a strong association between clonality and JAK2V617F in PV but not ET/MMM, and identifies a subset of JAK2V617F-negative ET and MMM patients with clonal hematopoiesis. *Blood*, **107**, 4139–4141.

92 Wilkins BS, Erber WN, Bareford D, Buck G, Wheatley K and East CL (2008) Bone marrow pathology in essential thrombocythemia: interobserver reliability and utility for identifying disease subtypes. *Blood*, **111**, 60–70.

93 Carneskog J, Kutti J, Wadenvik H, Lundberg P-A and Lindstedt G (1998) Plasma erythropoietin by high detectability immunoradiometric assay in untreated patients with polycythaemia rubra vera and essential thrombocythaemia. *Eur J Haematol*, **60**, 278–282.

94 Barosi G, Ambrosetti A, Finelli C, Grossi A, Leoni P, Liberato NL *et al.* (1999) The Italian Consensus Conference on Diagnostic Criteria for Myelofibrosis with Myeloid Metaplasia. *Br J Haematol*, **104**, 730–737.

95 Thiele J, Kvasnicka HM, Werden C, Zankovich R, Diehl V and Fischer R (1996) Idiopathic primary osteo-myelofibrosis: a clinico-pathological study on 208 patients with special emphasis on evolution of disease features, differentiation from essential thrombocythemia and variables of prognostic impact. *Leuk Lymphoma*, **22**, 303–317.

96 Cervantes F, Pereira A, Esteve J, Rafel M, Cobo F, Rozman C and Montserrat E (1997) Identification of 'short-lived' and 'long-lived' patients at presentation of idiopathic myelofibrosis. *Br J Haematol*, **97**, 635–640.

97 Kvasnicka HM, Thiele J, Werden C, Zankovich R, Diehl V and Fischer R (1997) Prognostic factors in idiopathic (primary) osteomyelofibrosis. *Cancer*, **80**, 708–719.

98 Lennert K, Nagai K and Schwarze EW (1975) Patho-anatomical features of the bone marrow. *Clin Haematol*, **4**, 331–351.

99 Pereira A, Cervantes F, Brugues R and Rozman C (1990) Bone marrow histopathology in primary myelofibrosis: clinical and haematologic correlations and prognostic evaluation. *Eur J Haematol*, **44**, 95–99.

100 Apaja-Sarkkinen M, Autio-Harmainen H, Alavaikko M, Risteli J and Risteli L (1986) Immunohistochemical study of basement membrane proteins and type III procollagen in myelofibrosis. *Br J Haematol*, **63**, 571–580.

101 Guardiola P, Anderson JE and Gluckman E (2000) Myelofibrosis with myeloid metaplasia. *N Engl J Med*, **343**, 659.

102 Lohmann TP and Beckman EN (1983) Progressive myelofibrosis in agnogenic myeloid metaplasia. *Arch Pathol Lab Med*, **107**, 593–594.

103 Laszlo J (1975) Myeloproliferative disorders (MPD): myelofibrosis, myelosclerosis, extramedullary hematopoiesis, undifferentiated MPD, and hemorrhagic thrombocythemia. *Semin Hematol*, **12**, 409–432.

104 Kreft A, Wiese B, Weiss M, Choritz H, Buhr T, Büsche G and Georgii A (2004) Analysis of risk factors of the evolution of myelofibrosis in pre-fibrotic chronic idiopathic myelofibrosis: a retrospective study based on follow up biopsies of 70 patients by using the RECPAM method. *Leuk Lymphoma*, **45**, 553–559.

105 Yoon SY, Li CY, Mesa RA and Tefferi A (1999) Bone marrow effects of anagrelide therapy in patients with myelofibrosis with myeloid metaplasia *Br J Haematol*, **106**, 682–688.

106 Elliott MA, Mesa RA, Li C-Y, Hook CC, Ansell SM, Levitt RM, Geyer SM and Tefferi A (2002) Thalidomide treatment in myelofibrosis with myeloid metaplasia. *Br J Haematol*, **117**, 288–296.

107 Tefferi A, Cortes J, Verstovsek S, Mesa RA, Thomas D, Lasho TL *et al.* (2006) Lenalidomide therapy in myelofibrosis with myeloid metaplasia. *Blood*, **108**, 1158–1164.

108 Akikusa B, Komatsu T, Kondo Y, Yokota T, Uchino F and Yonemitsu H (1987) Amyloidosis complicating idiopathic myelofibrosis. *Arch Pathol Lab Med*, **111**, 525–529.

109 Ferhanoğlu B, Erzin Y, Başlar Z and Tüzüner HAN (1997) Secondary amyloidosis in the course of idiopathic myelofibrosis. *Leuk Res*, **21**, 897–898.

110 Dingli D, Grand FH, Mahaffey V, Spurbeck J, Ross FM, Watmore AE *et al.* (2005) Der(6)t(1;6)(q21–23;p21.3): a specific cytogenetic abnormality in myelofibrosis with myeloid metaplasia. *Br J Haematol*, **130**, 229–232.

111 Al-Assar O, Ul-Hassan A, Brown R, Wilson GA, Hammond DW and Reilly JT (2005) Gains on 9p are common genomic aberrations in idiopathic myelofibrosis: a comparative genomic hybridization study. *Br J Haematol*, **129**, 66–71.

112 Strasse-Weippl K, Steurer M, Kees M, Augustin F, Tzankov A, Dirnhofer S *et al.* (2005) Chromosome 7 deletions are associated with unfavourable prognosis in myelofibrosis with myeloid metaplasia. *Blood*, **105**, 4146.

113 Bogani C, Guglielmelli P, Antonioli E, Pancrazzi A, Bosi A and Vannucchi AM (2007) B-, T-, and NK-cell lineage involvement in JAK2V617F-positive patients with idiopathic myelofibrosis. *Haematologica*, **92**, 258–259.

114 Campbell PJ, Griesshammer M, Dohner K, Dohner H, Kusec R, Hasselbalch HC *et al.* (2006) V617F mutation in *JAK2* is associated with poorer survival in idiopathic myelofibrosis. *Blood*, **107**, 2098–2100.

115 Guglielmelli P, Pancrazzi A, Bergamaschi G, Rosti V, Villani L, Antoniolo E *et al.* (2007) Anaemia characterises patients with myelofibrosis harbouring *MplW515L/K* mutation. *Br J Haematol*, **137**, 244–247.

116 Bain BJ, Gilliland DG, Vardiman JW and Horny H-P (2008) Chronic eosinophilic leukaemia, not otherwise specified. In: Swerdlow SH, Campo E, Harris NL, Jaffe ES, Pileri SA, Stein H, Thiele J and Vardiman JW (eds) *World Health Organization Classification of Tumours of Haematopoietic and Lymphoid Tissue*, 4th edn. IARC Press, Lyon, pp. 51–53.

117 Lyall H, O'Connor S and Clark D (2007) Charcot-Leyden crystals in the trephine biopsy of a patient with *FIP1L1-PDGFRA* – positive myeloproliferative disorder. *Br J Haematol*, **138**, 405.

118 Bain BJ (2003) Cytogenetic and molecular genetic aspects of eosinophilic leukaemia. *Br J Haematol*, **122**, 173–179.

119 Reiter A, Walz C, Watmore A, Schoch C, Blau I, Schlegelberger B *et al.* (2005) The t(8;9)(p22;p24) is a recurrent abnormality in chronic and acute leukemia that fuses *PCM1* to *JAK2*. *Cancer Res*, **65**, 2662–2667.

120 Simon HU, Plötz SG, Dummer R and Blaser K (1999) Abnormal clones of T cells producing interleukin-5 in idiopathic eosinophilia. *N Engl J Med*, **341**, 1112–1120.

121 Bain BJ (1999) Eosinophilia – idiopathic or not? *N Engl J Med*, **341**, 1141–1143.

122 Garcia-Montero AC, Jara-Acevedo M, Teodosio C, Sanchez ML, Nunez R, Prados A *et al.* (2006) KIT mutation in mast cells and other bone marrow hematopoietic cell lineages in systemic mast cell disorders: a prospective study of the Spanish Network on Mastocytosis (REMA) in a series of 113 patients. *Blood*, **108**, 2366–2372.

123 Horny H-P, Metcalfe DD, Bennett JM, Bain BJ, Akin C, Escribano L and Valent P (2008) Mastocytosis. In: Swerdlow SH, Campo E, Harris NL, Jaffe ES, Pileri SA, Stein H, Thiele J and Vardiman JW (eds) *World Health Organization Classification of Tumours of Haematopoietic and Lymphoid Tissue*, 4th edn. IARC Press, Lyon, pp. 54–63.

124 Webb TA, Li CY and Yam LT (1982) Systemic mast cell disease: a clinical and hematopathologic study of 26 cases. *Cancer*, **49**, 927–938.

125 Brunning RD, McKenna RW, Rosai J, Parkin JL and Risdall R (1983) Systemic mastocytosis. Extracutaneous manifestations. *Am J Surg Pathol*, **7**, 425–438.

126 Travis WD, Li CY, Bergstralh EJ, Yam LT and Swee RG (1988) Systemic mast cell disease. Analysis of 58 cases and literature review. *Medicine*, **67**, 345–368 [published erratum appears in *Medicine*, 1990, 69, 34].

127 Lennert K and Parwaresch MR (1979) Mast cells and mast cell neoplasia: a review. *Histopathology*, **3**, 349–365.

128 Horny HP, Ruck M, Wehrmann M and Kaiserling E (1990) Blood findings in generalized mastocytosis: evidence of frequent simultaneous occurrence of myeloproliferative disorders. *Br J Haematol*, **76**, 186–193.

129 Sperr WR, Escribano L, Jordan J-H, Schernthaner G-H, Kundi M, Horny H-P and Valent P (2001) Morphologic properties of neoplastic mast cells: delineation of stages of maturation and implication for cytological grading of mastocytosis. *Leuk Res*, **25**, 529–536.

130 Travis WD, Li CY, Yam LT, Bergstralh EJ and Swee RG (1988) Significance of systemic mast cell disease with associated hematologic disorders. *Cancer*, **62**, 965–972.

131 Parker RI (1991) Hematologic aspects of mastocytosis. I: Bone marrow pathology in adult and pediatric systemic mast cell disease. *J Invest Dermatol*, **96**, 47S–51S.

132 Parker RI (1991) Hematologic aspects of mastocytosis. II: Management of hematologic disorders in association with systemic mast cell disease. *J Invest Dermatol*, **96**, 52S–53S; discussion 53S–54S.

133 Stevens EC and Rosenthal NS (2001) Bone marrow mast cell morphologic features and hematopoietic dyspoiesis in systemic mast cell disease. *Am J Clin Pathol*, **116**, 177–182.

134 Jara-Acevado M, García-Montero AC, Teodosio C, Escribano L, Alvarex I, Sanchez-Muños L *et al.* (2008) Well differentiated systemic mastocytosis (WDSM): a novel form of systemic mastocytosis. *Haematologica*, **93** (Suppl. 1), 91.

135 Escribano L, Diaz-Agustin B, Bellas C, Navalon R, Nuñez R, Sperr W *et al.* (2001) Utility of flow cytometric analysis of mast cells in the diagnosis and classification of adult mastocytosis. *Leuk Res*, **25**, 563–570.

136 Horny HP, Parwaresch MR and Lennert K (1985) Bone marrow findings in systemic mastocytosis. *Hum Pathol*, **16**, 808–814.

137 Butterfield JH and Li C-Y (2004) Bone marrow biopsies for the diagnosis of systemic mastocytosis: is one biopsy sufficient? *Am J Clin Pathol*, **121**, 264–267.

138 Horny H-P and Valent P (2001) Diagnosis of masto-cytosis: general histopathological aspects, morpho-logical criteria, and immunohistochemical findings. *Leuk Res*, **25**, 543–551.

139 Fallon MD, Whyte MP and Teitelbaum SL (1981) Systemic mastocytosis associated with generalized osteopenia. Histopathological characterization of the skeletal lesion using undecalcified bone from two patients. *Hum Pathol*, **12**, 813–820.

140 Horny HP and Kaiserling E (1988) Lymphoid cells and tissue mast cells of bone marrow lesions in sys-temic mastocytosis: a histological and immunohisto-logical study. *Br J Haematol*, **69**, 449–455.

141 Akin C, Jaffe ES, Semere T, Daley T and Metcalfe DD (1999) Demonstration of stem cell factor associated with mast cells in the bone marrow of patients with systemic indolent mastocytosis. *Blood*, **94** (Suppl. 1), 37b.

142 Horny H-P, Lange K, Sotlar K and Valent P (2003) Increase of bone marrow lymphocytes in systemic mastocytosis: reactive lymphocytosis or malignant lymphoma? Immunohistochemical and molecular findings on routinely processed bone marrow biopsy specimens. *J Clin Pathol*, **56**, 575–578.

143 Horny HP, Reimann O and Kaiserling E (1988) Immunoreactivity of normal and neoplastic human tissue mast cells. *Am J Clin Pathol*, **89**, 335-40.

144 Horny H-P, Greschniok A, Jordan J-H, Menke DM and Valent P (2003) Chymase expressing bone marrow mast cells in mastocytosis and myelodysplas-tic syndromes: an immunohistochemical and mor-phometric study. *J Clin Pathol*, **56**, 103–106.

145 Hoyer JD, Li CY, Yam LT, Hanson CA and Kurtin PJ (1997) Immunohistochemical demonstration of acid phosphatase isoenzyme 5 (tartrate-resistant) in paraffin sections of hairy cell leukemia and other hematologic disorders. *Am J Clin Pathol*, **108**, 308–315.

146 Li C-Y (2001) Diagnosis of mastocytosis: value of cytochemistry and immunohistochemistry. *Leuk Res*, **25**, 537–541.

147 Toro TZ, Hsieh FH, Bodo J, Dong HY and His ED (2007) Detection of phospho-STAT5 in mast cells: a reliable phenotypic marker of systemic mast cell disease that reflects constitutive tyrosine kinase acti-vation. *Br J Haematol*, **139**, 31–40.

148 Bain BJ (1999) Systemic mastocytosis and other mast cell neoplasms *Br J Haematol*, **106**, 9–17.

149 Akin C, Fumo G, Yavuz AS, Lipsky PE, Neckers L and Metcalfe DD (2004) A novel form of mastocyto-sis associated with a transmembrane c-kit mutation and response to imatinib. *Blood*, **103**, 3222–3225.

150 Kettelhut BV, Parker RI, Travis WD and Metcalfe DD (1989) Hematopathology of the bone marrow in pediatric cutaneous mastocytosis. A study of 17 patients. *Am J Clin Pathol*, **91**, 558–562.

151 Topar G, Staudacher C, Geisen F, Gabl C, Fend F, Herold M *et al.* (1998) Urticaria pigmentosa: a clini-cal, hematopathologic, and serologic study of 30 adults. *Am J Clin Pathol*, **109**, 279–285.

152 Rywlin AM, Hoffman EP and Ortega RS (1972) Eosinophilic fibrohistiocytic lesions of bone marrow: a new morphologic finding probably related to drug hypersensitivity. *Blood*, **40**, 464–472.

153 Kvasnicka HM, Bain BJ, Thiele J, Orazi A Horny H-P and Vardiman JM (2008) Myeloproliferative neo-plasm, unclassifiable. In: Swerdlow SH, Campo E, Harris NL, Jaffe ES, Pileri SA, Stein H, Thiele J and Vardiman JW (eds) *World Health Organization Classification of Tumours of Haematopoietic and Lymphoid Tissue*, 4th edn. IARC Press, Lyon, pp. 64–65.

154 Pettit JE, Lewis SM and Nicholas AW (1979) Transitional myeloproliferative disorder *Br J Haematol*, **43**, 167–184.

155 Gupta R, Abdalla SH and Bain BJ (1999) Thrombocytosis with sideroblastic erythropoiesis: a mixed myeloproliferative myelodysplastic syndrome. *Leuk Lymphoma*, **34**, 615–619.

156 Bennett JM, Catovsky D, Daniel MT, Flandrin G, Galton DA, Gralnick HR and Sultan C (1982) Proposals for the classification of the myelodysplastic syndromes *Br J Haematol*, **51**, 189–199.

157 Orazi A, Bennett J, Germing U, Brunning RD, Bain BJ and Thiele J (2008) Chronic myelomonocytic leu-kaemia. In: Swerdlow SH, Campo E, Harris NL, Jaffe ES, Pileri SA, Stein H, Thiele J and Vardiman JW (eds) *World Health Organization Classification of Tumours of Haematopoietic and Lymphoid Tissue*, 4th edn. IARC Press, Lyon, pp. 76–79.

158 Chen Y-C, Chou J-M, Ketterling RP, Letendre L and Li C-Y (2003) Histologic and immunohistochemical study of bone marrow monocyte nodules in 21 cases with myelodysplasia. *Am J Clin Pathol*, **120**, 874–873.

159 Chen Y-C, Chou J-M, Letendre L and Li C-Y (2005) Clinical importance of bone marrow monocytic nodules in patients with myelodysplasia: retrospec-tive analysis of 21 cases. *Am J Hematol*, **79**, 329–331.

160 Orazi A, Chiu R, O'Malley DP, Czader M, Allen SL, An C and Vance GH (2006) Chronic myelomonocytic leukemia: the role of bone marrow biopsy immuno-histology. *Mod Pathol*, **19**, 1536–1545.

161 Kantarjian HM, Keating MJ, Walters RS, McCredie KB, Smith TL, Talpaz M *et al.* (1986) Clinical and prognostic features of Philadelphia chromosome-negative chronic myelogenous leukemia *Cancer*, **58**, 2023–2030.

162 Martiat P, Michaux JL and Rodhain J (1991) Philadelphia-negative (Ph-) chronic myeloid leuke-mia (CML): comparison with Ph+ CML and chronic myelomonocytic leukemia. The Groupe Francais

de Cytogenetique Hematologique. *Blood*, **78**, 205–211.

163 Vardiman J, Bennett JM, Bain BJ, Brunning RD and Thiele J (2008) Atypical chronic myeloid leukaemia, *BCR-ABL1*-negative. In: Swerdlow SH, Campo E, Harris NL, Jaffe ES, Pileri SA, Stein H, Thiele J and Vardiman JW (eds) *World Health Organization Classification of Tumours of Haematopoietic and Lymphoid Tissue*, 4th edn. IARC Press, Lyon, pp. 80–81.

164 Emanuel PD (1999) Myelodysplasia and myeloproliferative disorders in childhood: an update. *Br J Haematol*, **105**, 852–863.

165 Baumann I, Bennett JM, Niemeyer CM, Thiele J and Shannon K (2008) Juvenile myelomonocytic leukaemia. In: Swerdlow SH, Campo E, Harris NL, Jaffe ES, Pileri SA, Stein H, Thiele J and Vardiman JW (eds) *World Health Organization Classification of Tumours of Haematopoietic and Lymphoid Tissue*, 4th edn. IARC Press, Lyon, pp. 82–84.

166 Kondoh T, Ishii E, Aoki Y, Shimizu T, Zaitsu M, Matsubara Y and Moriuchi H (2003) Noonan syndrome with leukaemoid reaction and overproduction of catecholamines: a case report. *Eur J Pediat*, **162**, 548–549.

167 Bain BJ (1999) The relationship between the myelodysplastic syndromes and the myeloproliferative disorders. *Leuk Lymphoma*, **34**, 443–449.

168 Vardiman JW, Bennett JM, Bain BJ, Baumann I, Thiele J and Orazi A (2008) Myelodysplastic/myeloproliferative neoplasm, unclassified. In: Swerdlow SH, Campo E, Harris NL, Jaffe ES, Pileri SA, Stein H, Thiele J and Vardiman JW (eds) *World Health Organization Classification of Tumours of Haematopoietic and Lymphoid Tissue*, 4th edn. IARC Press, Lyon, pp. 85–86.

169 Gattermann N, Billiet J, Kronenwett R, Zipperer E, Germing U, Nollet F *et al.* (2007) High frequency of the JAK2 V617F mutation in patients with thrombocytosis (platelet count >600 × 10^9/L) and ringed sideroblasts more than 15% considered as MDS/MPD, unclassifiable. *Blood*, **109**, 1334–1335.

170 Schmitt-Graeff AH, Teo SS, Olschewski M, Schaub F, Haxelmans S, Kirn A *et al.* (2008) *JAK2*^{V617F} mutation status identifies subtypes of refractory anemia with ringed sideroblasts associated with marked thrombocytosis. *Haematologica*, **93**, 34–40.

171 Bain BJ and Fletcher S (2007) Chronic eosinophilic leukemias and the myeloproliferative variant of the hypereosinophilic syndrome. *Immunol Allergy Clin North Am*, **27**, 377–388.

172 Bain BJ, Gilliland DG, Horny H-P and Vardiman JW (2008) Myeloid and lymphoid neoplasms with eosinophilia and abnormalities of *PDGFRA*, *PDGFRB* and *FGFR1*. In: Swerdlow SH, Campo E, Harris NL, Jaffe ES, Pileri SA, Stein H, Thiele J and Vardiman JW (eds) *World Health Organization Classification of Tumours of Haematopoietic and Lymphoid Tissue*, 4th edn. IARC Press, Lyon, pp. 68–73.

173 Cools J, DeAngelo DJ, Gotlib J, Stover EH, Legare RD, Cortes J *et al.* (2003) A tyrosine kinase created by fusion of the *PDGFRA* and *FIP1L1* genes is a therapeutic target of imatinib in idiopathic hypereosinophilic syndrome. *N Engl J Med*, **348**, 1201–1214.

174 Granjo E, Guimaräes A, Mirand M, Vasconcelos C, Carduso L, Rocha S *et al.* (2000) Chronic eosinophilic leukaemia presenting with erythroderma. *Hematol J*, **1** (Suppl. 1), 74.

SIX

LYMPHOPROLIFERATIVE DISORDERS

In this chapter we shall discuss acute and chronic leukaemias of lymphoid lineage and Hodgkin and non-Hodgkin lymphomas. The disease entities will be classified according to the 2008 World Health Organization (WHO) classification of lymphoid neoplasms [1], which is based upon the Revised European American Lymphoma (REAL) classification proposed by the International Lymphoma Study Group [2], subsequently modified and incorporated into the 2001 WHO classification. The REAL classification was an attempt to harmonize European and North American classifications. It built on the Kiel classification [3,4] but simplified some aspects and incorporated several well-recognized entities, such as extranodal marginal zone B-cell lymphoma of mucosa-associated lymphoid tissue (MALT) type, that were not included in the Kiel classification. The 2008 WHO classification of B- and T/NK-lineage neoplasms (excluding Hodgkin lymphoma) is summarized in Tables 6.1 and 6.2 and that of Hodgkin lymphoma, (based on the earlier Rye classification [5]), in Table 6.3.

Bone marrow infiltration in lymphoproliferative disorders

Bone marrow infiltration is frequent in lymphoproliferative disorders. Such infiltration can be detected by a variety of procedures including microscopic examination of bone marrow aspirates and trephine biopsy sections, immunophenotyping and molecular biological techniques (see Chapter 2). Assessment of cytological details can be carried

out using films of aspirates, imprints from trephine biopsy specimens or thin sections of aspirated fragments or trephine biopsy specimens. Histological features can be assessed using sections of either trephine biopsy specimens or aspirated fragments. The pattern of infiltration can only be fully assessed using sections from trephine biopsy specimens. Six major patterns can be seen, either alone or in combination [6–9] (Fig. 6.1). Such patterns are important in the differential diagnosis of lymphoproliferative disorders and can also be of prognostic significance. They are designated: (1) interstitial, (2) nodular, (3) paratrabecular, (4) random focal, (5) intrasinusoidal, and (6) diffuse.

1 *Interstitial infiltration* indicates the presence of individual neoplastic cells interspersed between haemopoietic and fat cells. Although there is generalized marrow involvement there is considerable sparing of normal haemopoiesis and bone marrow architecture is not distorted.

2 *Nodular infiltration* indicates the presence of non-paratrabecular, round or oval aggregates of lymphoid cells with a well-defined border; they sometimes form or colonize lymphoid follicles. They may incidentally touch a trabecula but do not spread along it.

3 *Paratrabecular infiltration* indicates that the neoplastic cells are immediately adjacent to the bony trabeculae, either in the form of a band lining a trabecula or as an aggregate with a broad base abutting on a trabecula.

4 *Random focal infiltration* indicates irregularly distributed foci of neoplastic cells separated by residual haemopoietic marrow. The aggregates of neoplastic cells have no particular relationship to bony trabeculae and have irregular margins.

5 *Intrasinusoidal infiltration* indicates the presence of neoplastic cells within sinusoids, either alone

Bone Marrow Pathology. By Barbara Bain, David Clark and Bridget Wilkins. © 2010, Blackwell Publishing.

Table 6.1 WHO classification of B-cell neoplasms [1].

B-cell precursor neoplasms
B lymphoblastic leukaemia/lymphoma, not otherwise specified
B lymphoblastic leukaemia/lymphoma with recurrent genetic abnormalities

Mature B-cell neoplasms
B-cell chronic lymphocytic leukaemia/small lymphocytic lymphoma
B-cell prolymphocytic leukaemia
Splenic marginal zone lymphoma*
Hairy cell leukaemia
Splenic B-cell lymphoma/leukaemia, unclassifiable
   Splenic diffuse red pulp small B-cell lymphoma
   Hairy cell leukaemia variant
Lymphoplasmacytic lymphoma
Heavy chain diseases
Plasma cell neoplasms
Extranodal marginal zone lymphoma of mucosa-associated lymphoid tissue (MALT lymphoma)
Nodal marginal zone B-cell lymphoma
Follicular lymphoma
Primary cutaneous follicle centre lymphoma
Mantle cell lymphoma
Diffuse large B-cell lymphoma (DLBCL), not otherwise specified
DLBCL, specified types
   T-cell/histiocyte-rich large B-cell lymphoma
   Primary DLBCL of the central nervous system
   Primary cutaneous DLBCL, leg type
   Epstein–Barr virus (EBV)-positive DLBCL of the elderly
Other lymphomas of large B cells
   Primary mediastinal (thymic) B-cell lymphoma
   Intravascular large B-cell lymphoma
   DLBCL associated with inflammation
   Lymphomatoid granulomatosis
   ALK-positive large B-cell lymphoma
   Plasmablastic lymphoma
   Large B-cell lymphoma arising in HHV8-associated multicentric Castleman's disease
   Primary effusion lymphoma
B-cell lymphoma, unclassifiable, with features intermediate between DLBCL and Burkitt lymphoma
B-cell lymphoma, unclassifiable, with features intermediate between DLBCL and classical Hodgkin lymphoma
Burkitt lymphoma

*Includes splenic lymphoma with villous lymphocytes.

[10,11], which is rare, or in association with other patterns of infiltration. It is characteristic of several lymphoma subtypes. Unless extreme, it is difficult to recognize without immunohistochemistry and it is increasing use of the latter technique that has led to the appreciation of this pattern.

6 *Diffuse infiltration* indicates extensive replacement of normal marrow elements, both haemopoietic tissue and fat, so that marrow architecture is effaced. An alternative designation is a 'packed marrow' pattern [7]; this latter term could be preferred since it is unambiguous, whereas 'diffuse' could be taken to also include interstitial infiltration.

Various mixed patterns of infiltration occur, including interstitial–nodular, interstitial–diffuse and interstitial–intrasinusoidal. The presence of particular combinations can provide useful differential diagnostic information, since some are strongly associated with individual lymphoma

Table 6.2 WHO classification of T-cell and NK-cell neoplasms [1].

T-cell precursor neoplasms
T lymphoblastic leukaemia/lymphoma, not otherwise specified
T lymphoblastic leukaemia/lymphoma with recurrent genetic abnormalities

Mature T-cell and NK-cell neoplasms
T-cell prolymphocytic leukaemia
T-cell large granular lymphocytic leukaemia
Chronic lymphoproliferative disorders of NK lineage
Aggressive NK-cell leukaemia
Epstein–Barr virus (EBV)-positive T-cell lymphoproliferative diseases of childhood
Adult T-cell leukaemia/lymphoma
Extranodal NK/T-cell lymphoma, nasal type
Enteropathy-associated T-cell lymphoma
Hepatosplenic T-cell lymphoma
Subcutaneous panniculitis-like T-cell lymphoma
Mycosis fungoides
Sézary syndrome
Primary cutaneous CD30-positive T-cell lymphoproliferative disorders
Primary cutaneous peripheral T-cell lymphomas, rare subtypes
Angioimmunoblastic T-cell lymphoma
Anaplastic large cell lymphoma, ALK positive
Anaplastic large cell lymphoma, ALK negative
Peripheral T-cell lymphoma, not otherwise specified

Table 6.3 The WHO classification of Hodgkin lymphoma [1].

Category	Specific histological characteristics*
Nodular lymphocyte predominant Hodgkin lymphoma	Typical Reed–Sternberg cells are infrequent or absent; LP (lymphocyte predominant) cells are present; prominent proliferation of lymphocytes, histiocytes or both; usually nodular pattern in lymph nodes
Classical Hodgkin lymphoma	
Nodular sclerosis classical Hodgkin lymphoma	Typical Reed–Sternberg cells often very infrequent; lacunar cell variant of Reed–Sternberg cell present; collagen bands prominent in lymph nodes
Mixed cellularity classical Hodgkin lymphoma	Moderately frequent typical Reed–Sternberg cells; variable proliferation of reactive cells; there may be disorderly fibrosis; lymph node infiltrate is typically interfollicular or diffuse
Lymphocyte-rich classical Hodgkin lymphoma	Small numbers of typical Reed–Sternberg cells; background of small lymphocytes with infrequent plasma cells and eosinophils; in lymph nodes background follicular pattern is often preserved
Lymphocyte-depleted classical Hodgkin lymphoma	Patterns vary; nodularity absent; may resemble mixed cellularity subtype but with abundant Reed–Sternberg cells; neoplastic cells may be pleomorphic and confluent; reactive cells infrequent; fibrosis may be extensive

*Histological features are most clearly seen in lymph nodes and not all are apparent in trephine biopsy sections; in the bone marrow, infiltrates of classical Hodgkin lymphoma of all subtypes tend to show extensive fibrosis and few Reed–Sternberg cells.

Normal

Interstitial

Nodular

Paratrabecular

Random focal

Intrasinusoidal

Diffuse, 'packed
marrow' pattern

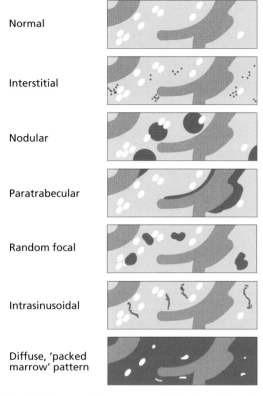

Fig. 6.1 Patterns of bone marrow infiltration observed in lymphoproliferative disorders.

subtypes or, alternatively, are rare in certain subtypes.

Further unusual patterns of infiltration include perivascular infiltration, reported in some T-cell lymphomas [9], and intravascular infiltration involving larger blood vessels in the marrow such as arterioles and venules.

Among B-lineage lymphomas, bone marrow infiltration is more common in low grade tumours than in high grade. Overall, infiltration is probably more common in B-cell lymphomas than in T-cell ones [12,13] but the frequency of infiltration detected in T-cell lymphomas has varied widely in reported series. The relative frequency of different patterns of infiltration varies between T and B lymphomas and between different histological categories but, in general, focal infiltration is more common than diffuse [14]. This is particularly so of B-cell lymphomas; diffuse infiltration is relatively

more common in T-cell lymphomas than in B-cell ones.

Increased reticulin deposition, restricted to the area of marrow infiltration, is common in lymphoma [15]. Collagen fibrosis is less common.

Trephine biopsy is generally more successful at detecting marrow infiltration by lymphoma than is bone marrow aspiration; this is a consequence of the frequency of focal infiltration and of fibrosis. However, occasionally cytologically distinctive lymphoma cells are detected in an aspirate but not in biopsy sections. In a series of 93 lymphoma cases, Foucar *et al.* [14] found that trephine sections and aspirate films were both positive in 79% of cases, trephine biopsy sections alone were positive in 18%, and films alone were positive in 3%. Similarly, Conlan *et al.* [12] reported that in 102 cases of non-Hodgkin lymphoma (NHL) with marrow involvement, the trephine biopsy section, marrow clot section and marrow aspirate films were positive in 94%, 65% and 46% of cases, respectively; in only 6% of cases was the bone marrow aspirate positive when the trephine biopsy was negative. The detection of bone marrow infiltration is increased when a larger volume of marrow is sampled; this can be achieved either by increasing the size of the trephine biopsy specimen or by performing multiple biopsies. Detection is also increased by serial sectioning of trephine biopsy specimens [16].

Immunohistochemical techniques performed on sections of paraffin-embedded tissue (see pages 68–80) are useful in establishing or confirming the nature of lymphoid infiltrates [17] and in assessing their extent. Flow cytometric immunophenotyping may demonstrate neoplastic cell populations, even small populations that cannot be detected in sections, but may also fail to reveal them when infiltration is focal or there is fibrosis. Molecular genetic analysis using the polymerase chain reaction (PCR) to detect immunoglobulin (Ig) heavy chain (*IGH*) and T-cell receptor (*TCR*) loci rearrangements, applied to aspirated cells or fixed tissue sections, can be useful in confirming clonality in difficult cases. However, reported sensitivity of a clonal *IGH* rearrangement by PCR on bone marrow aspirate samples has varied from 57% to 80% of cases with unequivocal morphological evidence of marrow infiltration by B-lineage NHL in trephine biopsy sections [18,19].

The above techniques are complementary and their sensitivity for the detection of bone marrow infiltration varies between lymphoma subtypes. Techniques used should therefore be selected according to the clinical circumstances.

There may be discordance between the type of lymphoma seen in the marrow and that present in the lymph node or other tissues. The frequency of such discordance has varied from 16% to 40% in reported series [12,20–22]. In a smaller number, varying between 6% and 21%, there is discordance as to grade of lymphoma. Discordance is most often seen in B-cell lymphomas. Although Conlan *et al.* [12] observed discordance in 25% of T-cell lymphomas, no discordance was found in two other series of T-cell lymphomas [23,24]. One surprising and relatively common occurrence is the presence of follicular lymphoma in the lymph node and lymphoplasmacytic lymphoma in the marrow [20,22]. This may represent altered differentiation of tumour in the marrow site, a phenomenon that is well recognized in follicular lymphomas in lymph nodes [25].

The clinical importance of marrow involvement varies with the type of NHL. In general, in low grade lymphomas the presence of marrow involvement does not adversely affect the clinical outcome. In patients with high grade lymphoma at an extramedullary site, the presence of high grade lymphoma in the marrow is a poor prognostic sign, often predictive of central nervous system involvement [26]. The presence of low grade lymphoma in the marrow of patients with high grade lymphoma has been considered to have no adverse effect on prognosis [21] but there is evidence to suggest that such patients have continuing risk of late relapse of low grade lymphoma [26].

Bone marrow infiltration may be concordant (the same histological type as elsewhere) or discordant (a different histological type). It needs to be remembered that discordant bone marrow infiltration sometimes represents a clonally unrelated neoplasm [27].

Problems and pitfalls

Lymphomatous infiltration of the marrow needs to be distinguished from infiltration by reactive lymphocytes. Flow cytometric immunophenotyping can provide evidence that an infiltrate is neoplastic but care in gating the correct cells and in interpretation is essential. For example, haematogones must be distinguished from leukaemic lymphoblasts.

In histological sections, consideration should be given both to the pattern of infiltration and to cytological characteristics. Interstitial infiltration can occur both in neoplastic and in reactive conditions. Paratrabecular infiltration and a 'packed marrow' (diffuse infiltration) are almost always indicative of neoplasia. Nodular lymphomatous infiltrates have to be distinguished from reactive nodular hyperplasia (see pages 132–134). Caution should be exercised in diagnosing lymphoma solely on the basis of the presence of nodules of small lymphocytes since there are no clear criteria at present for establishing whether infrequent small nodules are neoplastic. Reactive lymphoid nodules are usually small with well-defined margins and have a polymorphous cell population, made up predominantly of small lymphocytes with smaller numbers of immunoblasts, macrophages and plasma cells. A small feeder capillary may be seen leading towards the centre of such a reactive nodule and there is sometimes a reactive corona of eosinophils in the surrounding marrow. Neoplastic nodular lymphoid infiltrates are usually larger with less well-defined margins, often extending outwards around fat cells, and have a relatively homogeneous cellular composition. In some cases it is not possible to make a distinction between a reactive and neoplastic process on morphological grounds alone. Immunohistochemical staining is of limited value unless a distinctly abnormal B-cell immunophenotype (e.g. that of mantle cell lymphoma or B-cell chronic lymphocytic leukaemia) is found. Nodules composed entirely of B cells are usually neoplastic, whereas a mixed population of B and T cells may be seen in both reactive and neoplastic nodules. Although it was suggested that immunohistochemical staining for BCL2 may be helpful in distinguishing reactive from neoplastic lymphoid aggregates [28,29], another report did not confirm this finding [30] and, since BCL2 is expressed constitutively by most mature T and B lymphocytes, other than germinal centre cells, this is clearly not a reliable discriminatory technique.

In difficult cases, the use of PCR on a marrow aspirate sample to demonstrate clonal *IGH* or *TCR* loci rearrangements may be helpful [31]. PCR for detection of κ gene rearrangement increases the sensitivity above that which is achieved by *IGH* gene analysis alone [32]. Equivalent PCR techniques for detection of clonality can be applied successfully to trephine biopsy sections, particularly if ethylene diamine tetra-acetic acid (EDTA) or other non-acidic decalcification methods have been used in processing the tissue.⌐

B-lineage lymphomas and leukaemias

B lymphoblastic leukaemia/lymphoma

This condition has long been recognized by haematologists as acute lymphoblastic leukaemia (ALL), which has been subdivided according to lineage. About three quarters of cases of ALL are of B lineage and about one quarter of T lineage. In the WHO classification, B-lineage ALL has been amalgamated with B-lineage lymphoblastic lymphoma, designated in the 2001 classification precursor-B lymphoblastic leukaemia/lymphoma [33] but in the 2008 classification called B lymphoblastic leukaemia/lymphoma [1], and further divided into 'not otherwise specified' [34] and 'with recurrent genetic abnormalities' [35]. Cases of Burkitt lymphoma in leukaemic phase are not included in this category of precursor neoplasm, since they have a mature B immunophenotype. The incidence of B-lineage lymphoblastic lymphoma/leukaemia is highest in young children, has a nadir between 25 and 45 years and then rises again to a peak around 70 years of age [36].

Cases of ALL were divided by the French–American–British (FAB) group [37], on the basis of cytological features, into three categories designated L1, L2 and L3 ALL. The distinction between FAB L1 and L2 cases is now considered to be of little clinical significance. However, the cytological features of the FAB L3 category of ALL should be recognized since this often represents Burkitt lymphoma, a condition that should be identified and excluded from the group of B-precursor neoplasms.

The majority of cases of B lymphoblastic leukaemia/lymphoma present as ALL, a disease resulting from proliferation in the bone marrow of a neoplastic clone of immature lymphoid cells with the morphological features of lymphoblasts. A minority of cases present as B lymphoblastic lymphoma. These represent only 10–15% of cases of lymphoblastic lymphoma, the latter being more often of T lineage [38].

Common clinical features of B-lineage ALL are bruising, pallor, bone pain, lymphadenopathy, hepatomegaly and splenomegaly. The peak incidence is in childhood but the disease occurs at all ages. Common clinical features of B lymphoblastic lymphoma are lymphadenopathy, either localized or generalized, and skin and bone infiltration [39]. Bone lesions are usually lytic. B lymphoblastic lymphoma occurs in children and adults with a third of patients being more than 18 years old [39].

Peripheral blood

In the majority of cases of B-lineage ALL, leukaemic lymphoblasts, similar to those in the bone marrow (see below), are present in the peripheral blood; as a consequence, the total white blood cell count (WBC) is usually increased. Normocytic normochromic anaemia and thrombocytopenia are also common. In B lymphoblastic lymphoma the peripheral blood is usually normal; when lymphoblasts are present they are identical to those of ALL.

Bone marrow cytology

In B-lineage ALL the bone marrow is markedly hypercellular and is heavily infiltrated by leukaemic blasts. Normal haemopoietic cells are reduced in number but are morphologically normal. The blast cells vary cytologically between cases. In the FAB category of L1 ALL (Fig. 6.2) they are fairly small and relatively uniform in appearance with a round nucleus and a regular cellular outline. The nucleocytoplasmic ratio is high, the chromatin pattern is fairly homogeneous and nucleoli are inconspicuous or inapparent. In L2 ALL (Fig. 6.3) the blasts are generally larger and more pleomorphic. Cytoplasm is more plentiful, the nuclei vary in shape and nucleoli may be prominent. Bone marrow necrosis may complicate ALL and, rarely, an aspirate contains only necrotic cells.

In B lymphoblastic lymphoma the bone marrow is often normal. When there is infiltration, the cells cannot be distinguished cytologically from those of ALL. By convention, cases with fewer than 25% or 30% of bone marrow lymphoblasts are categorized

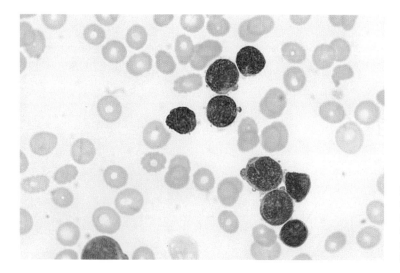

Fig. 6.2 Bone marrow (BM) aspirate, FAB L1 ALL, showing a uniform population of small and medium-sized blasts with a high nucleocytoplasmic ratio. May-Grünwald-Giemsa (MGG) ×100.

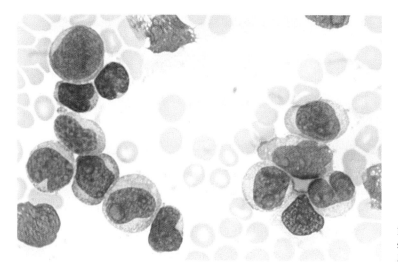

Fig. 6.3 BM aspirate, FAB L2 ALL, showing large pleomorphic blasts. MGG ×100.

as lymphoblastic lymphoma and cases with a heavier infiltration as ALL. The distinction is to some extent arbitrary since the cells are not only morphologically but also immunophenotypically indistinguishable from those of ALL.

Flow cytometric immunophenotyping

Cases of B lymphoblastic leukaemia/lymphoma express B-cell-associated antigens such as CD19, cytoplasmic CD22, CD24 and CD79a (Box 6.1). Most cases are positive for terminal deoxynucleotidyl transferase (TdT). Three immunophenotypic groups are recognized which are believed to be analogous to successive stages of maturation of normal B lymphocytes. They have been defined by the European Group for the Immunological Characterization of Leukaemia (EGIL) [40] as follows:

1 Cells of cases in the most immature group, designated pro-B-ALL, express one or more of the above-mentioned B-cell-associated antigens but do not express the common ALL antigen (CD10) or cytoplasmic or surface membrane immunoglobulin.

BOX 6.1

B lymphoblastic leukaemia/lymphoma

Flow cytometric immunophenotyping
CD19+, cCD22+, CD24+, CD79a+, TdT+, CD34+/–,
   variable expression of CD20
   Pro-B-ALL: cIg–, SmIg–, CD10–
   Common ALL: CD10+, cIg–, SmIg–
   Pre-B-ALL: CD10+, cIg (μ)+, SmIg–

Immunohistochemistry
CD10+/–, CD20–/+, CD34+/–, CD79a+, PAX5+, TdT+, BCL6–

Cytogenetic and molecular genetic analysis
Most cases have an abnormal karyotype
The most common abnormalities are hyperdiploidy
   and the translocations t(1;19)(q23;p13), t(12;21)
   (q12;q22) (cryptic) and t(9;22)(q34;q11). Less
   common, but of prognostic significance, is t(4;11)
   (q21;q23). The most common fusion genes include
   ETV6-RUNX1, TCF3-PBX1 and, in adults, *BCR-ABL1*

Percentages are approximate: +, >90% of cases
positive; +/–, >50% positive; –/+, <50% positive; –,
<10% positive. ALL, acute lymphoblastic leukaemia;
c, cytoplasmic; Ig, immunoglobulin; SmIg, surface
membrane immunoglobulin; TdT, terminal
deoxynucleotidyl transferase.

2 The next group, which includes the majority of cases, is designated common ALL; the cells express CD10. There is no expression of cytoplasmic or surface membrane immunoglobulin.

3 In the third group, designated pre-B-ALL, cells express B-lineage markers and CD10; they also express the μ chain of IgM in the cytoplasm but not surface membrane immunoglobulin.

It should be noted that the EGIL group's fourth category of mature B-ALL mainly represents Burkitt lymphoma and is classified by the WHO as a mature B-cell neoplasm rather than as lymphoblastic leukaemia/lymphoma.

The immunophenotype of precursor B lymphoblastic lymphoma is similar to that of ALL.

Cytogenetic and molecular genetic analysis

Up to 90% of cases of ALL have a demonstrable karyotypic abnormality, such cytogenetic abnormalities being of independent prognostic value [41]. The most common abnormalities among B-lineage cases are hyperdiploidy and the translocations t(1;19)(q23;p13.3), cryptic t(12;21) (p13;q22) and t(9;22)(q34;q11.2). Less common, but of considerable prognostic significance, is t(4;11)(q21;q23). In the 2008 WHO classification, genetic analysis is used to subdivide cases of B-ALL/lymphoblastic lymphoma [35] (Table 6.4).

Cases with a hyperdiploid karyotype are often divided into high hyperdiploidy (greater than 50 chromosomes) and low hyperdiploidy (47–50 chromosomes). High hyperdiploidy is the most common abnormality seen in childhood ALL (25% cases) and is associated with a relatively good prognosis. Low hyperdiploidy is seen in up to 15% of cases and is associated with an intermediate prognosis. Only the high hyperdiploid group are categorized as having hyperdiploidy in the WHO classification [35]. The translocation, t(1;19) (q23;p13.3), occurs in 2–5% of cases of childhood ALL. It was previously associated with a poor prognosis but, with modern intensive therapy, prognosis is now relatively good. The Philadelphia chromosome, formed as a result of the t(9;22) (q34;q11.2) translocation, is seen in 2–5% of cases of childhood ALL and 15–25% of cases in adults; it is associated with a poor prognosis. The t(4;11) (q21;q23) rearrangement is seen in less than 5% of cases of childhood ALL; it is associated with a pro-B immunophenotype and a poor prognosis. Other translocations with an 11q23 breakpoint are less common and generally indicate a poor prognosis. The t(12;21)(q12;q22) rearrangement is seen in 10–30% of cases of childhood ALL. It can be associated with a pro-B, common ALL or pre-B immunophenotype and an intermediate to good prognosis. This abnormality is not usually demonstrable by conventional cytogenetic analysis. A normal karyotype is associated with an intermediate prognosis.

Cytogenetic abnormalities can be detected by conventional cytogenetic analysis or by fluorescence *in situ* hybridization (FISH). Alternatively, the equivalent molecular genetic abnormality can be detected by DNA analysis (PCR or Southern blot) or RNA analysis (reverse transcriptase (RT)-PCR). The detection of t(12;21)(q12;q22) usually requires FISH or molecular analysis to detect the

Table 6.4 WHO categories of B lymphoblastic leukaemia/lymphoma with recurrent genetic abnormalities [35].

Genetic characteristics	Epidemiology and other features	Prognosis	Usual immunophenotype
t(9;22)(q34;q11.2) and BCR-ABL1	Increases markedly with age	Poor	CD10+, CD19+, TdT+ CD13 and CD33 may be aberrantly expressed CD25 often expressed
t(4;11)(q21;q23) and MLL-MLLT2 plus other cases with 11q23 and MLL rearrangement	Uncommon; often infants; WBC often high	Poor if MLL-MLLT2	CD10−, CD19+, CD24− CD15 may be aberrantly expressed
t(12;21)(p13;q22) and ETV6-RUNX1	Common; mainly children	Good	CD10+, CD19+, usually CD34+, CD9− CD13 may be aberrantly expressed
Hyperdiploidy (more than 50 chromosomes)	Common; mainly children	Good	CD10+, CD19+, usually CD34+
Hypodiploidy (less than 46 chromosomes)	Uncommon	Poor	CD10+, CD19+
t(5;14)(q31;q32) and IL3-IGH	Rare; eosinophilia; blast count may be low		CD10+, CD19+
t(1;19)(q23;p13.3) and TCF3-PBX1	Uncommon (6% of children)	Good with current treatment	CD10+, CD19+, cytoplasmic μ chain, CD9 strong

TdT, terminal deoxynucleotidyl transferase; WBC, white blood cell count.

ETV6-RUNX1 (*TEL-AML1*) fusion gene. Other fusion products that can be detected by molecular analysis include: *BCR-ABL1* associated with t(9;22), *TCF3-PBX1* (*E2A-PBX*) associated with t(1;19) and *MLL-MLLT2* (*MLL-AF4*) associated with t(4;11).

The cytogenetic and molecular genetic characteristics of B lymphoblastic lymphoma are believed to be similar to those of B-lineage ALL.

Bone marrow histology

In B-lineage ALL, the marrow is diffusely infiltrated by lymphoblasts, which replace most of the haemopoietic and fat cells. The infiltrating cells vary in size but are on average about twice the diameter of red blood cells. They are characterized by a large nucleus and minimal cytoplasm (Fig. 6.4). The chromatin is finely stippled with one or two small or medium-sized nucleoli. The number of mitotic figures is greater than in most mature B-cell neoplasms but is less than in Burkitt lymphoma/FAB L3 ALL. The number of mitoses in B lymphoblastic cases is less than in T lymphoblastic leukaemia [42]. Bone marrow necrosis is seen occasionally.

Reticulin fibrosis occurs to a varying degree in up to 57% of cases of ALL and collagen fibrosis (Fig. 6.5) in a quarter [43]. Reticulin fibrosis regresses slowly following remission of the leukaemia. Fibrosis is responsible for occasional failure to obtain an aspirate. Angiogenesis is increased but in ALL this is not of any prognostic significance [44]. Bone spicules may be thinned, indicating osteoporosis.

The diagnosis of ALL is usually made easily on the basis of the cytological features of neoplastic cells in bone marrow aspirates or peripheral blood films. Trephine biopsy is therefore not usually necessary. Occasionally, when there is minimal evidence of leukaemia in the peripheral blood and when bone marrow cannot be aspirated, the diagnosis is dependent on a trephine biopsy. In addition, treatment schedules are increasingly using the number of bone marrow lymphoblasts shortly after treatment, e.g. at 7 or 14 days, to plan further therapy; if the aspirate is inadequate, trephine biopsy, supplemented by immunohistochemistry, may be needed at this stage.

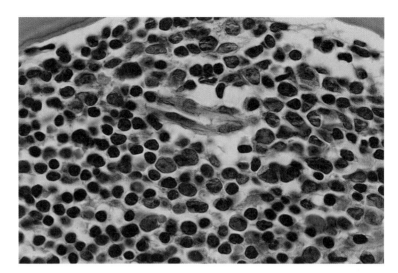

Fig. 6.4 BM trephine biopsy section, ALL, showing diffuse infiltration by predominantly small lymphoblasts. Note the high nucleocytoplasmic ratio and finely stippled chromatin pattern. Paraffin-embedded, haematoxylin and eosin (H&E) ×100.

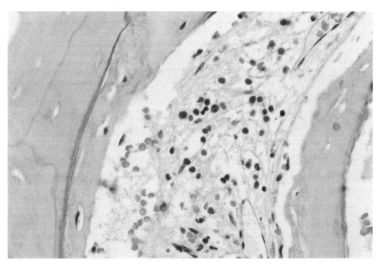

Fig. 6.5 BM trephine biopsy section, ALL, showing new bone formation and bone marrow fibrosis as a result of necrosis; there is new bone formation on the surface of a spicule of dead bone; leukaemic lymphoblasts are scattered through the fibrous tissue. Paraffin-embedded, H&E ×40.

If bone marrow infiltration occurs during the course of B lymphoblastic lymphoma, the cytological features are similar to those of ALL but the infiltration is initially patchy with intervening areas of surviving haemopoietic tissue and fat.

Immunohistochemistry

Cells of B lymphoblastic leukaemia/lymphoma express CD79a (also sometimes expressed in T-ALL) and PAX5 (see Box 6.1). They show variable expression of CD10, CD20 and TdT; TdT expression is more common in pro-B-ALL and common ALL. By definition, cells of common ALL express CD10 and expression of this antigen is usual in pre-B-

ALL; CD20 expression is more frequent in cases with a more mature phenotype. B lymphoblasts do not express CD1, CD3, CD4 or CD5 but there is occasional expression of myeloid antigens such as CD13 or CD33. CD45 is usually but not always positive, expression often being stronger in ALL blasts than would be expected in myeloblasts.

Problems and pitfalls

The most important differential diagnoses of B-lineage ALL are T-lineage ALL and acute myeloid leukaemia (AML). In general, ALL blasts have a very high nucleocytoplasmic ratio and are more regular in shape than the blasts of AML. There are no accompanying myelodysplastic features and the primitive cells do not usually contain granules. Cytochemistry and histochemistry can be important in confirming a diagnosis of AML but it must be noted that negative reactions are consistent with either ALL or AML with minimal evidence of myeloid differentiation (FAB M0 category). Immunophenotyping is therefore essential for establishing a diagnosis of B lymphoblastic leukaemia/lymphoma.

It may also be necessary to distinguish B lymphoblastic lymphoma from infiltration of the marrow by mature B-cell lymphomas. The distinction from Burkitt lymphoma is important and can be difficult. Cytological details and the high mitotic count are useful features in the recognition of Burkitt lymphoma; immunohistochemistry to demonstrate the high proliferation fraction is indicated and may be supplemented by genetic analysis for *MYC* rearrangement. In large cell lymphomas, the cells are larger and more pleomorphic than those of ALL/lymphoblastic lymphoma. In low grade lymphomas, infiltration is often focal and the nuclei show at least some degree of chromatin condensation; mitotic figures are quite uncommon. When there is heavy infiltration, chronic lymphocytic leukaemia can be confused with ALL, particularly if sections are too thick and cytological details are not readily assessable. The blastoid variant of mantle cell lymphoma poses a particular problem since the chromatin pattern resembles that of ALL; immunophenotyping will allow the distinction to be made.

A preleukaemic episode of marrow aplasia is a rare presentation of ALL, seen in about 2% of childhood cases and in some adults [45,46]. In contrast to aplastic anaemia, neutropenia is usually more marked than thrombocytopenia [47]. Trephine biopsy sections show a hypocellular marrow; haemopoietic cells are generally reduced but there may be some sparing of megakaryocytes. In most reported cases, increased lymphoblasts have not been detected. However, hypercellular areas with a lymphoid infiltrate have sometimes been noted, permitting distinction from aplastic anaemia [48]. A common feature is the presence of reticulin fibrosis and increased numbers of fibroblasts [45]. The expression of substance P by apparently normal lymphoid cells has been found predictive of transformation to ALL [49]. Two patients have been reported in whom an aplastic presentation of ALL was associated with acute parvovirus infection [50], but whether this is common or important in pathogenesis is not known. Recovery of haemopoiesis occurs, usually spontaneously, and after an interval of some weeks ALL is manifest in the marrow and the peripheral blood. In the absence of an apparent increase in lymphoid cells it can be difficult to distinguish an aplastic preleukaemic phase of ALL from aplastic anaemia, although the presence of increased reticulin and fibroblasts may suggest that the aplastic anaemia is not the correct diagnosis.

In making a diagnosis of both *de novo* and recurrent ALL, it should be noted that increased numbers of immature lymphoid cells resembling lymphoblasts of L1 ALL are often seen in children [47]. Such cells may also be present, but less often, even in adolescents and adults who do not have ALL. The term 'haematogone' has been used for these cells. The possibility of confusion with ALL is increased by the fact that they may be positive for CD34, CD10 and TdT. Such cells (Fig. 6.6) have been observed after cessation of chemotherapy for ALL, following bone marrow transplantation, in the acquired immune deficiency syndrome (AIDS), in aplastic anaemia, during infection, in children with non-haemopoietic neoplasms, in children with inherited conditions such as Blackfan–Diamond syndrome and Shwachman–Diamond syndrome, in transient erythroblastopenia of childhood, in congenital cytomegalovirus infection (up to 40% of cells) [51], in miscellaneous benign conditions and even in healthy children (found when acting as bone marrow donors). An increase of 'blast-like cells' (which the authors considered to be different from haematogones) appears to be particularly common after transplantation of cord blood stem cells [52]. Flow cytometric immunophenotyping shows that haematogones tend to express TdT strongly and CD10 and CD19 weakly, whereas the reverse pattern of reactivity is seen with ALL blast cells [53]. Haematogones are more heterogeneous than leukaemic lymphoblasts, there being a mixture of immature cells (expressing CD19, weak CD22, TdT and CD34), intermediate cells (expressing CD19, weak CD22 and CD10) and more mature cells (expressing CD19, CD20 and weak CD22 with or

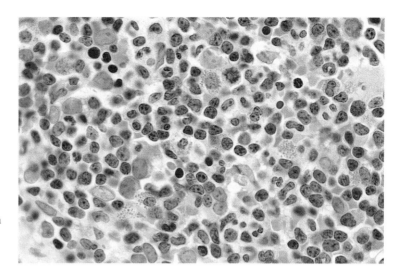

Fig. 6.6 BM trephine biopsy section from a 3-year-old child with an infection showing haematogones. Paraffin-embedded, H&E ×100.

without surface membrane Ig (SmIg)) [54,55]. The expression of adhesion molecules, such as CD44 and CD54, was also more heterogeneous than in ALL blast cells [54]. Haematogones do not show aberrant or asynchronous expression of surface antigens, both of which are common in leukaemic lymphoblasts [55]. In one histological study, cases with haematogones showed more cells expressing CD20 than cells expressing either CD34 or TdT and there were no clusters of more than five immature cells [54].

Acute lymphoblastic leukaemia can be confused with small cell tumours of childhood, e.g. neuroblastoma, Ewing's tumour and other primitive neuroectodermal tumours (PNET), rhabdomyosarcoma, medulloblastoma and retinoblastoma. It should be noted that leukaemic lymphoblasts may fail to express CD45, that neuroendocrine tumours can express PAX5 [56] and that blasts in a large proportion of ALL patients express CD99, an antigen commonly expressed in Ewing's tumour/PNET.

It is important that clinical and laboratory haematologists and haematopathologists use the same terminology or at least understand each other's terminology. It should be noted that the 2008 WHO [34] classification uses the abbreviation B-ALL for precursor B lymphoblastic leukaemia/lymphoma. Previously this abbreviation was used for mature 'B-ALL', which usually equates with Burkitt lymphoma. Since these two conditions require quite different management absolute clarity is necessary in communication.

B-cell chronic lymphocytic leukaemia/small lymphocytic lymphoma

B-cell chronic lymphocytic leukaemia (CLL) is a disease resulting from neoplastic proliferation of mature B lymphocytes that infiltrate the bone marrow and circulate in the peripheral blood. It is predominantly a disease of middle and old age. The incidence of CLL plus small lymphocytic lymphoma (SLL) (see below) is of the order of 5 per 100 000 per year, rising from negligible figures in young adults to more than 10 per 100 000 per year in those over 65 years of age [36,57]. The incidence of SLL is about a third that of CLL [57]. The incidence is higher in white Americans than in black or Asian Americans [36]. Familial occurrence, although rare, is more common in this disease than in any other type of lymphoproliferative disorder. Patients diagnosed in the early stages of the disease may have no abnormal physical findings. In those with more advanced disease, common clinical features are lymphadenopathy, hepatomegaly and splenomegaly. There is commonly an immune paresis, with impaired B- and T-cell function and reduced concentration of immunoglobulins. Autoimmune phenomena are also common.

Various arbitrary levels of peripheral blood lymphocyte count, for example more than $5 \times 10^9/l$ or more than $10 \times 10^9/l$, have been suggested as objective criteria to establish a diagnosis of CLL. The WHO classification requires at least $5 \times 10^9/l$ lymphocytes with a typical immunophenotype [58].

312   CHAPTER 6

In the WHO classification, CLL is grouped with SLL. Small lymphocytic lymphoma is a lymphoproliferative disorder characterized by lymphadenopathy in which the histological features of involved lymph nodes are identical to those of CLL. The major differences from CLL are that there is no more than a minor leukaemic component and the incidence of marrow infiltration is lower. Some patients have disease clinically confined to one lymph node group. Others have generalized lymphadenopathy which may be accompanied by hepatomegaly or splenomegaly. The immunophenotype is indistinguishable from that of CLL.

Examination of the peripheral blood is essential in the diagnosis of CLL. A bone marrow aspirate is of little importance in comparison with a trephine biopsy, which yields information important both for diagnosis and prognosis. Other neoplasms of mature lymphoid cells are easily confused with CLL/SLL if a trephine biopsy specimen is not examined and immunophenotyping is not employed.

In most patients, CLL has a relatively indolent course with a median survival of more than 10 years. However, in a minority there is transformation to a more aggressive form of disease. The most common transformation is characterized by a progressive rise in the numbers of prolymphocytes in the peripheral blood and is termed prolymphocytoid transformation. Transformation to a large B-cell lymphoma, Richter's syndrome, is much less common. Transformation of CLL [59] and SLL [60] to Hodgkin lymphoma has been reported.

Peripheral blood

The blood film often shows a uniform population of mature, small lymphocytes with round nuclei, clumped chromatin (often with a mosaic pattern), scanty cytoplasm and a regular cellular outline (Fig. 6.7). Cells in other patients are less distinctive or more pleomorphic. Broken cells, known as smear cells or smudge cells, are characteristic but not pathognomonic since they are occasionally seen in a variety of other conditions. With advanced disease there is anaemia and thrombocytopenia. Autoimmune haemolytic anaemia can occur, either early or late in the course of CLL. The blood film then shows spherocytes and the direct antiglobulin test is positive. When bone marrow reserve is adequate there is also polychromasia and the reticulocyte count is increased. Autoimmune destruction of platelets may also occur and, in patients with early disease, may be responsible for an isolated thrombocytopenia. Pure red cell aplasia is a less common complication; the peripheral blood shows morphologically normal red cells and a lack of polychromasia.

Patients with CLL may have a small proportion of cells with the morphology of prolymphocytes, i.e. with a prominent nucleolus and more abundant cytoplasm. Cases with more than 10% pro-

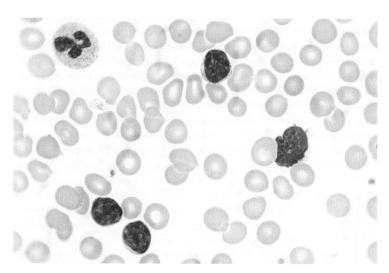

Fig. 6.7 Peripheral blood (PB) film, CLL, showing a uniform population of small mature lymphocytes. One smear cell is present. MGG ×100.

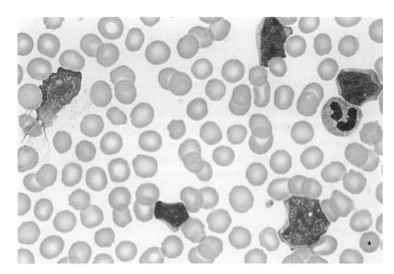

Fig. 6.8 PB film, CLL/mixed cell type, showing pleomorphic lymphocytes and one smear cell. MGG ×100.

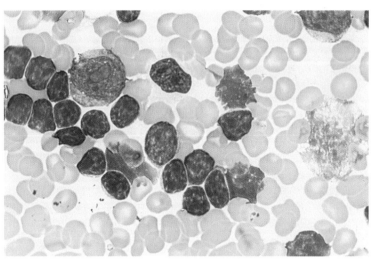

Fig. 6.9 PB film, Richter's syndrome, showing mature small lymphocytes, smear cells and a large cell with a giant nucleolus. MGG ×100.

lymphocytes at presentation have been included in the FAB category of CLL, mixed cell type (Fig. 6.8); in some patients the prolymphocyte count remains stable and the disease behaves like classic CLL [61]. Others have a progressively increasing prolymphocyte count and a more aggressive course, probably representing prolymphocytoid transformation. When CLL undergoes transformation to large cell lymphoma transformed cells are only rarely present in the peripheral blood (Fig. 6.9) but, when present, have the same cytological features as large cell lymphoma in leukaemic phase.

In patients with SLL the lymphocyte count is usually normal at presentation and the peripheral blood film shows no specific abnormalities. Many patients develop lymphocytosis during the course of the illness [58], usually during the first few years after presentation [62].

Bone marrow cytology

The bone marrow is hypercellular and contains increased numbers of mature lymphocytes which are generally uniform in appearance. Normal haemopoietic cells are reduced, there being a continued fall with disease progression. Various arbitrary percentages of bone marrow lymphocytes, for example more than 30% or more than 40%, have been suggested as necessary to establish the diagnosis of CLL. A figure of 30% is quite adequate for diagnosis if a good aspirate, not diluted with peripheral blood, is obtained and if other features are typical. In one study the percentage of lymphocytes in the aspirate showed independent prognostic significance [63].

In SLL the bone marrow is infiltrated in the majority of patients particularly, but not exclusively, in those who have clinically apparent generalized disease [62,64,65]. Cytological features of the infiltrating cells are the same as those of CLL.

When CLL is complicated by autoimmune haemolytic anaemia the bone marrow shows erythroid hyperplasia and in autoimmune thrombocytopenia there are increased megakaryocytes, at least in those patients with an adequate haemopoietic reserve. In pure red cell aplasia there is a lack of any red cell precursors beyond proerythroblasts.

When prolymphocytoid transformation of CLL occurs, increasing numbers of prolymphocytes are present in the bone marrow. Richter's transformation sometimes occurs in the bone marrow but more often occurs initially at an extramedullary site with bone marrow infiltration being a late event. When infiltration occurs, the cells usually have the morphology of a pleomorphic large B-cell lymphoma, often with immunoblastic features – immunoblasts being large cells with deeply basophilic cytoplasm and a large nucleus with a large prominent central nucleolus (Fig. 6.10).

Flow cytometric immunophenotyping

Cells of CLL show weak expression of monoclonal SmIg, commonly IgM with or without IgD (Box 6.2). They express other B-cell markers such as CD19 and CD24. CD22 is expressed in the cyto-

---

BOX 6.2

Chronic lymphocytic leukaemia

Flow cytometric immunophenotyping
CD5+, CD19+, CD23+, CD24+, weak SmIg (IgM+, IgD+/–)
CD10–, CD22–, CD79b–, FMC7–
Variable expression of CD38 and ZAP70; adverse prognostic significance if posititve

Immunohistochemistry
CD5+, CD20+/–, CD23+/–, CD43+, CD79a+, PAX5+
CD10–, CD11c–, cyclin D1–, BCL6–

Cytogenetic and molecular genetic analysis
No specific abnormality and many cases have normal karyotypes
The most common cytogenetic abnormalities are del(13)(q12-14), trisomy 12, del(6)(q21), del(11)(q22-23) and del(17)(p13)

Percentages are approximate: +, >90% of cases positive; +/–, >50% positive; –/+, <50% positive; –, <10% positive. Ig, immunoglobulin; SmIg, surface membrane immunoglobulin.

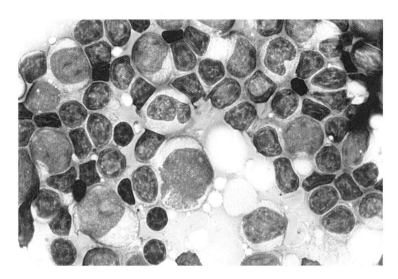

Fig. 6.10 BM aspirate, Richter's syndrome (same patient as Fig. 6.9), showing mature small lymphocytes admixed with frequent very large cells with large nucleoli. MGG ×100.

plasm but is expressed weakly, if at all, on the cell surface. CD20 is also weakly expressed. CD11c may be weakly expressed. FMC7 is usually negative and CD79b is weak or negative. There is cell surface expression of CD5 and CD23 in the majority of cases [66,67]. Expression of CD5 is weaker than on normal T cells. Coexpression of CD5 and CD19 can be shown using two-colour immunofluorescence. Clonality of the CD5-positive population can be demonstrated by showing light chain restriction. A scoring system has been described using immunophenotypic data to help discriminate between CLL and other B-cell lymphoproliferative disorders [66,67]. Cases score one point for each of the following five features: weak expression of SmIg, expression of CD5, expression of CD23, negativity with FMC7 and lack of expression of CD79b (or CD22). Most cases of CLL have a score of four or five points; a minority have a score of three points. CD38 is expressed by cells of 40–50% of cases. Expression of CD38 or ZAP70 indicates a worse prognosis; expression of either correlates with unmutated immunoglobulin variable region genes.

Cytogenetic and molecular genetic analysis
A normal karyotype has been reported in from 40% to 72% of cases in different series of patients [68–70]. The most common cytogenetic abnormalities are del(13)(q14.3) and trisomy 12, the latter often associated with additional changes. Other abnormalities include: deletion of 6q21, 11q22-23

or 17p13; other abnormalities of 17p; and 14q+. A normal karyotype, del(13q) and most cases with an isolated trisomy 12 are associated with classical morphology and a good prognosis. Trisomy 12 with additional abnormalities, 14q+, del(6q) and chromosome 17 abnormalities are associated with an atypical immunophenotype and a worse prognosis [70]. FISH shows a much higher proportion of cases with clonal abnormalities than conventional cytogenetic analysis [71,72]. There may be a different distribution of cytogenetic abnormalities between cases of CLL and cases of SLL; in one study del(13q) was significantly more common in CLL [73].

Molecular genetic analysis indicates that CLL may result from mutation in a pre-germinal centre B lymphocyte that lacks somatic hypermutation (40–50% of cases) or a post-germinal centre B lymphocyte that has undergone somatic hypermutation (50–60% of cases) [58]. Patients belonging to the former group have a worse prognosis. Cases with trisomy 12 have mainly unmutated immunoglobulin variable region genes whereas cases with 13q14 abnormalities more often have hypermutated genes [58].

Bone marrow histology
Usually at presentation, the vast majority of the neoplastic cells in the marrow are small lymphocytes (Fig. 6.11). These cells are slightly larger than the average normal lymphocyte. They have

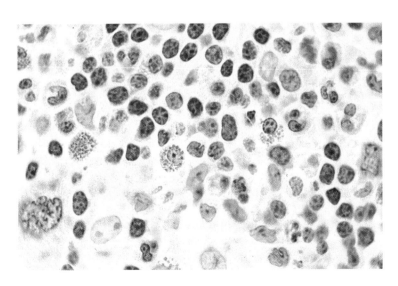

Fig. 6.11 BM trephine biopsy section, CLL, showing mature small lymphocytes infiltrating between residual normal haemopoietic cells. Resin-embedded, H&E ×100.

nuclei with coarsely clumped chromatin and insignificant nucleoli; there is little cytoplasm. The nuclear outline appears somewhat irregular in sections of paraffin- and resin-embedded specimens. In addition to the predominant small lymphocytes there are small numbers of prolymphocytes and para-immunoblasts. The latter are medium-sized cells with plentiful cytoplasm and a large nucleus with a prominent nucleolus. The cytoplasm of para-immunoblasts is less intensely basophilic than that of immunoblasts. Prolymphocytes are intermediate in size between small lymphocytes and para-immunoblasts; they have nuclei with dispersed chromatin and a nucleolus which is often large and prominent. Proliferation centres are seen in patients with nodular or diffuse infiltration. In cases with diffuse infiltration, focal proliferation centres sometimes give the infiltrate a 'pseudofollicular' pattern. The proliferation centres contain increased numbers of prolymphocytes and para-immunoblasts and, although less often observed in the bone marrow, are identical to those seen in lymph nodes of patients with CLL. Occasional cases of CLL have prominent non-neoplastic mast cells within and around the areas of infiltration. Small blood vessels are increased [74] and this has been found to be of prognostic significance in early stage disease [75].

Four histological patterns of marrow infiltration are seen in CLL: interstitial (Figs 6.12 and 6.13), nodular (Fig. 6.14), diffuse ('packed marrow') (Fig.

6.15) and mixed [6,76]. A mixed pattern represents a combination of nodular and interstitial infiltration. Paratrabecular infiltration is not seen unless previous treatment or coincidental disease has altered the stromal environment. An unusual pattern of infiltration is for there to be a marked increase in reactive germinal centres, either randomly distributed or paratrabecular, with the bone marrow otherwise showing a diffuse infiltrate of neoplastic cells [77]; this has been described as an interfollicular pattern of infiltration. There is usually little if any increase in reticulin [15].

Examination of bone marrow trephine biopsy sections in CLL provides a valuable prognostic indicator which is partly independent of clinical stage. Most investigators have demonstrated a statistically significant difference between the outcome in cases with a diffuse pattern (poor prognosis) and those with non-diffuse (nodular and interstitial) patterns (good prognosis) [6,76,78]. Some workers have further found cases with a mixed pattern to have a prognosis intermediate between that of the above two groups [6]. Somewhat divergent findings were reported by Frisch and Bartl [79]; they also found the shortest survival in those with diffuse infiltration, but those with an interstitial pattern had a shorter survival than those with a nodular infiltrate. Attempts have been made, with some success, to correlate the clinical staging systems with patterns of bone marrow infiltration. In general, within a single stage, patients in whom the bone

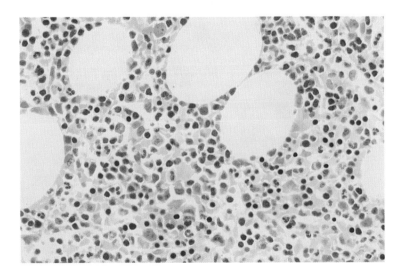

Fig. 6.12 BM trephine biopsy section, CLL, showing interstitial infiltration. Resin-embedded, H&E ×40.

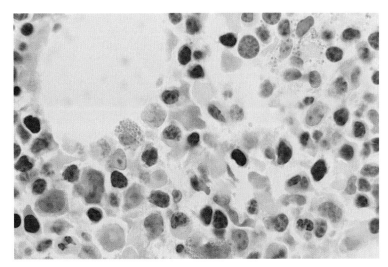

Fig. 6.13 BM trephine biopsy section, CLL, showing interstitial infiltration. Resin-embedded, H&E ×100.

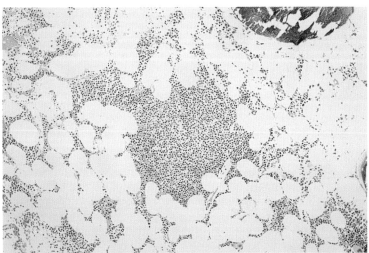

Fig. 6.14 BM trephine biopsy section, CLL, showing nodular infiltration. Resin-embedded, H&E ×10.

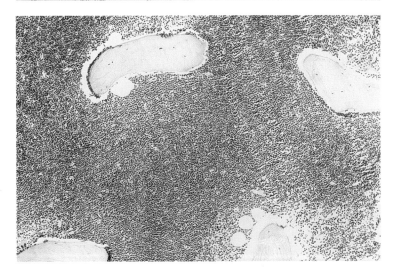

Fig. 6.15 BM trephine biopsy section, CLL, showing diffuse infiltration ('packed marrow' pattern). Resin-embedded, H&E ×10.

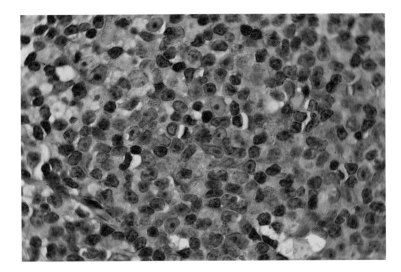

Fig. 6.16 BM trephine biopsy section, CLL, showing para-immunoblasts and prolymphocytes in a proliferation centre. Paraffin-embedded, Giemsa ×100.

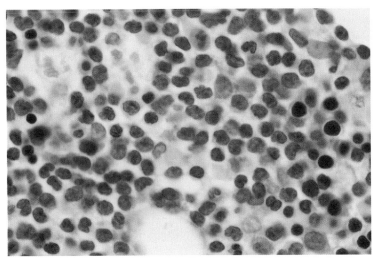

Fig. 6.17 BM trephine biopsy section, CLL/mixed cell type, showing pleomorphic small and medium-sized lymphocytes. Paraffin-embedded, H&E ×100.

marrow is diffusely infiltrated do worse than those with non-diffuse patterns of infiltration [76,78].

The trephine biopsy is also of importance in assessing response to treatment since there may be residual lymphoid nodules when the percentage of lymphocytes in the aspirate is no longer increased [63]. This is referred to as nodular partial remission.

In prolymphocytoid transformation of CLL [61] there are increased numbers of prolymphocytes and para-immunoblasts in the marrow (Fig. 6.16). This needs to be distinguished from CLL/mixed cell type (Fig. 6.17) (see above). In Richter's syndrome [80,81] the marrow is infiltrated only in a minority

of cases; the infiltrate is of immunoblasts admixed with bizarre giant cells, some of which resemble Reed–Sternberg cells (Fig. 6.18). In the majority of cases the marrow shows only the characteristic features of CLL. In rare cases of transformation to Hodgkin lymphoma the marrow may be involved.

The incidence of bone marrow involvement in patients with SLL, as determined from biopsy sections, varies from 30% to 90% in reported series [14,82,83]. Various patterns of infiltration have been reported. Pangalis and Kittas [83] found a nodular pattern in all of six patients with bone marrow infiltration but others [8,14,64] have observed focal, interstitial and occasionally diffuse

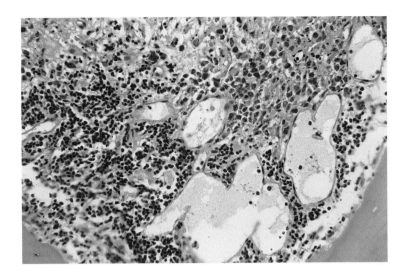

Fig. 6.18 BM trephine biopsy section, Richter's transformation of CLL; part of the section shows residual mature small lymphocytes (bottom left) and part shows infiltration by pleomorphic immunoblasts (top right). Paraffin-embedded, H&E ×40.

patterns. The cytological features of the infiltrate are similar to those seen in CLL; there are predominantly small lymphocytes with round or slightly irregular contours and occasional para-immunoblasts. No correlation has been found between the bone marrow findings and survival in SLL [83,84].

Immunohistochemistry

Cells of CLL express the B-cell markers CD20 and CD79a (see Box 6.2). Expression of CD20 is often weak. The markers CD5, CD23 and CD43 are usually positive and are useful in discriminating CLL from other small B-cell lymphoproliferative diseases. Expression of CD23 is sometimes weak on small CLL lymphocytes but this antigen is more strongly expressed by prolymphocytes and para-immunoblasts, highlighting the proliferation centres [85]. On occasions, only the cells within proliferation centres stain for CD23. Expression of the proliferation marker, Ki-67, is confined to the proliferation centres and scattered para-immunoblasts. Staining for CD10 is negative. Cyclin D1 is usually negative but is occasionally expressed in cells of proliferation centres [58]. ZAP70 expression, of adverse prognostic significance, can be detected by immunohistochemistry [86].

In large cell transformation the cells express CD79a but CD20 staining may be negative; the pleomorphic tumour cells resembling Reed–Sternberg cells often express CD30. There is little information regarding CD5 and CD23 but expres-

sion is lost in at least a proportion of cases. Staining for Ki-67 shows a high proliferative fraction.

Problems and pitfalls

In its earliest stages, CLL can be diagnosed in patients with clonal lymphocyte counts as low as $5 \times 10^9/l$ provided there is typical morphology and immunophenotype with evidence of monotypic Ig light chain expression by the CD5-positive B cells on flow cytometry. CLL needs to be distinguished from monoclonal B lymphocytosis, which is usually an incidental finding; it has fewer circulating clonal cells than CLL and no tissue manifestations of SLL. It can be a forerunner of CLL.

Polyclonal B-cell lymphocytosis is an uncommon condition that is usually associated with cigarette smoking in young or middle-aged women [87,88]. This condition has sometimes been confused with CLL. The lymphocytosis is usually mild and there are typical morphological abnormalities including binuclearity and deeply lobed nuclei. A minority of patients have lymphadenopathy and splenomegaly. No evidence of clonality is found on immunophenotypic or molecular genetic analysis, although there may be cytogenetic abnormalities and oligoclonal *BCL2-IGH* rearrangement [89].

Lymphoproliferative disorders that may be mistaken for CLL include B-cell prolymphocytic leukaemia, lymphoplasmacytic lymphoma, follicular lymphoma, mantle cell lymphoma, splenic lymphoma with villous lymphocytes, T-cell prolymphocytic leukaemia and T-cell large granular lymphocytic leukaemia. Correct diagnosis requires correlation of cytological features, immunophenotype and, in some cases, molecular genetic analysis. With careful assessment of cytological features and immunophenotype, distinction from other small B-cell lymphoproliferative disorders is usually not a problem. Cases with atypical cytological features (mixed cell type and cases undergoing prolymphocytoid transformation) may be confused with mantle cell lymphoma, which also expresses CD5. In these cases, immunophenotypic and molecular genetic analysis will usually enable the distinction to be made.

The histological features in trephine biopsy sections that are helpful in differentiating CLL from other small B-cell lymphoproliferative disorders are the non-paratrabecular pattern, the presence of para-immunoblasts within the infiltrate and, in some cases, the presence of proliferation centres. Care is needed in interpreting CD5 and CD23 immunohistochemistry when expression is very weak or restricted to subpopulations of CLL cells. CD5 is expressed strongly by T cells, which may be abundant, admixed with CLL cells. Interpretation of ZAP70 expression may similarly be difficult in infiltrates accompanied by abundant non-neoplastic T cells, since the latter are also strongly ZAP70 positive.

B-cell prolymphocytic leukaemia

B-cell prolymphocytic leukaemia (B-PLL) is a disease resulting from the proliferation of a clone of mature B cells with distinctive cytological characteristics. B-PLL differs clinically, cytologically, immunophenotypically and genetically from CLL and is recognized as a separate entity in the WHO classification [90]. It is much less common than CLL and, on average, occurs at an older age. There is an equal gender distribution [90]. Patients generally have marked splenomegaly but only minor lymphadenopathy. Its diagnosis requires exclusion of t(11;14)(q13;q32) [90] since features may overlap with mantle cell lymphoma.

Peripheral blood examination is most important in the diagnosis of B-PLL; bone marrow aspiration and trephine biopsy are less important.

Peripheral blood

The WBC is typically quite high, for example 50–100 × 10^9/l or even higher. Anaemia and thrombocytopenia may be present. Leukaemic cells are larger and in many cases less homogeneous than those of CLL. They vary in size with the larger cells having moderately abundant, weakly basophilic cytoplasm and a round nucleus containing a prominent nucleolus (Fig. 6.19). Smaller cells tend to have a somewhat higher nucleocytoplasmic ratio and the nucleolus is less prominent.

Bone marrow cytology

The bone marrow is infiltrated by cells of similar appearance to those in the peripheral blood. Often

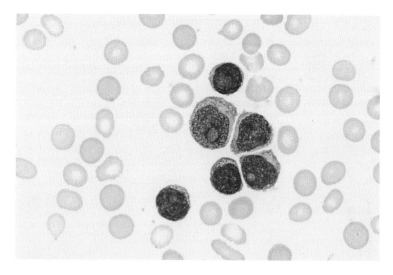

Fig. 6.19 PB film, B-PLL, showing prolymphocytes with plentiful cytoplasm and a single prominent nucleolus. MGG ×100.

the morphology is less characteristic than in the blood.

Flow cytometric immunophenotyping

The cells of B-PLL show strong expression of monoclonal SmIg, which is usually IgM with or without IgD. Pan-B-cell markers are expressed but the immunophenotype differs from that of CLL; CD5 and

CD23 are much less often expressed (20–30% and 10–20%, respectively) whereas CD22, CD79b and FMC7 are commonly positive [90] (Box 6.3).

Cytogenetic and molecular genetic analysis

There is no specific associated cytogenetic abnormality, but complex karyotypes, 14q+, trisomy 3, trisomy 12, del(6q) and del(17p) have been reported. *TP53* may be mutated. In the past, cases with similar cytology to that described above with t(11;14)(q13;q32) were considered to be B-PLL [91] but these are now thought to represent a leukaemic phase of mantle cell lymphoma.

Bone marrow histology

Recognition of prolymphocytes in tissue sections may be difficult although thin sections and techniques of resin embedding make this easier. The cells are slightly larger than those of CLL and have round nuclei [92]. The chromatin is coarsely clumped and there is a distinct and usually prominent nucleolus (Figs 6.20 and 6.21). The mitotic count is much lower than in diffuse large B-cell lymphoma, with which it may be confused. Some cases show increased eosinophils or plasma cells or sinusoidal dilation.

The following four patterns of marrow infiltration have been found: interstitial, interstitial–nodular, interstitial–diffuse (Fig. 6.20) and diffuse (Fig. 6.21). The commonest pattern is interstitial–nodular. The pure nodular form of infiltration which occurs in CLL is not seen in PLL. Proliferation

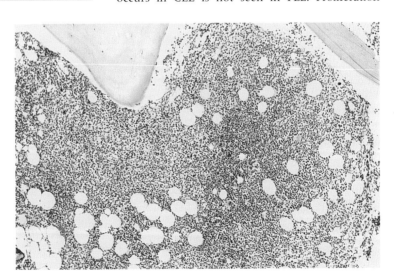

Fig. 6.20 BM trephine biopsy section, B-PLL, showing interstitial–diffuse infiltration. Resin-embedded, H&E ×10.

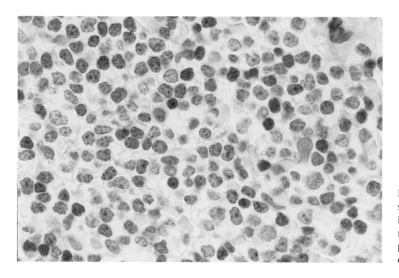

Fig. 6.21 BM trephine biopsy section, B-PLL, showing diffuse infiltration by medium-sized cells, many of which have a single prominent nucleolus. Resin-embedded, H&E ×100.

centres are not seen [90]. In contrast to CLL, all cases show increased reticulin.

Immunohistochemistry

Pan-B-cell markers CD20 and CD79a are positive (Box 6.3). Staining for CD5, CD10, CD23, CD43 and cyclin D1 is usually negative. Proliferative activity, represented by expression of Ki-67, is generally higher than in CLL, aound 20–30%, but without the areas of accentuation that are seen in the proliferation centres of CLL.

Problems and pitfalls

B-cell prolymphocytic leukaemia needs to be distinguished from CLL with mixed cell morphology (CLL/PL) and other B-cell lymphoproliferative disorders with a leukaemic component, particularly mantle cell lymphoma. Cytological features are more useful than histological features in making this distinction. The percentage of prolymphocytes in the peripheral blood is greater in B-PLL than CLL/PL, with most cases of B-PLL having more than 55% prolymphocytes. The immunophenotype is variable, but strong FMC7 reactivity will usually allow distinction from CLL.

Distinction between B-cell and T-cell prolymphocytic leukaemia (T-PLL) requires immunophenotypic analysis although cytological features usually indicate the correct diagnosis.

Hairy cell leukaemia

Hairy cell leukaemia is a rare disease consequent on the proliferation, particularly in the spleen, of a clone of post-germinal centre B cells with distinctive morphology and immunophenotype. This disease is more than three times as common in men (0.62/100000/year) as in women (0.16/100000/year) [36]. It is recognized as a specific entity in the WHO classification [93]. The common clinical features are splenomegaly and signs and symptoms resulting from anaemia and neutropenia. There may be defective immune responses.

The neoplastic cells almost always have tartrate-resistant acid phosphatase (TRAP) activity in the cytoplasm; such activity is very uncommon in other lymphoproliferative disorders.

The diagnosis can often be suspected from peripheral blood examination and confirmed by a bone marrow aspirate. However, hairy cells may be infrequent in the blood and the characteristic bone marrow reticulin fibrosis commonly renders aspiration difficult. Examination of trephine biopsy sections therefore plays an important role in diagnosis.

Peripheral blood

Hairy cells are usually present in the peripheral blood only in small numbers and in some cases none are detected. Pancytopenia is usual. Neutropenia and monocytopenia are particularly severe. The

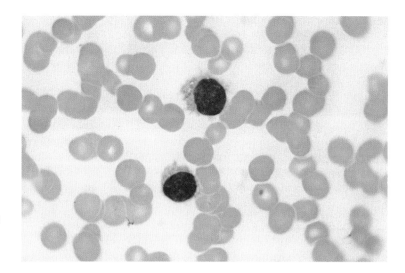

Fig. 6.22 PB film, hairy cell leukaemia, showing two hairy cells with weakly basophilic cytoplasm, which has irregular hair-like projections. MGG ×100.

leukaemic cells are larger than those of CLL and have abundant weakly basophilic cytoplasm with irregular cytoplasmic margins (Fig. 6.22). The nucleus may be round, oval, kidney or dumb-bell shaped or bilobed. There is some condensation of chromatin but no nucleolus is apparent. The demonstration of TRAP enzymatic activity can be important in confirming the diagnosis if appropriately targeted immunophenotyping is not available.

Bone marrow cytology

The bone marrow is often difficult or impossible to aspirate. When an aspirate is obtained the characteristic cell has the same morphological features as the few circulating neoplastic cells. Aspirates are often aparticulate but, when fragments are present, mast cells are often very prominent within them.

Rarely large cell transformation occurs, particularly in abdominal lymph nodes [94]. Sometimes transformed cells are also present in the bone marrow (Fig. 6.23).

Flow cytometric immunophenotyping

The cells show strong SmIg expression which, in about one third of cases, is IgM with or without IgD and, in the remaining two thirds, is IgA or IgG. The pan-B markers CD19, CD20, CD22 and CD24 are usually expressed but CD5 and CD23 are typically

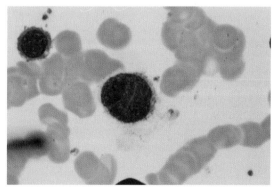

Fig. 6.23 BM film showing a large atypical cell in the bone marrow of a patient with transformation of hairy cell leukaemia. MGG ×100. (By courtesy of Professor D. Catovsky, London.)

negative (Box 6.4). There is usually FMC7 reactivity and, in addition, there is expression of several markers that are otherwise uncommon in chronic leukaemias of B lineage – CD11c, CD25, CD71, CD103, CD123, HC2 and several markers also expressed on plasma cells. Cyclin D1 is often expressed [56].

BOX 6.4

Hairy cell leukaemia

Flow cytometric immunophenotyping
CD11c+, CD19+, CD20+, CD22+, CD24+, CD25+,
   CD71+, CD79a+, CD79b+, CD103+, CD123+, strong
   SmIg, HC2+, FMC7+
CD5–, CD10–, CD23–

Immunohistochemistry
CD11c+, CD20+, CD79a+, CD72 (DBA.44)+, TRAP+,
   PAX5+, CD25+, CD123+
CD5–, CD10–/+, CD23–, CD25+, CD43–, BCL6–,
   cyclin D1–/+

Cytogenetic and molecular genetic analysis
No specific abnormality

Percentages are approximate: +, >90% of cases positive; +/–, >50% positive; –/+, <50% positive; –, <10% positive. SmIg, surface membrane immunoglobulin; TRAP, tartrate-resistant acid phosphatase.

Cytogenetic and molecular genetic analysis

No consistent cytogenetic or molecular genetic abnormality has been found. The neoplastic clone is derived from a post-germinal centre B cell with hypermutated immunoglobulin variable region genes.

Bone marrow histology

The degree of marrow involvement is very extensive in all but the earliest of cases [95–98]. Infiltration is usually either random focal or diffuse; focal involvement is generally extensive with large confluent patches involving up to 50% of the marrow. Distinct nodules or a predilection for specific areas of the marrow are not found. A third pattern of infiltration is that of interstitial infiltration in a severely hypoplastic marrow [97,99]. Rare cases occur in which no hairy cells are seen in the blood or in bone marrow biopsy sections but neoplastic cells are detectable in the spleen [100].

The infiltrates consist of widely spaced mononuclear cells, ranging in size from 10 to 25 µm, producing a striking appearance on low power examination (Fig. 6.24). The relatively wide separation of nuclei is due to a zone of abundant pale or water-clear cytoplasm and also in part, particularly in paraffin rather than resin-embedded sections, to cytoplasmic retraction (Fig. 6.25); this appearance is accentuated by underlying reticulin fibrosis, which holds the cells apart. The tumour cell nuclei appear bland with pale, stippled

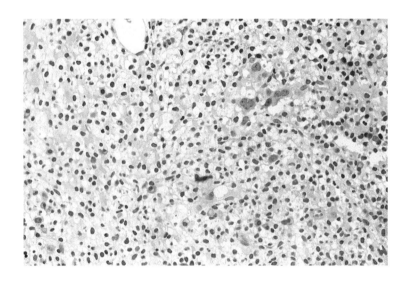

Fig. 6.24 BM trephine biopsy section, hairy cell leukaemia, showing diffuse infiltration by hairy cells; note the characteristic 'spaced' arrangement of the cells. Resin-embedded, H&E ×20.

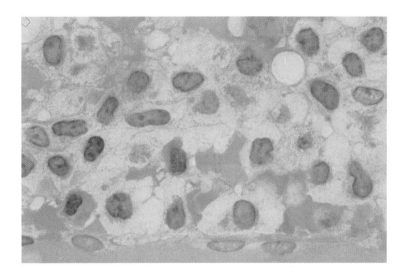

Fig. 6.25 BM trephine biopsy section, hairy cell leukaemia, showing bland nuclei of various shapes surrounded by shrunken cytoplasm with irregular margins; clear spaces surround the cells. Resin-embedded, H&E ×100.

chromatin; nucleoli are not prominent (Fig. 6.25). Nuclei vary in both size and shape and may include round, oval, indented, dumb-bell shaped and bilobed forms. The mitotic count is low. In resin-embedded specimens, a characteristic ribosome–lamellar complex can sometimes be identified within the cytoplasm of hairy cells and may aid in their identification [101]. In some cases there are foci of hairy cells with spindle-shaped or fusiform nuclei giving the cells a fibroblastic appearance; however, a fibrous or fusiform pattern may also be due to accompanying clusters of fibroblasts [97]. Red blood cells may be seen in infiltrated areas, either apparently extravasated or surrounded by a layer of hairy cells; this appearance resembles the red blood cell lakes seen in the spleen and liver [96,97]. Reactive plasma cells, lymphocytes and mast cells are also often prominent in areas of infiltration.

Residual haemopoiesis is observed in all but the most severely infiltrated areas. Haemopoietic elements are scattered among the infiltrating hairy cells and consist of isolated erythroid clusters and megakaryocytes; granulocyte precursors are particularly sparse [97,98].

When the marrow is hypocellular, small clusters of hairy cells and residual haemopoietic cells are identified between the fat cells.

Reticulin fibrosis occurs in the areas of marrow infiltration, producing a characteristic mesh-like pattern with fine reticulin fibres surrounding single cells and groups of cells (Fig. 6.26). This may result from the synthesis of fibronectin by hairy cells [102]. Collagen fibrosis is distinctly unusual [15,103]. Rare patients have osteosclerosis [104,105].

When large cell transformation occurs, large atypical cells may be noted in trephine biopsy sections (Fig. 6.27).

Much of the information on prognosis dates from the period when patients were treated by splenectomy or with interferon. Such data may not be relevant to patients treated with nucleoside analogues. Historically both the extent of infiltration [96,106] and cellular morphology were found to be of prognostic importance. A lesser degree of infiltration was found predictive of a good response to splenectomy [106] and of longer survival [96]. Nuclear form was found to be of prognostic significance, with patients whose cells had small, round or ovoid nuclei having a better survival than those with cells showing intermediate-sized, convoluted or large indented nuclei [96]. It was suggested that this prognostic relevance was related more to increasing nuclear size in these three types than to nuclear shape *per se* [107]. The presence of rod-like cytoplasmic inclusions, corresponding to ribosome–lamellar complexes, was also found to correlate with a worse prognosis [96].

Bone marrow histology may be modified by therapy. Splenectomy corrects hypersplenism but rarely has any effect on the bone marrow tumour

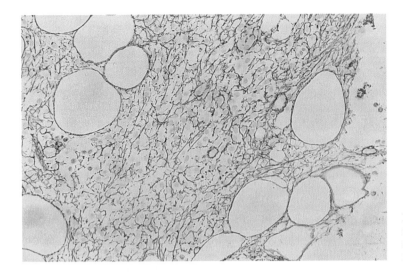

Fig. 6.26 BM trephine biopsy section, hairy cell leukaemia, showing increased reticulin. Resin-embedded, Gomori stain ×20.

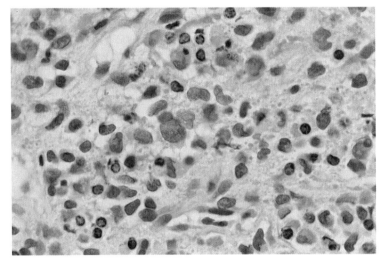

Fig. 6.27 BM trephine biopsy section, large cell transformation of hairy cell leukaemia, showing several large atypical cells. Paraffin-embedded, H&E ×40. (By courtesy of Professor D. Catovsky, London.)

burden. Alpha-interferon causes a slow but progressive decline in the number of bone marrow hairy cells over a period of several months with a response being seen in the great majority of patients [103,108,109]. This is accompanied by a slow increase in haemopoietic cells, but recovery of haemopoiesis, particularly granulopoiesis, may lag behind reduction of hairy cell infiltration [103]. Complete clearing of hairy cells from the marrow occurs in only a small minority of interferon-treated patients [110]. The loss of hairy cells can continue after cessation of therapy but, in general, there is subsequently a tendency for their numbers to rise slowly [103,109]. At the end of such therapy

the marrow often shows reduced cellularity and occasionally it is severely hypocellular [103,109].

The two chemotherapeutic agents now most frequently employed in treatment, pentostatin and cladribine, are more effective than α-interferon in clearing hairy cells from the marrow, complete remission being observed in about three quarters of cases with pentostatin [110,111]. With the clearing of hairy cells, the increased reticulin is lost progressively but, in general, loss of reticulin lags behind loss of hairy cells. Reticulin fibrosis may resolve completely when complete remission is achieved. The rare osteosclerotic lesions also resolve [104]. Following cladribine therapy a high prevalence of severely hypoplastic foci has been noted, often still present many years after treatment [112]. Immunohistochemistry is essential in identifying residual hairy cells in treated patients.

Immunohistochemistry

Hairy cells express the B-cell-associated antigens CD20, CD79a [113] and CD72 (monoclonal antibody DBA.44) (see Box 6.4). Annexin A1 is also positive [114]. Staining for CD5, CD10 and CD23 is negative. There may be cytoplasmic dot-positive staining for CD68. Cyclin D1 is often expressed but more weakly than in mantle cell lymphoma [93]. When interpreting CD20-stained sections, it is important to be sure that the positive cells have the characteristic morphology of hairy cells as this antigen is expressed by most B lymphocytes. CD72 is less often expressed on normal lymphocytes so again assessment of cytological features is important. Among B-lineage neoplasms, annexin A1 has a high degree of specificity for hairy cells; however its expression must be compared with a B-cell marker since myeloid cells and some T cells are also positive [93]. Monoclonal antibodies that identify TRAP are also of use in confirming a diagnosis of hairy cell leukaemia [115,116] but cross-reactivity with haemopoietic components makes their use unsatisfactory in minimally infiltrated marrows including those sampled post-treatment.

Problems and pitfalls

The differential diagnosis of hairy cell leukaemia includes other lymphoproliferative disorders, primary myelofibrosis, systemic mastocytosis, aplastic anaemia and hypoplastic myelodysplastic syndrome (MDS). The morphological features of marrow infiltration by hairy cell leukaemia are unlike those of other lymphoproliferative disorders. In particular, the spacing of the neoplastic cells and the regular meshwork of reticulin are useful in making the distinction from other lymphoproliferative disorders. Coexpression of CD22 and CD11c and strong TRAP positivity are the most useful markers. Distinction between hairy cell leukaemia and systemic mastocytosis is dependent on demonstration of B-cell markers and reactivity with CD72 in the former and confirmation of the identity of mast cells by mast cell tryptase immunostaining in the latter. In the past, some cases of hairy cell leukaemia were misdiagnosed as primary myelofibrosis. Since the distinctive histological features of hairy cell leukaemia are now well recognized, this diagnostic problem should no longer arise. The differential diagnosis between the hypoplastic variant of hairy cell leukaemia and aplastic anaemia and hypoplastic MDS depends on recognition of the infiltrating neoplastic cells. In difficult cases cytochemistry and immunophenotypic analysis are invaluable.

Lymphoplasmacytic lymphoma

The WHO category of lymphoplasmacytic lymphoma incorporates Waldenström macroglobulinaemia [117]. It excludes other specific lymphoma subtypes with plasmacytic differentiation. Gamma heavy chain disease may have similar histological features but is better regarded as a separate entity. The WHO-defined category of lymphoplasmacytic lymphoma has an incidence of 0.91 per 100 000 per year in white male Americans and 0.48 in white female Americans [36]. The median age of onset is in the seventh decade [118]. There is a familial clustering with other B-cell neoplasms [118]. Several series have been reported with a significant proportion of patients with hepatitis C infection [117,119].

Secretion of a monoclonal immunoglobulin is common; this is most often IgM but sometimes IgG, IgA or an immunoglobulin light chain. Clinical features are very variable. Some patients present with typical features of a lymphoma such as lymphadenopathy or splenomegaly. Others, however, present with signs and symptoms resulting from the presence of the abnormal monoclonal immunoglobulin without necessarily having any obvious signs of lymphoma. The clinical presentations include specific syndromes such as: (i) Waldenström macroglobulinaemia, when there is hyperviscosity due to production of large amounts of an IgM paraprotein; (ii) cold haemagglutinin disease (CHAD), when the paraprotein is a cold agglutinin with specificity against the I, or less often the i, antigen of the erythrocyte; (iii) idiopathic or essential cryoglobulinaemia, when the paraprotein is either itself a cryoglobulin or has antibody activity against another immunoglobulin, the immune complex being a cryoglobulin; (iv) acquired angiooedema due to C1 esterase inhibitor deficiency, when an immune reaction involving the parapro-

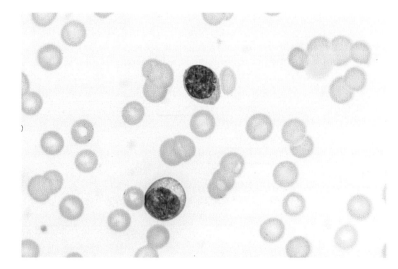

Fig. 6.28 PB film, lymphoplasmacytic lymphoma, showing a lymphocyte, a plasmacytoid lymphocyte, increased rouleaux formation and increased background staining. The patient had a high concentration of an IgM paraprotein and the clinical features of Waldenström macroglobulinaemia. MGG ×100.

tein leads to consumption of C1 esterase inhibitor with a consequent excessive complement activation and susceptibility to angio-oedema; (v) peripheral neuropathy; and (vi) light chain-associated amyloidosis. These specific entities and several other rare conditions which may be associated with the histological features of lymphoplasmacytic lymphoma are dealt with in more detail in Chapter 7. Rarely, diffuse large B-cell lymphoma supervenes in lymphoplasmacytic lymphoma with an associated worsening of prognosis.

Peripheral blood

In some patients the peripheral blood film is normal. In others there are circulating plasmacytoid lymphocytes (Fig. 6.28), usually present only in small numbers, with or without small numbers of plasma cells. Plasmacytoid lymphocytes are slightly larger than normal lymphocytes and show various combinations of features usually associated with plasma cell differentiation, such as more abundant and more basophilic cytoplasm, an eccentric nucleus, coarse chromatin clumping or the presence of a paler-staining area (a 'hof') adjacent to the nucleus which represents the Golgi zone. In some cases there is anaemia and increased background staining and rouleaux formation due to the presence of a paraprotein. Patients whose paraprotein is a cold agglutinin show red cell agglutination unless the blood specimen has been kept warm until the blood film is made. Occasionally, in patients with a cry-oglobulin, globular or fibrillar deposits of the paraprotein are seen in the blood film.

Bone marrow cytology

The bone marrow aspirate may be normal or abnormal (Fig. 6.29). When present, lymphoma cells in the bone marrow vary from infrequent to numerous. They have the same cytological features as those in the peripheral blood. Cells often contain cytoplasmic or apparently intranuclear inclusions due to immunoglobulin accumulation, but neither of these features is specific for a neoplastic proliferation; the inclusions are usually periodic acid–Schiff (PAS) positive, due to the high carbohydrate content of IgM. There is sometimes an increase in mast cells or macrophages.

Flow cytometric immunophenotyping

Cells express B-cell markers such as CD19, CD20, CD22, CD79a and CD79b; in the majority of patients there is FMC7 reactivity and often expression of CD38. CD5, CD10 and CD23 are usually negative (Box 6.5). There is usually expression of both membrane and cytoplasmic immunoglobulin, typically IgM but not IgD. Plasma cells express CD38, CD138 and monotypic Ig.

Cytogenetic and molecular genetic analysis

The neoplastic clone is derived from a post-germinal centre B cell with hypermutated immunoglobulin variable region genes.

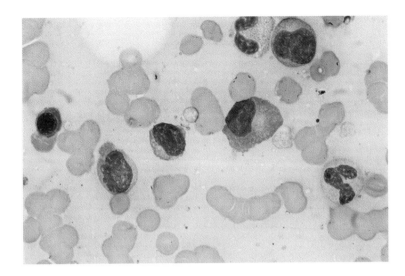

Fig. 6.29 BM aspirate, lymphoplasmacytic lymphoma. MGG ×100.

A translocation, t(9;14)(p13;q32), involving *IGH* and *PAX5*, which encodes a B-cell-specific activating protein, was reported as a frequent finding in lymphoplasmacytic lymphoma [120,121] but the association is not specific and other investigators have not found a strong association. Other abnormalities include del(6)(q21-22.1) and trisomy 4 [118]. Cytogenetic abnormalities are more often detected in patients whose cells have a greater degree of pleomorphism, often associated with a complex karyotype [122].

Bone marrow histology
Bone marrow involvement is frequent in lymphoplasmacytic lymphoma, the reported incidence varying from 50% to more than 80% of cases [62,65,123]. Nodules are often more ellipsoid and have less well-defined edges than those occurring in CLL. The patterns of infiltration seen are interstitial, nodular, paratrabecular, diffuse and mixed [14, 67,83,123,124]. In a series of 111 patients, in all of whom there was expression of IgM, diffuse and interstitial infiltration were common whereas nodular and paratrabecular infiltration were uncommon, being seen in 6% and 4%, respectively, of patients [125]. Many of the infiltrating cells are small mature lymphocytes. Other cells show varying degrees of plasma cell differentiation (Figs 6.30–6.32). In addition to the usual nuclear and cytoplasmic features of plasma cells there may be cells with intracytoplasmic or apparently intranuclear inclusions (Russell bodies and Dutcher bodies, respectively) (Figs 6.30–6.32). Rare cases have signet ring cells [126]. A small number of immunoblasts may be present. Some cases show a wide spectrum of lymphoid cells – lymphocytes, lymphoplasmacytoid cells, plasma cells and immunoblasts – and have frequent mitotic figures. An increase in mast cells (which over-express CD154,

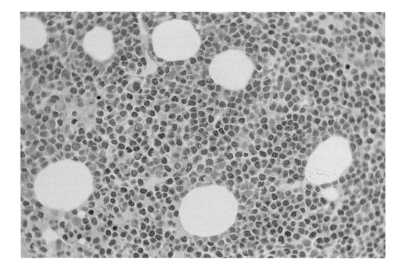

Fig. 6.30 BM trephine biopsy section, lymphoplasmacytic lymphoma, showing diffuse infiltration by lymphocytes, plasmacytoid lymphocytes and occasional plasma cells; note the cytoplasmic and intranuclear inclusions. Resin-embedded, H&E ×40.

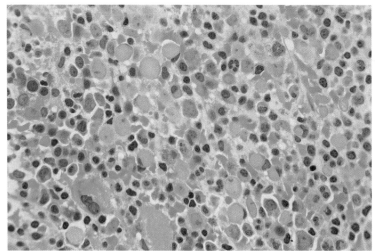

Fig. 6.31 BM trephine biopsy section, lymphoplasmacytic lymphoma, showing diffuse infiltration by lymphocytes, plasmacytoid lymphocytes and plasma cells; note the large cytoplasmic inclusions (Russell bodies) compressing the nuclei and giving some cells a 'signet ring' appearance. Resin-embedded, H&E ×40.

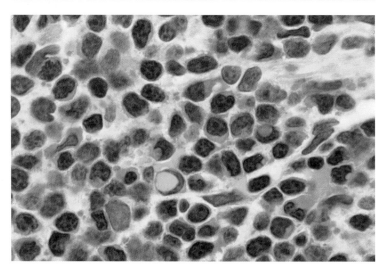

Fig. 6.32 BM trephine biopsy section, lymphoplasmacytic lymphoma, showing diffuse infiltration by lymphocytes and plasmacytoid lymphocytes; note the cytoplasmic and intranuclear inclusions. Resin-embedded, H&E ×100.

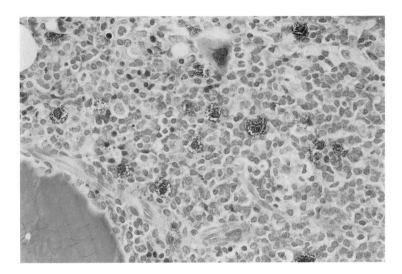

Fig. 6.33 BM trephine biopsy section, lymphoplasmacytic lymphoma, showing reactive mast cells. Resin-embedded, Giemsa ×40.

an inducer of B-cell expansion [118]) usually accompanies neoplastic infiltration (Fig. 6.33). Reticulin fibres are frequently increased in areas of infiltration [15]. In cases with a paraprotein, bone marrow vessels may contain homogeneous PAS-positive material [127] representing immunoglobulin. Paratrabecular and interstitial deposits of crystalline PAS-positive immunoglobulin may rarely be seen. Amyloid is present in rare cases.

Both the pattern of infiltration and cytological features have been found to be related to prognosis. Diffuse infiltration is associated with advanced disease and the worst prognosis [83,123]. A nodular infiltrate is associated with the best prognosis, while a mixed interstitial–nodular infiltrate is intermediate [123].

Immunohistochemistry

The small lymphocytes are CD20, CD45, CD79a and PAX5 positive. Staining for CD5, CD10 and CD43 is usually negative. CD23 may be positive or negative, a wide range in the proportion of positive cases being reported [118]. The plasma cells and cells with plasmacytoid features express CD38, CD138, p63 (antibody VS38c) [128], MUM1/IRF4 and monotypic cytoplasmic immunoglobulin. Clonality may be demonstrated not only by immunohistochemistry to show κ or λ light chain restriction but also by *in situ* hybridization to show κ or λ messenger RNA; κ is more commonly expressed than λ.

Problems and pitfalls

Lymphoplasmacytic lymphoma must be distinguished from other lymphomas with plasmacytic differentiation. As has been noted previously (see page 304), a proportion of patients with follicular lymphoma in lymph nodes have a bone marrow infiltrate with the histological features of lymphoplasmacytic lymphoma. Splenic and other marginal zone lymphomas can also have a mature plasma cell component and can resemble lymphoplasmacytic lymphoma (see pages 342–348). Bone marrow infiltrates of CLL cells can be confused with lymphoplasmacytic lymphoma. Useful distinguishing features include the lack of proliferation centres, the presence of paratrabecular infiltration, a mature plasma cell component and a prominent mast cell infiltrate, all of which favour a diagnosis of lymphoplasmacytic lymphoma rather than CLL. Intrasinusoidal infiltration is common in splenic marginal zone lymphoma and unusual in lymphoplasmacytic lymphoma. Immunophenotypic analysis will resolve most of these diagnostic problems except that distinction from marginal zone lymphomas remains a frequent difficulty since these entities share the same immunophenotype as that of lymphoplasmacytic lymphoma.

Follicular lymphoma

Follicular lymphoma, as defined in the WHO classification, is a lymphoma of follicle centre cells (centrocytes and centroblasts), with a growth pattern that is usually at least partly follicular [129]. In the bone marrow, follicles are rare even when lymph nodes show a follicular growth pattern. In the WHO classification, follicular lymphoma is divided into four grades on the basis of the proportion of centroblasts: grades 1, 2, 3a and 3b. If diffuse areas of any size are composed predominantly or entirely of centroblasts the patient is regarded as also having diffuse large B-cell lymphoma, regardless of the general grade [129]. A specific translocation, t(14;18)(q32;q21), is associated with a high percentage of neoplasms of follicle centre cell origin.

Follicular lymphoma is rare in childhood and quite uncommon during adolescence. Cases occur throughout adult life with the incidence in white Americans rising steadily from about 1 per 100 000 per year at the age of 40 years to more than 10 per 100 000 per year by the age of 70 years [36]. The incidence is lower in black and Asian Americans [36]. Unlike all other mature B-cell lymphomas, the incidence is somewhat higher in women. The most common clinical feature is lymphadenopathy, either localized or generalized. Some patients have hepatomegaly or splenomegaly. Patients with advanced disease may also have pleural effusions or ascites with neoplastic cells in the effusions. Follicular lymphoma is commonly widely disseminated (stage IV) at presentation. Transformation not only to diffuse large B-cell lymphoma but also to ALL or Burkitt lymphoma can occur. The latter two transformations are associated with a second chromosomal rearrangement leading to *MYC* rearrangement [130] and are associated with a particularly poor prognosis.

In the minority of patients who have circulating lymphoma cells, the diagnosis of follicular lymphoma can usually be suspected from the cytological and immunophenotypic characteristics of the peripheral blood cells. Bone marrow aspiration commonly fails to detect bone marrow involvement, as a consequence of both the focal nature of infiltration and of increased reticulin deposition in areas of infiltration. A trephine biopsy is therefore important if accurate staging is required. However, patients with stage III and stage IV disease are often treated with the same therapeutic protocols and, in such cases, bone marrow examination is not essential.

Peripheral blood

The blood count and film are often normal at presentation, even in patients with stage IV disease. When there is heavy bone marrow infiltration the haemoglobin concentration (Hb) and platelet and neutrophil counts may be reduced. A significant minority of patients have circulating neoplastic cells. These may be infrequent or may be present, rarely, in very large numbers. Cytological features vary between cases. In some patients, particularly those with high counts, the cells are smaller than normal lymphocytes with a very high nucleocytoplasmic ratio, condensed chromatin and narrow clefts in some nuclei (Fig. 6.34). In other patients

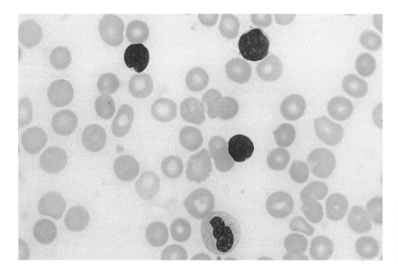

Fig. 6.34 PB film, follicular lymphoma, showing very small lymphocytes with dense, cleaved nuclei and very scanty cytoplasm. MGG ×100.

the cells are somewhat larger. Cytological features may include scanty cytoplasm, angular shape, homogeneous rather than clumped chromatin and narrow nuclear clefts. The lymphoma cells are more pleomorphic than the cells of most cases of CLL. Generally, only small lymphoid cells, corresponding to those recognized histologically as centrocytes, are present in the peripheral blood. Even cases with a large proportion of centroblasts in tissue sections usually have only centrocytes in the circulation.

Patients who do not have any peripheral blood abnormality at presentation may develop it during the course of the disease. In the minority of patients in whom transformation to a large B-cell lymphoma occurs, large cells corresponding to centroblasts may appear in the blood. These cells are rather pleomorphic with plentiful cytoplasm, little chromatin condensation and prominent, often peripheral, nucleoli; the nuclei may be predominantly round or may be cleft.

In multivariate analysis, an Hb of less than $120\,g/l$ and a lymphocyte count of less than $1.0 \times 10^9/l$ are associated with a worse prognosis [131].

Bone marrow cytology

The bone marrow is often infiltrated (more than 40% of patients) [129], even when the peripheral blood is normal. However, because infiltration is often patchy and there is associated reticulin fibrosis, the aspirate may be normal even when infiltration is detectable histologically. When the aspirate is abnormal, the cells may show the same morphological features as those in the peripheral blood but they are often less easy to recognize with certainty.

Flow cytometric immunophenotyping

The cells of follicular lymphoma show strong expression of SmIg (IgM with or without IgG, IgD being negative) and are positive for B-cell markers such as CD19, CD20, CD22, CD24 and CD79a (Box 6.6). They are usually CD5 negative and are sometimes positive for CD38. They usually express CD10, CD79b and the antigen detected by FMC7. Bone marrow flow cytometry and trephine biopsy with immunohistochemistry are complementary investigations for disease staging. In one study, of 60 patients with bone marrow infiltration, flow cytometry was falsely negative in 23% and histology falsely negative in 8% [132].

Cytogenetic and molecular genetic analysis

Most cases have a t(14;18)(q32;q21) translocation resulting in dysregulation of the *BCL2* oncogene (Box 6.6). The translocation can be detected by conventional cytogenetic analysis or FISH. Rearrangements involving the *BCL2* gene can also be detected by PCR or RT-PCR. A minority of cases show one of two variant translocations also involving the *BCL2* gene, t(2;18)(p12;q21) or t(18;22)(q21;q11.2). Secondary chromosomal abnormalities are common. These include trisomy 7, trisomy 18 and deletion of 6q23-26 or 17p. *BCL6* rearrangement (in approximately 15%) and 5' *BCL6* deletions (in approximately 40%) are seen [129]. A minority of patients do not have t(14;18) or either of the variant translocations. These patients appear to fall into two groups: (i) with *BCL2* expression and often with trisomy 18; and (ii) without *BCL2*

BOX 6.6

Follicular lymphoma

Flow cytometric immunophenotyping
CD10+/−, CD19+, CD20+, CD22+, CD24+, CD79a+, CD79b+, SmIg+
CD5−, CD23−

Immunohistochemistry
CD20+, CD79a+, PAX5+, BCL2+ (ranging from ~100% in grade 1 to ~75% in grade 3), BCL6+/− (in bone marrow), CD10−/+ (in bone marrow)
CD5−, CD23−, CD43−, cyclin D1−, MUM1/IRF4−

Cytogenetic and molecular genetic analysis
Most patients have t(14;18)(q32;q21) or a variant translocation – t(2;18)(p12;q21) or t(18;22)(q21;q11.2) – that also dysregulates *BCL2*
A minority lack *BCL2* rearrangement and expression and these patients often have t(3;14)(q27;q32) or a variant translocation associated with *BCL6* rearrangement

Percentages are approximate: +, >90% of cases positive; +/−, >50% positive; −/+, <50% positive; −, <10% positive. SmIg, surface membrane immunoglobulin.

expression and often with t(3;14)(q27;q32) or other 3q27 (*BCL6*) rearrangements [133]. The absence of t(14;18) is much more frequent among grade 3b follicular lymphoma [134]. The presence of t(3;14)(q27;q32) has also been associated with CD10 negativity, large follicles on histology, and advanced stage and bulky disease, but without a worse prognosis [135]. Over-expression of SOCS3 has been found to be an independent poor prognostic factor [136].

The neoplastic cells show hypermutated immunoglobulin variable region genes with extensive intraclonal heterogeneity, indicating a germinal centre origin with ongoing mutational activity [129].

DNA analysis indicates that healthy individuals have very small numbers of cells with t(14;18) [137], suggesting that further genetic events may be needed to induce development of follicular lymphoma.

Bone marrow histology

The bone marrow is infiltrated in 25–68% of cases [14,64,65,138]. On multivariate analysis, bone marrow infiltration is associated with a somewhat worse prognosis [131]. Infiltration is predominantly focal and very rarely interstitial or diffuse. The focal lesions are overwhelmingly paratrabecular in location (Figs 6.35 and 6.36) but there may be random focal infiltrates, generally in association with paratrabecular involvement. When infiltra-tion is heavy, individual focal lesions may coalesce and replace large areas of marrow; however, the paratrabecular concentration of lymphoma can usually still be appreciated. A follicular (nodular) pattern (Fig. 6.37), resembling that in the lymph node, is found in less than 5% of patients [12,14,139–142]; the neoplastic follicles are inter-trabecular, occasionally abutting on but not spreading along the trabecular margins. They usually occur in heavily infiltrated bone marrow with, in addition, extensive paratrabecular or diffuse infil-tration. Both the extent and pattern of infiltration have been found to be of prognostic significance [138]. A worse prognosis was associated with more than 10% of the intertrabecular space being occupied by lymphoma cells and with two different patterns of infiltration (e.g. paratrabecular and nodular) rather than a single pattern (mainly par-atrabecular) [138].

The predominant lymphoma cell in the bone marrow is a small cleft lymphocyte (small follicle centre cell or centrocyte) (Figs 6.38 and 6.39). These cells appear larger than small lymphocytes with a more variable amount of cytoplasm and nuclei which are irregular and often angular or elongated. The nuclear chromatin may be less dense and clumped than that of a normal small lymphocyte. The nuclear clefts may be difficult to recognize in paraffin-embedded tissue sections but can be seen in resin-embedded sections. Smaller but variable numbers of large cells, either cleft

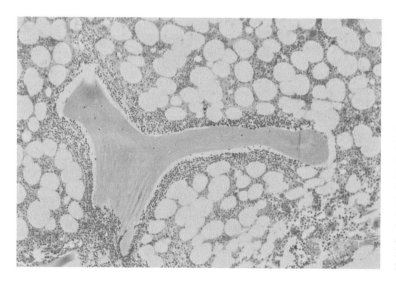

Fig. 6.35 BM trephine biopsy section showing paratrabecular infiltration by low grade follicular lymphoma. At low magnification, Giemsa staining helps to highlight such lymphoid infiltrates, which appear blue-green in comparison with the more lilac-blue tones of adjacent haemopoietic tissue. Paraffin-embedded, Giemsa stain ×4.

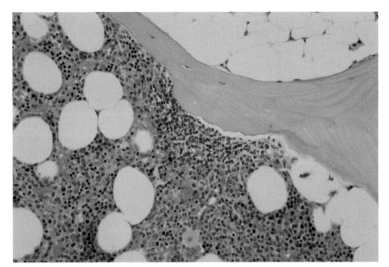

Fig. 6.36 BM trephine biopsy section showing minimal infiltration by low grade follicular lymphoma. The infiltrate is compact and crescent-shaped; even though small, it can be seen clearly to have its longest axis aligned along the trabecular margin. Paraffin-embedded, H&E ×10.

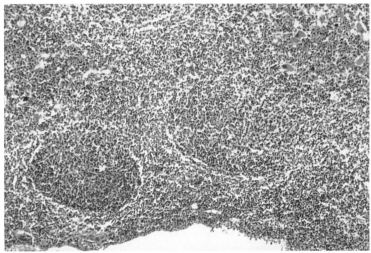

Fig. 6.37 BM trephine biopsy section, follicular lymphoma, showing diffuse infiltration with the formation of follicles. Paraffin-embedded, H&E ×10.

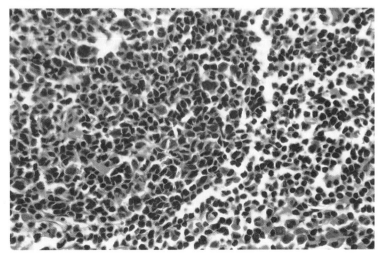

Fig. 6.38 BM trephine biopsy section, follicular lymphoma (same patient as Fig. 6.37), showing a follicle composed of centrocytes. Paraffin-embedded, H&E ×40.

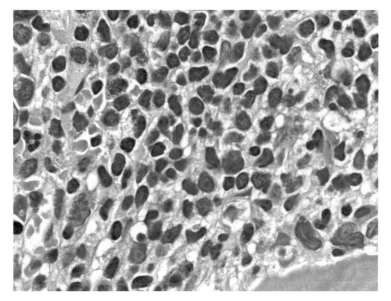

Fig. 6.39 BM trephine biopsy section, follicular lymphoma, showing an infiltrate composed predominantly of centrocytes (with occasional centroblasts); note also the eosinophils at the edge of the infiltrate. Reactive accumulation of eosinophils is a common finding at the periphery of neoplastic and non-neoplastic lymphoid aggregates in the bone marrow. Paraffin-embedded, H&E ×100.

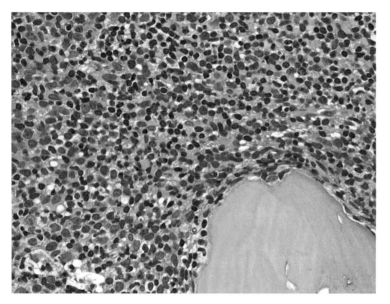

Fig. 6.40 BM trephine biopsy section from a patient with follicular lymphoma grade 3a on lymph node biopsy showing a paratrabecular lymphoid infiltrate in which there are centrocytes and larger numbers of centroblasts than are usually seen in the bone marrow in follicular lymphoma. Paraffin-embedded, H&E ×20.

(large centrocytes) or non-cleft (centroblasts), are present. Large centrocytes have irregular or cleft nuclei while centroblasts have round or ovoid nuclei; both cell types have a moderate amount of cytoplasm and small nucleoli abutting on the nuclear membrane. The nucleoli are more prominent in centroblasts than in large centrocytes. There may also be some large cells with large central nucleoli resembling immunoblasts. The proportions of these cells may differ considerably from those found in an accompanying lymph node specimen. Criteria have not been established for grading bone marrow infiltrates according to the WHO classification. However, in grade 3 disease, a significant proportion of larger cells may be seen (Fig. 6.40). A minority of patients have epithelioid granulomas (see Fig. 3.39), which are presumed to form as a reaction to the presence of neoplastic lymphoid cells. Abundant, reactive, small lymphocytes (predominantly T cells) are a more usual accompaniment of follicular lymphoma infiltrates in bone marrow. Reticulin fibres are significantly increased in infiltrated areas [15].

Following chemotherapy, the areas of previous infiltration may be recognized as hypocellular paratrabecular foci, containing increased reticulin, with or without recognizable neoplastic cells [141].

Bone marrow trephine biopsy is specifically indicated if apparently limited stage disease is to be treated by radiotherapy or if a stem cell harvest is to be done. A trephine biopsy should also be performed if radioimmunotherapy is planned since more than 25% infiltration is a contraindication to such therapy [143].

Immunohistochemistry

The neoplastic cells express CD20, CD79a and BCL2 protein (see Box 6.6). In contrast with the findings in lymph nodes, expression of CD10 and BCL6 is often negative. Staining for CD5, CD23, CD43, cyclin D1 and MUM1/IRF4 is usually negative. Falini and Mason [144] suggested that strong BCL2 staining could help to highlight the presence of cells with characteristic cleft nuclei, whereas West et al. [145] found BCL2 expression to be of diagnostic value only when it was negative. Interpretation of BCL2 staining is complicated by the frequent presence of a large number of reactive T cells that express this antigen (in addition to CD3 and CD5). Expression of BCL2 by the neoplastic cells is not generally useful in making the distinction from other lymphoproliferative disorders with similar histological features, which are often also positive. Cases with follicles in the bone marrow are an exception to this generalization. West et al. [145] found that helpful immunohistochemical features in distinguishing infiltration by follicular lymphoma from benign or atypical lymphoid aggregates were a higher percentage of CD20-positive B cells, a lower percentage of CD5-positive T cells and positivity for CD10. However, it should be noted that the latter is an uncommon finding since this antigen is often down-regulated in follicular lymphoma cells except those within well-formed follicle centres. Follicle-forming cells express pan-B-cell antigens, CD10, BCL2 and BCL6 and are supported by a network of follicular dendritic cells [142].

An unusual CD10-negative, MUM1/IRF4-positive phenotype correlates with higher grade, lack of BCL2 rearrangement and translocation or amplification of BCL6 [146].

Following treatment with anti-CD20 monoclonal antibodies (e.g. rituximab), the trephine biopsy sections may show disappearance of the B-cell infiltrate but persistence of reactive T cells [147]. In some patients, there is a change of immunophenotype shortly after such immunotherapy with B cells failing to express CD20 [148]; this may be persistent for several months and does not correlate with a failure of response.

Problems and pitfalls

A diffuse growth pattern is uncommon in follicular lymphoma and in these cases the diagnosis should be confirmed by demonstration of either a typical immunophenotype or a relevant translocation [129]. The lack of a follicular growth pattern in the bone marrow is of no consequence if this pattern has been demonstrated elsewhere.

Discordant bone marrow histopathology from that seen at other sites in the same patient is not uncommon in follicular lymphoma. Occasionally, patients with follicular lymphoma have infiltration of the bone marrow by diffuse large B-cell lymphoma. Although uncommon, this is clinically important since it alters management. More often patients presenting with diffuse large B-cell lymphoma at an extramedullary site are found to have low grade follicular lymphoma in the bone marrow. Discordant differentiation with bone marrow infiltrates resembling lymphoplasmacytic lymphoma has also been observed in patients with follicular lymphoma; this discordant pattern is probably of no clinical significance.

Infiltration of the marrow by follicular lymphoma can be confused with other small cell B-lineage lymphoproliferative disorders, particularly CLL, mantle cell lymphoma and splenic marginal zone lymphoma. Paratrabecular infiltration is not seen in CLL and a purely nodular infiltrate is very rare in follicular lymphoma. The distinction of follicular lymphoma from mantle cell lymphoma and splenic marginal zone lymphoma can be difficult on histological grounds alone and careful consideration of the morphology together with immunophenotypic and molecular genetic analysis may be required for diagnosis.

Mantle cell lymphoma

Mantle cell lymphoma is a distinct entity recognizable on the basis of morphological, clinical, immunophenotypic and molecular genetic features [149]. The lymphoma cells are analogous to lymphocytes of the mantle zone of the lymphoid follicle [150,151]. Mantle cell lymphoma is a disease of adult life. There is a marked male predominance (male:female ratio 2:1). The incidence rises from negligible figures at the age of 40 years to about 5 per 100000 per year in men and about 2 per 100000 per year in women in those over 75 years [36]. Common clinical features are generalized lymphadenopathy, splenomegaly (often marked), hepatomegaly and involvement of the gastro-intestinal tract and Waldeyer's ring. Gastro-intestinal involvement often takes the form of multiple lymphomatous polyposis, which is often but not always mantle cell lymphoma. Histological features in the lymph node include a diffuse or vaguely nodular growth pattern and a tendency for the lymphoma cells to grow in a mantle around residual normal lymphoid follicles. Rare cases have a true follicular pattern [149]. Some cases of mantle cell lymphoma have cells resembling lymphoblasts ('blastoid variant'). Others have highly pleomorphic cells ('pleomorphic variant'). Both are associated with an adverse prognosis.

Peripheral blood

In many patients the peripheral blood shows no abnormality. A leukaemic phase was reported in 20–30% of patients in two series of patients [151,152] but, in another large series, circulating lymphoma cells could be detected in the peripheral blood in 77% of cases at some point during the course of the disease [153]. A marked elevation of the WBC can occur but is uncommon [150,154]. In many cases the neoplastic cells are larger than those of CLL, varying from small to medium or large (Fig. 6.41). They are characteristically pleomorphic; some have prominent nucleoli and some have irregular, angular or cleft nuclei [154]. In comparison with the centrocytes of follicular lymphoma, cells tend to be more pleomorphic and less angular with broader nuclear clefts and more cytoplasm. Other patients have peripheral blood lymphocytes more like those of CLL, although possibly with some cleft cells, and the diagnosis is made only from lymph node histology [102]. In the leukaemic phase of the blastoid variant a spectrum of neoplastic cells is usually present in the peripheral blood, ranging from small lymphocytes with irregular nuclear contours to medium-sized lymphoid cells with a nuclear chromatin pattern similar to that seen in lymphoblasts [155] (Fig. 6.42). The pleomorphic variant is less common but, as the name implies, shows even greater variability and atypia of cells, which are generally large.

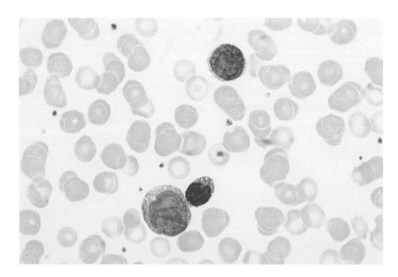

Fig. 6.41 PB film, mantle cell lymphoma, showing pleomorphic lymphocytes. MGG ×100.

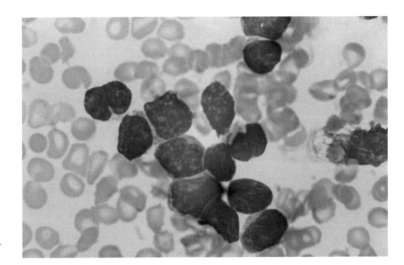

Fig. 6.42 PB film, blastoid mantle cell lymphoma, showing pleomorphic lymphocytes, some of which have a diffuse chromatin pattern and resemble lymphoblasts. MGG ×100.

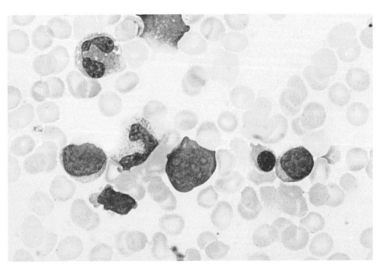

Fig. 6.43 BM aspirate, mantle cell lymphoma, showing pleomorphic lymphocytes varying from small, mature lymphocytes to large lymphoid cells with multiple nucleoli. MGG ×100.

Bone marrow cytology

The bone marrow is infiltrated in the majority of patients, including many who do not have lymphoma cells in the peripheral blood [151,152]. The infiltrating cells have the same cytological features as those in the blood (Fig. 6.43).

Flow cytometric immunophenotyping

Cells show strong expression of SmIg, usually IgM and sometimes also IgD; IgG is expressed in a minority (Box 6.7). Unusually for B-cell lymphomas, λ light chain expression is more common than κ. Cells are positive for B-cell markers CD19, CD20, CD79a and CD79b. They are usually positive for both CD5 and the antigen detected by FMC7 but do not express CD10 or CD23.

Cytogenetic and molecular genetic analysis

A characteristic translocation, t(11;14)(q13;q32), involving the *CCND1* (*BCL1*) gene, encoding cyclin D1, is detectable in almost all cases of mantle cell lymphoma if a FISH technique is used [156] (Box 6.7). The translocation is also detectable by conventional cytogenetic analysis and RT-PCR but these are less sensitive than FISH. This translocation is not specific for mantle cell lymphoma. Although cases with t(11;14) and a diagnosis of B-PLL are now thought to represent mantle cell lymphoma,

BOX 6.7

Mantle cell lymphoma

Flow cytometric immunophenotyping
CD5+, CD19+, CD20+, CD22+, CD79a+, CD79b+,
   SmIg+ (usually IgM, sometimes with IgD)
FMC7+/–, CD10–/+, CD23–

Immunohistochemistry
CD5+, CD20+, CD79a+, cyclin D1+, BCL2+, PAX5+
CD43+/–, CD10–/+
CD23–, BCL6–, MUM1/IRF4–

Cytogenetic and molecular genetic analysis
The majority of cases have t(11;14)(q13;q32)
A minority have a variant translocation t(11;22)
   (q13;q11)
CCND1 (BCL1) is rearranged

Percentages are approximate: +, >90% cases
positive; +/–, >50% positive; –/+, <50% positive; –,
<10% positive. Ig, immunoglobulin; SmIg, surface
membrane immunoglobulin.

---

the translocation is also seen in some cases of splenic marginal zone lymphoma and in plasma cell myeloma. A minority of cases of mantle cell lymphoma have a variant translocation t(11;22) (q13;q11.2) involving the *CCND1* gene and the λ light chain gene. In these translocations *CCND1* is dysregulated by its proximity to the *IGH* locus at 14q32 and the λ light chain gene at 22q11 respectively. In rare cases it is the gene encoding either cyclin D2 or cyclin D3 that is dysregulated. Secondary chromosomal abnormalities may include del(11)(q22-23), trisomy 12, 13q14 deletion and 17p deletion. Mutations and/or deletions of the *ATM* gene at 11q22-23 are common [149]. There may be loss or mutation of *TP53*, loss of expression of *CDKN2A* (*INK4A*) and *CDKN2B* (*INK4B*) (in the blastoid variant), reduced expression of *CDKN1B* (*KIP1*) and increased expression of *BMI1* [157]. *BCL2* is highly expressed and *MYC* is sometimes over-expressed [157]. Microarray analysis shows that expression of genes that are characteristically expressed in proliferating cells is associated with a considerably better prognosis [158].

In the majority of patients the neoplastic clone appears to be derived from a pre-germinal centre

(*IGH* unmutated) cell but, in a minority, the cell of origin appears to be a post-germinal centre (*IGH* hypermutated) cell [149,159]. In contrast to CLL, ZAP70 expression is relatively low and does not differ between patients with hypermutated or unmutated *IGH* genes [159].

Bone marrow histology

Bone marrow involvement is frequent, being found in more than three quarters of patients [12,151,152,160]. Infiltration may be interstitial, paratrabecular, random focal or diffuse [7,154,161,162]. However, in contrast to follicular lymphoma, paratrabecular infiltration is less common [162]. Morphology varies between cases. Typical cases have uniformly small lymphoid cells with nuclei being either mainly round or mainly irregular (Fig. 6.44); cells of the blastoid variant resemble lymphoblasts while the pleomorphic variant is characterized by cellular and nuclear pleomorphism. There may be an admixture of epithelioid macrophages [154]. Occasionally there are naked germinal centres similar to those that are seen in lymph nodes in some cases [163]. Reticulin fibres are increased in infiltrated areas. The number of mitotic figures is of prognostic significance [149].

Immunohistochemistry

The cells of mantle cell lymphoma express CD5, CD20, CD79a, CD43, BCL2 and PAX5 (see Box 6.7). Nuclear staining for cyclin D1 is often demonstrable, being reported in 72% of cases with bone marrow involvement in one series [164] (Fig. 6.44b). Technical improvements mean that positive staining can now be shown in the great majority of cases. It should be noted that a variable proportion of neoplastic cell nuclei stain positively. Staining for CD10, CD23 and BCL6 is usually negative. The percentage of cells expressing a proliferation marker such as Ki-67 varies widely and is of prognostic significance [165].

Problems and pitfalls

Mantle cell lymphoma needs to be distinguished from other small B-cell lymphoproliferative diseases, particularly CLL, B-PLL, follicular lymphoma and marginal zone lymphomas. Immunophenotypic analysis is essential for accurate diagnosis, with CD5 and cyclin D1 being the most useful markers.

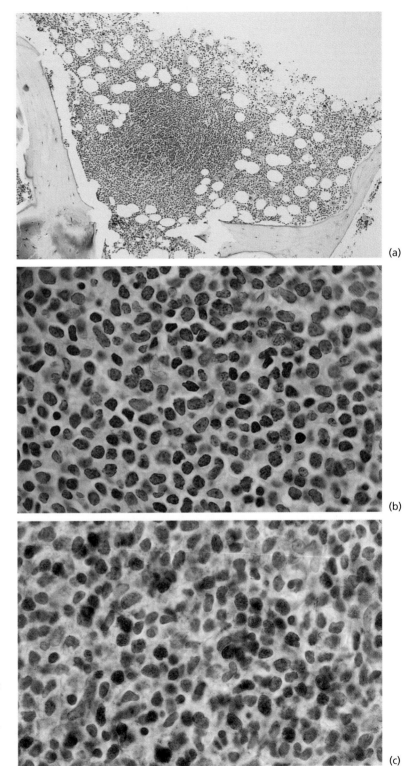

(a)

(b)

(c)

Fig. 6.44 Trephine biopsy sections, mantle cell lymphoma. (a) A mixed interstitial and nodular infiltrate; the nodule abuts on a trabecula. Paraffin-embedded, H&E ×5. (b) Very irregular small and medium-sized lymphocytes with little chromatin condensation in the larger cells. Paraffin-embedded, H&E ×100. (c) Nuclear staining for cyclin D1; note that not all the cells show positive staining. Paraffin-embedded, immunoperoxidase ×100.

The cells of CLL also express CD5 but they are negative for cyclin D1. In B-PLL, there is no expression of cyclin D1 and CD5 is usually negative. The neoplastic cells of follicular lymphoma may express CD10 and are negative for CD5 and cyclin D1. Marginal zone lymphomas can be distinguished from mantle cell lymphoma by the lack of CD5 and cyclin D1 expression.

Follicular lymphoma usually has a predominantly paratrabecular pattern of marrow infiltration, which is less common in mantle cell lymphoma. An additional interstitial infiltrate is usual in mantle cell lymphoma, whereas this is rare in follicular lymphoma. There may also be intrasinusoidal infiltration, which is rare in both CLL and follicular lymphoma although common in marginal zone lymphomas.

Extranodal marginal zone lymphoma of mucosa-associated lymphoid tissue (MALT lymphoma)

The WHO classification recognizes three types of lymphoma that are designated 'marginal zone lymphoma' – nodal, splenic and that involving mucosa-associated lymphoid tissue (MALT) – although there is some uncertainty as to the cell of origin of the splenic form [166]. Lymphomas of MALT type are relatively indolent neoplasms that occur at a number of extranodal sites including the gastro-intestinal tract, salivary gland, orbit, lung and skin. The most common primary site is the stomach, where there is an association with infection by *Helicobacter pylori* [167]. Immunoproliferative small intestinal disease, also known as α heavy chain disease, associated in at least some cases with infection by *Campylobacter jejuni*, is regarded as a variant of MALT lymphoma. MALT lymphomas at other sites also appear to be associated with chronic infections in at least a proportion of patients, with a variety of organisms being involved.

Peripheral blood
Peripheral blood involvement is rare. The cells of MALT lymphoma are small centrocyte-like cells with irregular nuclei and scanty cytoplasm.

Flow cytometric immunophenotyping
Cells express SmIg (IgM and less often IgG or IgA) and B-cell markers such as CD19, CD20, CD22, CD79a and CD79b but do not express CD5, CD10,

CD23 or cyclin D1 [166]. There is variable weak expression of CD11c.

Cytogenetic and molecular genetic analysis
Cytogenetic/molecular lesions differ in occurrence and frequency according to site [166]. Trisomy 3 has been reported in 20–75% of cases using FISH or comparative genomic hybridization techniques [166,168,169]. Trisomies 7, 12 and 18 are seen less frequently [168]. Extranodal lymphomas of MALT type are commonly associated with t(11;18) (q21;q21), resulting in the formation of an *API2-MALT1* (*AP12-MLT*) fusion gene. In one study, t(11;18) was observed in nine of 33 (27%) marginal zone lymphomas of MALT type but was not found in any cases of nodal or splenic marginal zone lymphomas [170]. Less common associations are t(1;14)(p22;q32), t(3;14)(p14.1;q32) and t(14;18)(q32;q21). Both t(11;18) and t(1;14) have been associated with a worse prognosis [171].

The putative cell of origin is a post-germinal centre marginal zone B cell showing hypermutated immunoglobulin variable region genes [166].

Bone marrow cytology and histology
The bone marrow has been considered to be infiltrated only rarely in MALT lymphoma. However, in one large series, 20% of 158 patients had infiltration [172] and in another study 10% of 72 patients with non-gastric MALT lymphoma showed infiltration [173]. Infiltration is reported to be more common with lung and ocular MALT lymphoma than with gastric MALT lymphoma [166]. In these series of patients the pattern of infiltration was not described. We have observed a mixture of nodules and paratrabecular infiltrates in some patients (about a quarter of patients) and large nodules (Fig. 6.45) in others. Interstitial infiltration sometimes accompanies other patterns [174]. Paratrabecular infiltration as the sole pattern has also been reported [175]. Neoplastic cells are predominantly small lymphocytes with variable monocytoid and plasma cell differentiation. Occasionally reactive germinal centres are observed within nodules (Fig. 6.46).

Immunohistochemistry
The neoplastic cells express CD20 and CD79a. Staining for CD5, CD10, CD23 and cyclin D1 is usually negative. BCL6 expression is also absent. CD43 expression is variable [166]. Nodules can

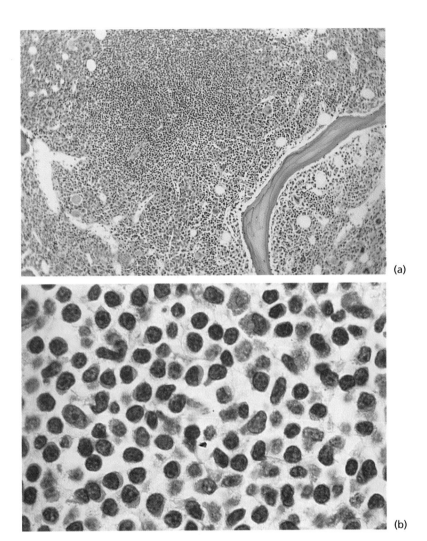

(a)

(b)

Fig. 6.45 BM trephine biopsy section, MALT lymphoma. (a) A large, ill-defined nodule. Paraffin-embedded, H&E ×10. (b) An infiltrate of small angular lymphocytes. Paraffin-embedded, H&E ×100. (By courtesy of Professor P. G. Isaacson, London.)

often be shown to be centred on lymphoid follicles with supporting meshworks of follicular dendritic cells expressing CD21, CD23 and CD35, suggesting that there is follicular colonization as is seen at primary extranodal sites. In the case of immuno-proliferative small intestinal disease, α heavy chain is expressed.

Problems and pitfalls
Marrow and peripheral blood involvement by MALT lymphoma is uncommon and seen only in late stages of the disease. If the clinical features are taken into account, it is unlikely to be confused with other lymphoproliferative disorders. However, reactive lymphoid nodules in staging bone marrow trephine biopsy specimens may be difficult to distinguish with certainty from involvement by MALT lymphoma. Careful evaluation of any additional infiltration (including examination of sections cut from multiple levels through the tissue), immuno-phenotype and immunoglobulin clonality analysis by PCR may be required in individual cases.

Splenic marginal zone lymphoma
The WHO classification recognizes splenic marginal zone lymphoma (SMZL) as a distinct entity

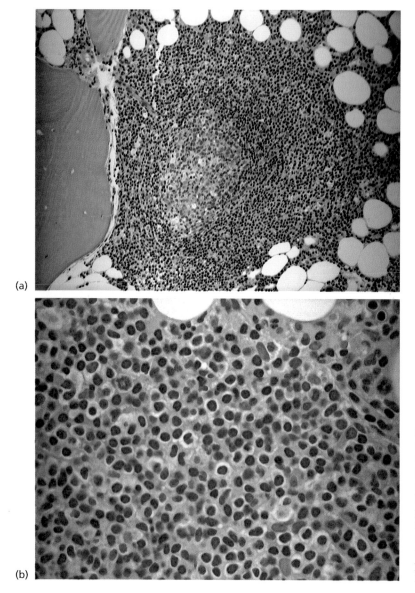

(a)

(b)

Fig. 6.46 BM trephine biopsy section from a patient with extranodal (pulmonary) marginal zone lymphoma. (a) There is a reactive germinal centre surrounded by a relatively monomorphic population of 'monocytoid' B cells. Paraffin-embedded, H&E ×10. (b) Surrounding the germinal centre there is a relatively monomorphic population of 'monocytoid' B cells. Paraffin-embedded, H&E ×60.

[176,177]. It may be diagnosed following splenectomy or from blood and bone marrow features. Cases presenting as splenic lymphoma with villous lymphocytes (SLVL) [178,179] often represent the same condition and are usually diagnosed on peripheral blood cytology and immunophenotype; however, some cases previously diagnosed as SLVL would now be regarded as examples of splenic

diffuse red pulp small B-cell lymphoma [180]. Patients with SMZL are usually over the age of 50 years with there being no gender difference. Some carry the hepatitis C virus.

SMZL is an indolent lymphoma with prominent splenomegaly and often no lymphadenopathy. Transformation to diffuse large B-cell lymphoma occurs occasionally [181] and the transformed

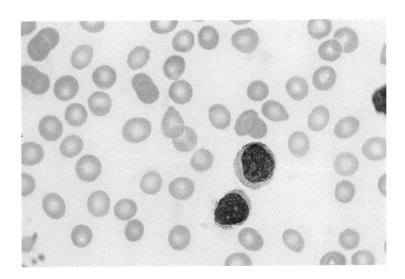

Fig. 6.47 PB film, splenic marginal zone lymphoma, showing two lymphocytes, one of which has 'villous' projections. MGG ×100.

lymphoma may have T-cell and histiocyte-rich histology.

Peripheral blood

The WBC ranges from normal to moderately elevated. In patients diagnosed by splenectomy, approaching 70% have peripheral blood involvement [182]. Circulating neoplastic cells are pleomorphic small lymphocytes, which may include 'villous' lymphocytes and some plasmacytoid lymphocytes (Fig. 6.47). There are usually also occasional plasma cells. In one study circulating cells were villous in a third of patients [182]. Villous lymphocytes are somewhat larger than CLL cells and have a round or oval nucleus with moderately condensed chromatin and, in about half of the cases, a small nucleolus. Their cytoplasm is moderately basophilic and may show short, fine cytoplasmic projections, often at one pole of the cell.

Some patients have autoimmune thrombocytopenia or anaemia [176]. Some have a paraprotein in low concentration.

Bone marrow cytology

The bone marrow aspirate is normal in about 50% of patients with SMZL, even though some such patients are found to have a nodular infiltrate on trephine biopsy [178]. The lymphoma cells are small lymphocytes, some of which show plasmacytoid differentiation. The bone marrow is infiltrated in those patients who present with SLVL.

Flow cytometric immunophenotyping

There is strong expression of SmIg (IgM and usually IgD) and expression of B-cell markers, such as CD19, CD20, CD22, CD79a and CD79b (Box 6.8). CD25 is positive in a third of cases, CD10 in a third and CD11c in a half [183]. The antigen recognized by FMC7 is expressed in most cases [184]. CD5 is usually negative; in the minority of patients with CD5 expression there may be a discrepancy between CD5-positive cells in the peripheral blood and bone marrow and CD5-negative cells in the spleen [185]. CD43, CD103, annexin A1, BCL6 and cyclin D1 are characteristically negative [176].

Cytogenetic and molecular genetic analysis

Trisomy 3 can be demonstrated by FISH in approximately 18% of patients [168,186] (Box 6.8), this being a considerably lower proportion of cases than is observed in MALT lymphoma. Trisomies 7 and 12 are found in smaller numbers of cases. Approximately 20% of cases have been reported to have t(11;14)(q13;q32) [187], correlating with cyclin D1 expression; at a molecular level this is not the same rearrangement that characterizes mantle cell lymphoma [188] but it is nevertheless considered possible that these cases do represent that disease [176]. Other recurrent translocations include t(6;14)(p12;q32) and t(9;14)(p13;q32). In contrast to MALT lymphoma, t(11;18) is not observed [176].

BOX 6.8

Splenic marginal zone lymphoma (including splenic lymphoma with villous lymphocytes)

Flow cytometric immunophenotyping
CD19+, CD20+, CD22+, CD79a+, CD79b+, strong
    SmIg (IgM, usually also IgD)
FMC7+/–, CD11c–/+, CD10–/+, CD25–/+
CD5–, CD23–, CD38-

Immunohistochemistry
CD20+, CD79a+, BCL2+
CD10–/+, CD11c–/+, CD72 (DBA.44)–/+, MUM1/
    IRF4–/+
CD5–, CD23–, CD43–, cyclin D1–, BCL6–

Cytogenetic and molecular genetic analysis
A minority of cases show cytogenetic abnormalities
    including trisomies 3, 7 and 12, t(6;14)(p12;q32)
    with *CCND3* (cyclin D3) dysregulation, and t(9;14)
    (p13;q32) with *PAX5* dysregulation
Cases with t(11;14)(q13;q32) and *CCND1* (*BCL1*)
    dysregulation may represent mantle cell
    lymphoma rather than SMZL

Percentages are approximate: +, >90% cases
positive; +/–, >50% positive; –/+, <50% positive; –,
<10% positive. Ig, immunoglobulin; SmIg, surface
membrane immunoglobulin; SMZL, splenic marginal
zone lymphoma.

Allelic loss at 7q31-32 is common [176] and loss or inactivation of *TP53* at 17p13 is found in around 10% of patients.

In about 50% of cases the cell of origin is a post-germinal centre B cell with somatic hypermutation of immunoglobulin variable region genes and some intraclonal variation [176,189,190]. One patient has been reported in whom cells initially had unmutated genes but somatic hypermutation was present when disease evolution occurred [189].

Bone marrow histology

In patients diagnosed by splenectomy, around 80% have bone marrow infiltration [182]. This is usually mixed, often with interstitial, nodular, intrasinusoidal and paratrabecular components; occasionally infiltration is diffuse (Fig. 6.48). Multiple nodules [191] and intrasinusoidal infiltration [181,192]

(Fig. 6.49) are most characteristic. The intrasinusoidal lymphocytes are CD27 negative whereas those in the interstitium and nodules are CD27 positive [193]. Nodules occasionally have germinal centres with a marginal zone [181], the germinal centres being reactive with encircling neoplastic cells [181,190,194]. An intrasinusoidal pattern is not unique to SMZL but, when it present as the predominant pattern, is believed to be highly suggestive of that diagnosis. However, a pure intrasinusoidal pattern is uncommon [191]. There may be an admixture of small lymphocytes with plasma cells and plasmacytoid lymphocytes. In about 40% of patients there is an infiltrate of monotypic plasma cells and these patients are more likely to have a paraprotein [181]. In a similar proportion of patients, there are polytypic, presumably reactive, plasma cells [181].

Immunohistochemistry

The neoplastic cells express the B-cell markers CD20 and CD79a. Staining for CD5, CD10, CD43 and cyclin D1 is negative. CD72 (reactive with DBA.44) was expressed in a third of patients in one study [181] and in most patients in another [184]. Immunohistochemical staining for CD20 or CD79a may be crucial in demonstrating intrasinusoidal infiltration. This pattern of infiltration can also be shown by using CD34 to identify endothelial cells. Reactive germinal centres in infiltrated areas can be highlighted by the lack of BCL2 expression by germinal centre B cells, whereas the surrounding lymphoma cells show expression [194].

Problems and pitfalls

Splenic marginal zone lymphoma needs to be distinguished from other small B-cell lymphoproliferative disorders that present with peripheral blood lymphocytosis and splenomegaly, particularly hairy cell leukaemia, CLL and mantle cell lymphoma. The circulating cells are larger than those of CLL and have a higher nucleocytoplasmic ratio than hairy cells. Lack of CD5 and CD23 staining further distinguishes SMZL from CLL. In contrast to the cells of hairy cell leukaemia, the neoplastic cells of SMZL are usually TRAP negative. Marginal zone lymphomas have a similar immunophenotype so this does not provide a basis for distinguishing between them.

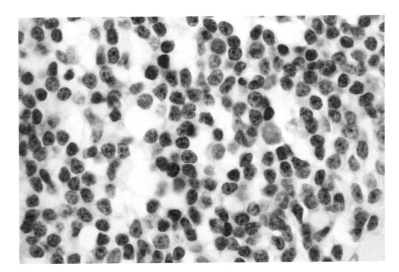

Fig. 6.48 BM trephine biopsy section, splenic marginal zone lymphoma, showing diffuse infiltration by mature small lymphocytes and occasional cells with plasmacytoid features. Resin-embedded, H&E ×100.

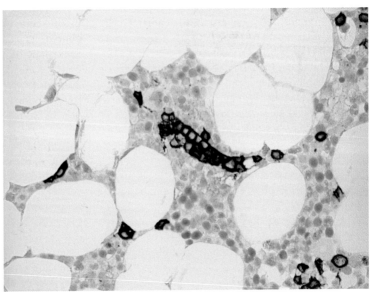

Fig. 6.49 BM trephine biopsy section showing intrasinusoidal infiltration by splenic marginal zone lymphoma. Although endothelial cells lining sinusoids are usually inapparent without additional immunostaining (e.g. for CD34) the linear array of CD20-positive lymphocytes is distinctive. There are also scattered interstitial CD20-positive lymphocytes. Paraffin-embedded, immunoperoxidase for CD20 ×40.

Intrasinusoidal infiltration by neoplastic cells is likely to be missed unless immunohistochemistry is used. A pure intrasinusoidal pattern of bone marrow infiltration by small B cells raises the possibility of an alternative diagnosis, e.g. splenic diffuse red pulp small B-cell lymphoma (see below) or smoking-associated polyclonal B lymphocytosis [89]. The pattern of marrow infiltration in trephine biopsy sections in hairy cell leukaemia is characteristic and is unlikely to be confused with SMZL unless minimal infiltrates mimic intrasinusoidal involvement. Because of the frequent occurrence of a monotypic plasma cell component within infiltrates of SMZL, distinction from lymphoplasmacytic lymphoma may not be possible [181]. Indeed, it is controversial how distinct these two conditions are, since patients may have disease features overlapping between the two.

Nodal marginal zone B-cell lymphoma

Nodal marginal zone lymphoma (which includes tumours previously classified as monocytoid B-cell lymphoma) is a rare condition [195] recognized as a distinct entity in the WHO classification [196]. It usually presents with lymphadenopathy and needs to be distinguished from nodal spread from an extranodal marginal zone lymphoma of MALT type and from follicular lymphoma lacking CD10 expression [146,197]. Some patients have hepatitis C infection. Bone marrow infiltration is rare.

Peripheral blood
Peripheral blood involvement is rare. The circulating neoplastic monocytoid B cells are small to medium-sized cells, which may have some similarities to hairy cells. They have been described as having homogeneous, round to reniform or irregular nuclei and relatively abundant, weakly basophilic cytoplasm, which may have a few hair-like projections [194,198].

Flow cytometric immunophenotyping
The lymphoma cells express SmIg and B-cell markers such as CD19, CD20, CD22, CD79a and CD79b. There is usually no expression of CD5, CD10, CD23 or cyclin D1. There is expression of CD11c in some cases.

Cytogenetic and molecular genetic analysis
Some cases have trisomy 3, 7 or 18 [168,186].

Bone marrow histology
The bone marrow is rarely infiltrated [198–201]. When infiltration occurs, the pattern may be focal and predominantly paratrabecular [198] or nodular [201]. The infiltrate may consist of loose polymorphic nodules made up of monocytoid B cells, small lymphocytes with irregular nuclei and plasma cells [202].

Immunohistochemistry
The lymphoma cells express B-cell markers CD20 and CD79a. Staining for CD5, CD10, CD23, CD43 and cyclin D1 is usually negative [203]. Approximately half of cases are CD43 positive [196].

Problems and pitfalls
Marrow infiltration by nodal marginal zone lymphoma needs to be distinguished from other small B-cell lymphoproliferative disorders, particularly CLL, follicular lymphoma and mantle cell lymphoma. The presence of a monocytoid B-cell component and the lack of expression of CD5, CD10 and CD23 by the cells of nodal marginal zone lymphoma are helpful in making this distinction. Separation from SMZL and marginal zone lymphoma of MALT type requires consideration of the clinical features and peripheral blood findings since marginal zone lymphomas of all three types share a similar immunophenotype.

Splenic B-cell lymphoma/leukaemia, unclassifiable

Splenic diffuse red pulp small B-cell lymphoma
The 2008 WHO classification has introduced two provisional entities under the heading of splenic B-cell lymphoma/leukaemia, unclassifiable. One of these is splenic diffuse red pulp small B-cell lymphoma. This condition has many similarities to SMZL but its splenic histology differs and is the basis of the diagnosis [180]. Clinically there is prominent splenomegaly without lymphadenopathy. Histologically there is diffuse red pulp infiltration in cords and sinusoids.

Peripheral blood
There is usually a relatively mild lymphocytosis with villous lymphocytes.

Bone marrow cytology
The bone marrow is infiltrated by small lymphoid cells, typically villous.

Flow cytometric immunophenotyping
There is expression of B-cell markers but CD5, CD10, CD23 and markers typical of hairy cell leukaemia are negative.

Cytogenetic and molecular genetic analysis
No characteristic cytogenetic association has been found but complex karyotypes and t(9;14)(p13;q32) have been observed.

Bone marrow histology
Intrasinusoidal infiltration is usual and sometimes, and most distinctively, this is the exclusive pattern. However, there may be accompanying nodular or interstitial infiltration or both. [204].

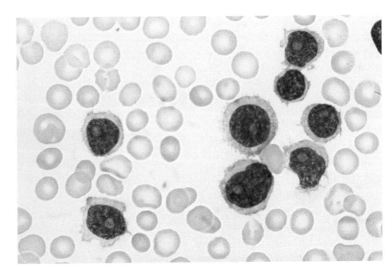

Fig. 6.50 PB film, variant form of hairy cell leukaemia; the nuclei have prominent nucleoli resembling those of prolymphocytes and the cytoplasm is weakly basophilic with hair-like projections. MGG ×100.

Immunohistochemistry

The lymphoma cells express B-cell markers. They may express CD72 but not TRAP or other markers typical of hairy cell leukaemia.

Problems and pitfalls

Awareness of this rare variant is necessary to ensure that it is considered in the differential diagnosis of small B-cell lymphoma presenting with splenomegaly.

Hairy cell leukaemia variant

The very rare 'variant form of hairy cell leukaemia' is not in fact a variant of hairy cell leukaemia although it is morphologically somewhat similar. It differs in cytological and haematological features and in its responsiveness to various therapeutic agents [205]. This is the second provisional entity introduced in the 2008 WHO classification [180] under the heading of splenic B-cell lymphoma/leukaemia, unclassifiable. Its relationship to splenic diffuse red pulp small B-cell lymphoma and SMZL is currently unknown. The major clinical feature is splenomegaly.

Peripheral blood

This condition differs from hairy cell leukaemia in that the WBC is usually moderately to markedly elevated and numerous neoplastic cells are present in the peripheral blood. Anaemia and thrombocy-topenia are each seen in about 50% of patients but pancytopenia is generally less pronounced than in hairy cell leukaemia and monocytopenia and neutropenia are not usual. The cells have somewhat more cytoplasmic basophilia than classical hairy cells but show the same irregular cytoplasmic margins. The nucleus, which shows moderate chromatin condensation, has a prominent nucleolus similar to that seen in B-PLL; this is the major distinguishing cytological feature from hairy cell leukaemia (Fig. 6.50). Variable numbers of binucleate cells and large cells with hyperchromatic nuclei are present [205].

Bone marrow cytology

Bone marrow aspiration is usually easier than in hairy cell leukaemia. The aspirate often contains numerous cells with the same features as those in the blood.

Flow cytometric immunophenotyping

The cytochemical and immunological markers differ in some respects from those of hairy cell leukaemia. TRAP reactivity is usually not detectable. There is usually expression of CD11c, CD19, CD20, CD22, CD72, the antigen recognized by FMC7 and various plasma cell markers. The hairy cell leukaemia markers, CD25, CD123, HC2 and annexin A1, are usually negative but there may be expression of CD103.

Cytogenetic and molecular genetic analysis

It is likely that the neoplastic clone is derived from a post-germinal centre B cell with hypermutated immunoglobulin variable region genes. Various clonal cytogenetic abnormalities have been described, among which those most often reported are trisomies (e.g. trisomy 5, 6 or 12), monosomies (e.g. 10, 12 or 17) and translocations with a 14q32 breakpoint.

Bone marrow histology

The trephine biopsy appearances [205] differ from those of hairy cell leukaemia. Infiltration is interstitial and less confluent than is usual in hairy cell leukaemia. Cells may form clumps without the intercellular spaces that are characteristic of hairy cell leukaemia or there may be a mixture of clumps of cells and spaced cells. Moderately condensed chromatin and prominent nucleoli are apparent. A dominant sinusoidal pattern of infiltration is common [191]. There is only a slight to moderate increase in reticulin fibres.

Diffuse large B-cell lymphoma and other large B-cell lymphomas

In the 2008 WHO classification, lymphomas of large B cells are further subdivided in a variety of different ways. Major categories are recognized as distinct clinicopathological entities and these are: (i) diffuse large B-cell lymphoma, not otherwise specified (DLBCL, NOS), which is the largest category and which remains heterogeneous; (ii) four specific subtypes of DLBCL; and (iii) eight other subtypes of lymphoma of large B cells [206] (see Table 6.1, page 301). In the 2008 WHO classification T-cell/histiocyte-rich DLBCL is a specific subtype of lymphoma categorized for the first time as a distinct subtype of DLBCL; it is one of the four specific subtypes referred to above. Intravascular large B-cell lymphoma, one of the eight other specified subtypes of large B-cell lymphoma, is a rare variant that may be first diagnosed by bone marrow biopsy [207]. In some subtypes of large B-cell lymphoma bone marrow infiltration has not been described. The 2008 WHO classification also recognizes 'grey zone' lymphomas in which features of

DLBCL overlap with those of either Burkitt lymphoma or classical Hodgkin lymphoma.

Diffuse large B-cell lymphoma (including diffuse large B-cell lymphoma, not otherwise specified)

Diffuse large B-cell lymphoma is the commonest subtype of lymphoma, accounting for about a fifth of all cases. It is uncommon in children and adolescents but rises steadily in incidence thereafter, reaching about 50 per 100 000 per year in those over 75 years [36]. DLBCL, NOS can be further subdivided on histological grounds into centroblastic, immunoblastic and anaplastic variants (see below). It can also be divided, on the basis of immunophenotyping or gene expression profiling, into germinal centre B-cell like, activated B-cell like and indeterminate (see below). The correlations between morphological, immunophenotypic and gene expression subclassifications are imperfect.

Bone marrow infiltration is much less common in DLBCL than in the other B-lineage lymphoproliferative diseases. Bone marrow involvement, particularly if there is a diffuse pattern of infiltration, is associated with a poor prognosis [208]. Concordant bone marrow infiltration is prognostically adverse, independently of the International Prognostic Index, whereas discordant infiltration, with low grade B-cell lymphoma in the bone marrow, is not [209]. Rarely patients with DLBCL have isolated bone marrow disease, detected following presentation with systemic symptoms and cytopenia [210]. Bone marrow trephine biopsy is indicated in those patients in whom detection of involvement would alter treatment. Biopsy should therefore be done in patients with apparently limited stage disease in whom the therapeutic plan is for brief chemotherapy followed by involved-field radiotherapy [143]. It need not necessarily be performed to indicate the requirement for central nervous system (CNS) prophylaxis since there is only 1% incidence of CNS relapse in the absence of bulky disease, high lactate dehydrogenase and high International Prognostic Index [143].

Cytogenetic and molecular genetic analysis

Typical cytogenetic abnormalities (Box 6.9) differ according to the specific subtype of DLBCL (see below). Translocations with a 3q27 breakpoint,

Diffuse large B-cell lymphoma

Flow cytometric immunophenotyping
CD19+, CD20+, CD22+, CD79a+, SmIg+
Variable expression of CD5, CD10, CD30
CD34–, TdT–

Immunohistochemistry
CD20+, CD79a+, PAX5+, OCT2+, BOB1+
Variable expression of CD5, CD10, CD23, CD30,
    MUM1/IRF4, BCL2 and BCL6
CD15–, CD34–, TdT–

Cytogenetic and molecular genetic analysis
Complex abnormalities are common. Frequently seen
    abnormalities include t(14;18)(q32;q21), t(3;14)
    (q27;q32), t(1;3)(q34;q27), t(2;3)(q35;q27), t(3;12)
    (q27;q13), t(3;22)(q27;q11), inv(3)(q13q27) and
    aneuploidy with loss of Y, 6, 13, 15 and 17 and
    gains of X, 3, 5, 7, 12 and 18; in those with a 3q27
    breakpoint there is generally dysregulation of *BCL6*
EBER may be positive

Percentages are approximate: +, >90% cases
positive; +/–, >50% positive; –/+, <50% positive; –,
<10% positive. EBER, Epstein–Barr virus early RNA;
SmIg, surface membrane immunoglobulin; TdT,
terminal deoxynucleotidyl transferase.

seen in all subtypes of DLBCL, include t(1;3)
(q34;q27),   t(2;3)(q35;q27),   t(3;12)(q27;q13),
t(3;22)(q27;q11) and inv(3)(q13q27).

Many cases of DLBCL, NOS have hypermutated
IGH with evidence of ongoing mutation and there
is often somatic hypermutation in unrelated genes
including *MYC* and *PAX5*. *MYC* rearrangements are
found in approximately 10% of cases, usually with
additional complex genetic abnormalities; there is
concurrent *IGH-BCL2* or *BCL6* rearrangement, or
both, in about 20% of cases with rearranged *MYC*.

Microarray analysis for gene expression divides
DLBCL, NOS, into three groups: those with a germinal centre B-cell-like phenotype, those with an
activated B-cell-like phenotype and those with
neither [211]. *BCL2* translocation and *REL* amplification were seen only in the first group, which has
a better prognosis than the latter two groups. The
first two microarray phenotypes can be related, to
some extent, to centroblastic and immunoblastic

morphological subgroups, respectively. The microarray phenotype also correlates with immunophenotypic features, e.g. expression of BCL6 and CD10
with a germinal centre pattern. The better prognostic significance of a germinal centre phenotype in
comparison with an activated B-cell-like phenotype was first described in patient cohorts pre-
dating the rituximab era but is also present in
patients who receive rituximab in addition to combination chemotherapy [212]. Gene expression
profiles that relate to the stromal response rather
than the tumour cells are also of prognostic significance in DLBCL. A gene expression signature that
relates to extracellular matrix deposition and macrophage infiltration is prognostically good, whereas
a signature that reflects tumour blood vessel density
is prognostically bad [212].

Immunohistochemistry

The tumour cells express the B-cell markers CD20
and CD79a (see Box 6.9). OCT2 and BOB1 are
expressed [56]. There is variable expression of CD5,
CD10, CD30, CD43, BCL2, BCL6 and MUM1/IRF4.
CD30 expression is preferentially associated with
the morphological anaplastic variant [206]. Cyclin
D1 is not expressed [206]. Some cases show p53
expression but reports vary as to how frequent this
is [206]. Staining for Ki-67 antigen shows a variable but often high proliferative fraction. TdT and
CD34 are not expressed.

A better prognosis has been associated with
BCL6 and CD10 expression and a worse prognosis
with expression of BCL2 or a high proliferative
fraction [206,213–216]. Expression of MUM1/IRF4
and cyclin D2 correlate with a worse prognosis
[216]. Over-expression of p53 in the absence of
equivalent over-expression of p21 is a surrogate for
a *TP53* mutation and correlates with a worse prognosis [217,218]. CD40 expression is prognostically
favourable [219].

Problems and pitfalls

Diffuse large B-cell lymphoma, NOS, can be easily
confused with various T-cell lymphomas so that
immunohistochemistry is essential for diagnosis. In
addition, the immunoblastic variant can be confused with plasmablastic variant of plasma cell
myeloma, the anaplastic variant with anaplastic
T-cell lymphoma and carcinoma. A distinction

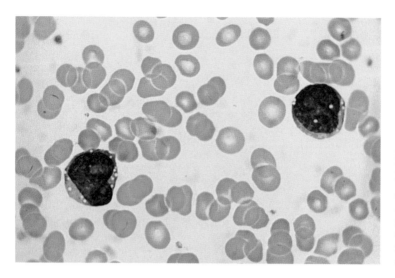

Fig. 6.51 PB film, diffuse large B-cell lymphoma (morphological variant, centroblastic lymphoma), showing large lymphoma cells with a high nucleocytoplasmic ratio, moderately basophilic vacuolated cytoplasm and medium-sized nucleoli sited towards the periphery of the nucleus. MGG ×100.

from aggressive variants of mantle cell lymphoma is also necessary.

Diffuse large B-cell lymphoma, not otherwise specified – morphological variant, centroblastic

The centroblastic variant of DLBCL, NOS [1,220] is a clinically aggressive lymphoma that may occur *de novo* or may represent transformation of a follicular lymphoma.

Peripheral blood

Lymphoma cells are rarely present in the peripheral blood. When the centroblastic variant occurs as a transformation of follicular lymphoma any circulating lymphoma cells are usually centrocytes. When peripheral blood dissemination of centroblasts does occur, the cells are very large and pleomorphic (Fig. 6.51). They have plentiful cytoplasm and an irregular, often lobated nucleus containing one or more fairly prominent nucleoli.

Bone marrow cytology

Bone marrow infiltration is uncommon but is considerably more common than peripheral blood spread; in one series, infiltration was detected in 15% of cases. In patients with preceding follicular lymphoma, the bone marrow is sometimes infiltrated by centroblasts but more often shows only centrocytes. A significant minority of patients with apparently *de novo* centroblastic lymphoma at an

extramedullary site also show infiltration of the bone marrow by centrocytes, indicative of underlying follicular lymphoma [21]. The presence of low grade follicular lymphoma in the bone marrow does not have the same poor prognostic significance as bone marrow infiltration by DLBCL, NOS.

Cytogenetic and molecular genetic analysis

In many cases the centroblastic variant of DLBCL, NOS arises in a germinal centre B cell that in some patients shows ongoing somatic *IGH* hypermutation. This variant shows t(14;18)(q32;q21) with *BCL2* rearrangement in about a third of patients and a fifth have gain of 12q12 [206]. Rearrangement of *MYC* worsens the prognosis in patients with t(14;18) [221]. The next most common group of abnormalities are t(3;14)(q27;q32) and other translocations with a 3q27 breakpoint resulting in rearrangement of the *BCL6* gene [222]. *REL* amplification is found in about 15% of patients [206,211]. Complex aberrant clones are common. Aneuploidy is a frequent finding with loss of Y, 6, 13, 15 and 17 and gains of X, 3, 5, 7, 12 and 18.

Bone marrow histology

Infiltration of the marrow is seen in 20–30% of patients with the centroblastic variant of DLBCL [12,14]. This may be concordant infiltration by centroblasts or discordant infiltration by low grade follicular lymphoma [12,14,22]. Discordance is relatively common. Low grade lymphoma may be

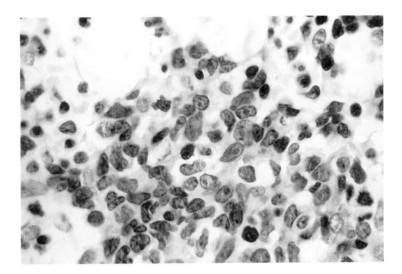

Fig. 6.52 BM trephine biopsy section, diffuse large B-cell lymphoma (morphological variant, centroblastic lymphoma), showing infiltration by pleomorphic centroblasts and occasional immunoblasts. Resin-embedded, H&E ×100.

seen both in those with and without a previous history of low grade disease. The pattern of centroblast infiltration may be either focal or diffuse. The infiltrate may be composed of relatively monomorphic centroblasts or may be pleomorphic with admixed immunoblasts (Fig. 6.52), multilobated cells and large cleft cells. By definition (WHO classification), immunoblasts do not exceed 90%.

Immunohistochemistry

There is expression of B-cell markers, which may include CD20, CD79a and PAX5. Immunohistochemical staining may demonstrate a germinal centre B-cell pattern with expression of CD10 or of BCL6 with no expression of MUM1/IRF4. However, it should be noted that centroblastic morphology does not correlate closely with a germinal centre immunophenotype or genotype.

Diffuse large B-cell lymphoma, not otherwise specified – morphological variant, immunoblastic

The immunoblastic variant of DLBCL is a clinically aggressive lymphoma that can develop in previously healthy subjects or in patients with immunodeficiency. The immunodeficiency may be either congenital or the result of HIV infection or immunosuppressive therapy. The Epstein–Barr virus (EBV) is implicated in the pathogenesis of many but not all cases in immunodeficient subjects. The immunoblastic variant of DLBCL may also occur following transformation of a low grade lymphoproliferative disease such as CLL or lymphoplasmacytic lymphoma. The immunoblastic variant occurs at all ages. Because of the relationship to underlying immune deficiency this subtype forms a significant proportion of childhood lymphomas. Prognosis appears to be worse than in the centroblastic variant [206]. The definition of this subtype in the WHO classification requires there to be more than 90% immunoblasts [206].

Peripheral blood

Neoplastic cells are rarely present in the peripheral blood. When present they are very large with plentiful, strongly basophilic cytoplasm and a large nucleus containing a prominent central nucleolus. In patients with underlying immune deficiency there may be marked lymphopenia or, in patients with AIDS, pancytopenia.

Bone marrow cytology

The bone marrow is not often infiltrated; in one series marrow infiltration was seen in less than a quarter of patients [65]. When lymphoma cells are present they have the same morphological features as those described above (Fig. 6.53). A significant minority of patients with the immunoblastic variant of DLBCL at an extramedullary site show low grade lymphoma in the bone marrow, usually follicular lymphoma, but occasionally small lymphocytic lymphoma with plasmacytoid differentiation [21]; this does not have the same grave prognostic import as marrow infiltration by immunoblasts.

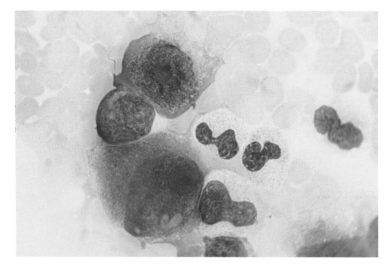

Fig. 6.53 BM aspirate, diffuse large B-cell lymphoma (morphological variant, immunoblastic lymphoma) in a patient with AIDS, showing lymphoma cells varying from medium-sized to very large; note the basophilic cytoplasm and, in the largest cell, a giant nucleolus. MGG ×100.

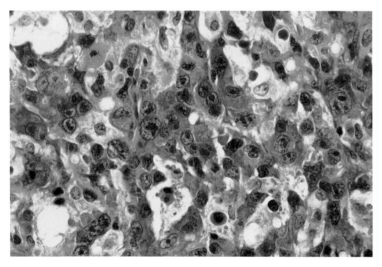

Fig. 6.54 BM trephine biopsy section, diffuse large B-cell lymphoma (morphological variant, immunoblastic lymphoma) in a patient with AIDS (same patient as Fig. 6.53), showing diffuse infiltration by pleomorphic immunoblasts; note the prominent central nucleoli. Paraffin-embedded, H&E ×40.

Cytogenetic and molecular genetic analysis

This variant arises in a B cell that does not show somatic hypermutation [223]. It is characterized by complex aberrant clones, t(3;14)(q27;q32) and other translocations with a 3q27 breakpoint and *BCL6* rearrangement. Other cytogenetic abnormalities include gains of 3q and 18q21-22 and losses of 6q21-22 [206]. There may also be loss of Y, 8, 10, 14 and 21 and gain of 3, 7, 12 and 18.

Bone marrow histology

The neoplastic cells of the immunoblastic variant are distinguished from centroblasts by virtue of their larger size, more plentiful cytoplasm and the presence of a very large, prominent and usually central nucleolus (Fig. 6.54). Some cases have marked nuclear lobation. Binucleated and multi-nucleated forms may be present. Some cells may show signs of plasma cell differentiation but it is usually not possible to distinguish between T- and B-lineage immunoblasts on the basis of morphology alone [224].

The marrow is infiltrated in 15–20% of cases [12,65]. The pattern of bone marrow infiltration may be random focal, paratrabecular or diffuse [12,14,127]. In some patients there is marrow infiltration by discordant low grade lymphoma.

Immunohistochemistry

There is expression of B-cell markers which may include CD20, CD79a and PAX5. Immunohistochemical staining usually demonstrates a non-germinal centre phenotype with no expression of CD10, BCL6 infrequently positive and MUM1/IRF4 more often positive [223].

Diffuse large B-cell lymphoma, not otherwise specified – morphological variant, anaplastic

The anaplastic morphological variant of DLBCL resembles T-lineage anaplastic large cell lymphoma (see page 384) histologically but is an unrelated condition.

Flow cytometric immunophenotyping

B-cell antigens such as CD19, CD20, CD22 and CD79a are expressed (see Box 6.9). SmIg (IgM or, less often IgG or IgA) is expressed in the majority of cases. Cytoplasmic immunoglobulin is present in some cells in cases showing plasmacytic differentiation. Expression of CD5, CD10 and CD30 is variable. There is no expression of TdT or CD34.

Cytogenetic and molecular genetic analysis

No specific genetic abnormalities have been recognized.

Bone marrow histology

Sinusoidal and cohesive growth patterns have been described in other tissues but we have not observed a sinusoidal pattern in the bone marrow.

Diffuse large B-cell lymphoma

Subtype T-cell/histiocyte-rich large B-cell lymphoma

Some cases of DLBCL have admixed reactive cells, sometimes in considerable numbers, to the extent that neoplastic cells are in a minority and may be obscured by the accompanying reaction. Such cases are designated T-cell/histiocyte-rich large B-cell lymphoma (Figs 6.55 and 6.56). The WHO classification requires that neoplastic cells are less than 10% of cells of the infiltrate [225]. Cases that are T-cell rich but lack histiocytes are also included in this category but EBV-positive cases are excluded [225]. There is a male predominance, median age is low, most patients present with advanced disease and prognosis is poor [226,227].

Bone marrow histology

Bone marrow infiltration has been reported in between 17% and 60% of cases [225]. One study showed a much higher incidence of involvement than is seen in other subtypes of DLBCL [228]. Infiltration may be focal or diffuse. There are dispersed, large, atypical B cells with prominent nucleoli, often with lobated nuclei, set in a background containing large numbers of small T lymphocytes and histiocytes. Neoplastic B cells, which are infrequent, may resemble centroblasts, mononuclear Hodgkin cells or Reed–Sternberg cells of classical Hodgkin lymphoma or LP cells (for lym-

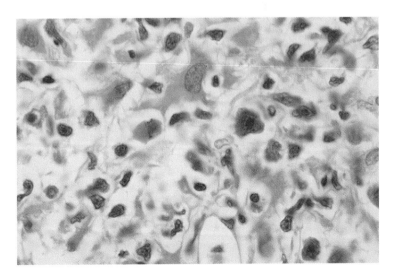

Fig. 6.55 BM trephine biopsy section, diffuse large B-cell lymphoma, subtype T-cell/histiocyte-rich B-cell lymphoma. Paraffin-embedded, H&E ×100. (By courtesy of Dr W. Erber and Dr L. Matz, Perth, Western Australia.)

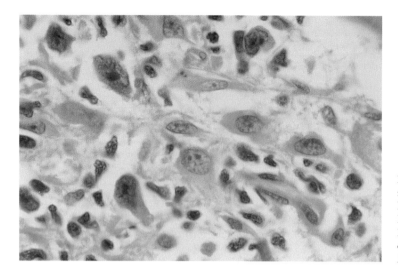

Fig. 6.56 BM trephine biopsy section, diffuse large B-cell lymphoma, subtype T-cell/histiocyte-rich B-cell lymphoma. Paraffin-embedded, H&E ×100. (By courtesy of Dr W. Erber and Dr L. Matz, Perth, Western Australia.)

phocyte predominant cells) of nodular lymphocyte-predominant Hodgkin lymphoma [206].

Immunohistochemistry

Immunohistochemical staining demonstrates that the large neoplastic cells are B cells (CD20 and CD79a positive) (Fig. 6.57a, b). They express CD45 and are negative for CD15, CD30 and CD138. There is usually expression of BCL6 and sometimes of BCL2 and epithelial membrane antigen. The smaller reactive lymphocytes are CD3-positive T cells (Fig. 6.57c, d). The reactive macrophages express CD68.

Problems and pitfalls

The marrow is often inaspirable but, if marrow is aspirated, flow cytometric immunophenotyping can be misleading since the majority of cells present are reactive T cells and the presence of small numbers of large monoclonal B cells may not be appreciated. Histologically there can be confusion with classical Hodgkin lymphoma or, in cases with only very rare large B cells, with T-cell lymphoma. It may be necessary to examine haematoxylin and eosin (H&E) and immunostained sections from several levels in order to demonstrate the neoplastic cells. However, it is very rare for this lymphoma to present primarily in the bone marrow and there is usually confirmatory diagnostic tissue from another site.

Subtype primary diffuse large B-cell lymphoma of the CNS

Not only central nervous system but also intra-ocular lymphomas are included in this subtype. Dissemination to the bone marrow is very rare.

Other lymphomas of large B cells

Primary mediastinal (thymic) large B-cell lymphoma

Primary mediastinal (thymic) large B-cell lymphoma is a distinct subtype of large B-cell lymphoma which characteristically presents as bulky mediastinal disease in young women [229]. The 2008 WHO classification requires absence of bone marrow disease to make the diagnosis [230]. However, bone marrow infiltration has been reported by others in a very small percentage of cases, in one series only 2% [229] and in another 4% [231]. Typically there is expression of CD20, CD23 and MUM1/IRF4 with CD30 and BCL2 often being positive and BCL6 being positive in about half of patients [56,230]. Reactions are typically negative for CD5, CD10 and SmIg [56,230].

Intravascular large B-cell lymphoma

Intravascular large B-cell lymphoma is a rare subtype of large cell B-cell lymphoma characterized by a tendency for the lymphoma cells to remain confined within the lumens of small and intermediate-sized blood vessels [232,233]. In European

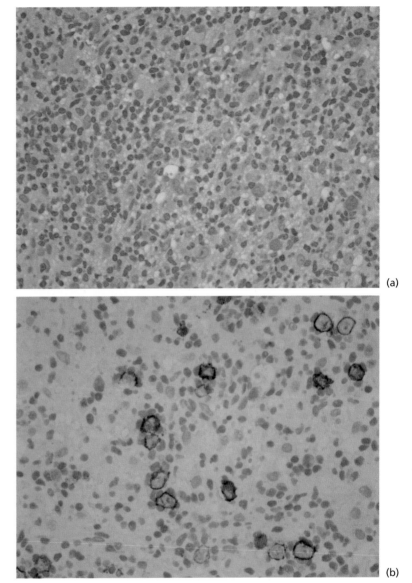

(a)

Fig. 6.57 BM trephine biopsy sections from a patient with diffuse large B-cell lymphoma, subtype T-cell/histiocyte-rich B-cell lymphoma. (a) H&E staining showing scattered large neoplastic cells, with prominent eosinophilic nucleoli, in a reactive background. Paraffin-embedded ×40. (b) Immunoperoxidase for CD20 showing that the large neoplastic cells are of B lineage and are accompanied by only rare small reactive B cells. Paraffin-embedded ×40.

(b)

continued

patients the most common involved sites are the skin and CNS. In the Asian variant these sites are not generally involved, whilst the bone marrow is the site most often involved and hepatosplenomegaly without lymphadenopathy is usual [234,235]. The disease has been reported to involve a number of other organs including, kidneys, liver, lungs and gastro-intestinal tract.

Peripheral blood

A single patient has been reported in whom diagnosis resulted from aspiration of a clump of lymphoma cells with a peripheral blood sample [236]. Usually circulating lymphoma cells are not a feature but there may be other peripheral blood abnormalities, which have included leucopenia, autoimmune haemolytic anaemia and pancytopenia.

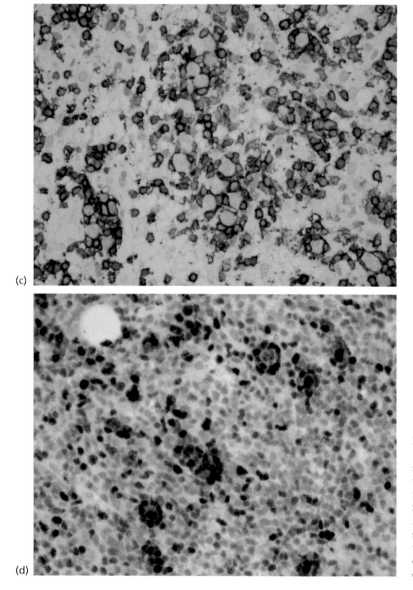

(c)

(d)

Fig. 6.57 (continued)
(c) Immunoperoxidase for CD3 showing small reactive T cells, which greatly outnumber the neoplastic B cells. Paraffin-embedded ×40. (d) Immunoperoxidase for MUM1/IRF4 showing positively stained reactive T cells encircling the neoplastic B cells, which also express this antigen. Paraffin-embedded ×40.

Anaemia, thrombocytopenia and pancytopenia are common in patients with the Asian variant [233,234,237]; isolated leucopenia is less common.

Bone marrow cytology
Lymphoma cells have been detected in bone marrow aspirates in the Asian variant of intravascular lymphoma. Cells are large with irregular nuclei and

moderate amounts of basophilic cytoplasm, which is sometimes vacuolated [237]. Reactive haemophagocytosis can be a feature, even in patients who lack bone marrow infiltration [238].

Bone marrow histology
Among European patients, bone marrow infiltration is uncommon. In one series it was found in

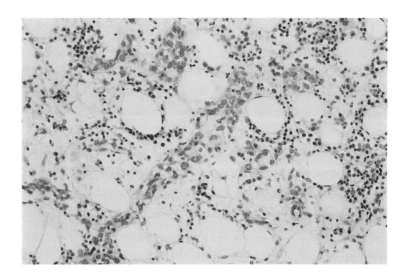

Fig. 6.58 BM trephine biopsy section, intravascular large B-cell lymphoma, showing sinusoids packed with atypical, large lymphoid cells. Paraffin-embedded, H&E ×20.

14% of patients [239]. However, among Asian patients bone marrow infiltration is usual and haemophagocytosis is common [234,237]. When the marrow is infiltrated, large atypical lymphoma cells with irregular, often lobulated nuclei, multiple prominent nucleoli and moderate amounts of basophilic cytoplasm are found, predominantly within sinusoids. A bone marrow trephine biopsy specimen or clotted aspirated marrow may be the initial diagnostic material (Fig. 6.58).

Immunohistochemistry
Identification of the infiltrating cells is facilitated by immunohistochemical staining for B-cell antigens (CD20 or CD79a) and CD34 staining to outline blood vessels. MUM1/IRF4 is expressed in the majority, CD5 in about 38% and CD10 in about 13% [235].

Large B-cell lymphoma arising in HHV8-associated multicentric Castleman's disease
This is an aggressive lymphoma that is cytologically plasmablastic, occurring mainly in HIV-infected persons who carry human herpesvirus 8 (HHV8). Leukaemic evolution can occur with appearance of plasmablasts in the peripheral blood [240,241].

Primary effusion lymphoma
Primary effusion lymphoma is a subtype of large cell B-cell lymphoma predominantly seen in patients with AIDS. It is associated with HHV8 and, usually, with co-infection by EBV. It presents typi-

cally with pleural or pericardial effusion or ascites in the absence of a tumour mass. The lymphoma usually remains localized to the body cavity in which it originated and bone marrow infiltration is not a feature [242]. However, a large cell extranodal lymphoma with a similar phenotype and herpesvirus association also occurs and occasionally such patients have had bone marrow infiltration [241,243].

Evidence of B-lineage differentiation in primary effusion lymphoma and its variants may be limited or undetectable by immunohistochemistry but there is usually detectable *IGH* rearrangement [243]. CD30 and HHV8 latency-associated nuclear antigen (LANA) are expressed and usually Epstein–Barr early RNA (EBER).

Burkitt lymphoma
Burkitt lymphoma is an aggressive lymphoma, the clinical features of which differ depending on whether cases are endemic, sporadic or immunodeficiency related. Endemic Burkitt lymphoma occurs in tropical Africa and New Guinea and is particularly a disease of childhood; tumour formation in the jaw is usually the most prominent clinical feature. Sporadic Burkitt lymphoma is worldwide in distribution and occurs at all ages; the commonest clinical features are abdominal tumour formation and malignant pleural or peritoneal effusions. Most cases of immunodeficiency-related Burkitt lymphoma occur among patients with AIDS but

cases also occur among other immunodeficient patients, particularly following organ transplantation. Clinically, immunodeficiency-related Burkitt lymphoma resembles sporadic disease more closely than endemic disease but meningeal and bone marrow involvement appear to be particularly common. EBV is an important pathogenetic factor in endemic Burkitt lymphoma and in a significant proportion of immunodeficiency-related cases but is much less often implicated in sporadic cases. EBV is more often implicated in AIDS-related cases in Africa than in developed countries [244]. The cell of origin appears to differ in EBV-positive and EBV-negative cases. EBV-related cases arise from a post-germinal centre memory B cell, whereas EBV-negative cases arise in a germinal centre B cell [244]. Except in the context of HIV infection, Burkitt lymphoma is rare in developed countries, less than 1 per 1 million per year; it is three times as common in men as in women [36].

Burkitt lymphoma can show plasmacytoid differentiation, particularly in immunodeficient patients, and these and others may show more pleomorphism; such cases do not differ in other features from morphologically typical cases [245].

The FAB L3 category of ALL is usually a leukaemic presentation of Burkitt lymphoma and, when this is so, is appropriately classified as Burkitt lymphoma rather than as ALL.

In the 2008 WHO classification, the category of Burkitt-like lymphoma has been abolished. Some of these cases are now included in the Burkitt lymphoma category while others are assigned to a new category of 'B-cell lymphoma, unclassifiable, with features intermediate between DLBCL and Burkitt lymphoma' [246]. This is seen as a heterogeneous group of diseases and includes cases with a mixture of small/medium-sized and large cells; some cases have BCL2 expression, some a low proliferation fraction and some have two mutations (e.g. of both *MYC* and *BCL2*). Some cases are likely to represent transformation of follicular lymphoma or other low grade lymphoma.

Peripheral blood

In the majority of patients with Burkitt lymphoma the peripheral blood shows no abnormality. Even when the bone marrow is infiltrated, circulating lymphoma cells are present in less than half of patients. Some patients whose peripheral blood is initially normal, subsequently show circulating lymphoma cells with disease progression or relapse. Circulating neoplastic cells are medium-sized, relatively uniform blasts with round nuclei, stippled chromatin, visible but delicate nucleoli, strongly basophilic cytoplasm and prominent cytoplasmic vacuolation. Peripheral blood dissemination appears to be particularly common in patients with underlying AIDS. Such patients are also commonly pancytopenic, even in the absence of bone marrow infiltration. A leukaemic phase is said not to be a feature of endemic disease, even when the bone marrow is infiltrated [246].

Bone marrow cytology

The bone marrow in Burkitt lymphoma is usually normal at presentation. The reported frequency of bone marrow infiltration has varied from 5% to 20% in different series. The frequency of infiltration appears to be similar in endemic [247,248] and in non-endemic [249–251] cases. In our experience, bone marrow infiltration is more common in AIDS-related Burkitt lymphoma than in other cases. When bone marrow infiltration occurs it is usually heavy and is readily detected by either an aspirate (Fig. 6.59) or a trephine biopsy. However, because of their striking cytological features, a low percentage of infiltrating cells may be detected in an aspirate when the trephine biopsy histology is apparently normal [252]. Some patients without infiltration of the marrow have an increase in non-neoplastic lymphocytes [250].

Heavy bone marrow infiltration is invariable in those patients who present with leukaemic manifestations.

Flow cytometric immunophenotyping

The tumour cells express the B-cell antigens CD19, CD20, CD22 and CD79a and show strong SmIg (IgM) expression (Box 6.10). There is usually expression of CD10 but not of CD5 or CD23. CD45 expression is stronger than in ALL [253]. CD34 and TdT are negative. CD21 may be positive in endemic cases but is usually negative in sporadic cases [253].

Cytogenetic and molecular genetic analysis

Burkitt lymphoma is characterized by translocations involving *MYC* at 8q24 and the *IGH*, κ and λ genes at 14q32, 2p12 and 22q11.2, respectively

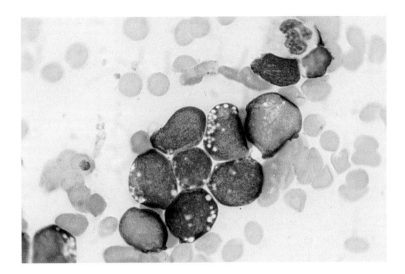

Fig. 6.59 BM aspirate, Burkitt lymphoma presenting as FAB L3 ALL in a patient with AIDS, showing blasts with marked cytoplasmic basophilia and heavy cytoplasmic vacuolation. MGG ×100.

BOX 6.10

Burkitt lymphoma

Flow cytometric immunophenotyping
CD19+, CD20+, CD22+, CD79a+, strong SmIg+
CD10+/–, CD5–, CD23–, TdT–, CD34–

Immunohistochemistry
CD20+, CD79a+, PAX5+, BCL6+, CD10+
CD43–/+, CD5–, CD23–, BCL2–, TdT–, CD34–
Ki-67+ proliferative fraction is usually greater than 99%

Cytogenetic and molecular genetic analysis
Most cases have t(8;14)(q24;q32). Smaller numbers
   of cases have variant translocations, t(2:8)
   (p12;q24) and t(8;22)(q24;q11.2); *MYC* is
   dysregulated
EBER may be positive, particularly in endemic and
   HIV-related cases

Percentages are approximate: +, >90% cases
positive; +/–, >50% positive; –/+, <50% positive;
–, <10% positive. EBER, Epstein–Barr virus early
RNA; HIV, human immunodeficiency virus; SmIg,
surface membrane immunoglobulin; TdT, terminal
deoxynucleotidyl transferase.

(Box 6.10). The *MYC* oncogene is brought into close proximity to one of the immunoglobulin genes as a result of t(8;14)(q24;q32), t(2:8)(p12;q24) or t(8;22)(q24;q11.2). Although the same three cytogenetic rearrangements are seen in all types of Burkitt lymphoma the precise breakpoints differ at a molecular level between sporadic and endemic cases, involving the heavy chain joining region in endemic cases (aberrant hypermutation, early B-cell origin) and the *IGH* switch region in sporadic Burkitt lymphoma (later stage of B-cell differentiation). *TP53* mutations are present in about a third of patients [253]. On microarray analysis, Burkitt lymphoma has a distinctive molecular signature which is, however, shared with a proportion of cases of diffuse large B-cell lymphoma [254,255]. If the diagnosis of Burkitt lymphoma is difficult it can be useful to demonstrate not only the presence of a *MYC* rearrangement but also the lack of a *BCL2* or *BCL6* rearrangement.

Bone marrow histology
Infiltration may be interstitial, nodular or diffuse [250–252]. Cells are uniform in appearance; they are medium-sized with a round or ovoid nuclear outline and a distinct, narrow rim of cytoplasm (Fig. 6.60). Cleft or folded nuclei are rare. Small nucleoli are usually present. Mitotic figures are numerous. Cytoplasmic vacuoles can sometimes be detected if specifically sought (Fig. 6.60). Tingible body macrophages, a characteristic feature in other tissues causing the so-called 'starry sky' appearance, are sometimes detected (Fig. 6.61) but are a less consistent feature than at other sites. Bone marrow necrosis can occur both before treatment is given and, to an even greater extent, after chem-

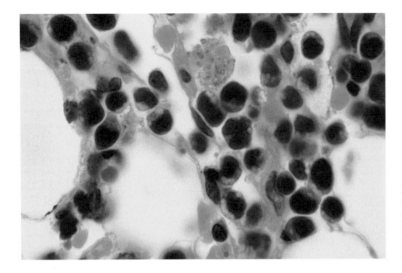

Fig. 6.60 BM trephine biopsy section, Burkitt lymphoma in a patient with AIDS, showing diffuse infiltration by lymphoma cells; note the prominent cytoplasmic vacuoles. Paraffin-embedded, H&E ×100.

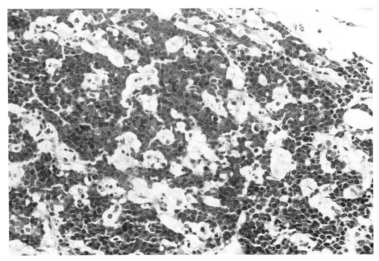

Fig. 6.61 BM trephine biopsy section, Burkitt lymphoma in a patient with AIDS, showing a 'starry sky' appearance. Paraffin-embedded, H&E ×20.

otherapy. Increased reticulin is frequent. In some cases, the lymphoma cells are more heterogeneous and the nuclear outlines are more irregular. There may be plasmacytoid differentiation.

Immunohistochemistry

Lymphoma cells express CD20, CD79a and CD10 although expression of CD20 may be weak. There may also be expression of CD38, CD43 and CD77 [245]. BCL2 is generally negative but a minority of cases show weak expression; all other disease characteristics should be typical before this diagnosis is made in a BCL2+ case [245]. Staining for Ki-67 antigen shows a very high proliferative fraction;

usually greater than 99% of tumour cell nuclei are positive. CD34 and TdT are not expressed. BCL6 is expressed. BCL2 is typically negative, but is weakly expressed in about a fifth of cases [245]. In cases with plasmacytic differentiation there is demonstrable cytoplasmic immunoglobulin [253]. In an appropriate histological context, a CD10-positive, BCL2-negative, BCL6-positive immunophenotype with a very high proliferative fraction gives reliable evidence for a diagnosis of Burkitt lymphoma.

Problems and pitfalls

The diagnosis of Burkitt lymphoma from a bone marrow aspirate is usually straightforward because of the distinctive cytological features of the neo-plastic cells. More difficulty may be experienced with a trephine biopsy section since cytoplasmic vacuolation may be inapparent and the 'starry-sky' appearance, which can provide a clue to this diag-nosis, is often absent. Correct assessment of cell size, nuclear features and the frequent mitoses are of critical importance in making this diagnosis. Immunohistochemistry is essential unless the immunophenotype has been established by flow cytometry. It can be useful in making a distinction between Burkitt lymphoma (CD5 and cyclin D1 negative and CD10 positive) and blastoid variant of mantle cell lymphoma (CD10 negative, CD5 and cyclin D1 positive). There are some cases of lym-phoma with a proliferative fraction approaching 100% but either the morphology or immunophe-notype is intermediate between DLBCL and Burkitt lymphoma. Such cases are classified in the 2008 WHO classification as a 'grey zone' lymphoma, 'B-cell lymphoma, unclassifiable, with features inter-mediate between DLBCL and Burkitt lymphoma'.

Small cell tumours of childhood, e.g. those with heavily vacuolated cells such as alveolar rhab-domyosarcoma, have been misdiagnosed and even treated as Burkitt lymphoma [256].

Lymphoproliferative disorders of T lineage and natural killer lineage

Prior to the publication of the 2001 WHO classifica-tion [33], the terminology and classification of T-cell and natural killer (NK)-cell leukaemias/ lymphomas was often unsatisfactory. Problems included: (i) failure of histopathologists and haematologists to recognize the same entities; (ii) difficulty in relating different histopathological classifications to each other; (iii) the use of a variety of terms for a single disease entity; (iv) the use of the same term (e.g. T chronic lymphocytic leukae-mia) to denote a variety of different diseases; (v) failure to recognize some disease entities (e.g. adult T-cell leukaemia/lymphoma); (vi) the assignment of a single specific entity (e.g. adult T-cell leukae-mia/lymphoma) to a number of different categories within a single classification; (vii) difficulty in devising a reproducible classification, as a conse-quence of the extreme histological diversity of

T-cell lymphomas; and (viii) difficulty in relating the histological diagnosis to the patient's prognosis.

The REAL and subsequently WHO classifications brought a degree of clarity to this field although knowledge of the pathogenesis of these diseases remains very limited in comparison with our understanding of B-cell lymphoproliferative dis-eases. The 2008 WHO classification, which we shall use as the framework for discussion of this group of disorders, is based on the premise that not only morphology but also clinical, immunophenotypic, cytogenetic and molecular genetic features are integral to the definition of specific entities [1,33]. T-cell neoplasms are divided into T-cell lympho-blastic leukaemia/lymphoma (analogous to thymic or pre-thymic cells) and mature T-cell neoplasms, sometimes referred to as 'peripheral T-cell lym-phoma', analogous to post-thymic cells. T-cell and NK-cell neoplasms are grouped together because of the clinical and immunophenotypic relationships of certain lymphomas of cytotoxic T cells and of NK cells.

The common patterns of bone marrow infiltra-tion in T-cell lymphoma differ from those most characteristic of B-cell lymphomas. Infiltration is usually interstitial, random focal, nodular or diffuse. Nodular infiltration differs from that seen in B-cell lymphomas and in reactive lymphoid hyperplasia in that the nodules often have ill-defined margins. Paratrabecular infiltration occurs [10,23] but is quite uncommon. T-cell lymphomas also differ from B-cell lymphomas in that reactive changes are more frequent; such changes include eosinophilia, vascular proliferation, polyclonal plasma cell prolif-eration, macrophage proliferation and activation, haemophagocytosis, epithelioid cell and granuloma formation, reactive follicular hyperplasia and reti-culin fibrosis.

The frequency with which marrow infiltration has been reported in peripheral T-cell lymphoma has varied from 10% [257] to 80% [23]. This wide disparity may be attributable in part to the occur-rence of histologically equivocal lesions that require immunophenotyping for confirmation [10] and in part to a variable mixture, in any series of patients reported in the past, of different disease entities with different probabilities of bone marrow spread.

Diagnosis and classification of T-lineage lymphomas and leukaemias is not always possible on the basis of lymph node histology alone. The immunophenotype and cytological features of peripheral blood and bone marrow cells can be of critical importance. Histological features in a trephine biopsy section are generally of less importance than lymph node histology and peripheral blood cytology. However, in some cases, a firm diagnosis can be established from the bone marrow when other diagnostic tissue is not available [10,23]. In other patients, lesions are suggestive of NHL but are non-diagnostic unless supplemented by immunophenotypic analysis or molecular genetic demonstration of a clonal *TCR* rearrangement. The differential diagnosis includes Hodgkin lymphoma, AIDS, autoimmune diseases, malignant histiocytosis and virus-associated haemophagocytosis.

Diagnosis of NK neoplasms is complicated by the lack of any readily applicable clonal marker in many patients. Patients with aggressive disease or with a clonal cytogenetic marker can be recognized as having a neoplastic condition. However for other patients with non-aggressive disease and no cytogenetic abnormality, it may not be possible to determine whether the condition is reactive or neoplastic.

T lymphoblastic leukaemia/lymphoma

About a quarter of cases of ALL are of T lineage. T-lineage ALL is closely related to T-cell lymphoblastic lymphoma, both being neoplasms of cells analogous to precursor T cells. In the WHO classification they constitute a single diagnostic category [258]. T lymphoblastic lymphoma, in which the bone marrow initially shows little or no infiltration, is less common than T-ALL. Before the routine use of chemotherapy, bone marrow infiltration usually supervened in those who initially had a normal marrow, giving historical insight into the nature of the disease. Both the leukaemic and lymphomatous forms of this disease are much more common in childhood than in adult life. About 80% of all lymphoblastic lymphomas, including the great majority of childhood lymphoblastic lymphoma, are of T lineage [38,259].

T lymphoblastic leukaemia/lymphoma shows a male preponderance. Thymic infiltration is very common and may be associated with pleural and pericardial effusions and superior vena cava obstruction. There may also be lymphadenopathy, hepatomegaly or splenomegaly.

Peripheral blood

The peripheral blood film in T-ALL often shows circulating blast cells. In T lymphoblastic lymphoma, the blood is often normal but some patients have small numbers of circulating neoplastic cells. T lymphoblasts may have FAB L1 or L2 cytological features. They cannot be distinguished reliably from B lymphoblasts on cytological grounds, although convoluted or hyperchromatic nuclei are sometimes noted.

Bone marrow cytology

In T-ALL the bone marrow is invariably infiltrated by lymphoblasts whereas, in T-lymphoblastic lymphoma, the bone marrow is often normal, with variable infiltration in some patients. By convention, cases with more than 25% of lymphoblasts in the marrow are classified as ALL and cases with a lower percentage as lymphoblastic lymphoma [258]. Patients with lymphoblastic lymphoma in whom the bone marrow is initially normal may later show infiltration if there is disease progression.

Flow cytometric immunophenotyping

T lymphoblasts express many antigens characteristic of T cells, such as CD2, CD3 (cytoplasmic with or without surface membrane expression), CD4, CD5, CD7 and CD8. In addition, they may show features of immaturity such as coexpression of CD4 and CD8 or expression of CD1a (Box 6.11). CD99 and TdT are usually expressed and CD34 may be expressed, any of these giving further evidence of the precursor nature of the neoplasm. CD10 may also be positive (although expression is weaker than in B-lineage ALL) and CD79a is expressed in about 10% of cases [258]. Aberrant CD13 or CD33 expression has been reported in a fifth to a third of cases [258].

Cases have been divided by the EGIL group into four immunophenotypic subtypes, all of which express cytoplasmic or surface membrane CD3:
1 Pro-T-ALL: this has the least mature immunophenotype. The cells do not express CD2, CD5 or CD8 but may express CD7.

2 Pre-T-ALL: the cells express CD2, CD5 or CD8 but not CD1a.

3 Cortical T-ALL: the cells show expression of CD1a with or without surface membrane CD3.

4 Mature T-ALL: the cells express surface membrane CD3 but not CD1a.

The immunophenotypic features of T lymphoblastic lymphoma are similar to those of T-ALL; although lymphoblastic lymphoma tends to have the more mature phenotype, the difference is not clear-cut so individual cases cannot be distinguished on this basis.

Cytogenetic and molecular genetic analysis

Cytogenetic abnormalities are common although no specific abnormalities occur at high frequency. However, several cryptic translocations and a cryptic deletion and their associated molecular abnormalities do occur at high frequency. Many of the more common abnormalities are translocations involving *TCR* loci, particularly the *TCRA/TCRD* locus at 14q11.2 and the *TCRB* locus at 7q35 but also the *TCRG* locus at 7p15-14 (Box 6.11). In addi-

tion, *TLX1* (*HOX11*) and *TLX3* (*HOX11L2*) rearrangement and *SIL-TAL1* fusion are common. Almost all cases show clonal rearrangement of *TCR* loci detectable by PCR analysis with *IGH* also being rearranged in about 20% [258].

Bone marrow histology

Bone marrow infiltration is invariable and extensive in T-ALL. In T lymphoblastic lymphoma there is marrow infiltration at diagnosis in approximately 60% of cases [14]; infiltration is initially focal but, with disease progression, focal deposits spread and coalesce to produce a diffuse pattern. The cytological features of the leukaemic and lymphomatous forms of the disease are very similar [42]. Lymphoblasts are of small or medium size, slightly larger than small lymphocytes, with scanty cytoplasm and relatively large, deeply staining nuclei. Nucleoli are usually relatively small and the chromatin is finely stippled. Mitotic figures are frequent and nuclear clefting, convolution or folding can be identified in some cases. Some cases also have small, hyperchromatic nuclei [42]. A tendency to perivascular infiltration by lymphoblasts may be pronounced [127]. When marrow involvement is minimal the lymphoblasts may be difficult to identify in trephine biopsy sections and may more easily be detected in aspirate films.

Immunohistochemistry

T lymphoblasts express CD3 (either in the cytoplasm or on the cell membrane) and usually CD5 and TdT (see Box 6.11). They may express CD4, CD8, CD34, CD43, CD45 and CD45RO. There may also be weak expression of CD10 and expression of CD79a but cells do not generally express other B-cell or myeloid antigens.

Problems and pitfalls

The main differential diagnoses of T-ALL/T lymphoblastic lymphoma are B lymphoblastic leukaemia/lymphoma and AML. These differential diagnoses have been discussed on pages 309–310.

It may be necessary to distinguish bone marrow accumulation of lymphoid cells in the autoimmune lymphoproliferative syndrome from infiltration by leukaemic cells. The immunophenotype in the former condition is distinctive with a heterogeneous lymphoid population including increased

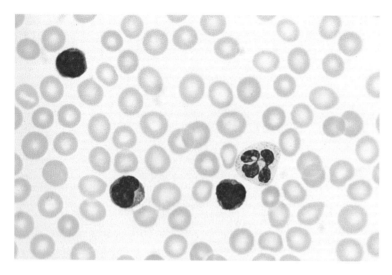

Fig. 6.62 PB film, T-PLL, showing dense irregular nuclei and, in one cell, a prominent medium-sized nucleolus. MGG ×100.

numbers of T cells that do not express either CD4 or CD8 [260].

T-cell prolymphocytic leukaemia

T-cell prolymphocytic leukaemia was initially recognized by Galton *et al.* [261] as a T-lineage neoplasm with cytological similarities to B-PLL. The term was accepted by the FAB group [262] who also recommended the inclusion in this category of cases with smaller cells that were less similar to those of B-PLL; the small cell variant was subsequently shown to have the same clinical, immunophenotypic, cytogenetic and molecular genetic abnormalities as other cases. T-PLL, including the small cell variant, is recognized as a distinct entity in the WHO classification [263].

T-cell prolymphocytic leukaemia is rare. It is mainly a disease of the elderly. Patients commonly present with marked splenomegaly, hepatomegaly and lymphadenopathy. Other clinical features may include skin infiltration and serous effusions.

Peripheral blood

The WBC is usually high and anaemia and thrombocytopenia are common [263]. In some cases the circulating neoplastic cells are similar in size to normal small lymphocytes while in others they are considerably larger, similar in size to B-PLL cells [264]. When cells are large there is usually relatively abundant cytoplasm and the nuclei have a prominent central nucleolus. Some cases are cyto-

logically indistinguishable from B-PLL cells but the majority differ. The cytoplasm is often more basophilic and the nucleus is irregular. In cases with predominantly small cells the nucleocytoplasmic ratio is higher and the nucleolus is smaller and less prominent (Fig. 6.62); the nucleus is often irregular ('knobby') and there may also be cytoplasmic blebs. In a minority of patients the neoplastic cells have cerebriform nuclei [263]. Overall, about 75% of patients have large cells, 20% have small cells and 5% have cells with cerebriform nuclei [263].

Bone marrow cytology

The bone marrow is infiltrated by cells of the same appearance as those in the blood but the morphology is usually less well preserved.

Flow cytometric immunophenotyping

The leukaemic cells express the T-cell-associated antigens, CD2, CD3 and CD5 (Box 6.12). The cells are characteristically CD7 positive, in contrast to most other leukaemias with a mature T-cell phenotype. In the majority of patients (about 60%), cells are CD4 positive and CD8 negative. In approximately a quarter of all cases, cells express both CD4 and CD8 [265]. Least often (in about 15% of patients), the cells are CD4 negative and CD8 positive. In most patients CD25 is not expressed. CD52 is strongly expressed, this being relevant to immunotherapy employing anti-CD52.

Cytogenetic and molecular genetic analysis

Approximately 75% of cases of T-PLL show abnormalities of chromosome 14, either inv(14)(q11q32) or t(14;14)(q11;q32) [91], leading to dysregulation of *TCL1A* (*TCL1*) and *TCL1B* by proximity to the *TCRAD* locus [263] (Box 6.12). Partial trisomy or multisomy of 8q is often present. Other abnormalities seen in a minority of patients are trisomy or partial trisomy of 7q and deletions of 6q and 12p13. Other molecular genetic lesions include mutations of the *ATM* gene.

Bone marrow histology

There may be only a modest degree of infiltration, even in those patients who have marked leucocytosis [163]. The patterns of infiltration seen are similar to those of B-PLL (see page 321). In many cases irregular nuclei and scanty cytoplasm suggest T lineage (Fig. 6.63) but some cases are indistinguishable from B-PLL. Reticulin fibrosis appears to be more common than in B-PLL [92].

Immunohistochemistry

The cells are CD3, CD5 and CD7 positive (Box 6.12). In most cases they are CD4 positive and CD8 negative. They show no expression of B-cell markers. TCL1A is expressed in about 70% of cases and monoclonal antibodies reactive with this antigen are potentially of use in diagnosis [266].

Problems and pitfalls

T-cell prolymphocytic leukaemia needs to be distinguished from B-PLL and from other leukaemias with a mature T-cell phenotype. Cases with cerebriform nuclei need to be distinguished from Sézary syndrome. Immunophenotypic analysis, correlation with the cytological features of the leukaemic cells and consideration of clinical features will enable these distinctions to be made.

T-cell large granular lymphocytic leukaemia

Large granular lymphocytes (LGL) of T-cell or NK-cell lineage comprise 10–15% of peripheral blood

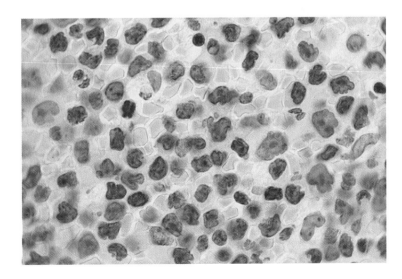

Fig. 6.63 BM trephine biopsy section, T-PLL, showing large and small prolymphocytes with prominent nucleoli, particularly in the larger cells; note the highly irregular nuclei. Resin-embedded, H&E ×100.

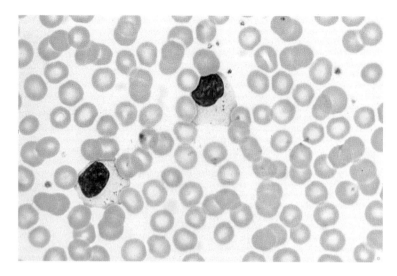

Fig. 6.64 PB film, T-cell large granular lymphocytic leukaemia, showing two large granular lymphocytes. MGG ×100.

lymphocytes [267]. The majority of cases of LGL leukaemia are of T lineage, the cells being CD3 positive and usually also expressing CD8 and other T-cell markers. There is clonal rearrangement of *TCR* loci. CD3 expression and *TCR* rearrangements distinguish these cases from the minority of cases that are of NK lineage (see below).

T-cell large granular lymphocytic leukaemia (T-LGL leukaemia) occurs predominantly in the elderly (median age 60 years) [268]. Approximately one third of patients are asymptomatic at the time of diagnosis [269,270]. However, many patients have cytopenia (most commonly neutropenia) and thus may present with recurrent bacterial infections affecting the skin, oropharynx and peri-anal region, or with symptoms of anaemia. There is a strong association with Felty's syndrome (rheumatoid arthritis with neutropenia and splenomegaly) [268,271]. Lymphadenopathy is uncommon, but hepatomegaly and splenomegaly are frequent findings. The disease typically has a prolonged survival with an actuarial median survival, in one series, of 166 months [269]. In a minority of patients, particularly those in whom cells coexpress CD3 and CD56, the disease has a more aggressive clinical behaviour similar to that of aggressive NK-cell leukaemia [272].

Peripheral blood

The WBC is increased due to an increased number of LGL [273,274]. In occasional patients there is a normal WBC although there are increased numbers of LGL. The neoplastic cells are morphologically very similar to normal LGL (Fig. 6.64). They have a round or oval nucleus with moderately condensed chromatin; the cytoplasm is voluminous and weakly basophilic and contains fine or coarse azurophilic granules. Smear cells are rare. Some patients have isolated neutropenia or thrombocytopenia or, less often, anaemia. Cyclical thrombocytopenia has been described [275]. These cytopenias are out of proportion to the degree of bone marrow infiltration and appear to have an immune basis. Macrocytosis is sometimes present.

Bone marrow cytology

The bone marrow shows a variable degree of infiltration by cells with the same cytological features as those in the blood. In early stage disease, infiltration may be minimal. In patients with marked neutropenia the bone marrow usually shows immature granulocytic cells in normal numbers but mature neutrophils are lacking. Patients with mild neutropenia may have apparently normal maturation. Patients with thrombocytopenia usually have normal numbers of megakaryocytes but amegakaryocytic thrombocytopenia has also been described [276]; in a reported patient with cyclical thrombocytopenia megakaryocytes disappeared from the bone marrow just before the nadir of the platelet count [275]. When anaemia is marked the marrow may show either a lack of maturing

T-cell large granular lymphocytic leukaemia

Flow cytometric immunophenotyping
CD2+, CD3+, CD5+, CD8+, TCRαβ+, CD16+/–, CD57+/–
CD4–, CD7–, CD56–

Immunohistochemistry
CD2+, CD3+, CD8+, CD5+/–, TIA-1+/–, perforin +/–,
    granzyme B+/–, CD7–/+
CD4–, CD56–, CD57–, CD25–

Cytogenetics and molecular genetics
No specific cytogenetic abnormality
Monoclonal *TCRB* or *TCRAD* loci rearrangements
    detectable in most cases

Percentages are approximate: +, >90% of cases
positive; +/–, >50% positive; –/+, <50% positive;
–, <10% positive. TCR, T-cell receptor.

erythroblasts (pure red cell aplasia) or megaloblastic erythropoiesis.

Flow cytometric immunophenotyping

Neoplastic cells are usually positive for CD2 and CD3, sometimes express CD5, CD16, CD57 and TCRαβ and are most often negative for CD7 [268] (Box 6.13). They are usually CD8 positive and CD4 negative. There is variable expression of CD11b. The NK-cell marker, CD56, is usually negative. In rare patients, cells express both CD3 and CD56, a phenotype that is associated with a more aggressive clinical behaviour [272]. Restricted or absent expression of CD94 (KIR, killer inhibitory receptor) isoforms provides surrogate evidence of clonality. A minority of cases have other aberrant or less usual phenotypes such as TCRγδ positive and either CD8 positive or CD4 negative/CD8 negative [277].

Cytogenetic and molecular genetic analysis

No consistent cytogenetic abnormalities have been observed (Box 6.13). Monoclonal rearrangements of *TCR* loci (most often *TCRB*, less often *TCRAD*) can be detected in most cases.

Bone marrow histology

The bone marrow is hypercellular in the majority of patients but may be normocellular or hypocellular [278]. There is infiltration in almost all cases,

although the degree of infiltration is usually not marked. Neoplastic cells are small and medium-sized lymphocytes (Fig 6.65), the nuclei of which have irregular contours, condensed nuclear chromatin and inconspicuous nucleoli [279]. There is a thin rim of cytoplasm in which granules are not visible. The pattern of infiltration is usually interstitial or intrasinusoidal; random focal or nodular infiltrates are reactive rather than part of the neoplastic infiltrate [279–281]. Some cases have plasmacytosis [279]. Severely neutropenic patients often show apparent maturation arrest at the myelocyte stage and increased numbers of apoptotic cells are present. Patients with thrombocytopenia usually have adequate or increased numbers of megakaryocytes although amegakaryocytic thrombocytopenia has been reported [282]. Anaemic patients often show the features of pure red cell aplasia with a reduction in late erythroid precursors. An association with trilineage myelodysplasia has been noted in a significant minority of patients.

Immunohistochemistry

The neoplastic cells express CD3 and CD8; CD5 is weakly expressed in the majority of patients whereas CD7 and CD56 are usually negative (Box 6.13). TIA-1 is expressed in three quarters of patients and granzyme B in half [278]. Granzyme M may be expressed [277]. CD95 (fas) and fas-ligand are usually positive [277]. CD57 is expressed only in a minority [278]. Immunohistochemistry highlights the presence of interstitial clusters and intrasinusoidal and intracapillary lymphocytes, the latter appearing as cells almost in single file.

Problems and pitfalls

The bone marrow infiltrate in T-LGL leukaemia may be subtle and does not have distinctive features. Without immunohistochemistry it can be missed completely or confused with that of various low grade B-cell lymphoproliferative disorders. Non-clonal disorders of LGL can also be confused with T-LGL leukaemia. Examination of peripheral blood and bone marrow aspirate films, together with immunophenotypic analysis, is essential if the nature of the infiltrate is to be recognized. In most cases it is the distinctive morphology of the LGL in the circulation that suggests the diagnosis, which is

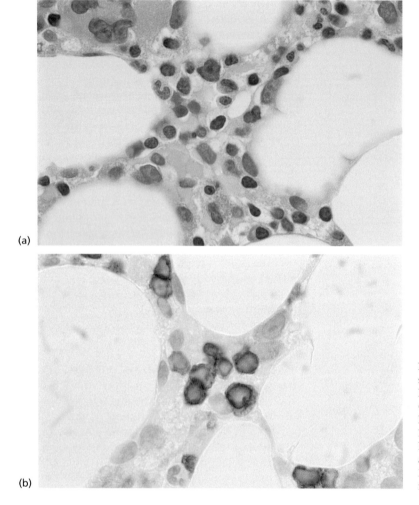

(a)

(b)

Fig. 6.65 BM trephine biopsy section, T-cell large granular lymphocytic leukaemia. (a) Occasional small and medium-sized lymphocytes. Paraffin-embedded, H&E ×100. (b) Infiltrating lymphoma cells are much more apparent by immunohistochemistry. Paraffin-embedded, immunoperoxidase for CD3 ×100.

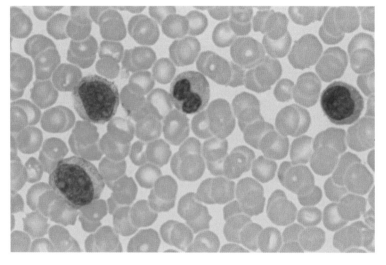

Fig. 6.66 PB film, aggressive NK-cell leukaemia, showing three lymphoma cells and a neutrophil. MGG ×100. (By courtesy of Dr K. F. Wong, Hong Kong.)

confirmed by immunophenotyping and clonality studies.

A reactive increase in LGL can be associated with a significant bone marrow infiltrate. This has been reported, for example, in association with rituximab-induced autoimmune neutropenia [283].

Chronic lymphoproliferative disorders of NK lineage

The 2008 WHO classification includes a provisional category for cases with a persistent unexplained increase of NK cells (>2 × 10^9/l for >6 months) [284]. In at least some patients this condition is neoplastic as evidenced by a clonal cytogenetic abnormality, skewed expression of X-chromosome genes, absent or restricted expression of CD94 (KIR) isoforms or subsequent transformation into a more aggressive condition. In other patients analysis of X-linked genes suggests that the disorder may not be clonal [285].

Aggressive NK-cell leukaemia

In contrast with indolent NK cell proliferation, aggressive NK-cell leukaemia can be recognized as neoplastic because of its clinical course. It is more common in Chinese than Caucasians and often occurs in teenagers and young adults [286]; in one series of patients, the median age was 39 years [268]. In more than 90% of cases the neoplastic cells show evidence of infection with EBV [286–288]. B symptoms and hepatosplenomegaly are common [268] but lymphadenopathy is less so [286]. There may be an associated coagulopathy or haemophagocytic syndrome [286]. The clinical course is aggressive with resistance to therapy and with survival being usually less than 2 months [268,286,288–290].

Peripheral blood

The peripheral blood shows variable numbers of LGL [286]. In some patients the circulating cells are similar to normal LGL. Cells may have various abnormal features, e.g. increased size, irregular or hyperchromatic nuclei, an open chromatin pattern or distinct nucleoli [286,288] (Fig. 6.66). There may be circulating normoblasts and myelocytes. Anaemia, thrombocytopenia and neutropenia are frequent [268].

Bone marrow cytology

Most cases show infiltration by cells similar to those seen in the peripheral blood [288] (Fig. 6.67). There may be increased macrophages and haemophagocytosis [286].

Flow cytometric immunophenotyping

The neoplastic cells are negative for CD3, CD4, TCRαβ and TCRγδ [268,288,291] (Box 6.14). They usually express CD2, CD16 (three quarters of cases), CD56, CD94 and CD161. There is variable expression of CD8, CD11b, CD57 (usually negative) and CD69.

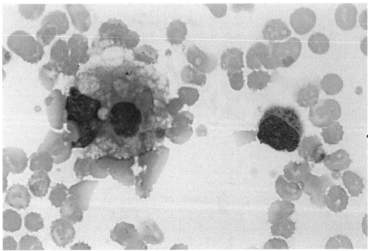

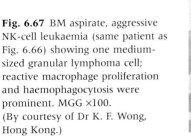

Fig. 6.67 BM aspirate, aggressive NK-cell leukaemia (same patient as Fig. 6.66) showing one medium-sized granular lymphoma cell; reactive macrophage proliferation and haemophagocytosis were prominent. MGG ×100. (By courtesy of Dr K. F. Wong, Hong Kong.)

BOX 6.14

Aggressive NK-cell leukaemia

Flow cytometric immunophenotyping
CD2+, CD16+, CD56+, CD8+/–, CD57–/+
CD3–, CD4–, TCRαβ–, TCRγδ–

Immunohistochemistry
CD2+, CD56+, TIA-1+/–, perforin +/–, granzyme B+/–,
   CD57–/+
CD3–, CD4–

Cytogenetic and molecular genetic analysis
Cytogenetic abnormalities common, but no
   consistent abnormality observed
TCR genes not rearranged
EBER+ in most cases

Percentages are approximate: +, >90% cases
positive; +/–, >50% positive; –/+, <50% positive;
–, <10% positive. EBER, Epstein–Barr virus early
RNA; TCR, T-cell receptor.

Cytogenetic and molecular genetic analysis

Many cases show clonal cytogenetic abnormalities although no consistent pattern has been reported [268] (Box 6.14). *TCR* genes are not rearranged. In most cases, EBV-EBER can be detected by *in situ* hybridization [288]. Clonality may be demonstrated in females by analysis of X-linked polymorphisms and in both males and females by the demonstration of a clonal episomal form of EBV [286].

Bone marrow histology

The degree of bone marrow infiltration is variable. The pattern of infiltration may be diffuse, interstitial or angiocentric. There is a monomorphic infiltrate of medium-sized cells with round nuclei and condensed chromatin [288]. Some patients have haemophagocytosis.

Immunohistochemistry

The neoplastic cells express CD56 and are negative for CD3 and CD4 (Box 6.14). Expression of CD3ε may lead to a positive reaction for CD3 with some antibodies.

Problems and pitfalls

This condition is readily distinguished from T-LGL leukaemia by immunophenotyping and *TCR* analysis. More significant problems occur in distinguishing NK-cell leukaemia from chronic NK-cell lymphocytosis (in WHO terminology, 'chronic lymphoproliferative disorders of NK lineage'), which result, in no small part, from the fact that the nature of the latter condition is often uncertain [292]. The distinction is made on the basis of the disease course. Aggressive NK-cell leukaemia is, by definition, an aggressive condition whereas chronic NK lymphocytosis is indolent with little tendency to progress.

Cases should not be interpreted as being aggressive NK-cell leukaemia purely on the basis of expression of CD56 since such expression can also be seen in other neoplasms, e.g. myeloma, blastic plasmacytoid dendritic cell neoplasm, acute myeloid leukaemia and some non-haemopoietic tumours.

Extranodal NK/T-cell lymphoma, nasal type

This condition differs from aggressive NK-cell leukaemia both clinically and pathologically [293]. Most cases are associated with EBV infection and the disease is much more common in the Far East, in Pacific islanders [294] and in Central and South America than in the rest of the world. It is twice as common in men as in women [294]. The incidence increases markedly above the age of 55 years [294]. Previous designations include angiocentric T-cell lymphoma, polymorphic reticulosis and lethal midline granuloma. It is an aggressive disease that typically presents with a destructive mass in the nose or palate. Although this tumour is most common in the nasopharynx, it can present at other sites, including the skin, without nasopharyngeal involvement [288]. The primary tumours are often extensively necrotic due to infiltration of blood vessel walls by neoplastic cells. Most cases express an NK phenotype, but some have a T-cell or hybrid T/NK phenotype. The prognosis is usually poor [290,295].

Peripheral blood

The minority of patients who present with disseminated disease have pancytopenia. Rarely, a leukaemic phase occurs. Circulating neoplastic cells have azurophilic granules, but they usually have a higher nucleocytoplasmic ratio and more diffuse chromatin pattern than the cells of T-LGL leukaemia [290].

Bone marrow cytology

In a small minority of patients the bone marrow is infiltrated by medium-sized cells with a high nucleocytoplasmic ratio, pleomorphic nuclear morphology and azurophilic cytoplasmic granules [290]. There may be haemophagocytosis [293].

Flow cytometric immunophenotyping

There is usually expression of CD56, CD69 and CD94 but not CD161; expression of CD16 is variable [291]. The neoplastic cells show variable expression of T-cell-associated antigens. CD3 is usually negative, CD2 is usually positive and there is often expression of CD5 and CD7. Cells may be CD4 or CD8 positive. Cytotoxic granule molecules, such as TIA-1, perforin and granzyme B, are often expressed [293], as are Fas (CD95) and Fas ligand [293].

Cytogenetic and molecular genetic analysis

No consistent cytogenetic abnormalities have been described. Those most commonly reported are del(6)(q21q25) [293], i(6)(p10) [283] and del(13)(q14q34) [296]. The *TCR* and *IGH* loci are in a germline pattern. EBV is present in a clonal episomal form [293].

Bone marrow histology

Bone marrow infiltration is uncommon; in one reported series it was found at diagnosis in two of 25 cases and during follow-up in another three [297]. Typically a subtle interstitial infiltrate is seen. Neoplastic cells are pleomorphic and medium-sized with a high nucleocytoplasmic ratio.

Immunohistochemistry

Immunohistochemistry for CD56 can be useful but *in situ* hybridization for the detection of EBV-EBER is a more sensitive technique for highlighting the presence of infiltrating lymphoma cells [297]. Detection of EBV-positive cells in the bone marrow is prognostically adverse [293]. Cytoplasmic CD3ε is expressed [293] so that immunohistochemistry for CD3 may be positive with some antibodies.

Problems and pitfalls

As for aggressive NK-cell leukaemia, expression of CD56 should not be overinterpreted.

Systemic EBV-positive T-cell lymphoproliferative disorder of childhood

The 2008 WHO classification has defined two EBV-positive T-cell lymphoproliferative disorders of children, of which the systemic form can involve the bone marrow [298]. This condition has a predilection for Chinese and Japanese and for Central and South American populations. It can arise in the context of either acute or chronic active EBV infection. It is an aggressive systemic disease with a very poor prognosis. There may be pancytopenia, haemophagocytosis and bone marrow infiltration. The infiltrating clonal T cells are small without clearly atypical features. They express CD2, CD3 and TIA-1; when the disease follows acute EBV infection they are usually CD8 positive whereas following chronic active EBV infection they are usually CD4 positive [298].

Mycosis fungoides/Sézary syndrome

Mycosis fungoides and Sézary syndrome are cutaneous T-cell lymphomas. These are rare conditions with an incidence of 0.64 per 100 000 per year in white American males and 0.36 in white American females [36]; the incidence is higher in black Americans. There is a steady rise in incidence above the age of 30 years. In both conditions there is infiltration of the dermis and the epidermis by neoplastic cells. The epidermal infiltrate is focal; the intra-epidermal accumulations of lymphocytes may form linear arrays, displacing basal epidermal cells from their basement membrane, or more distinctive clusters known as Pautrier's abscesses or micro-abscesses. Pautrier's abscesses are highly characteristic of primary cutaneous T-cell lymphoma of small cerebriform cells but they are not pathognomonic since they may also occur in adult T-cell leukaemia/lymphoma. Nor are they present in all patients [299]. In mycosis fungoides the initial manifestation is usually the presence of patchy erythematous lesions but, subsequently, plaques, nodules and fungating tumours may form. Spread to lymph nodes and transformation to large cell lymphoma occur late in the disease. Circulating neoplastic cells are sometimes, but not always,

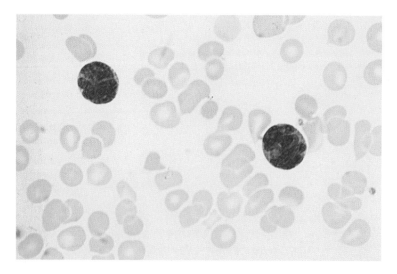

Fig. 6.68 PB film, Sézary syndrome, showing two cells with convoluted nuclei and scanty cytoplasm. MGG ×100.

apparent in mycosis fungoides. Sézary syndrome is characterized by both generalized erythroderma, consequent on infiltration of the skin by lymphoma cells, and circulating neoplastic cells, which may be numerous or scanty; these features are detectable at presentation although the skin histology may not be distinctive. In the 2008 WHO classification a diagnosis of Sézary syndrome requires erythroderma, generalized lymphadenopathy and the presence of clonal neoplastic T cells and, in addition, one or more of: (i) circulating Sézary cells at least $1 \times 10^9/l$; a ratio of CD4-positive T cells:CD8-positive T cells of >10:1; and (iii) loss of one or more T-cell antigens [299]. Although they are separate categories in the WHO classification, there is some overlap between Sézary syndrome and mycosis fungoides and they may be best regarded as different manifestations of a single disease; the circulating neoplastic cells of both are referred to as Sézary cells. Rare patients lack clinically detectable skin lesions but have circulating neoplastic cells with the cytological features of Sézary cells; this condition, which has been designated Sézary cell leukaemia, is now regarded as a variant of T-PLL.

Peripheral blood

The likelihood of Sézary cells being present in the peripheral blood can be related to the nature of the skin lesions. In one study, circulating neoplastic cells were not detectable in patients with localized skin plaques but were present in 9% of patients with generalized skin plaques, 27% of those with skin tumours and 90% of those with erythroderma [300]. Sézary cells vary in size from that of a normal small lymphocyte to two or three times this size. Individual patients may have predominantly small cells or predominantly large cells. Sézary cells have a high nucleocytoplasmic ratio. The chromatin is highly condensed and sometimes hyperchromatic. The nucleus is described as 'convoluted' or 'cerebriform', names indicative of the intertwined lobes resembling the convolutions of the brain (Fig. 6.68). This causes the surface of the nucleus to appear grooved. Lobes are often more readily discernible in large Sézary cells than in small forms. Nucleoli are usually inapparent but can sometimes be detected in large cells. Cytoplasm is scanty in small cells but more abundant in large cells; it is agranular and may contain a ring of vacuoles, which are PAS positive. When Sézary cells are infrequent and similar in size to normal lymphocytes they can be difficult to identify with certainty. Ultrastructural examination is very useful in those cases in which the characteristic cytological features cannot be discerned by light microscopy; demonstration of the characteristic form of the nucleus confirms the diagnosis (see Fig. 2.31).

Some patients have eosinophilia [300]. Except when disease is very advanced, anaemia and cytopenia is not usually features of Sézary syndrome or of mycosis fungoides.

Bone marrow cytology

The bone marrow aspirate is often normal, even in a high proportion of patients with circulating neoplastic cells [300]. However, a variable degree of infiltration by Sézary cells can occur, particularly in the advanced stages of the disease.

Flow cytometric immunophenotyping

Sézary cells are usually CD4 positive and CD8 negative; they express T-cell markers including CD2, CD3, CD5 and TCRαβ (Box 6.15); they are often CD7 negative [301]. In a minority of cases, cells are CD8 positive and CD4 negative. CD25 is usually not expressed.

Cytogenetic and molecular genetic analysis

A number of cytogenetic abnormalities have been reported and complex karyotypes are frequent (Box 6.15). Abnormalities of chromosomes 1 and 8 are common but no consistent or specific abnormality has been observed [302,303]. There is monoclonal rearrangement of *TCR* genes. However, detection of a dominant T-cell clone in the peripheral blood does not necessarily indicate the presence of neoplastic cells [304].

Bone marrow histology

In the first reported series of cases of cutaneous T-cell lymphomas bone marrow infiltration was detected in only 2–10% of patients and, even at autopsy, detection was no higher than 25% [305]. However, in two subsequent large series infiltration was detected in 18% [306] and 28% [307], respectively, of patients at presentation or early in the course of the disease. Infiltration is more common in Sézary syndrome than in mycosis fungoides [308] and shows some correlation with disease stage. However, not all patients with circulating Sézary cells have histologically detectable bone marrow infiltration [307].

Infiltrating cells are usually small and irregular in shape with convoluted and hyperchromatic nuclei (Fig. 6.69). In a minority of cases there is a population of large lymphoid cells with prominent nucleoli. Sometimes the infiltrate is pleomorphic and includes bizarre multinucleated cells. The presence of a significant proportion of transformed cells is of adverse prognostic significance [307]. Infiltrated bone marrows may also show an increase of eosinophils, macrophages or plasma cells and the presence of granulomas [307]. Reticulin is moderately increased.

When the bone marrow does not show any infiltrate of cytologically atypical cells there may nevertheless be increased eosinophils and macrophages, granulomas and aggregates of small round lymphocytes [307]. The presence of aggregates of cytologically normal lymphocytes does not have any adverse prognostic significance.

Bone marrow biopsy and clonality studies have been considered not clinically indicated since no extra prognostic information is gained beyond that available from peripheral blood examination [309].

Immunohistochemistry

The T-cell markers CD3 and CD5 are expressed (Box 6.15). Cells in most cases are CD4 positive and CD8 negative; in a minority of cases, cells are CD8 positive and CD4 negative. Rarely, staining for both CD4 and CD8 is negative. Cytotoxic granule-associated proteins are not usually expressed.

Subcutaneous panniculitis-like T-cell lymphoma

Bone marrow infiltration is not a feature of this skin lymphoma but reactive haemophagocytosis is common and cytopenia can occur [310].

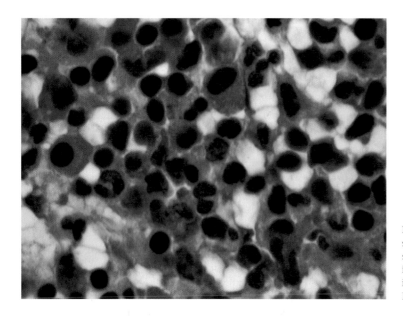

Fig. 6.69 BM trephine biopsy section from a patient with Sézary syndrome showing a mild interstitial infiltrate of lymphoid cells with irregular (cerebriform) nuclei. Paraffin-embedded, H&E ×100.

Primary cutaneous gamma-delta T-cell lymphoma

Bone marrow infiltration is not a feature of this skin lymphoma but a haemophagocytic syndrome can occur in patients with panniculitis-like tumours [311].

Angioimmunoblastic T-cell lymphoma

The nature of the condition previously designated angioimmunoblastic lymphadenopathy with dys-proteinaemia (AILD), immunoblastic lymphaden-opathy or AILD-like T-cell lymphoma has been controversial. With the greater availability of cytogenetic and DNA analysis, it has now become clear that this is a lymphoma of CD4-positive T cells [312], probably originating in a CD10-positive, BCL6-positive germinal centre helper T cell [313]. Not all cases have demonstrable rearrangement of *TCR* loci [257], possibly because the proportion of neoplastic cells can be very low. There is an early difference in survival curves between patients with and without demonstrable *TCR* rearrangement but they ultimately come together [257].

This is a rare lymphoma, the US incidence being 0.071 per 100 000 per year [294]. It is seen mainly in the elderly with a steady rise in incidence above the age of 55 years and with a male:female ratio of 1.5:1 [294]. Patients usually present with advanced symptomatic disease, which can include

skin infiltration and pleural effusions [314]. The diagnosis rests on lymph node histology. Typically there is effacement of nodal architecture with dis-appearance of germinal centres, a marked prolif-eration of venules and an infiltrate that is composed of a variable mixture of lymphocytes, plasma cells, immunoblasts, epithelioid macrophages and dendritic cells resembling follicular dendritic cells [4,257,315]. Many cases have extracellular PAS-positive deposits.

Characteristic clinical features are fever and lym-phadenopathy, autoimmune haemolytic anaemia and other autoimmune phenomena, allergic reac-tions to drugs and hypergammaglobulinaemia. Some patients have cold agglutinins and some have a cryoglobulin.

Transformation to a more aggressive T-cell lym-phoma occurs in 10–15% of cases. Some patients develop DLBCL, thought in most cases to result from reactivation of EBV infection followed by neoplastic transformation occurring in a context of disease-related immunodeficiency [312].

Peripheral blood

There is usually normocytic normochromic anaemia with increased rouleaux formation and an elevated erythrocyte sedimentation rate. Occasionally the anaemia is leucoerythroblastic. Complicating autoimmune haemolytic anaemia is common. Red cell agglutinates may be present in those with a cold agglutinin. Some patients have lymphopenia, thrombocytopenia, neutrophilia, eosinophilia or basophilia [315,316]. Plasma cells, plasmacytoid lymphocytes and atypical lymphocytes resembling those seen in viral infections or immunological reactions may be present. Striking polyclonal plasmacytosis (plasma cells $8.6 \times 10^9/l$) has been reported [317]; this may be transient.

Bone marrow cytology

The bone marrow aspirate may show non-specific changes such as the features of anaemia of chronic disease. There may be an infiltrate of small lymphocytes, sometimes with irregular nuclei, and of atypical lymphoid cells including immunoblasts. Inflammatory cells including eosinophils and plasma cells may be increased and the latter may be very numerous [317].

Flow cytometric immunophenotyping

The neoplastic cells express T-cell-associated antigens such as CD2 and usually CD5 (Box 6.16).

BOX 6.16

Angioimmunoblastic T-cell lymphoma

Flow cytometric immunophenotyping
CD2+, CD4+, CD5+, CD10+, CD57+, cCD3+, SmCD3
  varies, CD7+/–
CD8–, CD56–, TCRαβ+ or –, TCRγδ–

Immunohistochemistry
CD2+, CD3+, CD4+, CD5+, BCL6+
CD10+/–, CD57+/–, CXCL13+/–, CD7+/–
CD8–

Cytogenetic and molecular genetic analysis
Cytogenetic abnormalities with a complex karyotype
  common
The most frequent abnormalities are trisomy 3,
  trisomy 5 and additional copies of the X
  chromosome
Monoclonal *TCR* rearrangements detectable in most
  cases

Percentages are approximate: +, >90% of cases positive; +/–, >50% positive; –/+, <50% positive; –, <10% positive. c, cytoplasmic; Sm, surface membrane; TCR, T-cell receptor.

There may be expression of cytoplasmic CD3 without membrane CD3 in circulating neoplastic T cells [318–320]. CD7 is often not expressed. In most cases, cells express CD4 and are CD8 negative. CD10, CD57 and BCL6 are usually expressed [321]. CD56 is negative [320]. CXCL13 is expressed [322]. There may be failure to express TCRαβ and TCRγδ is usually negative [319,320].

Cytogenetic and molecular genetic analysis

Most cases show cytogenetic abnormalities with complex karyotypes and a high frequency of multiple, cytogenetically unrelated clones [323]. The most frequent abnormalities are trisomy 3, trisomy 5 and additional copies of the X chromosome (Box 6.16). Structural abnormalities of chromosome 1, additional X chromosomes and complex aberrant clones are associated with a worse prognosis [324]. Monoclonal rearrangements of *TCRB* and *TCRG* are seen in approximately 75% of cases and monoclonal *IGH* rearrangements are present in up to 25% of cases [325]. It is possible to detect EBV-EBER in B cells by *in situ* hybridization in many cases.

Bone marrow histology

The reported incidence of bone marrow infiltration varies widely, from 10% [257] to 60% [326,327]. The lesions may be single or multiple and the pattern of infiltration random focal, nodular, paratrabecular [24,322] or diffuse. The infiltrate is polymorphous, being composed of lymphocytes, plasma cells, immunoblasts, macrophages and sometimes eosinophils or neutrophils (Figs 6.70–6.72). Polyclonal plasma cells can be very numerous, e.g. 40–50% [322] and can be increased in the absence of infiltration [322]. The neoplastic lymphocytes have somewhat irregular nuclei and may be small and medium-sized or medium-sized and large. In some cases there are immunoblasts with clear cytoplasm and lymphoid cells resembling Hodgkin cells or Reed–Sternberg cells [24]. Because of the presence of epithelioid macrophages, focal lesions may resemble granulomas [327]. Some cases have increased numbers of capillaries, which are occasionally arborizing. Reticulin is usually increased.

Myeloid hyperplasia is common. Disorderly distribution and abnormal maturation may be found

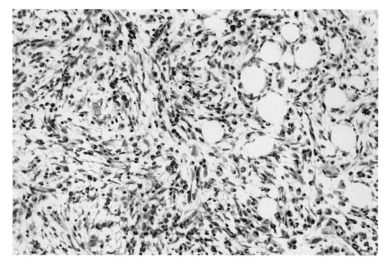

Fig. 6.70 BM trephine biopsy section, angioimmunoblastic T-cell lymphoma, showing a pleomorphic lymphoid infiltrate and irregular fibrosis. Paraffin-embedded, H&E ×10.

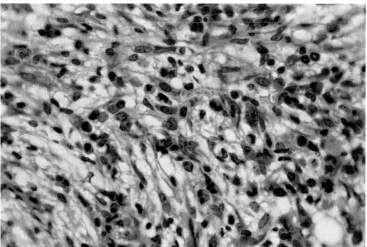

Fig. 6.71 BM trephine biopsy section, angioimmunoblastic T-cell lymphoma (same patient as in Fig. 6.70), showing that the infiltrate is composed of medium-sized lymphocytes admixed with fibroblasts, eosinophils, immunoblasts and plasma cells. Paraffin-embedded, H&E ×40.

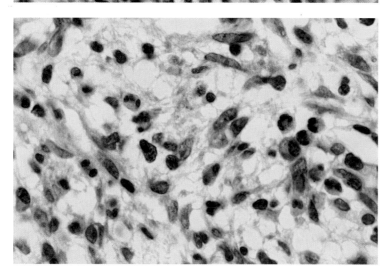

Fig. 6.72 BM trephine biopsy section, angioimmunoblastic T-cell lymphoma (same patient as in Fig. 6.70), showing fibroblasts, eosinophils and medium-sized lymphocytes with irregular nuclei. Paraffin-embedded, H&E ×100.

in any or all of the main haemopoietic lineages. Pure red cell aplasia has been reported [322]. Although angioimmunoblastic T-cell lymphoma may sometimes be suspected on bone marrow examination the diagnosis generally requires a lymph node biopsy. Two features that are particularly characteristic of the lymph node lesions, arborizing capillaries and PAS-positive extracellular deposits, are much less apparent (and sometimes completely inapparent) in bone marrow trephine biopsy sections.

Immunohistochemistry

Atypical lymphoid cells in the areas of infiltration usually express CD3 (Box 6.16). In most cases, cells are CD4 positive and CD8 negative. B-cell markers (CD20 and CD79a) are negative. Varying proportions of neoplastic cells of angioimmunoblastic lymphoma express CD10 (about 80% of cases), whereas CD10 expression is not seen in other T-cell lymphomas [328]; however, there is often failure to express CD10 in the bone marrow when nodal infiltrates are positive [322,329]. The neoplastic cells also express CXCL13 [322]. In about a third of cases there are numerous large B cells that are positive for EBV [330]. When plasma cell infiltration is heavy, immunohistochemistry can be useful to demonstrate the lack of light-chain restriction.

Problems and pitfalls

A similar pleomorphic infiltrate can occur in the bone marrow in Hodgkin lymphoma, in T-cell/histiocyte-rich large B-cell lymphoma and in inflammatory and autoimmune conditions. Close correlation with the clinical features, lymph node histology and cytogenetic and molecular genetic findings is required to establish a diagnosis of angioimmunoblastic T-cell lymphoma. In some patients the plasma cell infiltration is very marked, so that the differential diagnosis includes a plasma cell neoplasm [322,330]. The lesions of systemic mastocytosis may be confused with this condition if a Giemsa stain or immunohistochemical staining for mast cell tryptase is not performed. The myeloid hyperplasia may be sufficient to suggest a myeloproliferative neoplasm [322] or a myelodysplastic syndrome.

Adult T-cell leukaemia/lymphoma

Adult T-cell leukaemia/lymphoma (ATLL) is a specific neoplasm occurring in individuals whose T cells have earlier been infected by the retrovirus HTLV-I (human T-cell lymphotropic virus I). This virus integrates into host T cells at random sites but in the neoplastic T-cell clone of an individual patient is integrated at a consistent site. The lifetime risk of leukaemia/lymphoma in people infected by the virus has been estimated at about 1–2%. Cases of ATLL have mainly been observed in certain areas of known endemicity of the virus, specifically Japan and the West Indies, and in countries that have received immigrants from these two areas. Cases have also been reported from South America with a smaller number of cases being recognized in patients from Central and West Africa, the Middle East, Taiwan and other parts of the world [301,331–334]. ATLL occurs mainly in adults but rare childhood cases have been reported, particularly from South America. It is likely that co-factors are necessary for its development; these may differ in Japan and the West Indies since the disease usually has a later age of onset in Japan.

This condition may present as a lymphoma, without bone marrow and peripheral blood involvement, or as a leukaemia/lymphoma with both tissue infiltration and peripheral blood and bone marrow involvement. There is an acute course in the majority of patients, but chronic and smouldering forms are recognized [334,335] (Table 6.5). Cytologically and histologically, ATLL is very variable. Suchi et al. [4] have reported that a smouldering course is more likely in those with histologically low grade lymphoma but Jaffe et al. [332] did not observe any relationship between histological grade and outcome.

Prominent clinical features in the acute form are lymphadenopathy, skin infiltration and bone lesions associated with hypercalcaemia. Some patients have splenomegaly and hepatomegaly. The prognosis of the acute form is generally poor with a median survival of less than a year.

Examination of the peripheral blood is very important in diagnosis. Bone marrow aspiration and trephine biopsy are of less importance.

Peripheral blood

About three quarters of patients have circulating lymphoma cells, which are distinctive [301,331].

Table 6.5 Subclassification of adult T-cell leukaemia/lymphoma (ATLL) [334,335].*

Category	Peripheral blood lymphocytes	Tissue infiltration	Biochemistry
Smouldering ATLL	Lymphocyte count <4 × 10⁹/l and either ≥5% abnormal lymphocytes or histological proof of lung or skin infiltration	The lungs or skin may be infiltrated but there is no infiltration of lymph nodes, liver, spleen, gastrointestinal tract or CNS and no ascites or pleural effusion	LDH up to 1.5× the upper limit of normal No hypercalcaemia
Chronic ATLL	Lymphocyte count >4 × 10⁹/l and T lymphocytes >3.5 × 10⁹/l with morphologically abnormal cells and occasional frank ATLL cells (such as flower cells); in most cases there are >5% abnormal lymphocytes	The lungs, skin, lymph nodes, liver or spleen may be infiltrated, but there is no infiltration of the gastrointestinal tract or CNS and no ascites or pleural effusion	LDH up to twice the upper limit of normal No hypercalcaemia
Lymphoma-type ATLL	Lymphocyte count <4 × 10⁹/l and ≤1% abnormal lymphocytes	Histologically demonstrated lymphoma	There may be elevated LDH or hypercalcaemia
Acute ATLL		All other cases	

CNS central nervous system; LDH lactate dehydrogenase.
*Modified from reference [335].

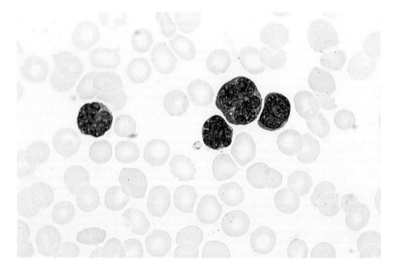

Fig. 6.73 PB film, ATLL, showing highly pleomorphic cells, the largest of which has a 'clover-leaf' or 'flower-like' lobulated nucleus containing prominent medium-sized nucleoli. MGG ×100.

They are extremely pleomorphic, varying in size, shape, nucleocytoplasmic ratio and degree of chromatin condensation (Fig. 6.73). Cytoplasm varies from scanty to moderately abundant and is sometimes basophilic. Some cells have nucleoli and a primitive open chromatin pattern while others, usually the majority, have condensed, sometimes hyperchromatic, chromatin. Nuclei are very variable in shape but some are deeply lobated, resembling clover leaves or flowers. Some cerebriform cells may be present but the degree of pleomorphism usually permits easy distinction from Sézary syndrome.

Because the marrow is not usually heavily infiltrated there may be little anaemia or thrombocytopenia at presentation. Eosinophilia is not infrequent [333].

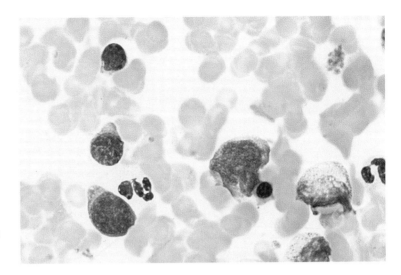

Fig. 6.74 BM aspirate, ATLL, showing an infiltrate of lymphoid cells; there is considerable variation in size: the largest cell has a lobulated nucleus. MGG ×100.

Bone marrow cytology

Patients who have leukaemia at presentation show a variable degree of bone marrow infiltration by cells similar to those described above (Fig. 6.74).

Flow cytometric immunophenotyping

The cells of ATLL are usually positive for CD2, CD3 and CD5 (Box 6.17). In most cases they lack CD7. Cells are most often CD4 positive and differ from the cells of other types of mature T-cell lymphoma in that CD25 is strongly expressed by all or most cells in the great majority of cases.

Cytogenetic and molecular genetic analysis

Most cases have an abnormal karyotype although no consistent abnormality has been reported (Box 6.17). The most common findings are trisomy 3, trisomy 7 and abnormalities of 6q [336]. There is monoclonal rearrangement of *TCR* loci.

Bone marrow histology

The bone marrow is infiltrated in about three quarters of patients. The pattern of marrow involvement may be interstitial, random focal or diffuse. Occasionally it is paratrabecular. The degree of infiltration at presentation is often slight.

The nature of the infiltrate varies considerably between cases. Many cases show considerable variation in cell size with nuclei varying from medium size to large (Figs 6.75 and 6.76). Other cases have predominantly small or predominantly large cells.

BOX 6.17

Adult T-cell leukaemia/lymphoma

Flow cytometric immunophenotyping
CD2+, CD3+, CD4+, CD5+, CD25+
CD7–, CD8–

Immunohistochemistry
CD2+, CD3+, CD4+, CD5+, CD25+
CD7–, CD8–

Cytogenetic and molecular genetic analysis
Most cases have cytogenetic abnormalities; trisomy 3, trisomy 7 and abnormalities of 6q are the most common
Monoclonal integration of HTLV-I

Percentages are approximate: +, >90% cases positive; +/–, >50% positive; –/+, <50% positive; –, <10% positive. HTLV-I, human T-cell lymphotropic virus I.

Cells are characteristically highly pleomorphic. In the larger cells, nuclei tend to be vesicular with a distinct nuclear membrane and two to five distinct nucleoli; smaller cells often show chromatin condensation. Nuclei vary in shape, being round, oval, indented, deeply lobated or convoluted. Giant cells may be present; some of these resemble Reed–Sternberg cells while others have nuclear convolutions, coarsely aggregated chromatin and prominent

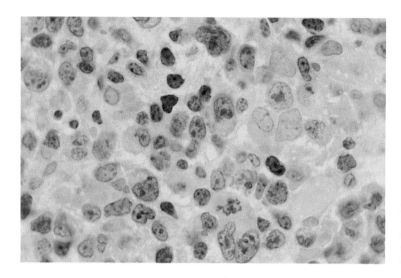

Fig. 6.75 BM trephine biopsy section, ATLL, showing diffuse infiltration by highly pleomorphic small, medium and large lymphoid cells. Resin-embedded, H&E ×100.

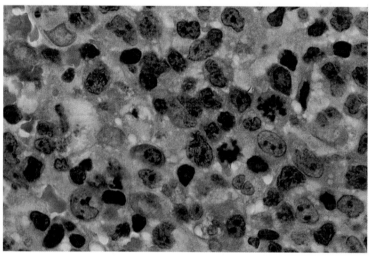

Fig. 6.76 BM trephine biopsy section, ATLL, showing diffuse infiltration by highly pleomorphic medium and large lymphoid cells. Note the high mitotic rate. Resin-embedded, H&E ×100.

nucleoli [4]. Mitotic figures are numerous (see Fig. 6.76). In addition to the neoplastic cells there are often large numbers of eosinophils and plasma cells. Marrow vascularity may be increased.

A characteristic but not invariable feature of ATLL is extensive bone resorption with large numbers of Howship's lacunae and numerous mononucleated and multinucleated osteoclasts (Fig. 6.77). There may be associated bone remodelling with a variable increase of osteoblast activity and paratrabecular fibrosis [332,337]. In some cases, increased osteoclasts are apparent when there is no detectable infiltration in biopsy sections [333].

Immunohistochemistry

The neoplastic cells are positive for CD2, CD3, CD5 and typically also CD25 (Box 6.17). In most cases, they are CD4 positive. Large cells may be CD30 positive [338].

Problems and pitfalls

The degree of marrow infiltration may be slight and difficult to recognize by morphology alone. Immunohistochemical staining for CD3 may be helpful in identifying a subtle interstitial infiltrate of atypical cells. Even in those with a heavy infiltrate, the histological features may closely resemble those of other peripheral T-cell lymphomas.

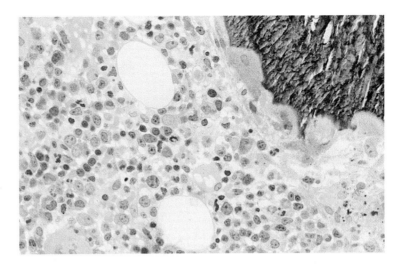

Fig. 6.77 BM trephine biopsy section, ATLL, showing heavy infiltration by pleomorphic medium and large lymphocytes; note the numerous osteoclasts in Howship's lacunae giving the bone trabecula a serrated appearance. Resin-embedded, H&E ×40.

Consequently close attention to the cytological features in bone marrow aspirate or blood films and a high index of suspicion are important in suggesting the diagnosis. The presence of increased osteoclastic activity is a useful pointer to a diagnosis of ATLL.

Hepatosplenic T-cell lymphoma

This is a clinically aggressive lymphoma that typically presents in young men with B symptoms, hepatosplenomegaly and cytopenia. Lymphadenopathy is not usual [339]. It is a rare lymphoma, the US incidence being 0.0004 per 100 000 per year, and is at least three times as common in black Americans as in white [294]. In most cases, the neoplastic cells express the γδ form of the TCR, which is normally expressed on a minor subset of peripheral blood T lymphocytes. In a small number of cases, with similar clinical and pathological features, the neoplastic cells express the αβ TCR as well as, or instead of, γδ TCR [340].

Peripheral blood
There is often a Coombs-negative haemolytic anaemia and thrombocytopenia as result of peripheral consumption. The WBC has usually been reported to be normal but in one series there were circulating lymphoma cells in the majority of patients [341].

Bone marrow cytology
The bone marrow is hypercellular with erythroid and megakaryocytic hyperplasia. The bone marrow is usually infiltrated by medium-sized lymphocytes, which may be in clumps [342]. The cells have moderately dispersed chromatin and moderate cytoplasmic basophilia [339] (Fig. 6.78). There may be fine cytoplasmic granules [341]. The infiltrate varies from scanty to moderate. There may be reactive haemophagocytosis. Lymphoma cells themselves can exhibit erythrophagocytosis [343].

Flow cytometric immunophenotyping
Cells in most cases express CD2 and CD3 and often CD7 but are negative for CD4, CD5 and CD8 (Box 6.18). CD7 is also often negative. In the majority of cases the cells express TCRγδ, but not TCRαβ; in a minority the reverse is true. CD56 is expressed in many cases [339,344] and CD16 in some [330].

Cytogenetic and molecular genetic analysis
The characteristic cytogenetic abnormalities are trisomy 8 and an isochromosome of 7q (Box 6.18). The majority of cases show a monoclonal rearrangement of *TCRG* or *TCRD*, but not of *TCRB*.

Bone marrow histology
The bone marrow is hypercellular with erythroid and megakaryocytic hyperplasia. Infiltration is present in most cases. The infiltrate may be interstitial, intrasinusoidal or both. The neoplastic cells are pleomorphic medium and large cells (Fig. 6.79) with irregular nuclear margins, coarse chromatin clumping in the smaller cells and a more diffuse chromatin pattern with small, conspicuous nucleoli in the larger cells [341]. Initially the infiltrate is

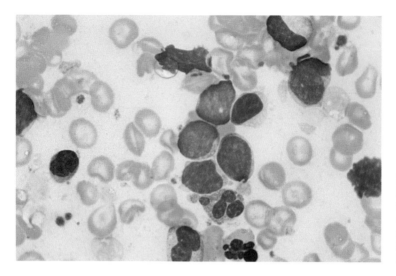

Fig. 6.78 BM aspirate, hepatosplenic T-cell lymphoma, showing medium-sized lymphoma cells with a high nucleocytoplasmic ratio and multiple small nucleoli. MGG ×100 (By courtesy of Dr Elizabeth Lombard, Cape Town.)

BOX 6.18

Hepatosplenic T-cell lymphoma

Flow cytometric immunophenotyping
CD2+, CD3+, TCRγδ+
CD7+/–, CD56+/–, CD8–/+
CD4–, CD5–, TCRαβ– (rarely TCRαβ+), CD57–

Immunohistochemistry
CD2+, CD3+, TIA-1+, granzyme M+
CD7+/–, CD11b+/–, CD16+, CD56+/–, CD8–/+
CD4–, CD5–,TCRαβ–, (rarely TCRαβ+), perforin –,
  granzyme B–

Cytogenetic and molecular genetic analysis
Trisomy 8 and an isochromosome of 7q – i(7)(q10)
  – are the most frequently seen abnormalities
In the majority of cases there is monoclonal
  rearrangement of *TCRG* but not *TCRB*

Percentages are approximate: +, >90% of cases
positive; +/–, >50% positive; –/+, <50% positive;
–, <10% positive. TCR, T-cell receptor.

---

subtle and may be more readily recognized with the aid of immunohistochemistry [341]. Plasma cells and small blood vessels are increased [341]. There may be reactive haemophagocytosis [341].

Immunohistochemistry
The tumour cells express CD3 and, in most cases, CD56 and CD11b (Box 6.18). In the majority of

patients CD4, CD5, CD8, CD57 and TCRαβ are not expressed. However about a quarter of patients do express CD8 [345] and a minority express TCRαβ; CD7 and CD16 are expressed in about 60% of patients [345]. The cytotoxic granule proteins, TIA-1 and granzyme M, are usually expressed but not perforin or granzyme B [346]. B-cell markers are not expressed.

Problems and pitfalls
The degree of infiltration may be very slight and, particularly in those cases with an exclusively intrasinusoidal pattern of infiltration, immunohistochemical staining for CD3 is important in identifying the neoplastic cells. Immunohistochemical staining for CD34 to highlight vascular endothelial cells is also useful in identifying the intrasinusoidal infiltrate.

Anaplastic large cell lymphoma, ALK positive
Anaplastic large cell lymphoma (ALCL) is an aggressive lymphoma, which is considered to be of T lineage even when lineage-associated lymphoid antigens are not expressed [347]. The majority of cases are associated with a specific translocation, t(2;5)(p23;q35), or variant translocations or other rearrangements involving chromosome 2 and the *ALK* gene, resulting in the formation of a fusion gene and expression of its product (ALK protein, CD246) [348,349].

Anaplastic large cell lymphoma has a wide age range, occurring in children, adolescents and

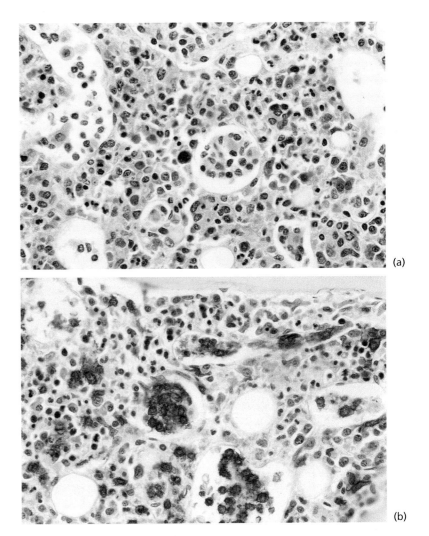

(a)

(b)

Fig. 6.79 BM trephine biopsy sections, hepatosplenic T-cell lymphoma (same patient as Fig. 6.78), showing intrasinusoidal and interstitial infiltrate. (a) Paraffin-embedded, H&E ×40. (b) Paraffin-embedded, immunoperoxidase for CD45RO ×40.

adults. Presentation is usually with nodal and extranodal, symptomatic, advanced stage disease [350], often with generalized lymphadenopathy, skin infiltration and systemic symptoms. Patients are young and there is a male preponderance (male:female ratio is 3:1). With effective treatment, prognosis is much better than that of most other T-cell lymphomas including ALK-negative ALCL (see below).

Peripheral blood
Circulation of lymphoma cells in the peripheral blood is uncommon and is indicative of a worse

prognosis [351]. When it occurs the lymphoma cells may be large and pleomorphic (Fig. 6.80). Pancytopenia may occur, resulting not only from bone marrow infiltration but also from haemophagocytosis.

Bone marrow cytology
Bone marrow infiltration has been reported in a quarter or more of patients [347,352]. Lymphoma cells are often infrequent (Fig. 6.81), usually less than 5% of marrow cells [353]. Neoplastic cells are large and pleomorphic, some being as large as megakaryocytes. They have weakly to strongly

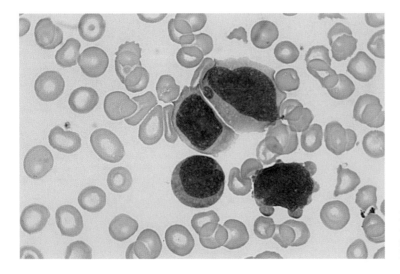

Fig. 6.80 PB film, anaplastic large cell lymphoma, ALK positive, showing large, pleomorphic lymphoma cells. MGG ×100.

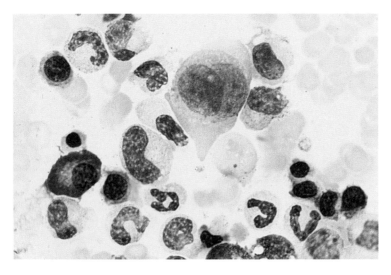

Fig. 6.81 BM aspirate, anaplastic large cell lymphoma, ALK positive, showing a single, large, binucleate lymphoma cell. MGG ×100.

basophilic cytoplasm, which may be finely vacuolated [353,354]; a Golgi zone may be apparent. Nuclei have irregular folds, a coarse open chromatin pattern and multiple prominent nucleoli [253]. Some cases have occasional phagocytic neoplastic cells. Associated macrophage proliferation and haemophagocytosis are common and may be conspicuous, overshadowing the neoplastic infiltrate. Macrophages are predominantly mature. Haemophagocytosis can be prominent even when lymphoma cells are not detectable in the bone marrow or are present in very small numbers [353].

Flow cytometric immunophenotyping

The tumour cells express CD30 (Box 6.19). In many cases they also express activation markers such as HLA-DR, CD25 and CD71. There is variable expression of CD2, CD3 (positive in only a minority of cases), CD4, CD5, CD7, CD8, CD15 (rarely), CD45 and CD45RO. B-cell markers are not expressed. CD56 is expressed in nearly 20% of cases and correlates with a worse prognosis [355]. Around half of cases show aberrant expression of CD13 [356]. TCRαβ is rarely expressed although the *TCRB* locus is often rearranged [357].

with very small clusters of lymphoma cells or even single cells) or diffuse. Sometimes the background marrow is fibrotic.

Cytological features are variable. In most cases tumour cells are very pleomorphic and include multinucleated giant cells and cells with lobated, wreath-shaped or embryo-shaped nuclei, sometimes abutting on the cell membrane [367] (Fig. 6.82). There may be cells resembling immunoblasts and others resembling Reed–Sternberg cells. In other cases tumour cells are less pleomorphic. Lymphohistiocytic and small cell variants have been described [348]. Mitotic figures are frequent [24]. Reticulin is increased in overtly infiltrated areas.

Immunohistochemistry

ALK protein is expressed in the nucleus and the cytoplasm (Golgi zone and surface membrane) in cases with t(2;5) but the location of the protein differs in cases with a variant chromosomal rearrangements [350,360,362] (Table 6.6). However, occasional cases with the classical translocation, particularly the small cell variant, show only cytoplasmic staining [349,368]. Monoclonal antibodies such as ALK-1 [369] or ALKc are preferred to polyclonal antibodies since the latter may give false-positive results [347]. The neoplastic cells express CD30 and, in many cases, epithelial membrane antigen (Box 6.19). Leucocyte common antigen (CD45) is expressed in only 50% of cases. There is variable expression of CD3 and CD45RO. CD43 is expressed in two thirds of cases [347] and cytotoxic granule proteins (TIA-1, granzyme B or perforin) may be expressed. B-cell markers are not expressed. CD68 expression may be detected with the KP1 monoclonal antibody but not with PG-M1 (CD68R) [347]. CD56 expression is prognostically adverse [350].

Problems and pitfalls

Subtle infiltration may be missed. Immunohistochemical staining for CD30, ALK and epithelial membrane antigen has been found very useful in identifying small clusters of lymphoma cells and single lymphoma cells scattered among haemopoietic cells [252]. Staining for ALK is particularly useful in this context as it is the most specific of the markers.

BOX 6.19

Anaplastic large cell lymphoma, ALK positive

Flow cytometric immunophenotyping
CD30+
Variable expression of CD2, CD3, CD4, CD5, CD7, CD8, CD15, CD45 and CD45RO
CD13 expressed in about half

Immunohistochemistry
CD30+, ALK(CD246)+ (see Table 6.6), CD56+/–
CD45+/–, EMA+/–, TIA-1+/–, perforin+/–, granzyme B+/–
Variable expression of CD2, CD3, CD4, CD5, CD7, CD15, CD43 and CD45RO
CD8–, BCL2– [144]

Cytogenetic and molecular genetic analysis
Most cases have t(2;5)(p23;q35) and *NPM1-ALK* fusion. Less common abnormalities include t(1;2)(q21;p23) with *TMP3-ALK* fusion, inv(2)(p23q35) with *ATIC-ALK* fusion, t(2;3)(p23;q21) with *TFG-ALK* fusion, t(2;5)(q37;q31), t(2;13)(p23;q34), *CLTC-ALK* fusion probably resulting from t(2;17)(p23;q23), t(2;22)(p23;q11) and *MSN-ALK* fusion resulting from t(X;2)(q11;p23)
Clonal *TCR* rearrangement

Percentages are approximate: +, >90% of cases positive; +/–, >50% positive; –/+, <50% positive; –, <10% positive. EMA, epithelial membrane antigen.

Cytogenetic and molecular genetic analysis

Most cases have t(2;5)(p23;q35) with the formation of an *NPM1-ALK* fusion gene detectable by conventional cytogenetic analysis, RT-PCR or FISH [358–360] (Box 6.19). Variant translocations and other rearrangements that have been reported are shown in Table 6.6 [347,360–366].

Bone marrow histology

Bone marrow involvement has been reported in up to a third of cases [347,353,354,367] and was found to correlate with worse prognosis [352] but most series have not separated this condition from ALK-negative ALCL (which is associated with a worse prognosis). The detection rate is significantly more common when immunohistochemistry is employed [352]. The pattern of infiltration by ALCL may be interstitial, random focal (sometimes

Table 6.6 Relationship between cytogenetic and molecular genetic abnormality and the pattern of distribution of the ALK protein [347,350,360].

Cytogenetic abnormality	Frequency	Fusion gene	ALK distribution
t(2;5)(p23;q35)	84%	NPM1-ALK	Nucleus and cytoplasm
t(1;2)(q22-23;p23)	13%	TPM3-ALK	Cytoplasmic with peripheral enhancement
inv(2)(p23q35)	1%	ATIC-ALK	Cytoplasmic
t(2;3)(p23;q11-12)	<1%	TFG-ALK	Cytoplasmic
t(2;17)(p23;q23)	<1%	CLTC-ALK	Cytoplasmic, granular
t(2;17)(p23;q25)	<1%	ALO17-ALK	Cytoplasmic
t(2;19)(p23;p13.1)	<1%	TPM4-ALK	Cytoplasmic
t(2;22)(p23;q11.2)	<1%	MYH9-ALK	Cytoplasmic, granular
t(X;2)(q11.2-12;p23)	<1%	MSN-ALK	Surface membrane

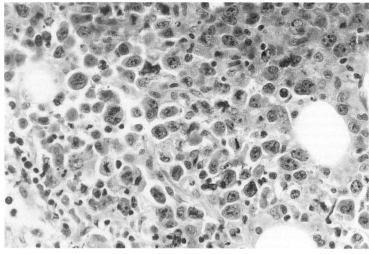

(a)

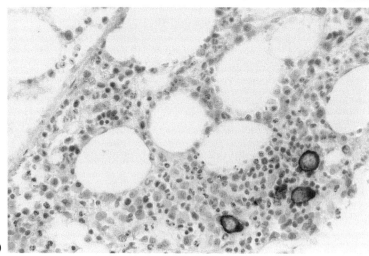

(b)

Fig. 6.82 BM trephine biopsy section, anaplastic large cell lymphoma, ALK positive. (a) A cohesive infiltrate of highly pleomorphic large lymphoma cells. Paraffin-embedded, H&E ×40. (b) An interstitial infiltrate of lymphoma cells identified by immunohistochemical staining for CD30. Paraffin-embedded, immunoperoxidase for anti-CD30 ×40. (By courtesy of Dr S. Juneja, Melbourne.)

Associated macrophage accumulation and hae-mophagocytosis may be so prominent and the lymphomatous infiltration so inconspicuous that a misdiagnosis of malignant histiocytosis is possible. The differential diagnosis also includes ALK-negative ALCL, Hodgkin lymphoma, pleomorphic variants of DLBCL, metastatic carcinoma and amelanotic melanoma. Since ALCL is often negative for CD45 and some non-lymphoid tumours (e.g. embryonal carcinoma) are CD30 positive, the diagnosis of ALCL requires careful assessment of both histological and immunophenotypic features. Those carcinomas that express CD30 almost invariably stain positively with anti-cytokeratin antibodies. Although early erythroid cells may be CD30 positive this should rarely cause any diagnostic problems as long as the cytological characteristics of such cells, compared to the pleomorphism of the neoplastic cells of this type of lymphoma, are remembered.

Anaplastic large cell lymphoma, ALK negative

Anaplastic large cell lymphoma, ALK negative, is a provisional entity in the 2008 WHO classification [370]. It lacks *ALK* rearrangement, occurs at an older age than ALK-positive ALCL and has a worse prognosis. Other clinical features are similar to those of ALK-positive ALCL. Apart from the lack of ALK expression and a lower frequency of epithelial membrane antigen positivity, the immunophenotype is similar to that of ALK-positive ALCL (Box 6.20). CD30 is strongly and uniformly expressed. CD56 expression is prognostically adverse [350]. There is bone marrow involvement in about a fifth of patients, a similar proportion to that observed in ALK-positive ALCL [371].

Enteropathy-associated T-cell lymphoma

Patients with adult-onset coeliac disease have a predisposition to this lymphoma, which shows a male predominance. Prognosis is poor, partly due to bleeding, perforation, fistula formation and poor nutritional status, with 5-year survival being about 20% [372]. This is a rare lymphoma, US incidence being 0.005 per 100 000 per year [294].

The bone marrow is not often infiltrated, in one series being seen in two of 24 patients (8%) [372]. Peripheral blood involvement is even less common. There may be anaemia and eosinophilia [373] and

---

BOX 6.20

Anaplastic large cell lymphoma, ALK negative

Flow cytometric immunophenotyping
CD30+
Variable expression of CD2, CD3, CD4, CD5, CD7, CD8, CD15, CD45 and CD45RO

Immunohistochemistry
CD30+
CD45+/–, CD43+/–, TIA-1+/–, granzyme B+/– and perforin +/–, CD15–/+, EMA–/+
Variable expression of CD2, CD3, CD4, CD5, CD7 and CD45RO
ALK (CD246)–

Cytogenetic and molecular genetic analysis
Clonal *TCR* rearrangement

Percentages are approximate: +, >90% of cases positive; +/–, >50% positive; –/+, <50% positive; –, <10% positive. EMA, epithelial membrane antigen.

---

there may be features of hyposplenism as a result of the associated coeliac disease.

The typical immunophenotype is that of a lamina propria lymphocyte: CD2+, CD3+, CD4–, CD8–, CD7+ and CD103+. Some cases show CD8 expression [372].

Peripheral T-cell lymphoma, not otherwise specified

This category represents a heterogeneous group of peripheral T-cell lymphomas that do not meet the criteria for categorization as one of the specific entities already described [374]. US incidence is 0.25 per 100 000 per year with a male:female ratio of 1.8:1 and an increasing incidence above the age of 45 years [294]. Morphological variants recognized are T-zone lymphoma, lymphoepithelioid (Lennert lymphoma) and follicular [374].

Patients usually have extensive nodal disease at the time of presentation and extranodal involvement is more common than in B-cell lymphomas. Systemic symptoms including fever are common. These lymphomas have an aggressive clinical course and, although potentially curable, they have a higher relapse rate and worse prognosis than aggressive B-cell lymphomas [375,376].

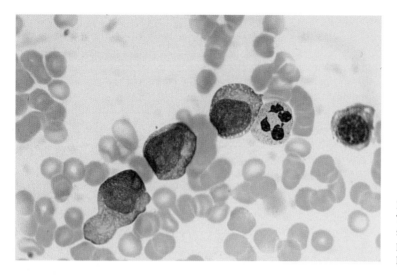

Fig. 6.83 BM aspirate, peripheral T-cell lymphoma, not otherwise specified, showing large cells with plentiful basophilic cytoplasm and prominent nucleoli. MGG ×100.

Most of the lymphomas in this category are neoplasms of mature CD4-positive cells expressing aberrant phenotypes which differ from those of normal peripheral blood T cells. Precise diagnosis usually depends on lymph node histology and immunophenotyping with bone marrow cytology and histology playing subsidiary roles. The neoplastic cells typically show marked variation in nuclear size and shape and there are often large numbers of reactive macrophages and eosinophils. There is often vascular proliferation.

Peripheral blood

Peripheral blood involvement is rare. In a minority of cases there are circulating neoplastic cells which may be medium-sized or large or a mixture of both. Cells are often highly pleomorphic. The nucleus may be round, oval or lobated with either a diffuse chromatin pattern or some chromatin condensation. One or more variably sited, prominent nucleoli are commonly present. The cytoplasm is usually moderately basophilic. There are no specific cytological features that allow T-cell lymphomas of this heterogeneous group to be distinguished from lymphomas of B lineage.

Bone marrow cytology

The bone marrow aspirate may be normal or contain abnormal lymphoid cells similar to those which may be seen in the peripheral blood (Fig. 6.83). A haemophagocytic syndrome can occur [374].

BOX 6.21

Peripheral T-cell lymphoma, not otherwise specified

Flow cytometric immunophenotyping
CD2+, CD3+, CD45RO+
CD4+/–, CD5+/–, CD7+/–, CD8–/+

Immunohistochemistry
CD2+, CD3+
CD4+/–, CD5+/–, CD7+/–, CD43+/–, CD45RO+/–, CD8–/+, CD30–/+
CD15–

Cytogenetic and molecular genetic analysis
Cytogenetic abnormalities are common, but no consistent or specific abnormality is described. Abnormalities of chromosomes 1, 2, 3, 8 and 14 are seen most frequently
Clonal *TCR* rearrangement

Percentages are approximate: +, >90% of cases positive; +/–, >50% positive; –/+, <50% positive; –, <10% positive.

Flow cytometric immunophenotyping

In most cases the cells express CD3, CD4 and TCRαβ and are CD8 negative [377] (Box 6.21). In a minority of cases, cells are CD8 positive or are negative for both CD4 and CD8. There is variable expression of CD2, CD5 and CD7. B-cell markers are not usually expressed, although rare cases of CD20-positive T-cell lymphoma have been reported [378]. CD52 is expressed in only 40% of patients [379].

Cytogenetic and molecular genetic analysis

Cytogenetic abnormalities are common but no consistent or specific abnormality has been observed (Box 6.21). Abnormalities of chromosomes 1, 2, 3, 8 and 14 [380–383] are seen most frequently. There is usually monoclonal rearrangement of one of the *TCR* loci.

Bone marrow histology

Bone marrow involvement is present in the majority of cases in most published series [10,23,24]. Infiltration may be interstitial, focal or diffuse [10,23,24,257]. We have observed paratrabecular involvement but this is quite uncommon. The neoplastic cells are often highly pleomorphic with marked variation in size, nuclear shape, chromatin pattern and the number and size of nucleoli. Some cells may have very atypical nuclear configurations, variously described as convoluted, hyperconvoluted, cerebriform or multilobated. There may be small lymphocytes, with round or irregular nuclei and a coarse chromatin pattern, and a variable admixture of medium-sized lymphocytes or immunoblasts (Figs 6.84 and 6.85). T immunoblasts typically have plentiful pale or clear cytoplasm. In some cases medium-sized or large cells predominate.

Multinucleated cells resembling Reed–Sternberg cells may be seen. Prominent reactive changes in the bone marrow are usually present [23]. Lymphoma cells may be only a minor part of an abnormal infiltrate, which may include non-neoplastic lymphocytes, plasma cells and haemo-phagocytic macrophages. There may be clusters of epithelioid cells (see Fig. 6.84). Stromal changes include increased vascularity, foci of haemorrhage and necrosis, and reticulin fibrosis. Reticulin is increased in the areas of neoplastic infiltration and, although often to a lesser extent, in non-infiltrated areas.

Immunohistochemistry

In the majority of cases the neoplastic cells express CD3 and CD45RO (see Box 6.21). Cells may express CD4 and CD43 but there is often loss of expression of CD5, CD7 and CD52. The neoplastic cells of Lennert lymphoma are often CD8 positive [374]. B-cell markers are generally negative, although aberrant expression of CD20 or CD79a can occur [374,378].

Problems and pitfalls

Bone marrow infiltrates of peripheral T-cell lymphoma need to be distinguished from reactive infiltrates such as the polymorphic lymphoid aggregates seen in HIV infection and some autoimmune conditions [23]. Close attention to the clinical features, histological appearances at other sites and

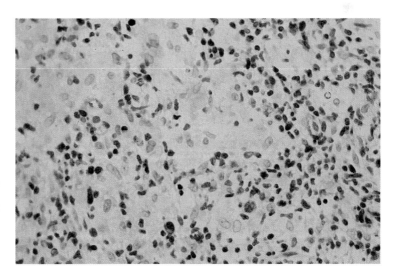

Fig. 6.84 BM trephine biopsy section, peripheral T-cell lymphoma, not otherwise specified (Lennert lymphoma), showing a pleomorphic lymphoid infiltrate and an admixture of epithelioid macrophages. Resin-embedded, H&E ×20.

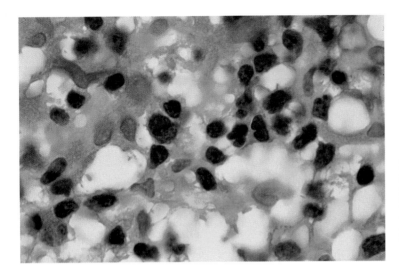

Fig. 6.85 BM trephine biopsy section, peripheral T-cell lymphoma, not otherwise specified (Lennert lymphoma) (same patient as Fig. 6.84), showing epithelioid macrophages and medium-sized lymphoid cells with irregular nuclei. Resin-embedded, H&E ×100.

immunophenotype and molecular genetic findings is required to establish the diagnosis. Hodgkin lymphoma and T-cell/histiocyte-rich DLBCL involving the marrow can resemble peripheral T-cell lymphoma; careful assessment of the immunophenotype of the neoplastic cells will usually allow the distinction to be made. Neutrophilic and eosinophilic hyperplasia are common and dysplastic changes are sometimes noted in haemopoietic cells so that confusion with a myeloproliferative or even a myelodysplastic disorder may occur [384]. When there is a marked reactive population of macrophages, eosinophils and fibroblasts, confusion with systemic mastocytosis can occur. A Giemsa stain plus immunohistochemical demonstration of mast cell tryptase will identify neoplastic mast cells in systemic mastocytosis.

Hodgkin lymphoma

Hodgkin lymphoma (previously widely known as Hodgkin's disease) encompasses a group of lymphomas, usually of nodal origin, that share some clinical and histological features. It is now recognized that this group of disorders should be divided into two distinct diagnostic categories: classical Hodgkin lymphoma, which comprises about 95% of cases, and nodular lymphocyte-predominant Hodgkin lymphoma (NLPHL) [5,385] (see Table 6.3). These two entities differ in their aetiology, epidemiology, histopathological features, immunophenotype, molecular genetic features and

disease course [386–388]. The immunophenotypic and genetic differences are summarized in Table 6.7. In NLPHL the neoplastic cells are clearly of B lineage whereas in classical Hodgkin lymphoma, although in the great majority of cases the neoplastic cells are also of B lineage, there is often a failure to express many of the usual immunophenotypic markers of B cells. The defective ability to synthesize immunoglobulin and lack of expression of typical B-cell-associated antigens has been attributed to crippling mutations in coding or regulatory regions of the immunoglobulin heavy chain gene, down-regulation of B-cell-specific transcription factors and epigenetic silencing of heavy chain genes as a result of methylation [389]. Very rare cases of classical Hodgkin lymphoma appear to be of T-cell origin [390].

Classical Hodgkin lymphoma (Hodgkin's disease)

In developed countries the incidence of classical Hodgkin lymphoma is of the order of 2–3 per 100 000 per year [36] with a peak in young adults and a second peak later in life. Some cases are aetiologically linked to EBV and incidence is increased in HIV-positive individuals. In developing countries cases in children and adolescents are much more common and an EBV association is more often found. The sex distribution and the median age of onset differ between different histological categories. The most common presenting

Table 6.7 A comparison of genotypic and phenotypic features of the neoplastic cells in nodular lymphocyte predominant Hodgkin lymphoma (NLPHL) with those in classical Hodgkin lymphoma.

	Nodular lymphocyte predominant Hodgkin lymphoma	Classical Hodgkin lymphoma
CD45	+	–
CD15	–	+/–
CD20	+	–/+
CD30	–	+
CD45	+	–
CD79a	+/–	–/+
BCL2	–	+/–
BCL6	+	–
BOB1	+	–
OCT2	+	–/+
PAX5*	+	+
MUM1/IRF4	+	+
EMA†	+/–	–
Immunoglobulin genes	Ongoing somatic hypermutation	Somatic hypermutation but not ongoing
Immunoglobulin J chain	+/–	–
Surface membrane immunoglobulin	+/–	–
EBV†	–	+ or –

EBV, Epstein–Barr virus; EMA: epithelial membrane antigen.
*The PAX5 gene encodes B-cell-specific activator protein (BSAP).
†Expression of EBV LMP1 (latent membrane protein 1) or detection, by *in situ* hybridization, of EBV-encoded early RNA (EBER).

feature is lymphadenopathy, most often involving cervical lymph nodes. Mediastinal lymphadenopathy is also common. Patients with advanced disease may have hepatomegaly and splenomegaly. Systemic symptoms such as fever, sweating and weight loss are common in those with advanced disease.

The neoplastic cells include distinctive polyploid cells designated Reed–Sternberg cells. These are giant cells, which may be binucleated or multinucleated or have lobated nuclei; they have very large inclusion-like nucleoli and abundant cytoplasm [385]. Also present are large cells of a similar appearance but with a single round nucleus and a very large nucleolus, designated mononuclear Hodgkin cells. Histological diagnosis requires not only the presence of characteristic neoplastic cells but also an appropriate cellular background, since cells morphologically resembling Reed–Sternberg cells may be seen in other lymphomas and in reac-

tive conditions such as infectious mononucleosis. There is a prominent inflammatory response so that the neoplastic cells are mixed with a variable number of lymphocytes, macrophages, eosinophils, plasma cells and fibroblasts. Some histological subtypes have prominent fibrosis.

Occasionally the primary diagnosis of classical Hodgkin lymphoma is made by examination of the bone marrow, particularly in HIV-positive patients and in other patients with lymphocyte-depleted subtype presenting with unexplained fever and pancytopenia [391]. More often bone marrow examination is done as part of a staging procedure in patients with a known diagnosis. The demonstration of infiltration usually requires a trephine biopsy. Detection rate is higher with bilateral biopsies or a single large biopsy [392]. Diagnostic cells are rarely present in films of aspirates although histological sections of aspirated fragments occasionally yield a diagnosis. Not all patients necessarily require investigation of the bone marrow as part of the staging procedure since a combination of clinical and laboratory features can be used as criteria to select those likely to have infiltration [393,394]. In one study, the results of trephine biopsy were found to influence management in less than 1% of patients [395] and in another the stage was altered from III to IV (a change unlikely to alter management) in only 2.2% of patients [396]. In a further study of more than 1000 patients there were 29% of patients with features predictive of the absence of bone marrow involvement: those who had neither B symptoms nor liver involvement nor other infra-diaphragmatic disease and who did not have lymphocyte-depleted or mixed cellularity histology had only a 0.3% prevalence of bone marrow infiltration [397]. Bone marrow infiltration is more likely in those with B symptoms, known stage III or IV disease, anaemia, age greater than 35 years, WBC less than $6.0 \times 10^9/l$ and iliac/inguinal involvement; a score based on these variables can indicate whether bone marrow biopsy is required [394].

Peripheral blood
The peripheral blood shows non-specific abnormalities. There may be anaemia, either normocytic normochromic or, less often, hypochromic microcytic. Rouleaux formation is often increased as is the erythrocyte sedimentation rate. Some patients have neutrophilia, eosinophilia or thrombocytosis.

Occasional patients have lymphocytosis. Lymphopenia is common, with severe lymphopenia being seen in patients with advanced disease or with unfavourable histological categories. Anaemia, leucopenia and pancytopenia are common in patients with bone marrow infiltration, but a leucoerythroblastic blood film is relatively uncommon. The neoplastic cells of classical Hodgkin lymphoma rarely if ever circulate in the peripheral blood; occasional instances of this phenomenon have been reported but not in recent decades and the diagnosis of the cases reported might therefore be doubted.

In multivariate analysis an increased WBC and a reduced lymphocyte count are of prognostic significance [398].

Bone marrow cytology
The bone marrow aspirate usually shows only reactive changes. The marrow is often hypercellular due to granulocytic (neutrophilic and eosinophilic) hyperplasia. Macrophages and plasma cells are often increased. Erythropoiesis is depressed and may show the features of the anaemia of chronic disease. Megakaryocytes are present in normal or increased numbers.

Even when the marrow is infiltrated it is uncommon for neoplastic cells to be present in the aspirate. When Reed–Sternberg cells are present they are very striking because of their large size, paired or multiple nuclei and large, prominent, usually centrally placed nucleoli (Fig. 6.86). With a May–

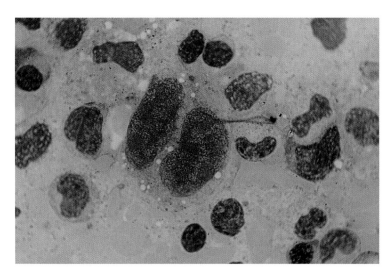

Fig. 6.86 BM aspirate, Hodgkin lymphoma in a patient with AIDS, showing a Reed–Sternberg cell – a binucleated giant cell with prominent inclusion-like nucleoli. MGG ×100.

Grünwald–Giemsa (MGG) stain, these cells and any mononuclear Hodgkin cells have moderately basophilic cytoplasm; the round, inclusion-like nucleoli stain deep blue.

Flow cytometric immunophenotyping

Neoplastic cells are very rarely seen in cytological preparations and flow cytometric analysis of the blood and bone marrow is unlikely to be of value [377].

Cytogenetic and molecular genetic analysis

Analysis of *TCR* and *IGH* loci by PCR usually shows a polyclonal pattern. However, PCR analysis of isolated neoplastic cells often shows that they have an identical *IGH* rearrangement, indicating that they belong to a single B-cell clone [399]. Very rare cases of classical Hodgkin lymphoma, when studied in the same way, have shown clonal *TCR* rearrangement without *IGH* rearrangement. There are no consistent cytogenetic abnormalities. Expression of EBV genes can be detected in up to 40% of cases of the nodular sclerosis subtype of Hodgkin lymphoma and 30–90% of the mixed cellularity subtype, with variations in incidence in different geographic regions and age groups.

Bone marrow histology

Bone marrow infiltration is present in 5–15% of patients. Infiltration is more frequent in males, in older patients, in HIV-positive individuals, in those with unfavourable histological types and in those with other evidence of advanced stage disease [393,400]. Infiltration is uncommon in nodular sclerosis disease (3–5%), is more common in mixed cellularity disease (around 10%) and has been reported in up to 50–60% of cases of those with lymphocyte-depleted histological features [228]. In HIV-positive patients, diagnosis is often made from a trephine biopsy.

With an H&E stain, Reed–Sternberg cells and mononuclear Hodgkin cells have acidophilic or amphophilic cytoplasm, a prominent nuclear membrane and an eosinophilic inclusion-like nucleolus (Figs 6.87–6.90). The features of the various variant forms of Reed–Sternberg cells have been described in detail [385]. Criteria to establish the presence of bone marrow infiltration differ according to whether or not a tissue diagnosis of classical Hodgkin lymphoma has already been established. Recommendations were drawn up at the Ann Arbor conference in 1971 [385,401]. Primary diagnosis requires the presence of Reed–Sternberg cells (Fig. 6.89) in an appropriate cellular background. The nodular sclerosis subtype is an exception to this diagnostic requirement, the presence of variant forms of Reed–Sternberg cells (lacunar cells) in an appropriate cellular background (Fig. 6.90) being considered sufficient to establish the diagnosis [402]. If the diagnosis has already been established in another tissue and a bone marrow biopsy is being performed for the purpose of staging, the

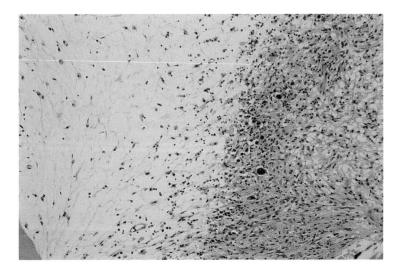

Fig. 6.87 BM trephine biopsy section, nodular sclerosis classical Hodgkin lymphoma, showing an abnormal infiltrate (right) and bone marrow hypoplasia (left). Paraffin-embedded, H&E ×4.

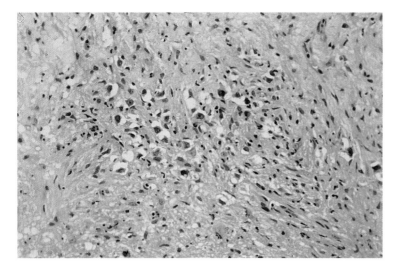

Fig. 6.88 BM trephine biopsy section, nodular sclerosis classical Hodgkin lymphoma (same patient as Fig. 6.87), showing fibrosis and a mixed infiltrate of mononuclear Hodgkin cells, eosinophils and small lymphocytes. Paraffin-embedded, H&E ×20.

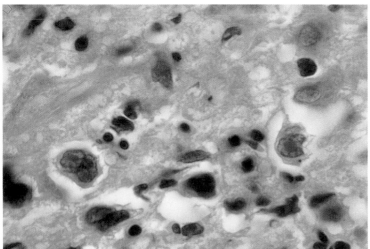

Fig. 6.89 BM trephine biopsy section, nodular sclerosis classical Hodgkin lymphoma (same patient as Fig. 6.87), showing a Reed–Sternberg cell (left) and a mononuclear Hodgkin cell (right). Paraffin-embedded, H&E ×100.

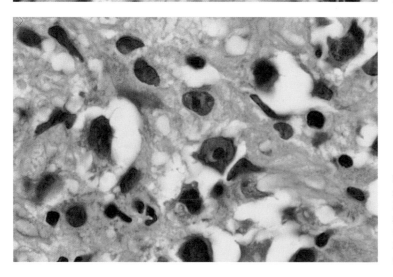

Fig. 6.90 BM trephine biopsy section, nodular sclerosis classical Hodgkin lymphoma (same patient as Fig. 6.87), showing a lacunar cell (left) and two mononuclear Hodgkin cells (centre). Paraffin-embedded, H&E ×100.

criteria for infiltration are less stringent. In this context the presence of mononuclear Hodgkin cells in an appropriate cellular background is sufficient [401]; the presence of large atypical cells or the presence of necrosis or focal or diffuse fibrosis with appropriate inflammatory cells is suggestive of classical Hodgkin lymphoma but is not diagnostic. When suspicious features are present, the examination of serial sections is indicated.

The pattern of infiltration is sometimes focal but more often diffuse. Focal lesions are mainly randomly distributed although some are paratrabecular [392,403]. Focal infiltration is most common in the nodular sclerosis subtype, whereas the lymphocyte-depleted subtype is characterized by diffuse infiltration. Focal lesions tend to be highly cellular with a mixed infiltrate of small lymphocytes with variable numbers of eosinophils, plasma cells, macrophages and Reed–Sternberg cells and their variants. The lymphoid infiltrate does not show features of cellular atypia. When infiltration is diffuse, the pattern is more variable [392,403–405]. Four patterns may be recognized:

1 In the majority of patients the marrow is hypercellular with a mixed cellular infiltrate as described above.

2 In other patients the bone marrow is very hypercellular with a predominant population of Reed–Sternberg cells and variant forms; reactive cells are not numerous.

3 In a third pattern there is focal replacement of the bone marrow by dense fibrous tissue with small numbers of macrophages and lymphocytes; neoplastic cells embedded in collagen may be relatively sparse.

4 In the fourth pattern the bone marrow is generally hypocellular with loose, sparsely cellular connective tissue through which are scattered more cellular foci containing lymphocytes, macrophages, Reed–Sternberg cells and variant forms.

Various combinations of these patterns may be seen in the same biopsy specimen or in different biopsy specimens from the same patient. In addition, amorphous eosinophilic background material may be apparent. Necrosis is occasionally detected prior to treatment [405] but is more common in treated patients. Granulomas are sometimes associated with infiltration, but also occur in the absence of bone marrow infiltration. Reticulin is increased in areas of infiltration and collagen is often present. There is sometimes osteolysis or osteosclerosis; increased bone remodelling is usual [392]. Histological appearances in the bone marrow often differ from those in lymph nodes. Sub-classification of the disease cannot be made on the basis of bone marrow histology alone. When infiltration is focal, the residual bone marrow is usually hypercellular as a consequence of granulocytic hyperplasia. Both eosinophils and neutrophils may be increased, at the margin of infiltrates and diffusely in non-involved marrow. Non-infiltrated marrow may also show increased megakaryocytes and plasma cells.

The bone marrow of patients in whom infiltration is not detected usually shows reactive changes. These often include increased granulopoiesis (neutrophilic and eosinophilic), reduced erythropoiesis, increased megakaryocytes, plasmacytosis, lymphoid infiltration including formation of lymphoid aggregates, increased and enlarged macrophages, haemophagocytosis, oedema, extravasation of erythrocytes, increased storage iron and occasionally the presence of sarcoid-like granulomas [392,403]; asteroid bodies may be seen in the giant cells of the granulomas. Bone marrow hypoplasia has been observed in some patients with lymphocyte-depleted classical Hodgkin lymphoma in whom infiltration was not detected [391].

Following successful treatment, the lymphomatous infiltrate disappears and reactive changes, including fibrosis, regress. When only reticulin fibrosis is present complete regression occurs. When there has been collagen deposition some patients show complete regression and others partial.

Immunohistochemistry

Classical Reed–Sternberg cells and their mononuclear variants are usually positive for CD30; in most cases the cells are CD15 positive but negative for CD45 (Box 6.22). In a proportion of cases Reed–Sternberg cells and mononuclear variants express CD20 and in a lower proportion CD79a is expressed. Expression of CD20 has been reported to be of adverse prognostic significance [398]. Expression of BCL2 protein has been reported in a third to three quarters of cases, whereas BCL6 protein is not usually expressed [406,407]. PAX5 is expressed [406]. MUM1/IRF4 is expressed in the majority of

BOX 6.22

Classical Hodgkin lymphoma

Flow cytometric immunophenotyping
Not usually of diagnostic value

Immunohistochemistry
CD30+, PAX5+, MUM1/IRF4+
CD15+/–, BCL2+/–, CD20–/+, CD79a–/+, EBV LMP1–/+
  or +/– depending on subtype (see Table 6.8)
CD2–, CD3–, CD5–, CD7–, CD45–, CD45RO–, BCL6–,
  OCT2–, BOB1–, EMA–, ALK(CD246)–

Cytogenetic and molecular genetic analysis
No consistent cytogenetic abnormality is described
Monoclonal *IGH* rearrangements are only detectable
  if isolated tumour cells are analysed
EBER may be positive

Percentages are approximate: +, >90% of cases
positive; +/–, >50% positive; –/+, <50% positive; –,
<10 % positive. EBER, Epstein–Barr virus early RNA;
EBV, Epstein–Barr virus; EMA, epithelial membrane
antigen; LMP1, latent membrane protein 1.

cases [406,407] and the minority of cases that are negative appear to have a worse prognosis [407]. The neoplastic cells are almost always CD3 negative.

The reactive lymphocytes are T cells expressing CD3 and CD45RO and sometimes CD57.

Problems and pitfalls
Marrow infiltration by classical Hodgkin lymphoma can be confused with infiltration by peripheral T-cell lymphoma and DLBCL (particularly the T-cell/histiocyte-rich B-cell variant), both of which can have neoplastic cells resembling Reed–Sternberg cells. Immunohistochemical staining will usually permit the correct diagnosis to be made. However, there are 'grey zone' cases recognized in the 2008 WHO classification as 'B cell lymphoma, unclassifiable, with features intermediate between DLBCL and classical Hodgkin lymphoma' where assignment to a more specific category is impossible.

A particular problem occurs in recognizing infiltration when there is a very pronounced fibroblastic response [408]. Primary myelofibrosis is easily

simulated since such patients often have splenomegaly, pancytopenia and radiologically demonstrable osteosclerosis. The large neoplastic cells in classical Hodgkin lymphoma can occasionally be mistaken for megakaryocytes or carcinoma cells. Megakaryocytes can be identified with CD42b and CD61 monoclonal antibodies. Staining for cytokeratin is useful in identifying carcinoma cells.

It should be noted that histological subtypes of classical Hodgkin lymphoma cannot be reliably differentiated from each other on bone marrow histology.

Nodular lymphocyte-predominant Hodgkin lymphoma

Nodular lymphocyte-predominant Hodgkin lymphoma (NLPHL) is an uncommon B-cell neoplasm defined by characteristic large neoplastic cells in an inflammatory background. The neoplastic cells have scanty cytoplasm and single multilobated nuclei with multiple small nucleoli; they were previously designated L&H cells (for lymphocytic and/ or histiocytic Reed–Sternberg cell variants) or 'popcorn cells' but the designation LP cells is now preferred [387,388]. NLPHL is considered to be of germinal centre B-cell origin [386].

Presentation is usually with localized lymphadenopathy. Patients are more often male with a peak incidence between 30 and 50 years. Prognosis is good but late relapses can occur. Sometimes relapse is as DLBCL.

Peripheral blood
The peripheral blood shows no specific features.

Bone marrow cytology
The bone marrow aspirate is usually normal.

Flow cytometric immunophenotyping
Since neoplastic cells are absent from the blood and very rarely present in the marrow aspirate, flow cytometric immunophenotyping is not indicated.

Cytogenetic and molecular genetic analysis
Immunoglobulin genes are clonally rearranged. There are no consistent cytogenetic abnormalities but translocations with a 3q27 breakpoint and *BCL6* rearrangement are common [386] (Box 6.23). EBV is not detected in neoplastic cells.

Bone marrow histology

Bone marrow infiltration is rare and, when present, the infiltrate often resembles that of T-cell/histiocyte-rich large B-cell lymphoma and may represent disease progression; it is prognostically adverse [409].

Immunohistochemistry

The neoplastic LP cells are CD15 and CD30 negative (see Table 6.7 and Box 6.23). They are CD45, CD20 and CD79a positive and immunoglobulin may be expressed. BCL2 protein is not expressed [406], whereas BCL6 protein is strongly expressed [406].

Problems and pitfalls

Since bone marrow infiltration is very rare in NLPHL the diagnosis should be critically reappraised if it is found. When there is infiltration, the features can be very similar to those of T-cell/histiocyte-rich DLBCL (see Fig. 6.57, in which large neoplastic B cells are ringed by MUM1/IRF4-positive T cells; disease evolution in NLPHL could produce a similar appearance). A distinction between these two alternatives may be impossible if no primary diagnosis has been established from another tissue.

Post-transplant and other immunodeficiency-related lymphoproliferative disorders and their relationship to the Epstein–Barr virus

Many of the entities already discussed have an increased incidence in, or are largely confined to, immunodeficient individuals. In this section we shall bring together lymphoproliferative disorders, non-neoplastic and lymphomatous, that are related to immune deficiency, many of which are also related to EBV.

Epstein–Barr virus has the ability to infect B lymphocytes *in vivo* and *in vitro*. *In vitro* it can transform and immortalize B lymphocytes. Primary infection usually occurs in childhood and, in the vast majority of individuals, is asymptomatic. In more prosperous countries primary infection is often delayed until adolescence or early adult life, resulting in infectious mononucleosis.

Epstein–Barr virus has been implicated in the pathogenesis of a number of distinct types of lymphoma and other non-neoplastic lymphoproliferative disorder [410] (Table 6.8). Many EBV-associated lymphomas occur in immunocompromised individuals. Evidence of latent EBV infection can be detected within tumour cells using *in situ* hybridization for EBV-EBER. Sometimes EBV latent proteins (LMP-1 and EBNA-2) are expressed and can be detected using immunohistochemistry.

Post-transplant lymphoproliferative disorders related to immunosuppression have been observed particularly following solid organ transplantation (renal, heart, heart/lung, thymus and liver) [411] and, to a lesser extent, following bone marrow transplantation [412]. The incidence following solid organ transplantation is related to the degree of immune suppression and in some series of patients has been as high as 20–25%. It is highest following heart/lung and intestinal transplantation. Following bone marrow transplantation, the cumulative incidence is around 1% by 10 years with the majority of cases occurring within the first 6 months [413]. Although the incidence is low, EBV-related lymphoproliferation is responsible for more than half of the cases of malignant disease following bone marrow transplantation [412]. The incidence is greater in children because of the greater risk associated with primary EBV infection. The onset of EBV-related lymphoproliferation typically occurs 6 months or more after solid organ transplantation.

Table 6.8 Epstein–Barr virus-related lymphomas and non-neoplastic lymphoproliferative disorders.

Type of lymphoma or lymphoproliferative disorder	Comment
Non-neoplastic lymphoproliferative disorder	
Fatal infectious mononucleosis	There is often an associated haemophagocytic syndrome
Polyclonal post-transplant or immunosuppression-related lymphoproliferative disorders	
Non-Hodgkin lymphoma	
Burkitt lymphoma	Almost all endemic cases, about a third of HIV-related cases, about 10% of sporadic cases, cases in X-linked lymphoproliferative syndrome, some cases in ALPS
Diffuse large B-cell lymphoma	40–50% of cases of DLBCL in HIV-positive patients and some cases in other immune deficiency syndromes, some cases in ALPS, occasionally in individuals with apparently normal immunity
Primary effusion lymphoma	HHV8 as co-factor and usually also HIV
Lymphomatoid granulomatosis	Higher incidence in inherited and acquired immunodeficiency
DLBCL associated with inflammation	Usually related to pyothorax due to *Mycobacterium tuberculosis*
EBV-positive DLBCL of the elderly	Age-related decline in immune function is presumed risk factor
Plasmablastic lymphoma, mainly of oral cavity	Mainly HIV-positive patients
Plasmacytoma or plasma cell myeloma	Post-transplant (some cases)
Large cell transformation of CLL or low grade non-Hodgkin lymphoma	Some cases
T/NK-cell lymphoma, nasal type	Particularly, but not only, in individuals of Chinese ethnic origin or from Central or South America
Aggressive NK-cell leukaemia	More prevalent among Chinese
EBV-positive T-cell lymphoproliferative disorders of childhood	Can emerge following primary infection by EBV or in patients with chronic active EBV infection
Hodgkin lymphoma	
Classical Hodgkin lymphoma (nodular sclerosis and mixed cellularity subtypes)	Up to 50% cases in developed countries, the majority of cases in the developing world and almost 100% of cases in HIV-positive patients; recognized in 10–50% of cases of nodular sclerosis subtype and 32–96% of cases of mixed cellularity subtype; EBV association is more common in paediatric cases; some cases of Hodgkin lymphoma occurring in primary immunodeficiency syndromes, post-transplantation and following iatrogenic immune suppression

ALPS, autoimmune lymphoproliferative syndrome; CLL, chronic lymphocytic leukaemia; DLBCL, diffuse large B-cell lymphoma; EBV, Epstein–Barr virus; HHV8, human herpesvirus 8; HIV, human immunodeficiency virus; NK, natural killer.

Similar lymphoproliferative disorders can occur in congenital and other acquired immune deficiency states including severe combined immune deficiency, ataxia telangiectasia, Wiskott–Aldrich syndrome, adenosine deaminase deficiency, X-linked lymphoproliferative disorder (Duncan's syndrome), hyperimmunoglobulin M syndrome, Chédiak–Higashi syndrome, common variable immunodeficiency, HIV infection and following methotrexate or ciclosporin therapy for rheumatoid arthritis, dermatomyositis or Wegener's granulomatosis or infliximab or related monoclonal antibody therapy for Crohn's disease. EBV-related lymphoproliferation can result from primary infection (virus acquired from donor tissue or from blood or blood products) or from reactivation of a latent viral infection. Primary infection at the time of transplantation carries the highest risk. The proliferating virus-infected B cells may be of donor or host origin. Following solid organ transplantation they are usually, but not always, of host origin whereas following bone marrow transplantation they are often of donor origin [414–416].

The lymphoproliferative disorders observed range from polyclonal through oligoclonal proliferations to monoclonal lymphomas [417–420]. Lymphoproliferative disorders observed post-transplant are often multifocal and extranodal. They often develop in the gut, central nervous system or transplanted organ, suggesting that micro-environmental factors contribute to their development. At one extreme, polyclonal proliferations may resemble severe infectious mononucleosis clinically and pathologically (with fever, pharyngitis and cervical lymphadenopathy) while at the other extreme they are high grade, monoclonal, clinically very aggressive lymphomas.

Classification of post-transplant lymphoproliferative disorders is based on the morphology of the proliferating cell population and whether there is immunohistochemical, cytogenetic or molecular genetic evidence of monoclonality. Clonality can be demonstrated by investigation of *IGH* rearrangement or by showing clonality of the episomal form of EBV within the tumour cells [421].

Polymorphic post-transplant lymphoproliferative disorder is characterized by a destructive infiltrate made up of a mixed population of cells representing the full spectrum of B-cell maturation from immunoblasts to plasma cells [422]. Most cases of polymorphic post-transplant lymphoproliferative disorder show evidence of monoclonality although a minority of cases appear to be polyclonal. Approximately half the patients have lesions in the bone marrow with aggregates of polymorphic lymphoid cells, including lymphocytes, plasmacytoid lymphocytes and plasma cells [423] (Figs 6.91 and 6.92). Bone marrow aspirates sometimes show considerable numbers of plasma cells and atypical lymphocytes may also be present [423]. Virus-infected (EBER-positive) cells are demonstrable in trephine biopsy sections in the majority of patients

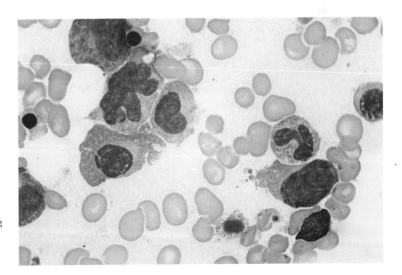

Fig. 6.91 BM aspirate from an immunosuppressed patient who developed fatal polyclonal EBV-related lymphoproliferation showing normal myeloid cells, a plasma cell and three atypical lymphoid cells. MGG ×100.

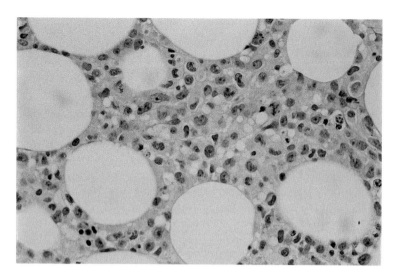

Fig. 6.92 BM trephine biopsy section, polymorphic post-transplant lymphoproliferative disorder. H&E ×40.

Table 6.9 The 2008 WHO classification of immunodeficiency-associated lymphoproliferative disorders.

Underlying condition	Comment
Primary immune disorder	May be non-neoplastic (e.g. tissue infiltration by phenotypically abnormal, CD4-negative/CD8-negative polyclonal T cells in ALPS or by plasma cells expressing immunoglobulins M and D in hyperimmunoglobulin M syndrome) or neoplastic (NHL or, less often, classical HL)
HIV infection	Mainly B-lineage NHL (DLBCL, BL, PEL, plasmablastic lymphoma), also classical HL
Transplantation	Polyclonal and oligoclonal lymphoproliferative disorders, plasma cell hyperplasia and lymphomas – mainly B-lineage NHL (DLBCL, BL) but also plasma cell myeloma, hepatosplenic T-cell and other T/NK-cell lymphomas and HL
Other iatrogenic immune deficiency	Mainly B-lineage NHL but similar spectrum to post-transplantation, related to methotrexate, ciclosporin and anti-tumour necrosis factor α monoclonal antibodies

ALPS, autoimmune lymphoproliferative syndrome; BL, Burkitt lymphoma; DLBCL, diffuse large B-cell lymphoma; HIV, human immunodeficiency virus; HL, Hodgkin lymphoma; NHL, non-Hodgkin lymphoma; NK, natural killer; PEL, primary effusion lymphoma.

with morphological changes in the marrow but not in patients lacking such changes [423]. Polyclonal plasmacytosis may also occur as an EBV-associated lymphoproliferative condition.

Monomorphic post-transplant lymphoproliferative disorders are usually B-cell proliferations although a small number of T-cell and NK-cell lymphomas have been reported. Most cases are DLBCL (immunoblastic or plasmablastic morphological variants) with a small number of cases being Burkitt lymphoma. In cases with bone marrow infiltration the disease is morphologically similar to that seen in these types of lymphoma occurring in non-immunocompromised patients. A classical Hodgkin

lymphoma-type post-transplant lymphoproliferative disorder also occurs.

In the 2008 WHO classification lymphoproliferative disorders associated with immune deficiency are categorized as shown in Table 6.9. Not all are EBV related.

References

1 Jaffe ES, Harris NL, Stein H, Campo E, Pileri SA and Swerdlow SH (2008) Introduction and overview of the classification of the lymphoid neoplasms. In: Swerdlow SH, Campo E, Harris NL, Jaffe ES, Pileri SA, Stein H, Thiele J and Vardiman JW (eds) *World*

Health Organization Classification of Tumours of Haematopoietic and Lymphoid Tissues. IARC Press, Lyon, pp. 158–166.

2 Harris NL, Jaffe ES, Stein H, Banks PM, Chan JK, Cleary ML *et al.* (1994) A revised European–American classification of lymphoid neoplasms: a proposal from the International Lymphoma Study Group. *Blood,* **84,** 1361–1392.

3 Stansfeld AG, Diebold J, Noel H, Kapanci Y, Rilke F, Kelényi G *et al.* (1988) Updated Kiel classification for lymphomas. *Lancet,* **i,** 292–293.

4 Suchi T, Lennert K, Tu LY, Kikuchi M, Sato E, Stansfeld AG and Feller AC (1987) Histopathology and immunohistochemistry of peripheral T cell lymphomas: a proposal for their classification. *J Clin Pathol,* **40,** 995–1015.

5 Lukes RJ, Craver LH, Hall TC, Rappaport H and Ruben P (1966) Report of the nomenclature committee. *Cancer Res,* **26,** 1311.

6 Rozman C, Hernandez Nieto L, Montserrat E and Brugues R (1981) Prognostic significance of bone-marrow patterns in chronic lymphocytic leukaemia. *Br J Haematol,* **47,** 529–537.

7 Bartl R, Frisch B, Burkhardt R, Jäger K, Pappenberger R and Hoffmann Fezer G (1984) Lymphoproliferations in the bone marrow: identification and evolution, classification and staging. *J Clin Pathol,* **37,** 233–254.

8 McKenna RW and Hernandez JA (1988) Bone marrow in malignant lymphoma. *Hematol Oncol Clin North Am,* **2,** 617–635.

9 Frisch B and Bartl R (1999) *Biopsy Interpretation of Bone and Bone Marrow,* 2nd edn. Arnold, London.

10 Gaulard P, Kanavaros P, Farcet JP, Rocha FD, Haioun C, Divine M *et al.* (1991) Bone marrow histologic and immunohistochemical findings in peripheral. T-cell lymphoma: a study of 38 cases. *Hum Pathol,* **22,** 331–338.

11 Tateyama H, Eimoto T, Tada T, Kamiya M, Fujiyoshi Y and Kajiura S (1991) Congenital angiotropic lymphoma (intravascular lymphomatosis) of the T-cell type. *Cancer,* **67,** 2131–2136.

12 Conlan MG, Bast M, Armitage JO and Weisenburger DD (1990) Bone marrow involvement by non-Hodgkin's lymphoma: the clinical significance of morphologic discordance between the lymph node and bone marrow. Nebraska Lymphoma Study Group. *J Clin Oncol,* **8,** 1163–1172.

13 Thaler J, Dietze O, Denz H, Demuth R, Nachbaur D, Stauder R and Huber H (1991) Bone marrow diagnosis in lymphoproliferative disorders: comparison of results obtained from conventional histomorphology and immunohistology. *Histopathology,* **18,** 495–504.

14 Foucar K, McKenna RW, Frizzera G and Brunning RD (1982) Bone marrow and blood involvement by lymphoma in relationship to the Lukes–Collins classification. *Cancer,* **49,** 888–897.

15 Thiele J, Langohr J, Skorupka M and Fischer R (1990) Reticulin fibre content of bone marrow infiltrates of malignant non-Hodgkin's lymphomas (B-cell type, low malignancy) – a morphometric evaluation before and after therapy. *Virchows Arch A Pathol Anat Histopathol,* **417,** 485–492.

16 Campbell JK, Juneja SK and Wolf MM (1999) Serial sectioning of the trephine biopsy increases the diagnostic accuracy of bone marrow involvement in diffuse large cell lymphoma. *Blood,* **94** (Suppl. 1), 243b.

17 Pezzella F, Munson PJ, Miller KD, Goldstone AH and Gatter KC (2000) The diagnosis of low-grade peripheral B-cell neoplasms in bone marrow trephines. *Br J Haematol,* **108,** 369–376.

18 Pittaluga S, Tierens A, Dodoo YL, Delabie J and De Wolf-Peeters C (1999) How reliable is histologic examination of bone marrow trephine biopsy specimens for the staging of non-Hodgkin lymphoma? A study of hairy cell leukemia and mantle cell lymphoma involvement of the bone marrow trephine specimen by histologic, immunohistochemical, and polymerase chain reaction techniques. *Am J Clin Pathol,* **111,** 179–184.

19 Coad JE, Olson DJ, Christensen DR, Lander TA, Chibbar R, McGlennen RC and Brunning RD (1997) Correlation of PCR-detected clonal gene rearrangements with bone marrow morphology in patients with B-lineage lymphomas. *Am J Surg Pathol,* **21,** 1047–1056.

20 Bartl R, Hansmann ML, Frisch B and Burkhardt R (1988) Comparative histology of malignant lymphomas in lymph node and bone marrow. *Br J Haematol,* **69,** 229–237.

21 Fisher DE, Jacobson JO, Ault KA and Harris NL (1989) Diffuse large cell lymphoma with discordant bone marrow histology. Clinical features and biological implications. *Cancer,* **64,** 1879–1887 [published erratum appears in *Cancer* 1990, **65,** 64].

22 Kluin PM, van Krieken JH, Kleiverda K and Kluin-Nelemans HC (1990) Discordant morphologic characteristics of B-cell lymphomas in bone marrow and lymph node biopsies. *Am J Clin Pathol,* **94,** 59–66.

23 Hanson CA, Brunning RD, Gajl-Peczalska KJ, Frizzera G and McKenna RW (1986) Bone marrow manifestations of peripheral T-cell lymphoma. A study of 30 cases. *Am J Clin Pathol,* **86,** 449–460.

24 Caulet S, Delmer A, Audouin J, Le Tourneau A, Bernadou A, Zittoun R and Diebold J (1990) Histopathological study of bone marrow biopsies in 30 cases of T-cell lymphoma with clinical, biological and survival correlations. *Hematol Oncol,* **8,** 155–168.

25 Frizzera G, Anaya JS and Banks PM (1986) Neoplastic plasma cells in follicular lymphomas. Clinical and pathologic findings in six cases. *Virchows Arch A Pathol Anat Histopathol*, **409**, 149–162.

26 Robertson LE, Redman JR, Butler JJ, Osborne BM, Velasquez WS, McLaughlin P *et al.* (1991) Discordant bone marrow involvement in diffuse large-cell lymphoma: a distinct clinical-pathologic entity associated with a continuous risk of relapse. *J Clin Oncol*, **9**, 236–242.

27 Kremer M, Spitzer M, Mandl-Weber S, Stecker K, Schmidt B, Höfler H *et al.* (2003) Discordant bone marrow involvement in diffuse large B-cell lymphoma: comparative molecular analysis reveals a heterogeneous group of disorders. *Lab Invest*, **83**, 107–114.

28 Chetty R, Echezarreta G, Comley M and Gatter K (1995) Immunohistochemistry in apparently normal bone marrow trephine specimens from patients with nodal follicular lymphoma. *J Clin Pathol*, **48**, 1035–1038.

29 Ben-Ezra JM, King BE, Harris AC, Todd WM and Kornstein MJ (1994) Staining for Bcl-2 protein helps to distinguish benign from malignant lymphoid aggregates in bone marrow biopsies. *Mod Pathol*, **7**, 560–564.

30 Skálová A and Fakan F (1997) Bcl-2 protein does not help to distinguish benign from malignant lymphoid nodules in bone marrow biopsy specimens. *J Clin Pathol*, **50**, 87–88.

31 Kröber SM, Horny HP, Greschniok A and Kaiserling E (1999) Reactive and neoplastic lymphocytes in human bone marrow: morphological, immunohistological, and molecular biological investigations on biopsy specimens. *J Clin Pathol*, **52**, 521–526.

32 Gong JZ, Zheng S, Chiarle R, De Wolf-Peeters C, Palestro G, Frizzera G and Inghirami G (1999) Detection of immunoglobulin kappa light chain rearrangements by polymerase chain reaction: an improved method for detecting clonal B-cell lymphoproliferative disorders. *Am J Clin Pathol*, **155**, 355–363.

33 Jaffe ES, Harris NL, Stein H and Vardiman JW (eds) (2001) *World Health Organization Classification of Tumours: Pathology and Genetics of Tumours of Haematopoietic and Lymphoid Tissues*. IARC Press, Lyon.

34 Borowitz MJ and Chan JKC (2008) B lymphoblastic leukaemia/lymphoma, not otherwise specified. In: Swerdlow SH, Campo E, Harris NL, Jaffe ES, Pileri SA, Stein H, Thiele J and Vardiman JW (eds) *World Health Organization Classification of Tumours of Haematopoietic and Lymphoid Tissues*. IARC Press, Lyon, pp. 168–170.

35 Borowitz MJ and Chan JKC (2008) B lymphoblastic leukaemia/lymphoma with recurrent genetic abnor-malities. In: Swerdlow SH, Campo E, Harris NL, Jaffe ES, Pileri SA, Stein H, Thiele J and Vardiman JW (eds) *World Health Organization Classification of Tumours of Haematopoietic and Lymphoid Tissues*. IARC Press, Lyon, pp. 171–175.

36 Morton LM, Wang SS, Devesa SS, Hartge P, Weisenburger DD and Linet MS (2006) Lymphoma incidence patterns by WHO subtype in the United States, 1992–2001. *Blood*, **107**, 265–276.

37 Bennett JM, Catovsky D, Daniel MT, Flandrin G, Galton DA, Gralnick HR and Sultan C (1976) Proposals for the classification of the acute leukaemias. French–American–British (FAB) co-operative group. *Br J Haematol*, **33**, 451–458.

38 Picozzi VJ and Coleman CN (1990) Lymphoblastic lymphoma. *Semin Oncol*, **17**, 96–103.

39 Maitra A, McKenna RW, Weinberg AG, Schneider NR and Kroft SH (2001) Precursor B-cell lymphoblastic lymphoma: a study of nine cases lacking blood and bone marrow involvement and review of the literature. *Am J Clin Pathol*, **115**, 868–875.

40 Bene MC, Castoldi G, Knapp W, Ludwig WD, Matutes E, Orfao A and Van't Veer MB (1995) Proposals for the immunological classification of acute leukemias. European Group for the Immunological Characterization of Leukemias (EGIL). *Leukemia*, **9**, 1783–1786.

41 Chessels JM, Swansbury GJ, Reeves B, Bailey CC and Richards SM (1997) Cytogenetics and prognosis in childhood lymphoblastic leukaemia: results of MRC UKALL X. Medical Research Council Working Party in Childhood Leukaemia. *Br J Haematol*, **99**, 93–100.

42 McKenna RW, Parkin J and Brunning RD (1979) Morphologic and ultrastructural characteristics of T-cell acute lymphoblastic leukemia. *Cancer*, **44**, 1290–1297.

43 Hann IM, Evans DI, Marsden HB, Jones PM and Palmer MK (1978) Bone marrow fibrosis in acute lymphoblastic leukaemia of childhood. *J Clin Pathol*, **31**, 313–315.

44 Pulè MA, Gullman C, Dennis D, McMahon C, Jeffers M and Smith OP (2002) Increased angiogenesis in bone marrow of children with acute lymphoblastic leukaemia has no prognostic significance. *Br J Haematol*, **118**, 991–998.

45 Breatnach F, Chessells JM and Greaves MF (1981) The aplastic presentation of childhood leukaemia: a feature of common-ALL. *Br J Haematol*, **49**, 387–393.

46 Dharmasena F, Littlewood T, Gordon-Smith EC, Catovsky D and Galton DA (1986) Adult acute lymphoblastic leukaemia presenting with bone marrow aplasia. *Clin Lab Haematol*, **8**, 361–364.

47 Chessells JM (2001) Pitfalls in the diagnosis of childhood leukaemia. *Br J Haematol*, **114**, 506–511.

48 Reid MM and Summerfield GP (1992) Distinction between aleukaemic prodrome of childhood acute lymphoblastic leukaemia and aplastic anaemia. *J Clin Pathol*, **45**, 697–700.

49 Nowicki M, Ostalska-Nowicka D, Konwerska A and Miskowiak B (2006) The predictive role of substance P in the neoplastic transformation of the hypoplastic bone marrow. *J Clin Pathol*, **59**, 935–941.

50 Savansan S and Özdeir Ö (2003) Parvovirus B19 infection and acute lymphoblastic leukaemia. *Br J Haematol*, **120**, 168–169.

51 Intermesoli T, Mangili G, Salvi A, Biondi A and Bassan R (2007) Abnormally expanded pro-B hematogones associated with congenital cytomegalovirus infection. *Am J Hematol*, **82**, 934–936.

52 McKenna D, Rupp C, Wagner J, McGlennen R, Hirsch B, Dolan M *et al.* (2000) Increased blast-like cells following cord blood transplantation do not predict recurrent acute leukemia. *Am J Clin Pathol*, **114**, 315–316.

53 Farahat N, Lens D, Zomas A, Morilla R, Matutes E and Catovsky D (1995) Quantitative flow cytometry can distinguish between normal and leukaemic B-cell precursors. *Br J Haematol*, **91**, 640–646.

54 Rimsza LM, Larson RS, Winter SS, Foucar K, Chong Y-Y, Garner KW and Leith CP (2000) Benign hematogone-rich lymphoid proliferations can be distinguished from B-lineage acute lymphoblastic leukemia by integration of morphology, immunophenotype, adhesion molecule expression, and architectural features. *Am J Clin Pathol*, **114**, 66–75.

55 McKenna RW, Washington LT, Aquino DB, Picker LJ and Kroft SH (2001) Immunophenotypic analysis of hematogones (B-lymphocyte precursors) in 662 consecutive bone marrow specimens by 4-color flow cytometry). *Blood*, **98**, 2498–2507.

56 Prakash P and Swerdlow SH (2007) Nodal aggressive B-cell lymphomas: a diagnostic approach. *J Clin Pathol*, **60**, 1076–1085.

57 Dores GM, Anderson WF, Curtis RE, Landgren O, Ostroumova E, Bluhm EC *et al.* (2007) Chronic lymphocytic leukaemia and small lymphocytic lymphoma: overview of the descriptive epidemiology. *Br J Haematol*, **139**, 809–819.

58 Müller-Hermelink HK, Montserrat E, Catovsky D, Harris NL and Stein H (2008) Chronic lymphocytic leukaemia/small lymphocytic lymphoma. In: Swerdlow SH, Campo E, Harris NL, Jaffe ES, Pileri SA, Stein H, Thiele J and Vardiman JW (eds) *World Health Organization Classification of Tumours of Haematopoietic and Lymphoid Tissues*. IARC Press, Lyon, pp. 180–182.

59 Ohno T, Smir BN, Weisenburger DD, Gascoyne RD, Hinrichs SD and Chan WC (1998) Origin of the Hodgkin/Reed–Sternberg cells in chronic lymphocytic leukaemia with 'Hodgkin's transformation'. *Blood*, **91**, 1757–1761.

60 Roddie C, Cwynarski K, Craig C, Diss T and McNamara C (2007) Hodgkin transformation of newly diagnosed small lymphocytic lymphoma in the gastrointestinal tract. *Leuk Lymphoma*, **48**, 1644–1646.

61 Enno A, Catovsky D, O'Brien M, Cherchi M, Kumaran TO and Galton DA (1979) 'Prolymphocytoid' transformation of chronic lymphocytic leukaemia. *Br J Haematol*, **41**, 9–18.

62 Pangalis GA, Nathwani BN and Rappaport H (1977) Malignant lymphoma, well differentiated lymphocytic: its relationship with chronic lymphocytic leukemia and macroglobulinemia of Waldenström. *Cancer*, **39**, 999–1010.

63 Montserrat E and Rozman C (1993) Chronic lymphocytic leukaemia: prognostic factors and natural history. *Baillières Clin Haematol*, **6**, 849–866.

64 Dick F, Bloomfield CD and Brunning RD (1974) Incidence cytology, and histopathology of non-Hodgkin's lymphomas in the bone marrow. *Cancer*, **33**, 1382–1398.

65 Mazza P, Gherlinzoni F, Kemna G, Poletti G, Zinzani PL, Verlicchi F *et al.* (1987) Clinicopathological study on non-Hodgkin's lymphomas. *Haematologica*, **72**, 351–357.

66 Moreau EJ, Matutes E, A'Hern RP, Morilla AM, Morilla RM, Owusu-Ankomah KA *et al.* (1997) Improvement of the chronic lymphocytic leukemia scoring system with the monoclonal antibody SN8 (CD79b). *Am J Clin Pathol*, **108**, 378–382.

67 Matutes E, Owusu-Ankomah K, Morilla R, Garcia-Marco J, Houlihan A, Que TH and Catovsky D (1994) The immunological profile of B-cell disorders and proposal of a scoring system for the diagnosis of CLL. *Leukemia*, **8**, 1640–1645.

68 Finn WG, Thangavelu M, Yelavarthi KK, Goolsby CL, Tallman MS, Traynor A and Peterson LC (1996) Karyotype correlates with peripheral blood morphology and immunophenotype in chronic lymphocytic leukemia. *Am J Clin Pathol*, **105**, 458–467.

69 Matutes E, Oscier D, Garcia-Marco J, Ellis J, Copplestone A, Gillingham R *et al.* (1996) Trisomy 12 defines a group of CLL with atypical morphology: correlation between cytogenetic, clinical and laboratory features in 544 patients. *Br J Haematol*, **92**, 382–388.

70 Geisler CH, Philip P, Christensen BE, Hou-Jensen K, Pedersen NT, Jensen OM *et al.* (1997) In B-cell chronic lymphocytic leukaemia chromosome 17 abnormalities and not trisomy 12 are the single most important cytogenetic abnormalities for the prognosis: a cytogenetic and immunophenotypic study of 480 unselected newly diagnosed patients. *Leuk Res*, **21**, 1011–1023.

71 Gahn B, Wendenburg B, Troff C, Neef J, Grove D, Haferlach T *et al.* (1999) Analysis of progenitor cell

involvement in B-CLL by simultaneous immunophenotypic and genotypic analysis at the single cell level. *Br J Haematol*, **105**, 955–959.

72 Garcia-Marco J, Matutes E, Morilla R, Ellis J, Oscier D, Fantes J *et al.* (1994) Trisomy 12 in B-cell chronic lymphocytic leukaemia: assessment of lineage restriction by simultaneous analysis of immunophenotype and genotype in interphase cells by fluorescence in situ hybridization. *Br J Haematol*, **87**, 44–50.

73 Dimopoulou MN, Vassilakopoulos TP, Siakantaris MP, Kyrtsonis MC, Kontopidou FN, Kokoris SI *et al.* (2007) Cytogenetic differences between B-chronic lymphocytic leukemia (B-CLL) and small lymphocytic lymphoma (SLL). *Leuk Lymphoma*, **48** (Suppl. 1), S142.

74 Peterson L-A, Kini AR and Kay N (2001) Angiogenesis is increased in B-cell chronic lymphocytic leukemia. *Blood*, **97**, 2529.

75 Molica S, Vacca A, Ribatti D, Cuneo A, Cavazzini F, Levato D *et al.* (2002) Prognostic value of enhanced bone marrow angiogenesis in early B-cell chronic lymphocytic leukemia. *Blood*, **100**, 3344–3351.

76 Rozman C, Montserrat E, Rodríguez-Fernández JM, Ayats R, Vallespí T, Parody R *et al.* (1984) Bone marrow histologic pattern – the best single prognostic parameter in chronic lymphocytic leukemia: a multivariate survival analysis of 329 cases. *Blood*, **64**, 642–648.

77 Kim YS, Ford RJ, Faber JA, Bell RH, Elenitoba-Johnson KSJ and Medeiros LJ (2000) B-cell chronic lymphocytic leukemia/small lymphocytic lymphoma involving bone marrow with an interfollicular pattern. *Am J Clin Pathol*, **114**, 41–46.

78 Geisler C, Ralfkiær E, Hansen MM, Hou-Jensen K and Larsen SO (1986) The bone marrow histological pattern has independent prognostic value in early stage chronic lymphocytic leukaemia. *Br J Haematol*, **62**, 47–54.

79 Frisch B and Bartl R (1988) Histologic classification and staging of chronic lymphocytic leukemia. A retrospective and prospective study of 503 cases. *Acta Haematol*, **79**, 140–152.

80 Trump DL, Mann RB, Phelps R, Roberts H and Conley CL (1980) Richter's syndrome: diffuse histiocytic lymphoma in patients with chronic lymphocytic leukemia. A report of five cases and review of the literature. *Am J Med*, **68**, 539–548.

81 Foucar K and Rydell RE (1980) Richter's syndrome in chronic lymphocytic leukemia. *Cancer*, **46**, 118–134.

82 Adelstein DJ, Henry MB, Bowman LS and Hines JD (1991) Diffuse well differentiated lymphocytic lymphoma: a clinical study of 22 patients. *Oncology*, **48**, 48–53.

83 Pangalis GA and Kittas C (1988) Bone marrow involvement in chronic lymphocytic leukemia, small

lymphocytic (well differentiated) and lymphoplasmacytic (macroglobulinemia of Waldenström) non-Hodgkin's lymphomas. In: Polliack A and Catovsky D (eds) *Chronic Lymphocytic Leukaemia*. Harwood Academic Publishers, Chur.

84 Pangalis GA, Roussou PA, Kittas C, Mitsoulis-Mentzikoff C, Matsouka-Alexandridis P, Anagnostopoulos N *et al.* (1984) Patterns of bone marrow involvement in chronic lymphocytic leukemia and small lymphocytic (well differentiated) non-Hodgkin's lymphoma. Its clinical significance in relation to their differential diagnosis and prognosis. *Cancer*, **54**, 702–708.

85 Lampert IA, Wotherspoon A, Van Noorden S and Hasserjian RP (1999) High expression of CD23 in the proliferation centers of chronic lymphocytic leukemia in lymph nodes and spleen. *Hum Pathol*, **30**, 648–654.

86 Sup SJ, Domiati-Saad R, Kelley TW, Steinle R, Zhao X and Hsi ED (2004) ZAP-70 expression in B-cell hematologic malignancy is not limited to CLL/SLL. *Am J Clin Pathol*, **122**, 582–587.

87 Gordon DS, Jones BM, Browning SW, Spira TJ and Lawrence DN (1982) Persistent polyclonal lymphocytosis of B lymphocytes. *N Engl J Med*, **307**, 232–236.

88 Bain B, Matutes E and Catovsky D (1998) Teaching cases from the Royal Marsden and St Mary's Hospitals. Case 14: persistent lymphocytosis in a middle aged smoker. *Leuk Lymphoma*, **28**, 623–625.

89 Feugier P, De March AK, Lesesve JF, Monhoven N, Dorvaux V, Braun F *et al.* (2004) Intravascular bone marrow accumulation in persistent polyclonal lymphocytosis: a misleading features for B-cell neoplasm. *Mod Pathol*, **17**, 1087–1096.

90 Campo E, Catovsky D, Montserrat E, Müller-Hermelink HK, Harris NL and Stein H (2008) B-cell prolymphocytic leukaemia. In: Swerdlow SH, Campo E, Harris NL, Jaffe ES, Pileri SA, Stein H, Thiele J and Vardiman JW (eds) *World Health Organization Classification of Tumours of Haematopoietic and Lymphoid Tissues*. IARC Press, Lyon, pp. 183–184.

91 Brito-Babapulle V, Pomfret M, Matutes E and Catovsky D (1987) Cytogenetic studies on prolymphocytic leukaemia. II. T cell prolymphocytic leukemia. *Blood*, **70**, 926–931.

92 Nieto LH, Lampert IA and Catovsky D (1989) Bone marrow histological patterns in B-cell and T-cell prolymphocytic leukemia. *Hematol Pathol*, **3**, 79–84.

93 Foucar K, Falini B, Catovsky D and Stein H (2008) Hairy cell leukaemia. In: Swerdlow SH, Campo E, Harris NL, Jaffe ES, Pileri SA, Stein H, Thiele J and Vardiman JW (eds) *World Health Organization Classification of Tumours of Haematopoietic and Lymphoid Tissues*. IARC Press, Lyon, pp. 189–190.

94 Mercieca J, Matutes E, Moskovic E, MacLennan K, Matthey F, Costello C et al. (1992) Massive abdominal lymphadenopathy in hairy cell leukaemia: a report of 12 cases. Br J Haematol, 82, 547–554.

95 Vykoupil KF, Thiele J and Georgii A (1976) Hairy cell leukemia. Bone marrow findings in 24 patients. Virchows Arch A Pathol Anat Histopathol 370, 273–289.

96 Bartl R, Frisch B, Hill W, Burkhardt R, Sommerfeld W and Sund M (1983) Bone marrow histology in hairy cell leukemia. Identification of subtypes and their prognostic significance. Am J Clin Pathol, 79, 531–545.

97 Burke JS and Rappaport H (1984) The diagnosis and differential diagnosis of hairy cell leukemia in bone marrow and spleen. Semin Oncol, 11, 334–346.

98 Naeim F (1988) Hairy cell leukemia: characteristics of the neoplastic cells. Hum Pathol, 19, 375–388.

99 Lee WM and Beckstead JH (1982) Hairy cell leukemia with bone marrow hypoplasia. Cancer, 50, 2207–2210.

100 Bouroncle BA (1987) Unusual presentations and complications of hairy cell leukemia. Leukemia, 1, 288–293.

101 Lazzaro B, Munger R, Flick J and Moriber-Katz S (1991) Visualization of the ribosome–lamella complex in plastic-embedded biopsy specimens as an aid to diagnosis of hairy-cell leukemia. Arch Pathol Lab Med, 115, 1259–1262.

102 Burthem J and Cawley JC (1994) The bone marrow fibrosis of hairy cell leukemia is caused by the synthesis and assembly of a fibronectin matrix by the hairy cells. Blood, 83, 497–504.

103 Flandrin G, Sigaux F, Castaigne S, Billard C, Aguet M, Boiron M et al. (1986) Treatment of hairy cell leukemia with recombinant alpha interferon: I. Quantitative study of bone marrow changes during the first months of treatment. Blood, 67, 817–820.

104 Verhoef GE, De Wolf-Peeters C, Zachee P and Boogaerts MA (1990) Regression of diffuse osteosclerosis in hairy cell leukaemia after treatment with interferon. Br J Haematol, 76, 150–151.

105 VanderMolen LA, Urba WJ, Longo DL, Lawrence J, Gralnick H and Steis RG (1989) Diffuse osteosclerosis in hairy cell leukemia. Blood, 74, 2066–2069.

106 Golomb HM and Vardiman JW (1983) Response to splenectomy in 65 patients with hairy cell leukemia: an evaluation of spleen weight and bone marrow involvement. Blood, 61, 349–352.

107 Katayama I (1988) Bone marrow in hairy cell leukemia. Hematol Oncol Clin North Am, 2, 585–602.

108 Naeim F and Jacobs AD (1985) Bone marrow changes in patients with hairy cell leukemia treated by recombinant alpha$_2$-interferon. Hum Pathol, 16, 1200–1205.

109 Ratain MJ, Golomb HM, Bardawil RG, Vardiman JW, Westbrook CA, Kaminer LS et al. (1987) Durability of responses to interferon alpha-2b in advanced hairy cell leukemia. Blood, 69, 872–877.

110 Doane LL, Ratain MJ and Golomb HM (1990) Hairy cell leukemia. Current management. Hematol Oncol Clin North Am, 4, 489–502.

111 Catovsky D, Golde DW and Golomb HM (1990) The third international workshop on hairy cell leukemia, Laguna Miguel, California, 19–20 October, 1989. Br J Haematol, 74, 378–379.

112 Gillis S, Amir G, Bennett M and Polliack A (2001) Unexpectedly high incidence of hypoplastic/aplastic foci in bone marrow biopsies of hairy cell leukemia patients in remission following 2-chlorodeoxyadenosine therapy. Eur J Haematol, 66, 7–10.

113 Falini B, Pileri SA, Flenghi L, Liberati M, Stein H, Gerli R et al. (1990) Selection of a panel of monoclonal antibodies for monitoring residual disease in peripheral blood and bone marrow of interferon-treated hairy cell leukaemia patients. Br J Haematol, 76, 460–468.

114 Hounieu H, Chittal SM, al Saati T, de Mascarel A, Sabattini E, Pileri S et al. (1992) Hairy cell leukemia. Diagnosis of bone marrow involvement in paraffin-embedded sections with monoclonal antibody DBA.44. Am J Clin Pathol, 98, 26–33.

115 Janckila AJ, Cardwell EM, Yam LT and Li C-Y (1995) Hairy cell identification by immunohistochemistry of tartrate-resistant acid phosphatase. Blood, 85, 2839–2844.

116 Hoyer JD, Li CY, Yam LT, Hanson CA and Kurtin PJ (1997) Immunohistochemical demonstration of acid phosphatase isoenzyme 5 (tartrate-resistant) in paraffin sections of hairy cell leukemia and other hematologic disorders. Am J Clin Pathol, 108, 308–315.

117 Swerdlow SH, Berger F, Pileri SA, Harris NL, Jaffe ES and Stein H (2008) Lymphoplasmacytic lymphoma. In: Swerdlow SH, Campo E, Harris NL, Jaffe ES, Pileri SA, Stein H, Thiele J and Vardiman JW (eds) World Health Organization Classification of Tumours of Haematopoietic and Lymphoid Tissues. IARC Press, Lyon, pp. 194–195.

118 Vijay A and Gertz MA (2007) Waldenström macroglobulinaemia. Blood, 109, 5096–5103.

119 Pozzato G, Mazzaro C, Crovatto M, Modolo ML, Ceselli S, Mazzi G et al. (1994) Low-grade malignant lymphoma, hepatitis C virus infection, and mixed cryoglobulinemia. Blood, 84, 3047–3053.

120 Iida S, Rao PH, Nallasivam P, Hibshoosh H, Butler M, Louie DC et al. (1996) The t(9;14)(p13;q32) chromosomal translocation associated with lymphoplasmacytoid lymphoma involves the PAX-5 gene. Blood, 88, 4110–4117.

121 Ohno H, Ueda C and Akasaka T (2000) The t(9;14)(p13;q32) translocation in B-cell non-

Hodgkin's lymphoma. *Leuk Lymphoma*, **36**, 435–445.

122 Mansoor A, Medeiros LJ, Weber DM, Alexanian R, Hayes K, Jones D *et al.* (2001) Cytogenetic findings in lymphoplasmacytic lymphoma/Waldenström macroglobulinemia: chromosomal abnormalities are associated with the polymorphous subtype and an aggressive clinical course. *Am J Clin Pathol*, **116**, 543–549.

123 Bartl R, Frisch B, Mahl G, Burkhardt R, Fateh-Moghadam A, Pappenberger R *et al.* (1983) Bone marrow histology in Waldenström's macroglobulinaemia. Clinical relevance of subtype recognition. *Scand J Haematol*, **31**, 359–375.

124 Brunning RD (1989) Bone marrow. In: Rosai J (ed) *Ackerman's Surgical Pathology*, 7th edn. vol **2**. Mosby, St Louis.

125 Owen RG, Barrans SL, Richards SJ, O'Connor SJM, Child JA, Parapia LA *et al.* (2001) Waldenstrom's macroglobulinemia: development of criteria and identification of prognostic factors. *Am J Clin Pathol*, **116**, 420–428.

126 Molero T, De La Iglesia S, Santana C, Lemes A and Matutes E (1998) Signet-ring cells in a Waldenström's macroglobulinaemia. *Leuk Lymphoma*, **32**, 175–177.

127 Frisch B, Lewis SM, Burkhardt R and Bartl R (1985) *Biopsy Pathology of Bone and Bone Marrow*. Chapman & Hall, London.

128 Banham AH, Turley H, Pulford K, Gatter K and Mason DY (1997) The plasma cell associated antigen detectable by antibody VS38 is the p63 rough endoplasmic reticulum protein. *J Clin Pathol*, **50**, 485–489.

129 Harris NL, Swerdlow SH, Jaffe AS, Ott G, Nathwani BN, de Jong G, Yoshino T and Spagnolo D (2008) Follicular lymphoma. In: Swerdlow SH, Campo E, Harris NL, Jaffe ES, Pileri SA, Stein H, Thiele J and Vardiman JW (eds) *World Health Organization Classification of Tumours of Haematopoietic and Lymphoid Tissues*. IARC Press, Lyon, pp. 220–226.

130 Young KH, Xie Q, Zhou G, Eickhoff JC, Sanger WG, Aoun P and Chan WC (2008) Transformation of follicular lymphoma to precursor B-cell lymphoblastic lymphoma with c-*myc* gene rearrangement as a critical event. *Am J Clin Pathol*, **129**, 157–166.

131 Solal-Celigny P, Roy P, Colombat P, White J, Armitage JO, Arranz-Saez R *et al.* (2004) Follicular lymphoma international prognostic index. *Blood*, **104**, 1258–1265.

132 Schmidt B, Kremer M, Gotze K, John K, Peschel C, Höfler H and Fend F (2006) Bone marrow involvement in follicular lymphoma: comparison of histology and flow cytometry as staging procedures. *Leuk Lymphoma*, **47**, 1857–1862.

133 Horsman DE, Okamoto I, Ludkovski O, Le N, Harder L, Gesk S *et al.* (2003) Follicular lymphoma lacking the t(14;18)(q32;q21): identification of two disease subtypes. *Br J Haematol*, **120**, 424–433.

134 Bosga-Bouwer AG, van Imhoff GW, Boonstra R, van der Veen A, Haralambieva E, van den Berg A *et al.* (2003) Follicular lymphoma grade 3B includes three cytogenetically defined subgroups with primary t(14;18), 3q27, or other translocations: t(14;18) and 3q27 are mutually exclusive. *Blood*, **101**, 1149–1154.

135 Jardin F, Gaulard P, Buchonnet G, Contentin N, Lepretre S, Lenain P *et al.* (2002) Follicular lymphoma without t(14;18) and with BCL-6 rearrangement: a lymphoma subtype with distinct pathological, molecular and clinical characteristics. *Leukemia*, **16**, 2309–2317.

136 Krishnadasan R, Bifulco C, Kim J, Rodov S, Zieske AW and Vanasse GJ (2006) Overexpression of SOCS3 is associated with decreased survival in a cohort of patients with de novo follicular lymphoma. *Br J Haematol*, **135**, 72–75.

137 Roulland S, Lebailly P, Lecluse Y, Heutte N, Nadel B and Gauduchon P (2006) Long-term clonal persistence and evolution of t(14;18)-bearing B cells in healthy individuals. *Leukemia*, **20**, 158–162.

138 Canioni D, Brice P, Lepage E, Chababi M, Meignin V, Salles B *et al.* for the Groupe d'Etude des Lymphomes Folliculaires (2004) Bone marrow histological patterns can predict survival of patients with grade 1 or 2 follicular lymphoma: a study from the Groupe d'Etude des Lymphomes Folliculaires. *Br J Haematol*, **126**, 364–371.

139 Kim H and Dorfman RF (1974) Morphological studies of 84 untreated patients subjected to laparotomy for the staging of non-Hodgkin's lymphomas. *Cancer*, **33**, 657–674.

140 Vykoupil KF and Georgii A (1984) Non Hodgkin's lymphomas in bone marrow: diagnosis according to the Kiel classification and their growth patterns and relations to survival. In: Lennert K and Hübner K (eds) *Pathology of the Bone Marrow*. Gustav Fischer Verlag, Stuttgart.

141 Osborne BM and Butler JJ (1989) Hypocellular paratrabecular foci of treated small cleaved cell lymphoma in bone marrow biopsies. *Am J Surg Pathol*, **13**, 382–388.

142 Torlakovic E, Torlakovic G and Brunning RD (2002) Follicular pattern of bone marrow involvement by follicular lymphoma. *Am J Clin Pathol*, **118**, 780–786.

143 Bairey O and Shpilberg O (2007) Is bone marrow biopsy obligatory in all patients with non-Hodgkin's lymphoma? *Acta Haematol*, **118**, 61–64.

144 Falini B and Mason DY (2002) Proteins encoded by genes involved in chromosomal alterations in lymphoma and leukemia: clinical value of their detection by immunocytochemistry. *Blood*, **99**, 409–426.

145 West RB, Warnke RA and Natkunam Y (2002) The usefulness of immunohistochemistry in the diagnosis of follicular lymphoma in bone marrow biopsy specimens. *Am J Clin Pathol*, **117**, 636–643.

146 Karube K, Guo Y, Suzumiya J, Sugita Y, Nomura Y, Yamamoto K *et al.* (2007) CD10-MUM1+ follicular lymphoma lacks BCL2 gene translocation and shows characteristic biologic and clinical features. *Blood*, **109**, 3076–3079.

147 Raynaud P, Caulet-Maugendre S, Foussard C, Salles G, Moreau A, Rossi JF *et al.* for the GOELAMS Group (2008) T-cell lymphoid aggregates in bone marrow after rituximab therapy for B-cell follicular lymphoma: a marker of therapeutic efficacy? *Hum Pathol*, **39**, 194–200.

148 Foran JM, Norton AJ, Micallef INM, Taussig DC, Amess JAL, Rohatiner AZS and Lister TA (2001) Loss of CD20 expression following treatment with rituximab (chimaeric monoclonal anti-CD20): a retrospective cohort analysis. *Br J Haematol*, **114**, 881–883.

149 Swerdlow SH, Campo E, Seto M and Müller-Hermelink HK (2008) Mantle cell lymphoma. In: Swerdlow SH, Campo E, Harris NL, Jaffe ES, Pileri SA, Stein H, Thiele J and Vardiman JW (eds) *World Health Organization Classification of Tumours of Haematopoietic and Lymphoid Tissues*. IARC Press, Lyon, pp. 229–232.

150 Raffeld M and Jaffe ES (1991) bcl-1, t(11;14), and mantle cell-derived lymphomas. *Blood*, **78**, 259–263.

151 Jaffe ES, Bookman MA and Longo DL (1987) Lymphocytic lymphoma of intermediate differentiation – mantle zone lymphoma: a distinct subtype of B-cell lymphoma. *Hum Pathol*, **18**, 877–880.

152 Perry DA, Bast MA, Armitage JO and Weisenburger DD (1990) Diffuse intermediate lymphocytic lymphoma. A clinicopathologic study and comparison with small lymphocytic lymphoma and diffuse small cleaved cell lymphoma. *Cancer*, **66**, 1995–2000.

153 Cohen PL, Kurtin PJ, Donovan KA and Hanson CA (1998) Bone marrow and peripheral blood involvement in mantle cell lymphoma. *Br J Haematol*, **101**, 302–310.

154 de Oliveira MS, Jaffe ES and Catovsky D (1989) Leukaemic phase of mantle zone (intermediate) lymphoma: its characterisation in 11 cases. *J Clin Pathol*, **42**, 962–972.

155 Singleton TP, Anderson MM, Ross CW and Schnitzer B (1999) Leukemic phase of mantle cell lymphoma, blastoid variant. *Am J Clin Pathol*, **111**, 495–500.

156 Vaandrager JW, Schuuring E, Zwikstra E, de Boer CJ, Kleiverda KK, van Krieken JH *et al.* (1996) Direct visualization of dispersed 11q13 chromosomal translocations in mantle cell lymphoma by multicolor DNA fiber fluorescence in situ hybridization. *Blood*, **88**, 1177–1182.

157 Bertoni F, Zucca E and Cotter FE (2004) Molecular basis of mantle zone lymphoma. *Br J Haematol*, **124**, 130–140.

158 Wright G, Tan B, Rosenwald A, Hurt EH, Wiestner A and Staudt LM (2003) A gene expression-based method to distinguish clinically subgroups of diffuse large B-cell lymphoma. *Proc Natl Acad Sci USA*, **100**, 9991–9996.

159 Kienle D, Kröber A, Katzenberger T, Ott G, Leupolt E, Barth TFE *et al.* (2003) V_H mutation status and *VDJ* rearrangement structure in mantle cell lymphoma; correlation with genomic aberrations, clinical characteristics, and outcome. *Blood*, **102**, 3003–3009.

160 Swerdlow SH, Habeshaw JA, Murray LJ, Dhaliwal HS, Lister TA and Stansfeld AG (1983) Centrocytic lymphoma: a distinct clinicopathologic and immunologic entity. A multiparameter study of 18 cases at diagnosis and relapse. *Am J Pathol*, **113**, 181–197.

161 Weisenburger DD, Kim H and Rappaport H (1982) Mantle-zone lymphoma: a follicular variant of intermediate lymphocytic lymphoma. *Cancer*, **49**, 1429–1438.

162 Obeso G, Sanz ER, Rivas C, Marcos B, García-Delgado R, Echezarreta G *et al.* (1994) B-cell follicular lymphomas: clinical and biological characteristics. *Leuk Lymphoma*, **16**, 105–111.

163 Brunning R and McKenna RW (1994) *Tumors of the Bone Marrow*. Armed Forces Institute of Pathology, Washington.

164 Vasef MA, Medeiros LJ, Koo C, McCourty A and Brynes RK (1997) Cyclin D1 immunohistochemical staining is useful in distinguishing mantle cell lymphoma from other low-grade B-cell neoplasms in bone marrow. *Am J Clin Pathol*, **108**, 302–307.

165 Katzenberger T, Petzoldt C, Holler S, Mader U, Kalla J, Adam P *et al.* (2006) The Ki67 proliferation index is a quantitative indicator of clinical risk in mantle cell lymphoma. *Blood*, **107**, 3407.

166 Isaacson PG, Chott A, Nakamura S, Müller-Hermelink HK, Harris NL and Swerdlow SH (2008) Extranodal marginal zone B-cell lymphoma of mucosa-associated lymphoid tissue (MALT lymphoma). In: Swerdlow SH, Campo E, Harris NL, Jaffe ES, Pileri SA, Stein H, Thiele J and Vardiman JW (eds) *World Health Organization Classification of Tumours of Haematopoietic and Lymphoid Tissues*. IARC Press, Lyon, pp. 214–217.

167 Wotherspoon AC, Doglioni C, Diss TC, Pan L, Moschini A, de Boni M and Isaacson PG (1993) Regression of primary low-grade B-cell gastric lymphoma of mucosa-associated lymphoid tissue type after eradication of Helicobacter pylori. *Lancet*, **342**, 575–577.

168 Brynes RK, Almaguer PD, Leathery KE, McCourty A, Arber DA, Medeiros LJ and Nathwani BN (1996) Numerical cytogenetic abnormalities of chromo-

somes 3, 7, and 12 in marginal zone B-cell lymphomas. *Mod Pathol*, **9**, 995–1000.

169 Dierlamm J, Rosenberg C, Stul M, Pittaluga S, Wlodarska I, Michaux L *et al.* (1997) Characteristic pattern of chromosomal gains and losses in marginal zone B cell lymphoma detected by comparative genomic hybridization. *Leukemia*, **11**, 747–758.

170 Rosenwald A, Ott G, Stilgenbauer S, Kalla J, Bredt M, Katzenberger T *et al.* (1999) Exclusive detection of the t(11;18) (q21;q21) in extranodal marginal zone B cell lymphomas (MZBL) of MALT type in contrast to other MZBL and extranodal large B cell lymphomas. *Am J Pathol*, **155**, 1817–1821.

171 Isaacson PG and Du MQ (2004) MALT lymphoma: from morphology to molecules. *Nat Rev Cancer*, **4**, 644–653

172 Thieblemont C, Berger F, Dumontet C, Moullet I, Bouafia F, Felon P *et al.* (2000) Mucosa-associated lymphoid tissue lymphoma is a disseminated disease in a third of 158 patients analysed. *Blood*, **95**, 802–806.

173 de Boer JP, Hiddink RF, Raderer M, Antonini N, Aleman BMP, Boot H and de Jong D (2008) Dissemination patterns in non-gastric MALT lymphoma. *Haematologica*, **93**, 201–206.

174 Griesser H, Kaiser U, Augener W, Tiemann M and Lennert K (1990) B-cell lymphoma of the mucosa-associated lymphatic tissue (MALT) presenting with bone marrow and peripheral blood involvement. *Leuk Res*, **14**, 617–622.

175 Diss TC, Peng H, Wotherspoon AC, Pan L, Speight PM and Isaacson PG (1993) Brief report: a single neoplastic clone in sequential biopsy specimens from a patient with primary gastric-mucosa-associated lymphoid-tissue lymphoma and Sjogren's syndrome. *N Engl J Med*, **329**, 172–175.

176 Isaacson PG, Piris MA, Berger F, Swerdlow SH, Thieblemont C, Pittaluga S and Harris NL (2008) Splenic B-cell marginal zone lymphoma. In: Swerdlow SH, Campo E, Harris NL, Jaffe ES, Pileri SA, Stein H, Thiele J and Vardiman JW (eds) *World Health Organization Classification of Tumours of Haematopoietic and Lymphoid Tissues*. IARC Press, Lyon, pp. 185–187.

177 Franco V, Florena AM and Iannitto E (2003) Splenic marginal zone lymphoma. *Blood*, **101**, 2464–2472.

178 Melo JV, Hegde U, Parreira A, Thompson I, Lampert IA and Catovsky D (1987) Splenic B cell lymphoma with circulating villous lymphocytes: differential diagnosis of B cell leukaemias with large spleens. *J Clin Pathol*, **40**, 642–651.

179 Isaacson PG, Matutes E, Burke M and Catovsky D (1994) The histopathology of splenic lymphoma with villous lymphocytes. *Blood*, **84**, 3828–3834.

180 Piris M, Foucar K, Mollejo M, Campo E and Falini B (2008) Splenic B-cell lymphoma/leukaemia, unclas-

sifiable. In: Swerdlow SH, Campo E, Harris NL, Jaffe ES, Pileri SA, Stein H, Thiele J and Vardiman JW (eds) *World Health Organization Classification of Tumours of Haematopoietic and Lymphoid Tissues*. IARC Press, Lyon, pp. 191–193.

181 Audouin J, Le Tourneau A, Molina T, Camilleri-Broët S, Adida C, Comperat E *et al.* (2003) Patterns of bone marrow involvement in 58 patients presenting primary splenic marginal zone lymphoma with or without circulating villous lymphocytes. *Br J Haematol*, **122**, 404–412.

182 Chacón JI, Mollejo M, Muñoz E, Algara P, Mateo M, Lopez L *et al.* (2002) Splenic marginal zone lymphoma: clinical characteristics and prognostic factors in a series of 60 patients, *Blood*, **100**, 1648–1654.

183 Matutes E, Morilla R, Owusu-Ankomah K, Houlihan A and Catovsky D (1994) The immunophenotype of splenic lymphoma with villous lymphocytes and its relevance to the differential diagnosis with other B-cell disorders. *Blood*, **83**, 1558–1562.

184 Troussard X, Valensi F, Duchayne E, Garand R, Felman P, Tulliez M *et al.* (1996) Splenic lymphoma with villous lymphocytes: clinical presentation, biology and prognostic factors in a series of 100 patients. Groupe Francais d'Hematologie Cellulaire (GFHC). *Br J Haematol*, **93**, 731–736.

185 Giannouli S, Paterakis G, Ziakas PD, Anagnostou D and Voulgarelis M (2004) Splenic marginal zone lymphomas with peripheral CD5 expression. *Haematologica*, **89**, 113–114.

186 Gruszka-Westwood AM, Matutes E, Coignet LJ, Wotherspoon A and Catovsky D (1999) The incidence of trisomy 3 in splenic lymphoma with villous lymphocytes: a study by FISH. *Br J Haematol*, **104**, 600–604.

187 Oscier DG, Matutes E, Gardiner A, Glide S, Mould S, Brito-Babapulle V *et al.* (1993) Cytogenetic studies in splenic lymphoma with villous lymphocytes. *Br J Haematol*, **85**, 487–491.

188 Troussard X, Mauvieux L, Radford-Weiss I, Rack K, Valensi F, Garand R *et al.* (1998) Genetic analysis of splenic lymphoma with villous lymphocytes: a Groupe Francais d'Hématologie Cellulaire (GFHC) study. *Br J Haematol*, **101**, 712–721.

189 Zhu D, Orchard J, Oscier DG, Wright DH and Stevenson FK (2002) V_H gene analysis of splenic marginal zone lymphomas reveals diversity in mutational status and initiation of somatic mutation in vivo. *Blood*, **100**, 2659–2661.

190 Piris MA, Mollejo M, Chacón I, García JF, Camacho F and Cruz MA (2003) Splenic B-cell lymphomas. *Hematol J*, **4** (Suppl. 3), 53–55.

191 Wotherspoon A and Matutes E (2004) Recent advances in understanding small B-cell leukaemias and lymphomas. *Curr Diag Pathol*, **10**, 374–384.

192 Franco V, Florena AM and Campesi G (1996) Intrasinusoidal bone marrow infiltration: a possible hallmark of splenic lymphoma. *Histopathology*, **29**, 571–575.

193 Franco V, Florena AM, Ascani S, Paulli M, Salvato M and Pileri SA (2004) CD27 distinguished two phases in bone marrow infiltration of splenic marginal zone lymphoma. *Histopathology*, **44**, 381–386.

194 Foucar K (2001) *Bone Marrow Pathology*, 2nd edn. ASCP Press, Chicago.

195 Nathwani BN, Drachenberg MR, Hernandez AM, Levine AM and Sheibani K (1999) Nodal monocytoid B-cell lymphoma (nodal marginal-zone B-cell lymphoma). *Semin Hematol*, **36**, 128–138.

196 Campo E, Pileri SA, Jaffe ES, Müller-Hermelink HK and Nathwani BN (2008) Nodal marginal zone lymphoma. In: Swerdlow SH, Campo E, Harris NL, Jaffe ES, Pileri SA, Stein H, Thiele J and Vardiman JW (eds) *World Health Organization Classification of Tumours of Haematopoietic and Lymphoid Tissues*. IARC Press, Lyon, pp. 218–219.

197 Naresh KN (2008) Nodal marginal zone B-cell lymphoma with prominent follicular colonization – difficulties in diagnosis: a study of 15 cases. *Histopathology*, **52**, 331–339.

198 Sheibani K (1992) Monocytoid B cell lymphoma. In: Knowles DM (ed) *Neoplastic Hematopathology*. Williams & Wilkins, Baltimore.

199 Carbone A, Gloghini A, Pinto A, Attadia V, Zagonel V and Volpe R (1989) Monocytoid B-cell lymphoma with bone marrow and peripheral blood involvement at presentation. *Am J Clin Pathol*, **92**, 228–236.

200 Traweek ST and Sheibani K (1990) Regarding the article entitled 'Monocytoid B-cell lymphoma with bone marrow and peripheral blood involvement at presentation' [letter; comment]. *Am J Clin Pathol*, **94**, 117–118.

201 Fend F, Kraus-Huonder B, Müller-Hermelink HK and Feller AC (1993) Monocytoid B-cell lymphoma: its relationship to and possible cellular origin from marginal zone cells. *Hum Pathol*, **24**, 336–339.

202 Henrique R, Achten R, Maes B, Verhoef G and De Wolf-Peeters C (1999) Guidelines for subtyping small B-cell lymphomas in bone marrow biopsies. *Virchows Arch*, **435**, 549–558.

203 Kurtin PJ, Hobday KS, Ziesmer S and Caron BL (1999) Demonstration of distinct antigenic profiles of small B-cell lymphomas by paraffin section immunohistochemistry. *Am J Clin Pathol*, **112**, 319–329.

204 Traverse-Glehen A, Baseggio L, Bauchu EC, Morel D, Gazzo S, Ffrench M et al. (2008) Splenic red pulp lymphoma with numerous basophilic villous lymphocytes: a distinct clinicopathologic and molecular entity? *Blood*, **111**, 2253–2260.

205 Sainati L, Matutes E, Mulligan S, de Oliveira MP, Rani S, Lampert IA and Catovsky D (1990) A variant form of hairy cell leukemia resistant to alpha-interferon: clinical and phenotypic characteristics of 17 patients. *Blood*, **76**, 157–162.

206 Stein H, Warnke RA, Chan WC, Jaffe ES, Chan JKC, Gatter KB and Campo E (2008) Diffuse large B-cell lymphoma, not otherwise specified. In: Swerdlow SH, Campo E, Harris NL, Jaffe ES, Pileri SA, Stein H, Thiele J and Vardiman JW (eds) *World Health Organization Classification of Tumours of Haematopoietic and Lymphoid Tissues*. IARC Press, Lyon, pp. 233–237.

207 Estalilla OC, Koo CH, Brynes RK and Medeiros LJ (1999) Intravascular large B-cell lymphoma. A report of five cases initially diagnosed by bone marrow biopsy. *Am J Clin Pathol*, **112**, 248–255.

208 Yan Y, Chan WC, Weisenburger DD, Anderson JR, Bast MA, Vose JM et al. (1995) Clinical and prognostic significance of bone marrow involvement in patients with diffuse aggressive B-cell lymphoma. *J Clin Oncol*, **13**, 1336–1342.

209 Chung R, Lai R, Wei P, Lee J, Hanson J, Belch AR et al. (2007) Concordant but not discordant bone marrow involvement in diffuse large B-cell lymphoma predicts a poor clinical outcome independent of the International Prognostic Index. *Blood*, **110**, 1278–1282.

210 Alvares CL, Matutes E, Scully MA, Swansbury J, Min T, Gruszka-Westwood AM et al. (2004) Isolated bone marrow involvement in diffuse large B cell lymphoma: a report of three cases with review of morphologic, immunophenotypic and cytogenetic findings. *Leuk Lymphoma*, **45**, 769–775.

211 Rosenwald A, Wright G, Chan WC, Connors JM, Campo E, Fisher RI et al. for the Lymphoma/Leukemia Molecular Profiling Group (2002) The use of molecular profiling to predict survival after chemotherapy for diffuse large B-cell lymphoma. *N Engl J Med*, **346**, 1937–1947.

212 Lenz G, Wright G, Dave SS, Xiao W, Powell J, Zhao et al. for the Lymphoma/Leukemia Molecular Profiling Project (2008) Stromal gene signatures in large B-cell lymphomas. *N Engl J Med*, **359**, 2313–2323.

213 Hill ME, MacLennan KA, Cunningham DC, Vaughan Hudson B, Burke M, Clarke P et al. (1996) Prognostic significance of BCL-2 expression and bcl-2 major breakpoint region rearrangement in diffuse large cell non-Hodgkin's lymphoma: a British National Lymphoma Investigation Study. *Blood*, **88**, 1046–1051.

214 Gaidano G (1996) Clinical implications of the molecular pathogenesis of non-Hodgkin's lymphomas. *Cancer J*, **9**, 187–191.

215 Gascoyne RD, Adomat SA, Krajewski S, Krajewska M, Horsman DE, Tolcher AW et al. (1997) Prognostic

significance of Bcl-2 protein expression and Bcl-2 gene rearrangement in diffuse aggressive non-Hodgkin's lymphoma. *Blood*, **90**, 244–251.

216 Kocjan G (2005) Cytological and molecular diagnosis of lymphoma. *J Clin Pathol*, **58**, 561–567.

217 Møller MB, Gerdes AM, Skjødt K, Mortensen LS and Pedersen NT (1999) Disrupted p53 function as predictor of treatment failure and poor prognosis in B- and T-cell non-Hodgkin's lymphoma. *Clin Cancer Res*, **5**, 1085–1091.

218 Leroy K, Haioun C, Lepage E, Le Métayer N, Berger F, Labouyrie E *et al.* for the Groupe d'Etude des Lymphomes de l'Adulte (2002) p53 gene mutations are associated with poor survival in low and low-intermediate risk diffuse large B-cell lymphomas. *Ann Oncol*, **13**, 1108–1115.

219 Linderoth J, Ehinger M, Jerkeman M, Bendahl PO, Akerman M *et al.* (2007) CD40 expression identifies a prognostically favourable subgroup of diffuse large B-cell lymphoma. *Leuk Lymphoma*, **48**, 1774–1779.

220 Hui PK, Feller AC and Lennert K (1988) High-grade non-Hodgkin's lymphoma of B-cell type. I. Histopathology. *Histopathology*, **12**, 127–143.

221 Le Gouill S, Talmant P, Touzeau C, Moreau A, Garand R, Juge-Morineau N *et al.* (2007) The clinical presentation and prognosis of diffuse large B-cell lymphoma with t(14;18) and 8q24/c-MYC rearrangement. *Haematologica*, **92**, 1335–1342.

222 Schlegelberger B, Zwingers T, Harder L, Nowotny H, Siebert R, Vesely M *et al.* (1999) Clinicopathogenetic significance of chromosomal abnormalities in patients with blastic peripheral B-cell lymphoma. Kiel-Wien-Lymphoma Study Group. *Blood*, **94**, 3114–3120.

223 Camara DA, Stefanoff CG, Pires AR, Soares F, Biasoli I, Zalcberg I *et al.* (2007) Immunoblastic morphology in diffuse large B-cell lymphoma is associated with a nongerminal center immunophenotypic profile. *Leuk Lymphoma*, **48**, 892–896.

224 Bain B, Matutes E, Robinson D, Lampert IA, Brito-Babapulle V, Morilla R and Catovsky D (1991) Leukaemia as a manifestation of large cell lymphoma. *Br J Haematol*, **77**, 301–310.

225 De Wolf-Peeters C, Delabie J, Campo E, Jaffe ES and Delsol G (2008) T cell/histiocyte-rich large B-cell lymphoma. In: Swerdlow SH, Campo E, Harris NL, Jaffe ES, Pileri SA, Stein H, Thiele J and Vardiman JW (eds) *World Health Organization Classification of Tumours of Haematopoietic and Lymphoid Tissues.* IARC Press, Lyon, pp. 238–239.

226 Achten R and De Wolf-Peeters C (2004) Nodular lymphocyte-predominant Hodgkin's lymphoma and T-cell/histiocyte-rich large B-cell lymphoma: near neighbours or distant cousins? *Curr Diagn Pathol*, **10**, 385–393.

227 El Weshi A, Akhtar S, Mourad WA, Ajarim D, Abdelsalm M, Khafaga Y *et al.* (2007) T-cell/histio-cyte-rich B-cell lymphoma: clinical presentation, management and prognostic factors: report on 61 patients and review of literature. *Leuk Lymphoma*, **48**, 1764–1773.

228 Skinnider BF, Connors JM and Gascoyne RD (1997) Bone marrow involvement in T-cell-rich B-cell lymphoma. *Am J Clin Pathol*, **108**, 570–578.

229 Cazals-Hatem D, Lepage E, Brice P, Ferrant A, d'Agay MF, Baumelou E *et al.* (1996) Primary mediastinal large B-cell lymphoma. A clinicopathologic study of 141 cases compared with 916 nonmediastinal large B-cell lymphomas, a GELA ('Groupe d'Etude des Lymphomes de l'Adulte') study. *Am J Surg Pathol*, **20**, 877–888.

230 Gaulard P, Harris NL, Pileri SA, Kutok JL, Stein H, Kovrigina AM, Jaffe ES and Möller P (2008) Primary mediastinal (thymic) large B-cell lymphoma. In: Swerdlow SH, Campo E, Harris NL, Jaffe ES, Pileri SA, Stein H, Thiele J and Vardiman JW (eds) *World Health Organization Classification of Tumours of Haematopoietic and Lymphoid Tissues.* IARC Press, Lyon, pp. 250–251.

231 Hamlin PA, Portlock CS, Straus DJ, Noy A, Singer A, Horwitz SM *et al.* (2005) Primary mediastinal large B-cell lymphoma: optimal therapy and prognostic factor analysis in 141 consecutive patients treated at Memorial Sloan Kettering from 1980 to 1999. *Br J Haematol*, **130**, 691–699.

232 Parrens M, Dubus P, Agape P, Rizcallah E, Marit G, de Mascarel A and Merlio JP (2000) Intrasinusoidal bone marrow infiltration revealing intravascular lymphomatosis. *Leuk Lymphoma*, **37**, 219–223.

233 Nakamura S. Ponzoni M and Campo E (2008) Intravascular large B-cell lymphoma. In: Swerdlow SH, Campo E, Harris NL, Jaffe ES, Pileri SA, Stein H, Thiele J and Vardiman JW (eds) *World Health Organization Classification of Tumours of Haematopoietic and Lymphoid Tissues.* IARC Press, Lyon, pp. 252–253.

234 Murase T, Nakamura S, Kawauchi K, Matsuzaki H, Sakai C, Inaba T *et al.* (2000) An Asian variant of intravascular large B-cell lymphoma: clinical, pathological and cytogenetic approaches to diffuse large B-cell lymphoma associated with haemophagocytic syndrome. *Br J Haematol*, **111**, 826–834.

235 Nakamura S, Murase T and Kinoshita T (2007) Intravascular large B-cell lymphoma: the heterogeneous clinical manifestations of its classical and hemophagocytosis-related forms. *Haematologica*, **92**, 434–436.

236 Cobcroft R (1999) Diagnosis of angiotropic large B-cell lymphoma from a peripheral blood film. *Br J Haematol*, **104**, 429.

237 Narimatsu H, Morishita Y, Saito SA, Shimada K, Ozeki K, Kohno A et al. (2004) Usefulness of bone marrow aspiration for definite diagnosis of Asian variant of intravascular lymphoma: four autopsied cases. *Leuk Lymphoma*, **45**, 1611–1616.

238 Bhagwati NS, Oiseth SJ, Abebe LS and Wiernik PH (2004) Intravascular lymphoma associated with hemophagocytic syndrome: a rare but aggressive clinical entity. *Ann Hematol*, **83**, 247–250.

239 Wick MR, Mills SE, Scheithauer BW, Cooper PH, Davitz MA and Parkinson K (1986) Reassessment of malignant 'angioendotheliomatosis'. Evidence in favor of its reclassification as 'intravascular lymphomatosis. *Am J Surg Pathol*, **10**, 112–123.

240 Dupin N, Diss TL, Kellam P, Tulliez M, Du M-Q, Sicard D et al. (2000) HHV-8 is associated with a plasmablastic variant of Castleman disease that is linked to HHV-8-positive plasmablastic lymphoma. *Blood*, **95**, 1406–1412.

241 Oksenhendler E, Boulanger E, Galicier L, Du M-Q, Dupin N, Diss TC et al. (2002) High incidence of Kaposi's sarcoma-associated herpesvirus-related non-Hodgkin lymphoma in patients with HIV infection and multicentric Castleman disease. *Blood*, **99**, 2331–2336.

242 Cesarman E and Knowles DM (1997) Kaposi's sarcoma-associated herpesvirus: a lymphotropic human herpesvirus associated with Kaposi's sarcoma, primary effusion lymphoma, and multicentric Castleman's disease. *Semin Diagn Pathol*, **14**, 54–66.

243 Song Y, Yoshida A, Yamamoto Y, Katano H, Hagihara K, Oka S et al. (2004) Viral load of human herpes virus 8 (HHV-8) in the circulatory blood cells correlates with clinical progression in a patient with HHV-8-associated solid lymphoma with AIDS-associated Kaposi's sarcoma. *Leuk Lymphoma*, **45**, 2343–2347.

244 Bellan C, Lazzi S, Hummel M, Palumno N, de Santi M, Amato T et al. (2005) Immunoglobulin gene analysis reveals 2 distinct cells of origin for EBV-positive and EBV-negative Burkitt lymphomas. *Blood*, **106**, 1031–1036.

245 Leoncini L, Raphael M, Stein H, Harris NL, Jaffe ES and Pileri S (2008) Burkitt lymphoma. In: Swerdlow SH, Campo E, Harris NL, Jaffe ES, Pileri SA, Stein H, Thiele J and Vardiman JW (eds) *World Health Organization Classification of Tumours of Haematopoietic and Lymphoid Tissues*. IARC Press, Lyon, pp. 262–264.

246 Kluin PL, Harris NL, Stein H, Leoncini L, Raphael M, Campo E and Jaffe ES (2008) B-cell lymphoma, unclassifiable, with features intermediate between diffuse large B-cell lymphoma and Burkitt lymphoma. In: Swerdlow SH, Campo E, Harris NL, Jaffe ES, Pileri SA, Stein H, Thiele J and Vardiman JW (eds) *World Health Organization Classification of Tumours*

of *Haematopoietic and Lymphoid Tissues*. IARC Press, Lyon, pp. 265–266.

247 Wright DH and Pike PA (1968) Bone marrow involvement in Burkitt's tumour. *Br J Haematol*, **15**, 409–416.

248 Bluming AZ, Ziegler JL and Carbone PP (1972) Bone marrow involvement in Burkitt's lymphoma: results of a prospective study. *Br J Haematol*, **22**, 369–376.

249 Arseneau JC, Canellos GP, Banks PM, Berard CW, Gralnick HR and DeVita VT (1975) American Burkitt's lymphoma: a clinicopathologic study of 30 cases. I. Clinical factors relating to prolonged survival. *Am J Med*, **58**, 314–321.

250 Banks PM, Arseneau JC, Gralnick HR, Canellos GP, DeVita VT and Berard CW (1975) American Burkitt's lymphoma: a clinicopathologic study of 30 cases. II. Pathologic correlations. *Am J Med*, **58**, 322–329.

251 Levine AM, Pavlova Z, Pockros AW, Parker JW, Teitelbaum AH, Paganini-Hill A et al. (1983) Small noncleaved follicular center cell (FCC) lymphoma: Burkitt and non-Burkitt variants in the United States. I. Clinical features. *Cancer*, **52**, 1073–1079.

252 Brunning RD, McKenna RW, Bloomfield CD, Coccia P and Gajl-Peczalska KJ (1977) Bone marrow involvement in Burkitt's lymphoma. *Cancer*, **40**, 1771–1779.

253 Diebold J, Jaffe ES, Raphaël M and Warnke RA (2001) Burkitt lymphoma. In: Jaffe ES, Harris NL, Stein H and Vardiman JW (eds) *World Health Organization Classification of Tumours: Pathology and genetics of tumours of haematopoietic and lymphoid tissues*. IARC Press, Lyon, pp. 181–184.

254 Hummel M, Bentink S, Berger H, Klapper W, Wessendorf S, Barth TFE et al. (2006) A biologic definition of Burkitt's lymphoma from transcriptional and genomic profiling. *N Engl J Med*, **354**, 2419–2430.

255 Dave SS, Fu K, Wright GW, Lam LT, Kluin P, Boerma E-J et al. (2006) Molecular diagnosis of Burkitt's lymphoma. *N Engl J Med*, **354**, 2431–2442.

256 Reinecke P, Gerharz CD, Thiele K-P, Jänig U, Schäfer K-L, Aul C and Gabbert HE (2000) Temporary remission of an alveolar rhabdomyosarcoma diagnosed and treated as acute leukaemia. *Leuk Lymphoma*, **36**, 405–409.

257 Nakamura S and Suchi T (1991) A clinicopathologic study of node-based, low-grade, peripheral T-cell lymphoma, angioimmunoblastic lymphoma, T-zone lymphoma, and lymphoepithelioid lymphoma. *Cancer*, **67**, 2566–2578.

258 Borowitz MJ and Chan JKC (2008) T lymphoblastic leukaemia/lymphoma. In: Swerdlow SH, Campo E, Harris NL, Jaffe ES, Pileri SA, Stein H, Thiele J and Vardiman JW (eds) *World Health Organization Classification of Tumours of Haematopoietic and Lymphoid Tissues*. IARC Press, Lyon, pp. 176–178.

259 Weiss LM, Bindl JM, Picozzi VJ, Link MP and Warnke RA (1986) Lymphoblastic lymphoma: an immunophenotype study of 26 cases with comparison to T cell acute lymphoblastic leukemia. *Blood*, **67**, 474–478.

260 Bleesing JJH, Brown MR, Straus SE, Dale JK, Siegel RM, Johnson M *et al.* (2001) Immunophenotypic profiles in families with autoimmune lymphoproliferative syndrome. *Blood*, **98**, 2466–2473.

261 Galton DAG, Goldmann JM, Wiltshaw E, Catovsky D, Henry K and Goldenberg GJ (1974) Prolymphocytic leukaemia. *Br J Haematol*, **27**, 7–23.

262 Bennett JM, Catovsky D, Daniel MT, Flandrin G, Galton DA, Gralnick HR and Sultan C (1989) Proposals for the classification of chronic (mature) B and T lymphoid leukaemias. French–American–British (FAB) Cooperative Group. *J Clin Pathol*, **42**, 567–584.

263 Catovsky D, Müller-Hermelink HK and Ralfkiaer E (2008) T-cell prolymphocytic leukaemia. In: Swerdlow SH, Campo E, Harris NL, Jaffe ES, Pileri SA, Stein H, Thiele J and Vardiman JW (eds) *World Health Organization Classification of Tumours of Haematopoietic and Lymphoid Tissues*. IARC Press, Lyon, pp. 270–271.

264 Matutes E, Garcia Talavera J, O'Brien M and Catovsky D (1986) The morphological spectrum of T-prolymphocytic leukaemia. *Br J Haematol*, **64**, 111–124.

265 Matutes E, Brito-Babapulle V, Swansbury J, Ellis J, Morilla R, Dearden C *et al.* (1991) Clinical and laboratory features of 78 cases of T-prolymphocytic leukaemia. *Blood*, **78**, 3269–3274.

266 Herling M, Khoury JD, Washington LT, Duvic M, Keating MJ and Jones D (2004) A systematic approach to diagnosis of mature T-cell leukemias reveals heterogeneity among WHO categories. *Blood*, **104**, 328–335.

267 Timonen T, Ortaldo JR and Herberman RB (1981) Characteristics of human large granular lymphocytes and relationship to natural killer and K cells. *J Exp Med*, **153**, 569–582.

268 Lamy T and Loughran TP (1999) Current concepts: large granular lymphocyte leukemia. *Blood Rev*, **13**, 230–240.

269 Dhodapkar MV, Li CY, Lust JA, Tefferi A and Phyliky RL (1994) Clinical spectrum of clonal proliferations of T-large granular lymphocytes: a T-cell clonopathy of undetermined significance? *Blood*, **84**, 1620–1627.

270 Pandolfi F, Loughran TP, Starkebaum G, Chisesi T, Barbui T, Chan WC *et al.* (1990) Clinical course and prognosis of the lymphoproliferative disease of granular lymphocytes. A multicenter study. *Cancer*, **65**, 341–348.

271 Prochorec-Sobieszek M, Rymkiewicz G, Makuch-Łasica H, Majewski M, Michalak K, Rupiński R *et al.* (2008) Characteristics of T-cell large granular lymphocyte proliferations associated with neutropenia and inflammatory arthropathy. *Arthritis Res Ther*, **10**, R55.

272 Gentile TC, Uner AH, Hutchison RE, Wright J, Ben-Ezra J, Russell EC and Loughran TP (1994) CD3+, CD56+ aggressive variant of large granular lymphocyte leukemia. *Blood*, **84**, 2315–2321.

273 Reynolds CW and Foon KA (1984) T-γ-lymphoproliferative disease and related disorders in humans and experimental animals: a review of the clinical, cellular, and functional characteristics. *Blood*, **64**, 1146–1158.

274 Loughran TP, Kadin ME, Starkebaum G, Abkowitz JL, Clark EA, Disteche C *et al.* (1985) Leukemia of large granular lymphocytes: association with clonal chromosomal abnormalities and autoimmune neutropenia, thrombocytopenia, and hemolytic anemia. *Ann Intern Med*, **102**, 169–175.

275 Fogarty PF, Stetler-Stevenson M, Pereira A and Dunbar CE (2005) Large granular lymphocytic proliferation-associated cyclic thrombocytopenia. *Am J Hematol*, **79**, 334–336.

276 Kouides PA and Rowe JM (1995) Large granular lymphocyte leukemia presenting with both amegakaryocytic thrombocytopenic purpura and pure red cell aplasia: clinical course and response to immunosuppressive therapy. *Am J Hematol*, **49**, 232–236.

277 Chan WC, Foucar K, Morice WG, Catovsky D and Montserrat E (2008) T-cell large granular lymphocytic leukaemia. In: Swerdlow SH, Campo E, Harris NL, Jaffe ES, Pileri SA, Stein H, Thiele J and Vardiman JW (eds) *World Health Organization Classification of Tumours of Haematopoietic and Lymphoid Tissues*. IARC Press, Lyon, pp. 272–273.

278 Morice WG, Kurtin PJ, Tefferi A and Hanson CA (2002) Distinct bone marrow findings in T-cell granular lymphocytic leukemia revealed by paraffin section immunoperoxidase stains for CD8, TIA-1, and granzyme B. *Blood*, **99**, 268–274.

279 Agnarsson BA, Loughran TP, Starkebaum G and Kadin ME (1989) The pathology of large granular lymphocyte leukemia. *Hum Pathol*, **20**, 643–651.

280 Brouet JC, Sasportes M, Flandrin G, Preud'Homme JL and Seligmann M (1975) Chronic lymphocytic leukaemia of T-cell origin. Immunological and clinical evaluation in eleven patients. *Lancet*, **ii**, 890–893.

281 Palutke M, Eisenberg L, Kaplan J, Hussain M, Kithier K, Tabaczka P *et al.* (1983) Natural killer and suppressor T-cell chronic lymphocytic leukemia. *Blood*, **62**, 627–634.

282 Kouides PA and Rowe JM (1995) Large granular lymphocyte leukemia presenting with both amegakaryocytic thrombocytopenic purpura and pure red cell aplasia: clinical course and response to

immunosuppressive therapy. *Am J Hematol*, **49**, 232–236.

283 Papadaki T, Stamatopoulos K, Stavroyianni N, Paterakis G, Phisphis M and Stefanoudaki-Sofianatou K (2002) Evidence for T-large granular lymphocyte-mediated neutropenia in Rituximab-treated lymphoma patients: report of two cases. *Leuk Research*, **26**, 597–600.

284 Villamor N, Morice WG, Chan WC and Foucar K (2008) Chronic lymphoproliferative disorders of NK cells. In: Swerdlow SH, Campo E, Harris NL, Jaffe ES, Pileri SA, Stein H, Thiele J and Vardiman JW (eds) *World Health Organization Classification of Tumours of Haematopoietic and Lymphoid Tissues.* IARC Press, Lyon, pp. 274–275.

285 Nash R, McSweeney P, Zambello R, Semenzato D and Loughran TP (1993) Clonal studies of CD3– lymphoproliferative disease of granular lymphocytes. *Blood*, **81**, 2363–2368.

286 Chan JKC, Jaffe ES, Ralfkiaer E and Ho Y-H (2008) Aggressive NK-cell leukaemia. In: Swerdlow SH, Campo E, Harris NL, Jaffe ES, Pileri SA, Stein H, Thiele J and Vardiman JW (eds) *World Health Organization Classification of Tumours of Haematopoietic and Lymphoid Tissues.* IARC Press, Lyon, pp. 276–277.

287 Kawa-Ha K, Ishihara S, Ninomiya T, Yumura-Yagi K, Hara J, Murayama F *et al.* (1989) CD3-negative lymphoproliferative disease of granular lymphocytes containing Epstein–Barr viral DNA. *J Clin Invest*, **84**, 51–55.

288 Chan JK, Sin VC, Wong KF, Ng CS, Tsang WY, Chan CH *et al.* (1997) Nonnasal lymphoma expressing the natural killer marker CD56: a clinicopathological study of 49 cases of an uncommon aggressive neoplasm. *Blood*, **89**, 4501–4513.

289 Imamura N, Kusunoki Y, Kawa-Ha K, Yumura K, Hara J, Oda K *et al.* (1990) Aggressive natural killer cell leukaemia/lymphoma: report of four cases and review of the literature. Possible existence of a new clinical entity originating from the third lineage of lymphoid cells. *Br J Haematol*, **75**, 49–59.

290 Kwong YL, Chan AC and Liang RH (1997) Natural killer cell lymphoma/leukemia: pathology and treatment. *Hematol Oncol*, **15**, 71–79.

291 Mori KL, Egashira M and Oshimi K (2001) Differentiation stage of natural killer cell-lineage lymphoproliferative disorders based on phenotypic analysis. *Br J Haematol*, **115**, 225–228.

292 Rabbani GR, Phyliky RL and Tefferi A (1999) A long-term study of patients with chronic natural killer cell lymphocytosis. *Br J Haematol*, **106**, 960–966.

293 Chan JKC, Quintanilla-Martinez L, Ferry JA and Peh S-C (2008) Extranodal NK/T cell lymphoma, nasal type. In: Swerdlow SH, Campo E, Harris NL, Jaffe ES, Pileri SA, Stein H, Thiele J and Vardiman JW (eds)

World Health Organization Classification of Tumours of Haematopoietic and Lymphoid Tissues. IARC Press, Lyon, pp. 285–288.

294 Abouyabis AN, Shenoy PJ, Lechowicz MJ and Flowers C (2008) Incidence and outcomes of the peripheral T-cell lymphoma subtypes in the United States. *Leuk Lymphoma*, **49**, 2099–2107.

295 Oshimi K (1996) Lymphoproliferative disorders of natural killer cells. *Int J Hematol*, **63**, 279–290.

296 Siu LL, Wong KF, Chan JK and Kwong YL (1999) Comparative genomic hybridization analysis in natural killer cell lymphoma/leukemia: recognition of consistent pattern of genetic alterations. *Am J Pathol*, **155**, 1419–1425.

297 Wong K-F, Chan JKC, Cheung MMC and So JCC (2001) Bone marrow involvement by nasal NK cell lymphoma at diagnosis is uncommon. *Am J Clin Pathol*, **115**, 266–270.

298 Quintanilla-Martinez L, Kimura H and Jaffe ES (2008) EBV-positive T-cell lymphoproliferative disorders of children. In: Swerdlow SH, Campo E, Harris NL, Jaffe ES, Pileri SA, Stein H, Thiele J and Vardiman JW (eds) *World Health Organization Classification of Tumours of Haematopoietic and Lymphoid Tissues.* IARC Press, Lyon, pp. 278–280.

299 Ralfkiaer E and Jaffe ES (2001) Mycosis fungoides and Sézary syndrome. In: Jaffe ES, Harris NL, Stein H and Vardiman JW (eds) *World Health Organization Classification of Tumours: Pathology and genetics of tumours of haematopoietic and lymphoid tissues.* IARC Press, Lyon, pp. 216–220.

300 Schechter GP, Sausville EA, Fischmann AB, Soehnlen F, Eddy J, Matthews M *et al.* (1987) Evaluation of circulating malignant cells provides prognostic information in cutaneous T cell lymphoma. *Blood*, **69**, 841–849.

301 Matutes E and Catovsky D (1991) Mature T-cell leukemias and leukemia/lymphoma syndromes: review of our experience of 175 cases. *Leuk Lymphoma*, **4**, 81–91.

302 Karenko L, Hyytinen E, Sarna S and Ranki A (1997) Chromosomal abnormalities in cutaneous T-cell lymphoma and in its premalignant conditions as detected by G-banding and interphase cytogenetic methods. *J Invest Dermatol*, **108**, 22–29.

303 Thangavelu M, Finn WG, Yelavarthi KK, Roenigk HH, Samuelson E, Peterson L *et al.* (1997) Recurring structural chromosome abnormalities in peripheral blood lymphocytes of patients with mycosis fungoides/Sézary syndrome. *Blood*, **89**, 3371–3377.

304 Delfau-Larue M-H, Laroche L, Wechsler J, Lepage E, Lahet C, Asso-Bonnet M *et al.* (2000) Diagnostic value of dominant T-cell clones in peripheral blood in 363 patients presenting consecutively with a clinical suspicion of cutaneous lymphoma. *Blood*, **96**, 2987–2992.

305 Rappaport H and Thomas LB (1974) Mycosis fungoides: the pathology of extracutaneous involvement. *Cancer*, **34**, 1198–1229.

306 Salhany KE, Greer JP, Cousar JB and Collins RD (1989) Marrow involvement in cutaneous T-cell lymphoma. A clinicopathologic study of 60 cases. *Am J Clin Pathol*, **92**, 747–754.

307 Graham SJ, Sharpe RW, Steinberg SM, Cotelingam JD, Sausville EA and Foss FM (1993) Prognostic implications of a bone marrow histopathologic classification system in mycosis fungoides and the Sézary syndrome. *Cancer*, **72**, 726–734.

308 Carbone A, Tirelli U, Volpe R, Sulfaro S and Manconi R (1986) Assessment of bone marrow histology in patients with cutaneous T-cell lymphomas (CTCL) at presentation and during the follow-up. *Br J Haematol*, **62**, 789–790.

309 Sibaud V, Beylot-Barry M, Thiébault R, Parrens M, Vergier B, Delaunay M *et al.* (2003) Bone marrow histopathologic and molecular staging in epidermotropic T-cell lymphomas. *Am J Clin Pathol*, **119**, 414–423.

310 Jaffe ES, Gaulard P, Ralfkiaer E, Cerroni L and Meijer CJLM (2008) Subcutaneous panniculitis-like T-cell lymphoma. In: Swerdlow SH, Campo E, Harris NL, Jaffe ES, Pileri SA, Stein H, Thiele J and Vardiman JW (eds) *World Health Organization Classification of Tumours of Haematopoietic and Lymphoid Tissues*. IARC Press, Lyon, pp. 294–295.

311 Gaulard P, Berti E, Willemze R and Jaffe ES (2008) Primary cutaneous peripheral T-cell lymphomas, rare subtypes. In: Swerdlow SH, Campo E, Harris NL, Jaffe ES, Pileri SA, Stein H, Thiele J and Vardiman JW (eds) *World Health Organization Classification of Tumours of Haematopoietic and Lymphoid Tissues*. IARC Press, Lyon, pp. 302–305.

312 Dogan A, Gaulard P, Jaffe ES, Ralfkiaer E and Müller-Hermelink HK (2008) Angioimmunoblastic T-cell lymphoma. In: Swerdlow SH, Campo E, Harris NL, Jaffe ES, Pileri SA, Stein H, Thiele J and Vardiman JW (eds) *World Health Organization Classification of Tumours of Haematopoietic and Lymphoid Tissues*. IARC Press, Lyon, pp. 309–311.

313 Warnke RA, Jones D and His ED (2007) Morphologic and immunophenotypic variants of nodal T-cell lymphomas and T-cell lymphoma mimics. *Am J Clin Pathol*, **127**, 511–527.

314 Park B-B, Ryoo B-Y, Lee J-H, Kwon H-C, Yang S-H, Kang H-J *et al.* (2007) Clinical features and treatment outcomes of angioimmunoblastic T-cell lymphoma. *Leuk Lymphoma*, **48**, 16–22.

315 Patsouris E, Noël H and Lennert K (1989) Angioimmunoblastic lymphadenopathy – type of T-cell lymphoma with a high content of epithelioid cells. Histopathology and comparison with lymphoepithelioid cell lymphoma. *Am J Surg Pathol*, **13**, 262–275.

316 Knecht H (1989) Angioimmunoblastic lymphadenopathy: ten years' experience and state of current knowledge. *Semin Hematol*, **26**, 208–215.

317 Yamane A, Awaya N, Shimizu T, Ikeda Y and Okamoto S (2007) Angioimmunoblastic T-cell lymphoma with polyclonal proliferation of plasma cells in peripheral blood and marrow. *Acta Haematol*, **117**, 74–77.

318 Todd T and Erber W (2006) Diagnosis of leukaemic phase of angioimmunoblastic T-cell lymphoma from the peripheral blood. *Br J Haematol*, **134**, 124.

319 Diaz-Alderete A, Menarguez J, Alvarez-Doval A, Sabin P, Escudero A, Fernández-Cruz E and Gil J (2006) Lymphocyte immunophenotype of circulating angioimmunoblastic T-cell lymphoma cells. *Br J Haematol*, **134**, 347–348.

320 Stacchini A, Demurtas A, Alibert S, Francia di Celle P, Godio L, Palestro G and Novero D (2007) The usefulness of flow cytometric CD10 detection in the differential diagnosis of peripheral T-cell lymphomas. *Am J Clin Pathol*, **128**, 854–864.

321 Dogan A, Atyegalle AD and Kyriakou C (2003) Angioimmunoblastic T-cell lymphoma. *Br J Haematol*, **121**, 681–691.

322 Grogg KL, Morice WG and Macon WR (2007) Spectrum of bone marrow findings in patients with angioimmunoblastic T-cell lymphoma. *Br J Haematol*, **137**, 416–422.

323 Schlegelberger B, Zwingers T, Hohenadel K, Henne-Bruns D, Schmitz N, Haferlach T *et al.* (1996) Significance of cytogenetic findings for the clinical outcome in patients with T-cell lymphoma of angioimmunoblastic lymphadenopathy type. *J Clin Oncol*, **14**, 593–599.

324 Schlegelberger B, Zhang Y, Weber-Matthiesen K and Grote W (1994) Detection of aberrant clones in nearly all cases of angioimmunoblastic lymphadenopathy with dysproteinemia-type T-cell lymphoma by combined interphase and metaphase cytogenetics. *Blood*, **84**, 2640–2648.

325 Smith JL, Hodges E, Quin CT, McCarthy KP and Wright DH (2000) Frequent T and B cell oligoclones in histologically and immunophenotypically characterized angioimmunoblastic lymphadenopathy. *Am J Pathol*, **156**, 661–669.

326 Schnaidt U, Vykoupil KF, Thiele J and Georgii A (1980) Angioimmunoblastic lymphadenopathy. Histopathology of bone marrow involvement. *Virchows Arch A Pathol Anat Histopathol*, **389**, 369–380.

327 Ghani AM and Krause JR (1985) Bone marrow biopsy findings in angioimmunoblastic lymphadenopathy. *Br J Haematol*, **61**, 203–213.

328 Attygalle A, Al-Jehani R, Diss TC, Munson P, Liu H, Du M-Q, Isaacson PG and Dogan A (2002) Neoplastic

T cells in angioimmunoblastic T-cell lymphoma express CD10. *Blood*, **99**, 627–633.

329 Attygalle A, Diss TC, Munson P, Isaacson PG, Du MO and Dogan A (2004) CD10 expression in extranodal dissemination of angioimmunoblastic T-cell lymphoma. *Am J Surg Pathol*, **28**, 54–61.

330 Dogan A and Morice WG (2004) Bone marrow histopathology in peripheral T-cell lymphomas. *Br J Haematol*, **127**, 140–154.

331 Uchiyama T, Yodoi J, Sagawa K, Takatsuki K and Uchino H (1977) Adult T-cell leukemia: clinical and hematologic features of 16 cases. *Blood*, **50**, 481–492.

332 Jaffe ES, Blattner WA, Blayney DW, Bunn PA, Cossman J, Robert-Guroff M and Gallo RC (1984) The pathologic spectrum of adult T-cell leukemia/lymphoma in the United States. Human T-cell leukemia/lymphoma virus-associated lymphoid malignancies. *Am J Surg Pathol*, **8**, 263–275.

333 Shih LY, Kuo TT, Dunn P and Liaw SJ (1991) Human T-cell lymphotropic virus type I associated adult T-cell leukaemia/lymphoma in Taiwan Chinese. *Br J Haematol*, **79**, 156–161.

334 Shimoyama M (1991) Diagnostic criteria and classification of clinical subtypes of adult T-cell leukaemia-lymphoma. A report from the Lymphoma Study Group (1984–87). *Br J Haematol*, **79**, 428–437.

335 Bain BJ (1998) Morphology and classification of leukaemias. In: Whittaker JA and Holmes JA (eds) *Leukaemia and Related Disorders*. Blackwell Science, Oxford.

336 Fujita K, Yamasaki Y, Sawada H, Izumi Y, Fukuhara S and Uchino H (1989) Cytogenetic studies on the adult T-cell leukemia in Japan. *Leuk Res*, **13**, 535–543.

337 Swerdlow SH, Habeshaw JA, Rohatiner AZ, Lister TA and Stansfeld AG (1984) Caribbean T-cell lymphoma/leukemia. *Cancer*, **54**, 687–696.

338 Kikuchi M, Jaffe ES and Ralfkiaer E (2001) Adult T-cell leukaemia/lymphoma. In: Jaffe ES, Harris NL, Stein H and Vardiman JW (eds) *World Health Organization Classification of Tumours: Pathology and genetics of tumours of haematopoietic and lymphoid tissues*. IARC Press, Lyon, pp. 200–203.

339 Cooke CB, Krenacs L, Stetler-Stevenson M, Greiner TC, Raffeld M, Kingma DW *et al.* (1996) Hepatosplenic T-cell lymphoma: a distinct clinicopathologic entity of cytotoxic gamma delta T-cell origin. *Blood*, **88**, 4265–4274.

340 Lai R, Larratt LM, Etches W, Mortimer ST, Jewell LD, Dabbagh L and Coupland RW (2000) Hepatosplenic T-cell lymphoma of αβ lineage in a 16-year-old boy presenting with hemolytic anemia and thrombocytopenia. *Am J Surg Pathol*, **24**, 459–463.

341 Vega F, Medeiros LJ, Bueso-Ramos C, Jones D, Lai R, Luthra R and Abruzzo LV (2001) Hepatosplenic

gamma/delta T-cell lymphoma in bone marrow: a sinusoidal neoplasm with blastic cytological features. *Am J Clin Pathol*, **116**, 410–419.

342 Yao M, Tien HF, Lin MT, Su IJ, Wang CT, Chen YC *et al.* (1996) Clinical and hematological characteristics of hepatosplenic T gamma/delta lymphoma with isochromosome for long arm of chromosome 7. *Leuk Lymphoma*, **22**, 495–500.

343 Rizvi MA, Evens AM, Nelson BP and Rosen ST (2007) T-cell lymphoma. In: Marcus R, Sweetenham JW and Williams ME (eds) *Lymphoma: Pathology, diagnosis and treatment*. Cambridge University Press, Cambridge, p. 226.

344 Salhany KE, Feldman M, Kahn MJ, Peritt D, Schretzenmair RD, Wilson DM *et al.* (1997) Hepatosplenic γδ T-cell lymphoma: ultrastructural, immunophenotypic, and functional evidence for cytotoxic T lymphocyte differentiation. *Hum Pathol*, **28**, 674–685.

345 Khan WA, Yu L, Eisenbrey AB, Crisan D, Al Saadi A, Davis BH *et al.* (2001) Hepatosplenic gamma/delta T-cell lymphoma in immunocompromised patients. *Am J Clin Pathol*, **116**, 41–50.

346 Gaulard P, Jaffe ES, Krenacs L and Macon WR (2008) Hepatosplenic T-cell lymphoma. In: Swerdlow SH, Campo E, Harris NL, Jaffe ES, Pileri SA, Stein H, Thiele J and Vardiman JW (eds) *World Health Organization Classification of Tumours of Haematopoietic and Lymphoid Tissues*. IARC Press, Lyon, pp. 292–293.

347 Delsol G, Falini B, Müller-Hermelink HK, Campo E, Jaffe ES, Gascoyne RD, Stein H and Kinney MC (2008) Anaplastic large cell lymphoma (ALCL), ALK-positive. In: Swerdlow SH, Campo E, Harris NL, Jaffe ES, Pileri SA, Stein H, Thiele J and Vardiman JW (eds) *World Health Organization Classification of Tumours of Haematopoietic and Lymphoid Tissues*. IARC Press, Lyon, pp. 312–316.

348 Falini B, Pileri S, Zinzani PL, Carbone A, Zagonel V, De Wolf-Peeters C *et al.* (1999) ALK+ lymphoma: clinico-pathological findings and outcome. *Blood*, **93**, 2697–2706.

349 Falini B, Pulford K, Pucciarini A, Carbone A, De Wolf-Peeters C, Cordell J *et al.* (1999) Lymphomas expressing ALK fusion protein(s) other than NPM-ALK. *Blood*, **94**, 3509–3515.

350 Rizvi MA, Evens AM, Tallman MS, Nelson BP and Rosen ST (2006) T-cell non-Hodgkin lymphoma. *Blood*, **107**, 1255–1264.

351 Takahashi D, Nagatoshi Y, Nagayama J, Inagaki J, Itonoaga N, Takeshita M and Okamura J (2008) Anaplastic large cell lymphoma: a case report and a review of the literature. *J Pediatr Hematol Oncol*, **30**, 696–700.

352 Fraga M, Brousset P, Schlaifer D, Payen C, Robert A, Rubie H *et al.* (1995) Bone marrow involvement in

anaplastic large cell lymphoma. Immunohistochemical detection of minimal disease and its prognostic significance. *Am J Clin Pathol*, **103**, 82–89.

353 Wong KF, Chan JK, Ng CS, Chu YC, Lam PW and Yuen HL (1991) Anaplastic large cell Ki-1 lymphoma involving bone marrow: marrow findings and association with reactive hemophagocytosis. *Am J Hematol*, **37**, 112–119.

354 Agnarsson BA and Kadin ME (1988) Ki-1 positive large cell lymphoma. A morphologic and immunologic study of 19 cases. *Am J Surg Pathol*, **12**, 264–274.

355 Suzuki R, Kagami Y, Takeuchi K, Kami M, Okamoto M, Ichinohasama R *et al.* (2000) Prognostic significance of CD56 expression for ALK-positive and ALK-negative anaplastic large-cell lymphoma of T/null cell phenotype. *Blood*, **96**, 2993–3000.

356 Juco J, Holden JT, Mann KP, Kelley LG and Li S (2003) Immunophenotypic analysis of anaplastic large cell lymphoma by flow cytometry. *Am J Clin Pathol*, **119**, 205–212.

357 Bonzheim I, Geissinger E, Roth S, Zettl A, Marx A, Rosenwald A *et al.* (2004) Anaplastic large cell lymphomas lack the expression of T-cell receptor molecules or molecules of proximal T-cell receptor signalling. *Blood*, **104**, 3358–3360.

358 Downing JR, Shurtleff SA, Zielenska M, Curcio-Brint AM, Behm FG, Head DR *et al.* (1995) Molecular detection of the (2;5) translocation of non-Hodgkin's lymphoma by reverse transcriptase-polymerase chain reaction. *Blood*, **85**, 3416–3422.

359 Kadin ME and Morris SW (1998) The t(2;5) in human lymphomas. *Leuk Lymphoma*, **29**, 249–256.

360 Falini B (2001) Anaplastic large cell lymphoma: pathological, molecular and clinical features. *Br J Haematol*, **114**, 741–760.

361 Wlodarska I, De Wolf-Peeters C, Falini B, Verhoef G, Morris SW, Hagemeijer A and Van den Berghe H (1998) The cryptic inv(2)(p23q35) defines a new molecular genetic subtype of ALK-positive anaplastic large-cell lymphoma. *Blood*, **92**, 2688–2695.

362 Stein H, Foss HD, Dürkop H, Marafioti T, Delsol G, Pulford K *et al.* (2000) CD30(+) anaplastic large cell lymphoma: a review of its histopathologic, genetic, and clinical features. *Blood*, **96**, 3681–3695.

363 Sainati L, Montaldi A, Stella M, Putti MC, Zanesco L and Basso G (1990) A novel variant translocation t(2;13)(p23;q34) in Ki-1 large cell anaplastic lymphoma. *Br J Haematol*, **75**, 621–622.

364 Rosenwald A, Ott G, Pulford K, Katzenberger T, Kühl J, Kalla J *et al.* (1999) t(1;2)(q21;p23) and t(2;3)(p23;q21): two novel variant translocations of the t(2;5)(p23;q35) in anaplastic large cell lymphoma. *Blood*, **94**, 362–364.

365 Lamant L, Dastugue N, Pulford K, Delsol G and Mariamé B (1999) A new fusion gene *TPM3-ALK*

in anaplastic large cell lymphoma created by a (1;2)(q25;p23) translocation. *Blood*, **93**, 3088–3095.

366 Morris SW, Xue L, Ma Z and Kinney MC (2001) ALK⁺ CD30⁺ lymphomas: a distinct molecular genetic subtype of non-Hodgkin's lymphoma. *Br J Haematol*, **113**, 275–295.

367 Chott A, Kaserer K, Augustin I, Vesely M, Heinz R, Oehlinger W *et al.* (1990) Ki-1-positive large cell lymphoma. A clinicopathologic study of 41 cases. *Am J Surg Pathol*, **14**, 439–448.

368 Benharroch D, Meguerian-Bedoyan Z, Lamant L, Amin C, Brugières L, Terrier-Lacombe MJ *et al.* (1998) ALK-positive lymphoma: a single disease with a broad spectrum of morphology. *Blood*, **91**, 2076–2084.

369 Pulford K, Lamant L, Morris SW, Butler LH, Wood KM, Stroud D *et al.* (1997) Detection of anaplastic lymphoma kinase (ALK) and nucleolar protein nucleophosmin (NPM)-ALK proteins in normal and neoplastic cells with the monoclonal antibody ALK1. *Blood*, **89**, 1394–1404.

370 Mason DY, Harris NL, Delsol G, Stein H, Campo E, Kinney MC, Jaffe ES and Falini B (2008) Anaplastic large cell lymphoma (ALCL), ALK-negative. In: Swerdlow SH, Campo E, Harris NL, Jaffe ES, Pileri SA, Stein H, Thiele J and Vardiman JW (eds) *World Health Organization Classification of Tumours of Haematopoietic and Lymphoid Tissues*. IARC Press, Lyon, pp. 317–319.

371 Weinberg OK, Seo K and Arber DA (2008) Prevalence of bone marrow involvement in systemic anaplastic large cell lymphoma: are immunohistochemical studies necessary? *Hum Pathol*, **39**, 1331–1340.

372 Gale J, Simmonds PD, Mead GM, Sweetenham JW and Wright DH (2000) Enteropathy-type intestinal T-cell lymphoma: clinical features and treatment of 31 patients in a single center. *J Clin Oncol*, **18**, 795–803.

373 Jayakar V, Goldin RD and Bain BJ (2007) Teaching cases: Case 31, eosinophilia and pruritus. *Leuk Lymphoma*, **47**, 2404–2405.

374 Pileri S, Weisenburger DG, Sng I, Jaffe ES, Ralfkiaer E, Nakamura S and Müller-Hermelink HK (2008) Peripheral T-cell lymphoma, not otherwise specified. In: Swerdlow SH, Campo E, Harris NL, Jaffe ES, Pileri SA, Stein H, Thiele J and Vardiman JW (eds) *World Health Organization Classification of Tumours of Haematopoietic and Lymphoid Tissues*. IARC Press, Lyon, pp. 306–308.

375 Lopez-Guillermo A, Cid J, Salar A, Lopez A, Montalban C, Castrillo JM *et al.* (1998) Peripheral T-cell lymphomas: initial features, natural history, and prognostic factors in a series of 174 patients diagnosed according to the R.E.A.L. classification. *Ann Oncol*, **9**, 849–855.

376 Shimoyama M, Oyama A, Tajima K, Tobinai K, Minato K, Takenaka T et al. (1993) Differences in clinicopathological characteristics and major prognostic factors between B-lymphoma and peripheral T-lymphoma excluding adult T-cell leukemia/lymphoma. Leuk Lymphoma, 10, 335–342.

377 Jennings CD and Foon KA (1997) Recent advances in flow cytometry: application to the diagnosis of hematologic malignancy. Blood, 90, 2863–2892.

378 Quintanilla-Martinez L, Preffer F, Rubin D, Ferry JA and Harris NL (1994) CD20+ T-cell lymphoma. Neoplastic transformation of a normal T-cell subset. Am J Clin Pathol, 102, 483–489.

379 Piccaluga PP, Agostinelli C, Righi S, Zinzani PL and Pileri SA (2007) Expression of CD52 in peripheral T-cell lymphoma. Haematologica, 92, 566–567.

380 Inwards DJ, Habermann TM, Banks PM, Colgan JP and Dewald GW (1990) Cytogenetic findings in 21 cases of peripheral T-cell lymphoma. Am J Hematol, 35, 88–95.

381 Montaldi A, Chisesi T, Stracca-Pansa V, Celli P, Vespignani M and Stella M (1990) Recurrent chromosomal aberrations in peripheral T-cell lymphoma. Cancer Genet Cytogenet, 48, 39–48.

382 Lakkala-Paranko T, Franssila K, Lappalainen K, Leskinen R, Knuutila S, de la Chapelle A and Bloomfield CD (1987) Chromosome abnormalities in peripheral T-cell lymphoma. Br J Haematol, 66, 451–460.

383 Sanger WG, Weisenburger DD, Armitage JO and Purtilo DT (1986) Cytogenetic abnormalities in noncutaneous peripheral T-cell lymphoma. Cancer Genet Cytogenet, 23, 53–59.

384 Auger MJ, Nash JR and Mackie MJ (1986) Marrow involvement with T cell lymphoma initially presenting as abnormal myelopoiesis. J Clin Pathol, 39, 134–137.

385 Lukes RJ (1971) Criteria for involvement of lymph node, bone marrow, spleen, and liver in Hodgkin's disease. Cancer Res, 31, 1755–1767.

386 Wlodarska I, Nooyen P, Maes B, Martin-Subero JI, Siebert R, Pauwels P et al. (2003) Frequent occurrence of BCL6 rearrangements in nodular lymphocyte predominance Hodgkin lymphoma but not in classical Hodgkin lymphoma. Blood, 101, 706–711.

387 Poppema S, Delsol G, Pileri SA, Stein H, Swerdlow SH, Warnke RA and Jaffe ES (2008) Nodular lymphocyte predominant Hodgkin lymphoma. In: Swerdlow SH, Campo E, Harris NL, Jaffe ES, Pileri SA, Stein H, Thiele J and Vardiman JW (eds) World Health Organization Classification of Tumours of Haematopoietic and Lymphoid Tissues. IARC Press, Lyon, pp. 323–325.

388 Stein H, Delsol G, Pileri SA, Weiss LM, Poppema S and Jaffe ES (2008) Classical Hodgkin lymphoma, introduction. In: Swerdlow SH, Campo E, Harris NL, Jaffe ES, Pileri SA, Stein H, Thiele J and Vardiman JW (eds) World Health Organization Classification of Tumours of Haematopoietic and Lymphoid Tissues. IARC Press, Lyon, pp. 326–327.

389 Ushmorov A, Ritz O, Hummel M, Leithauser F, Moller P, Stein H and Wirth T (2004) Epigenetic silencing of the immunoglobulin heavy-chain gene in classical Hodgkin lymphoma-derived cell lines contributes to the loss of immunoglobulin expression. Blood, 104, 3326–3334.

390 Willenbrock K, Ichinohasama R, Kadin ME, Miura I, Terui T, Meguro K et al. (2002) T-cell variant of classical Hodgkin's lymphoma with nodal and cutaneous manifestations demonstrated by single-cell polymerase chain reaction. Lab Invest, 82, 1103–1109.

391 Neiman RS, Rosen PJ and Lukes RJ (1973) Lymphocyte-depletion Hodgkin's disease. A clinicopathological entity. N Engl J Med, 288, 751–755.

392 Bartl R, Frisch B, Burkhardt R, Huhn D and Pappenberger R (1982) Assessment of bone marrow histology in Hodgkin's disease: correlation with clinical factors. Br J Haematol, 51, 345–360.

393 Ellis ME, Diehl LF, Granger E and Elson E (1989) Trephine needle bone marrow biopsy in the initial staging of Hodgkin disease: sensitivity and specificity of the Ann Arbor staging procedure criteria. Am J Hematol, 30, 115–120.

394 Vassilakopoulos TP, Angelopoulou MK, Constantinou N, Karmiris T, Repoussis P and Roussou P (2005) Development and validation of a clinical prediction rule for bone marrow involvement in patients with Hodgkin lymphoma. Blood, 105, 1875–1880.

395 Macintyre EA, Vaughan Hudson B, Linch DC, Vaughan Hudson G and Jelliffe AM (1987) The value of staging bone marrow trephine biopsy in Hodgkin's disease. Eur J Haematol, 39, 66–70.

396 Gómez-Almaguer D, Ruiz-Argüelles GJ, López-Martinez B, Estrada E, Lobato-Mendizábal E and Jaime-Pérez JC (2002) Role of bone marrow examination in staging Hodgkin's disease: experience in México. Clin Lab Haematol, 24, 221–223.

397 Levis A, Pietrasanta D, d'Andrea E, Betinin M, Botto B, Di Vito F et al. (2001) A study of bone marrow involvement in 1161 consecutive Hodgkin's lymphoma patients. Blood, 98, 129a.

398 Portlock CS, Donnelly GB, Qin J, Straus D, Yahalom J, Zelenetz A et al. (2004) Adverse prognostic significance of CD20 positive Reed–Sternberg cells in classical Hodgkin's disease. Br J Haematol, 125, 701–708.

399 Marafioti T, Hummel M, Foss HD, Laumen H, Korbjuhn P, Anagnostopoulos I et al. (2000) Hodgkin and Reed–Sternberg cells represent an expansion of a single clone originating from a germinal center B-cell with functional immunoglobulin gene rear-

rangements but defective immunoglobulin transcription. *Blood*, **95**, 1443–1450.

400 Rosenberg SA (1971) Hodgkin's disease of the bone marrow. *Cancer Res*, **31**, 1733–1736.

401 Rappaport H, Berard CW, Butler JJ, Dorfman RF, Lukes RJ and Thomas LB (1971) Report of the Committee on Histopathological Criteria Contributing to Staging of Hodgkin's Disease. *Cancer Res*, **31**, 1864–1865.

402 Banks PM (1990) The pathology of Hodgkin's disease. *Semin Oncol*, **17**, 683–695.

403 O'Carroll DI, McKenna RW and Brunning RD (1976) Bone marrow manifestations of Hodgkin's disease. *Cancer*, **38**, 1717–1728.

404 Myers CE, Chabner BA, De Vita VT and Gralnick HR (1974) Bone marrow involvement in Hodgkin's disease: pathology and response to MOPP chemotherapy. *Blood*, **44**, 197–204.

405 Kinney MC, Greer JP, Stein RS, Collins RD and Cousar JB (1986) Lymphocyte-depletion Hodgkin's disease. Histopathologic diagnosis of marrow involvement. *Am J Surg Pathol*, **10**, 219–226.

406 Falini B and Mason DY (2002) Proteins encoded by genes involved in chromosomal alterations in lymphoma and leukemia: clinical value of their detection by immunocytochemistry. *Blood*, **99**, 409–426.

407 Valsami S, Pappa V, Rontogianni D, Kontsioti F, Papageorgiou E, Dervenoulas J *et al.* (2007) A clinicopathological study of B-cell differentiation markers and transcription factors in classical Hodgkin's lymphoma: a potential prognostic role of MUM1/IRF4. *Haematologica*, **92**, 1343–1350.

408 Meadows LM, Rosse WR, Moore JO, Crawford J, Laszlo J and Kaufman RE (1989) Hodgkin's disease presenting as myelofibrosis. *Cancer*, **64**, 1720–1726.

409 Khoury JD, Jones D, Yared MA, Manning JT, Abruzzo LV, Hagemeister FB and Medeiros LJ (2004) Bone marrow involvement in patients with nodular lymphocyte predominant Hodgkin lymphoma. *Am J Surg Pathol*, **28**, 489–295.

410 Jarrett RF and MacKenzie J (1999) Epstein–Barr virus and other candidate viruses in the pathogenesis of Hodgkin's disease. *Semin Hematol*, **36**, 260–269.

411 Cohen JI (1991) Epstein–Barr virus lymphoproliferative disease associated with acquired immunodeficiency. *Medicine (Baltimore)*, **70**, 137–160.

412 Hopwood P and Crawford DH (2000) The role of EBV in post-transplant malignancies: a review. *J Clin Pathol*, **53**, 248–254.

413 Curtis RE, Travis LB, Rowlings PA, Socie G, Kingma DW, Banks PM *et al.* (1999) Risk of lymphoproliferative disorders after bone marrow transplantation: a multi-institutional study. *Blood*, **94**, 2208–2216.

414 Shapiro RS, McClain K, Frizzera G, Gajl-Peczalska KJ, Kersey JH, Blazar BR *et al.* (1988) Epstein–Barr virus associated B cell lymphoproliferative disorders following bone marrow transplantation. *Blood*, **71**, 1234–1243.

415 Spiro IJ, Yandell DW, Li C, Saini S, Ferry J, Powelson J *et al.* (1993) Brief report: lymphoma of donor origin occurring in the porta hepatis of a transplanted liver. *N Engl J Med*, **329**, 27–29.

416 Baumforth KR, Young LS, Flavell KJ, Constandinou C and Murray PG (1999) The Epstein–Barr virus and its association with human cancers. *Mol Pathol*, **52**, 307–322.

417 Hanto DW, Sakamoto K, Purtilo DT, Simmons RL and Najarian JS (1981) The Epstein–Barr virus in the pathogenesis of posttransplant lymphoproliferative disorders. Clinical, pathologic, and virologic correlation. *Surgery*, **90**, 204–213.

418 Hanto DW, Gajl-Peczalska KJ, Frizzera G, Arthur DC, Balfour HH, McClain K *et al.* (1983) Epstein–Barr virus (EBV) induced polyclonal and monoclonal B-cell lymphoproliferative diseases occurring after renal transplantation. Clinical, pathologic, and virologic findings and implications for therapy. *Ann Surg*, **198**, 356–369.

419 Craig FE, Gulley ML and Banks PM (1993) Posttransplantation lymphoproliferative disorders. *Am J Clin Pathol*, **99**, 265–276.

420 Knowles DM, Cesarman E, Chadburn A, Frizzera G, Chen J, Rose EA and Michler RE (1995) Correlative morphologic and molecular genetic analysis demonstrates three distinct categories of posttransplantation lymphoproliferative disorders. *Blood*, **85**, 552–565.

421 Cleary ML, Nalesnik MA, Shearer WT and Sklar J (1988) Clonal analysis of transplant-associated lymphoproliferations based on the structure of the genomic termini of the Epstein–Barr virus. *Blood*, **72**, 349–352.

422 Harris NL, Ferry JA and Swerdlow SH (1997) Posttransplant lymphoproliferative disorders: summary of Society for Hematopathology Workshop. *Semin Diagn Pathol*, **14**, 8–14.

423 Koeppen H, Newell K, Baunoch DA and Vardiman JW (1998) Morphologic bone marrow changes in patients with posttransplantation lymphoproliferative disorders. *Am J Surg Pathol*, **22**, 208–214.

SEVEN

PLASMA CELL NEOPLASMS

Plasma cell myeloma (multiple myeloma)

Plasma cell myeloma, multiple myeloma, or myelomatosis is a disease resulting from the proliferation in the bone marrow of a clone of neoplastic cells that are closely related, both morphologically and functionally, to plasma cells. The World Health Organization (WHO) classification uses the term 'plasma cell myeloma' [1]. In the great majority of cases, the neoplastic cells secrete a protein that is either a complete immunoglobulin (Ig) or an immunoglobulin light chain. Clinical features result either directly from the effects of the neoplastic proliferation or indirectly from effects of the protein, often designated a paraprotein, which the myeloma cells produce.

Myeloma is a disease predominantly of the middle-aged and elderly. The median age of presentation is around 70 years [2]. The reported incidence is 2–4 per 100 000 per year and the incidence is higher in men; a population survey in the UK found an incidence of 7.8 per 100 000 per year in adults, representing an age standardized incidence of 4.8 per 100 000 per year (standardized for the European population) [3]. The age-standardized incidence in white Americans is 6 per 100 000 per year for males and 4 per 100 000 per year for females [4]. The disease is more common in Afro-Americans and UK Afro-Caribbeans than in Caucasians; the incidence in black Americans is twice that in white Americans with the same male predominance being seen (around 12 and 10/100 000/year, respectively) [4]. Familial cases occur [5].

Characteristic clinical features are anaemia, bone pain, pathological fractures, hypercalcaemia, renal failure and recurrent infection. A minority of patients have hepatomegaly or lymphadenopathy. Splenomegaly is occasionally present. Patients with symptomatic bone lesions usually have either generalized osteoporosis or discrete osteolytic lesions but occasional patients have osteosclerosis. The paraprotein secreted is IgG in about 60% of cases and IgA in about 20%; in some patients there is secretion of excess monoclonal light chain (Bence–Jones protein) in addition to complete immunoglobulin and, in about 15–20% of patients, only light chain is produced (Bence–Jones myeloma). A minority of patients produce an IgM, IgD or IgE paraprotein. Occasional patients have two distinct paraproteins. A small minority of patients have no paraprotein in serum or urine (non-secretory myeloma). Any paraprotein secreted will, since it arises from a single clone of cells, contain only a single light chain type, either κ or λ. Monoclonal immunoglobulins, being of high molecular weight, are usually detected only or mainly in the serum whereas, unless there is coexisting renal failure, the low molecular weight Bence–Jones protein is detected only in the urine. The concentration of normal serum immunoglobulins is reduced in about 90% of patients.

Plasma cell myeloma can be diagnosed with reasonable certainty if two of the following three criteria are met:
- More than 10% plasma cells in a bone marrow aspirate.
- A paraprotein in serum or urine.
- Osteolytic bone lesions or osteoporosis [6].

The diagnostic criteria of the WHO classification [1] are shown in Table 7.1 and those of the International Myeloma Working Group [7] in Table 7.2. The probability of myeloma is high if concentration of an IgG paraprotein exceeds 30 g/l, an IgA parapro-

Bone Marrow Pathology. By Barbara Bain, David Clark and Bridget Wilkins. © 2010, Blackwell Publishing.

Table 7.1 WHO diagnostic criteria for symptomatic and smouldering plasma cell myeloma [1].

Symptomatic myeloma
M-protein in serum or urine (lower level not specified)
Bone marrow clonal plasma cells increased (lower level not specified) or plasmacytoma
Related organ or tissue impairment (e.g. hypercalcaemia, renal insufficiency, anaemia, bone lesions, hyperviscosity, recurrent infection)
Asymptomatic (smouldering) multiple myeloma
Serum M-protein greater than 30 g/l
and/or
10% or more of clonal plasma cells in bone marrow No related organ or tissue impairment or myeloma-related symptoms

Table 7.2 International Myeloma Working Group criteria for the diagnosis of monoclonal gammopathy of undetermined significance, asymptomatic (smouldering) myeloma and symptomatic multiple myeloma [7]. (Reprinted by permission of *Br J Haematol*, **12**, 749–757, 2003.)

Monoclonal gammopathy of undetermined significance	Asymptomatic (smouldering) myeloma	Symptomatic* multiple myeloma
Serum paraprotein less than 30 g/l	Serum paraprotein at least 30 g/l	Paraprotein in serum or urine
	and/or	
Bone marrow clonal plasma cells less than 10% and low level infiltration in trephine biopsy specimen	Bone marrow clonal plasma cells at least 10%	Bone marrow clonal plasma cells or plasmacytoma
No evidence of other B-lineage lymphoproliferative disorder		
No related organ damage or tissue impairment†	No related organ damage or tissue impairment†	Related organ damage or tissue impairment†

* Includes asymptomatic patients who have evidence of organ damage.
† Such as bone lesions, light chain-associated amyloidosis, paraprotein-associated neurological damage, hypercalcaemia, renal impairment, anaemia, symptomatic hyperviscosity, or more than two bacterial infections in 12 months.

tein exceeds 25 g/l or urine light chain exceeds 1 g in 24 hours, but some patients with this disease meet none of these criteria. It is useful to distinguish smouldering or asymptomatic myeloma from other cases [1,7]. 'Symptomatic' myeloma includes all cases with either symptoms or tissue or end-organ impairment.

The median survival in myeloma is 3–4 years. The condition usually terminates in refractory disease, sometimes with a leukaemic phase. In some cases there is transformation to immunoblastic lymphoma. A significant minority of patients (about 10% of those who survive 5–10 years after treatment) succumb to a secondary myelodysplastic syndrome or to acute myeloid leukaemia (AML); it is likely that these complications result from the administration of alkylating agents.

Peripheral blood
The great majority of patients have anaemia which is either normocytic normochromic or, less often, macrocytic. In most patients there is increased rouleaux formation and increased background basophilic staining due to the presence of the paraprotein in the blood. These features do not occur in the minority of patients whose cells secrete only Bence–Jones protein or are non-secretory. The blood film is occasionally leucoerythroblastic and it is often possible to find a small number of plasma cells or plasmacytoid lymphocytes. In patients with more advanced disease, there may be thrombocytopenia and neutropenia. Occasionally there are large numbers of circulating neoplastic cells, showing mild to marked atypia, either at presentation or during the terminal phase of the disease. The designation plasma cell leukaemia is then used (see page 438). Occasional patients have a neutrophilic leukaemoid reaction.

Bone marrow cytology
The bone marrow features are very variable. Plasma cells are usually increased, often constituting between 30% and 90% of bone marrow nucleated

cells. The myeloma cells may be morphologically fairly normal, showing the eccentric nucleus, clumped chromatin and Golgi zone typical of a normal plasma cell, or may be moderately or severely dysplastic. A common cytological abnormality is nucleocytoplasmic asynchrony; the cytoplasm is mature but the nucleus either has a diffuse chromatin pattern or contains a prominent nucleolus (Figs 7.1 and 7.2). Other cytological abnormalities include marked pleomorphism, increased size of cells, a high nucleocytoplasmic ratio, multinu-

clearity (Fig. 7.3), nuclear lobation (Fig. 7.4), phagocytosis by myeloma cells (Fig. 7.4) and the presence of mitotic figures. Occasionally multinuclearity is extreme with up to 40 nuclei per cell [8]. Sometimes there are giant dysplastic plasma cells. Cytoplasmic abnormalities include uniform basophilia without a distinct Golgi zone, cytoplasmic eosinophilia and 'flaming' eosinophilic margins (Fig. 7.3). The cytoplasm may be voluminous or may contain azurophilic granules or crystals (Fig. 7.5), vacuoles or dilated sacs of endoplasmic reticu-

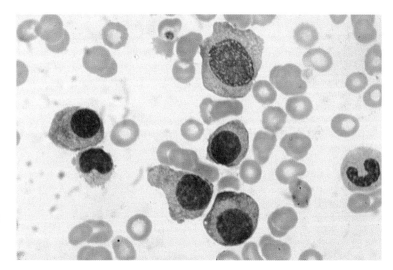

Fig. 7.1 Bone marrow (BM) aspirate, myeloma, showing a range of cells from a plasmablast to mature plasma cells. May–Grünwald–Giemsa (MGG) ×100.

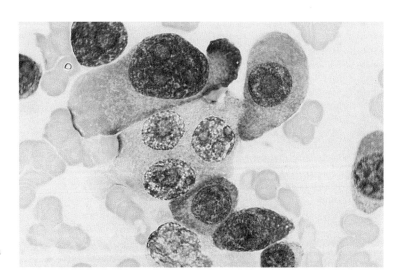

Fig. 7.2 BM aspirate, myeloma, showing plasmablasts, one of which is trinucleated. MGG ×100.

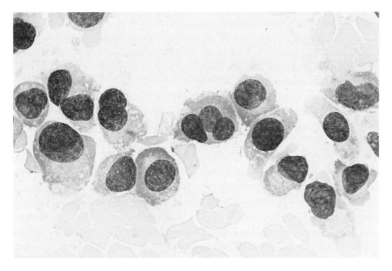

Fig. 7.3 BM aspirate, myeloma, showing bi- and trinucleated myeloma cells and myeloma cells with flaming cytoplasm. MGG ×100.

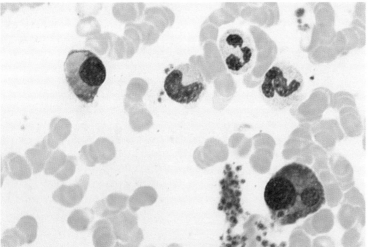

Fig. 7.4 BM aspirate, myeloma, showing one myeloma cell with a bilobed nucleus and another which has ingested an erythrocyte. MGG ×100.

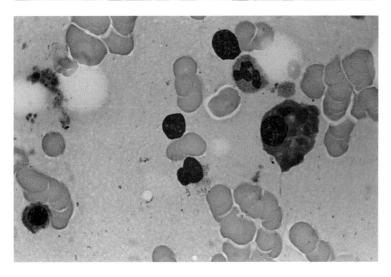

Fig. 7.5 BM aspirate, myeloma, showing a myeloma cell containing crystals of immunoglobulin. MGG ×100.

lum (Fig. 7.6). Myeloma cells may have small, large or giant spherical inclusions, referred to as Russell bodies (Fig. 7.7). They may have multiple small vacuoles or spherical inclusions containing weakly basophilic material (Fig. 7.8), the term 'Mott cell' then being used (with the apparent vacuoles or spherical inclusions being Russell bodies). Inclusions that appear to be intranuclear (Dutcher bodies) may be present (Fig. 7.9). Occasionally myeloma cells form rosettes around macrophages [9]. Haemosiderin is occasionally present in myeloma cells [10]. Rarely the bone marrow aspirate con-

tains amyloid (see Fig. 7.32, below). Occasionally there are macrophages laden with immunoglobulin crystals [11] and extracellular crystals have also been reported [12].

It is not always possible to make a diagnosis of myeloma on the basis of bone marrow morphology alone. The bone marrow is characteristically affected in a patchy manner and an aspirate will not necessarily contain a large number of plasma cells; nor will the morphology of the myeloma cells necessarily be very abnormal. Non-diagnostic aspirates are obtained in about 5% of patients. There

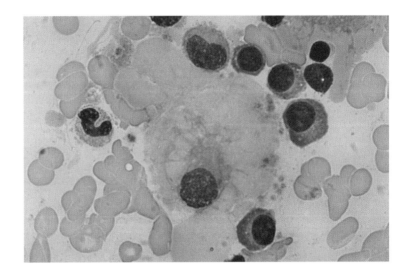

Fig. 7.6 BM aspirate, myeloma, showing myeloma cells, one of which has gross distension of the endoplasmic reticulum by immunoglobulin. MGG ×100.

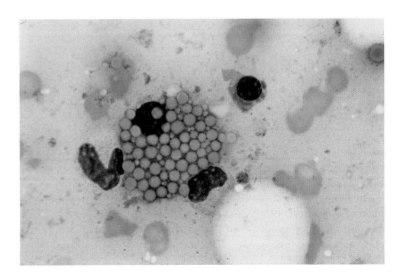

Fig. 7.7 BM aspirate, myeloma, showing numerous Russell bodies within a Mott cell. MGG ×100.

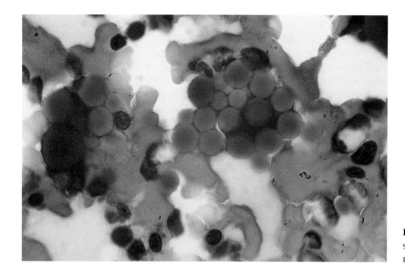

Fig. 7.8 BM aspirate, myeloma, showing a Mott cell containing multiple Russell bodies. MGG ×100.

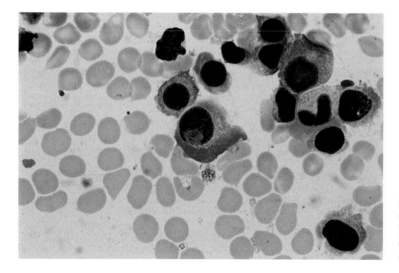

Fig. 7.9 BM aspirate, myeloma, showing formation of a Dutcher body by invagination from the cytoplasm. There are also 'flame cells'. MGG ×100.

is no particular percentage of plasma cells that reliably separates myeloma from reactive plasmacytosis or from monoclonal gammopathy of undetermined significance (MGUS) (see below). It is necessary, in doubtful cases, to assess not only the bone marrow cytology and histology but also the clinical, radiological and biochemical features.

The bone marrow aspirate is of value not only in making a diagnosis of myeloma but also in determining the prognosis. Both the percentage of plasma cells in the aspirate [13–15] and their degree of dysplasia [15–18] correlate with progno-

sis. In smouldering myeloma the presence of 20% or more plasma cells has been found predictive of progression [19].

Flow cytometric immunophenotyping

Myeloma cells give negative reactions with most B-cell markers but positive reactions are often obtained with CD79a. In addition, both normal plasma cells and myeloma cells express CD38 and CD138. Normal plasma cells usually express CD19 and CD45 and not CD56 whereas myeloma cells often over-express CD56 and fail to express CD19 and CD45 is negative or weak [20,21]. CD117 is expressed in a proportion of cases of myeloma and MGUS but is not expressed by normal plasma cells [22]. Other antigens that are not expressed in normal plasma cells but may show aberrant expression in myeloma cells include CD20, CD28 and CD33. Surface membrane Ig (SmIg) may be expressed whereas normal plasma cells express only cytoplasmic Ig [20]. CD86 expression by plasma cells correlates with worse prognosis [23]. CD56 negativity correlates with plasmablastic morphology and more aggressive disease [23]. In the rare entity of IgM myeloma the immunophenotype is somewhat different. There is expression of CD38 and CD138 but not CD56 or CD117 [24].

Flow cytometry can be used for monitoring minimal residual disease after intensive treatment. In patients with the usual CD19-negative, CD56-positive phenotype, cells are initially gated if they show strong expression of CD38 and CD138 and weak expression of CD45. Among the gated cells, normal plasma cells (CD19 positive, CD56 negative or weak) are then distinguished from the neoplastic plasma cells. Using a larger group of antibodies (CD19, CD27, CD45, CD56 and CD117) an aberrant immunophenotype, suitable for identifying minimal residual disease, is detectable in more than 99% of patients [25].

Bone marrow histology

Bone marrow biopsy can be of use both in the diagnosis of myeloma and in assessing the prognosis. A trephine biopsy at diagnosis is recommended, even if an adequate aspirate is obtained, since it may be needed as a baseline to assess a post-treatment biopsy when no adequate aspirate is obtained [2]. Biopsy is non-diagnostic in 5–10% of cases, either because of early disease or because the pattern of infiltration is nodular rather than diffuse and the biopsy has included only non-infiltrated marrow [26]. In addition, increased reticulin may mean that myeloma cells are not readily aspirated. Because a larger volume of tissue is sampled than in an aspirate and since the pattern of infiltration can be ascertained, a biopsy may confirm a diagnosis of myeloma when the aspirate has not done so. However, on occasions, more diagnostic information is obtained from the aspirate than from the trephine biopsy, so the two investigations should be regarded as complementary. Three major patterns of infiltration are seen: (i) interstitial, with or without paratrabecular seams of plasma cells; (ii) nodules or broad bands; and (iii) a packed marrow [26]. When infiltration is interstitial, myeloma cells are dispersed among haemopoietic and fat cells (Fig. 7.10), whereas in a 'packed marrow' (Fig. 7.11) the normal architecture of the marrow is obliterated. In reactive plasmacytosis, infiltration is interstitial and

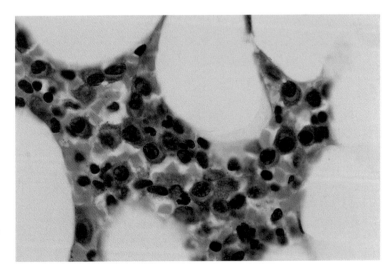

Fig. 7.10 BM trephine biopsy section, myeloma, showing interstitial infiltration of the marrow by plasma cells. Paraffin-embedded, H&E ×100.

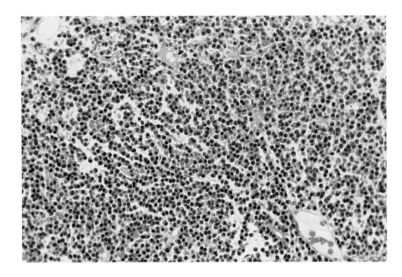

Fig. 7.11 BM trephine biopsy section, myeloma, showing diffuse infiltration by plasma cells (packed marrow). Paraffin-embedded, H&E ×20.

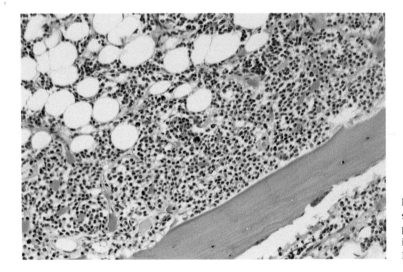

Fig. 7.12 BM trephine biopsy section, myeloma, showing a paratrabecular myelomatous infiltrate. Paraffin-embedded, H&E ×20.

large accumulations of plasma cells are not seen. Some histopathologists have considered that plasma cells sited around capillaries are indicative of reactive plasmacytosis rather than myeloma [26] but others have observed this feature also when plasma cells are neoplastic [27]. A paratrabecular pattern of infiltration (Fig. 7.12) may occur but is uncommon. Myeloma cells show varying degrees of dysplasia. In some cases they are morphologically very similar to normal plasma cells. In other cases the myeloma cells are very large, have nucleoli, are pleomorphic (Fig. 7.13) or are frankly blastic with a diffuse chro-matin pattern and a prominent nucleolus (Fig. 7.14). Nucleocytoplasmic asynchrony is common. Dutcher bodies (Fig. 7.13), Russell bodies (Fig. 7.15), cytoplasmic crystals (Figs 7.16 and 7.17) and Mott cells (Fig. 7.18) may be apparent. Dutcher bodies, although apparently intranuclear, result from invagination of cytoplasm into the nucleus.

Additional changes that may be associated with myeloma include reduced haemopoiesis, even in the absence of heavy infiltration, increased reticulin deposition, lymphoid infiltrates and, occasionally, the presence of granulomas (see Fig. 3.40).

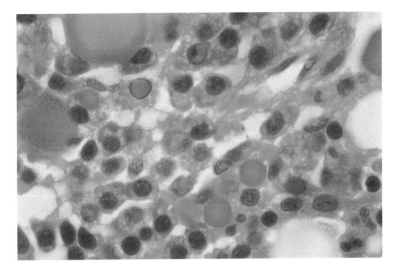

Fig. 7.13 BM trephine biopsy section, myeloma, showing plasma cells with moderate nuclear pleomorphism and numerous eosinophilic intranuclear (Dutcher) and intracytoplasmic (Russell) inclusion bodies. Paraffin-embedded, H&E ×100.

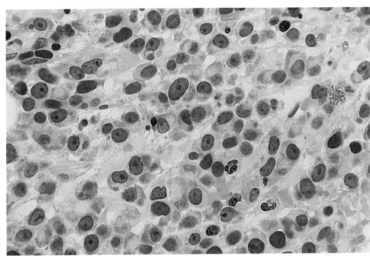

Fig. 7.14 BM trephine biopsy section, myeloma (plasmablastic), showing plasmablasts with marked variation in nuclear size and shape and prominent central nucleoli. Resin-embedded, H&E ×100.

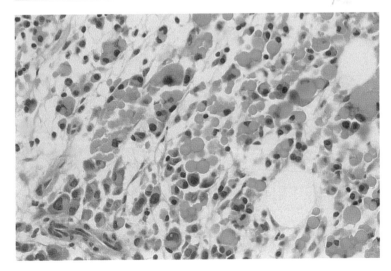

Fig. 7.15 BM trephine biopsy section, myeloma, showing abundant Russell bodies. Paraffin-embedded, H&E ×40.

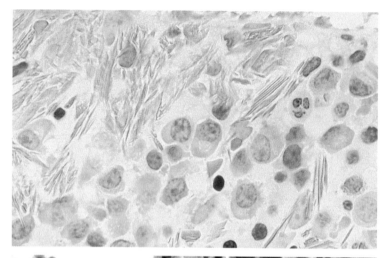

Fig. 7.16 BM trephine biopsy section, myeloma, showing a striking deposition of crystals of immunoglobulin. Paraffin-embedded, H &E ×100. (By courtesy of Dr P. Hayes, Chatham.)

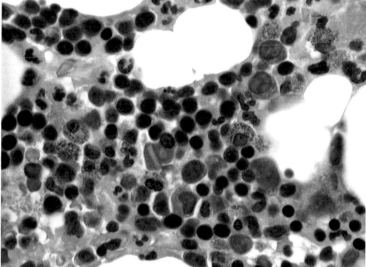

Fig. 7.17 BM trephine biopsy section from a patient with treated myeloma (follow-up biopsy). There is a plasma cell with a crystalline immunoglobulin inclusion within the cytoplasm. Paraffin-embedded, H&E ×60.

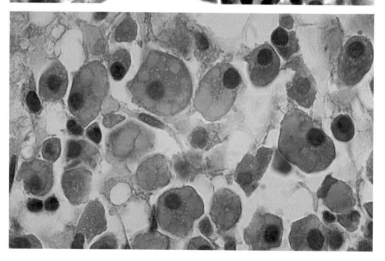

Fig. 7.18 BM trephine biopsy section, myeloma, showing myeloma cells with endoplasmic reticulum distended by immunoglobulin (Mott cells). Paraffin-embedded, H&E ×100.

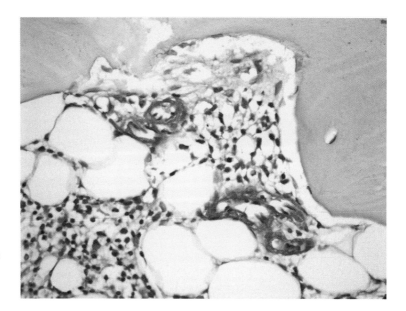

Fig. 7.19 Bone marrow trephine biopsy section from a patient with light chain-only plasma cell myeloma. Small interstitial blood vessels have mildly thickened walls staining intensely with a PAS stain due to light chain deposition. Paraffin-embedded, PAS ×40.

Bone marrow vascularity is increased, the increase correlating with a worse prognosis [28,29]; this may be because of an association between neovascularization and adverse cytogenetic abnormalities [30] and between neovascularization and an advanced clinical stage, higher cytological grade and higher proliferative fraction [31]. Increased vascularity correlates with expression of vascular endothelial growth factor by myeloma cells [31]. In patients with a neutrophilic leukaemoid reaction there is striking granulocytic hyperplasia and there may also be macrophages containing large numbers of neutrophils [32]. Occasionally reticulin deposition is markedly increased and there is also collagen deposition; this appears to be particularly associated with IgD myeloma [33,34]. Collagen deposition is preferentially type II rather than type I [35], as occurs also in primary myelofibrosis. If systematic evaluation is carried out, amyloid deposition is demonstrated in the bone marrow in up to 10% of patients [36]. Occasionally the walls of small blood vessels show increased periodic acid–Schiff (PAS) positivity resulting from deposition of light chain (Fig. 7.19). Occasionally there are macrophages laden with immunoglobulin crystals; these stain pink with haematoxylin and eosin (H&E) and deep blue with Giemsa in resin-embedded sections but stain only weakly in sections of paraffin-embedded

tissue [11]. Extracellular rhomboidal and hexagonal crystals have also been reported [12].

The bone changes usually associated with myeloma are diffuse osteoporosis, with thinning of all trabeculae, and osteolytic lesions with resorption of bone by osteoclasts. There is no relationship between osteoclastic and osteoblastic activity [37]. Diffuse osteoporosis has been found to be associated with a packed marrow pattern of infiltration, while osteolytic lesions are found particularly in those with nodular infiltration [26]. Osteoclastic activity correlates with the degree of plasma cell infiltration. Occasional patients have osteosclerosis (Fig. 7.20). Changes of secondary hyperparathyroidism may be seen in patients with renal insufficiency, particularly in those treated with bisphosphonates [38].

The prognosis in myeloma can be related to: (i) the extent of plasma cell infiltration (histological stage); (ii) the pattern of infiltration; and (iii) the cytological features of the cells (histological grade) [26]. Bartl *et al.* [26] found that a nodular pattern of infiltration correlated with more aggressive disease and with a worse prognosis than was seen when the pattern of infiltration was interstitial, with or without paratrabecular seams of plasma cells; a packed marrow indicated a worse prognosis than either of the other patterns. This has been

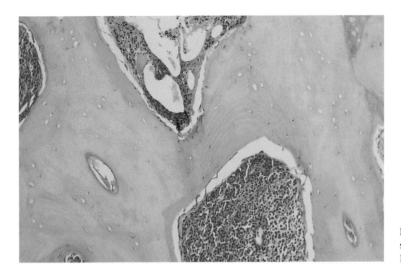

Fig. 7.20 BM trephine biopsy section in osteosclerotic myeloma. Paraffin-embedded, H&E ×10.

confirmed by Pich *et al.* [39]. These two groups and a number of other investigators have been able to relate prognosis also to the degree of dysplasia of the myeloma cells [37,39–41]. Bartl and Frisch [37] have suggested a classification that divides myeloma into three groups: (i) low grade, in which the plasma cells are mature with minimal dysplasia; (ii) intermediate grade, in which the plasma cells are dysplastic but not frankly blastic; and (iii) high grade, comprising plasmablasts. The three grades have median survivals of 60, 32 and 10 months, respectively [17,26]. The minority of cases of myeloma that show a high count of mitotic figures (more than one per high power field) have a shorter survival [42]; however a high mitotic rate is not necessarily present in patients with high grade histology. Angiogenesis correlates with adverse prognosis [43]. The best prognosis is found in those with 'smouldering' disease. Histologically, these patients have minimal interstitial infiltration by mainly mature plasma cells [37]. In smouldering myeloma the presence of sheets of plasma cells spanning the marrow spaces has been found predictive of progression [19]. The presence of amyloid deposits in the bone marrow or elsewhere has been found not to influence prognosis in patients who are treated with intensive chemotherapy followed by autologous stem cell transplantation [36]. It should be noted that much of the available infor-

mation on prognostic factors predates current, more effective, methods of treatment.

During follow-up, trephine biopsy sections reflect disease burden more accurately than do bone marrow aspirate films [44]. Response to treatment is associated with a reduction of plasma cell burden and reduced osteoclastic activity. Corticosteroid-treated patients may have aggravation of osteoporosis. Patients treated with bisphosphonates may show new bone formation with extensive osteoid seams [37].

Immunohistochemistry
Neoplastic cells in the great majority of cases of myeloma express monotypic immunoglobulin, i.e. there is expression of κ or λ light chains but not both (Fig. 7.21). There is usually expression of CD38, CD138 and MUM1/IRF4 and reactions with VS38c are positive [45–47]. Cells from cases with plasmacytic morphology, but rarely those with plasmablastic features, express the CD38 ligand, CD31 [48]. Expression of CD79a is usual but, in a substantial proportion of cases, cells fail to express this antigen. Cells in a proportion of cases express CD45, CD19 or CD20 but most do not. In one study CD20 was expressed in about 10% of patients at diagnosis and correlated with small mature plasma cell morphology and t(11;14) [49]. CD56 is usually expressed [50] and as it is not expressed by normal

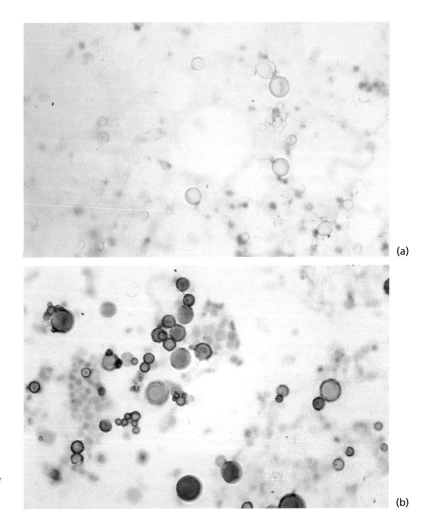

(a)

(b)

Fig. 7.21 BM trephine biopsy sections from a patient with multiple myeloma with abundant Russell bodies. (a) Immunoperoxidase for κ light chains; the Russell bodies are refractile but show no reaction. Paraffin-embedded ×50. (b) Immunoperoxidase for λ light chains showing positivity in the Russell bodies and strong positivity in the encircling cytoplasm. Paraffin-embedded ×50.

plasma cells this can be diagnostically useful. A variety of other antigens, including CD10, CD22, CD45RO, CD30, CD52, CD117 and non-haemopoietic antigens, such as epithelial membrane antigen and vimentin, are sometimes expressed [51]. However, in contrast to normal plasma cells, the expression of CD30 and epithelial membrane antigen is not at all common in myeloma. Nuclear expression of cyclin D1 (encoded by *CCND1*) is observed in the majority of patients in whom t(11;14)(q13;q32) is detected and in a minority of other patients [52]; in one study expression was detected in 24% of patients and correlated with

high grade and higher stage disease [53]. Immunohistochemistry for FGFR3 has been used to identify patients with *FGFR3* dysregulation as a result of a t(4;14)(p16;q32) translocation [54]. Expression of cyclin D1 correlates with a higher proliferation fraction and a worse prognosis [23]. Expression of CD45RO also correlates with a worse prognosis [55]. In IgM myeloma there is expression of MUM1/IRF4 and often cyclin D1 but not CD20, PAX5 or CD117 [24].

In low level residual disease, clusters of monotypic plasma cells can be found whereas normal plasma cells are scattered; the neoplastic plasma cells often express CD56 and sometimes cyclin D1 [44].

Cytogenetic and molecular genetic analysis

Because of the low proliferation rate of myeloma cells, cytogenetic analysis demonstrates a clonal abnormality in only 30–50% of cases whereas fluorescence *in situ* hybridization (FISH) techniques demonstrate an abnormality in the great majority. Aneuploidy and chromosomal translocations involving the *IGH* locus at 14q32 are both common. Translocations with a 14q32 breakpoint are demonstrable by FISH in more than 95% of patients [56] suggesting that these are early events in disease evolution. More than 20 different partner chromosomes have been described. These translocations include t(4;14)(p16;q32), t(6;14)(p25;q32), t(8;14) (q24;q32), t(9;14)(p13;q32), t(11;14)(q13;q32) (the commonest translocation demonstrated) and t(14;16)(q32;q22-23). Among these translocations, t(4;11) and t(14;16) are associated with a worse prognosis and t(11;14) with a somewhat better prognosis. The t(11;14) translocation is associated with lymphoplasmacytoid morphology, up-regulation of cyclin D1, a relatively low paraprotein concentration, a low rate of hyperdiploidy and a prognosis that is at least no worse than average for this disease [57]; it has a much greater prevalence among cases of IgE, IgM and non-secretory myeloma [58]. At a molecular level, the breakpoint in the *IGH* gene in t(11;14) differs from that in t(11;14) associated with mantle cell lymphoma, being in the switch region [59]. Other translocations demonstrated have sometimes had a 22q11 breakpoint related to the λ light chain gene, e.g. t(8;22)(q24;q11) and t(16;22)(q23;q11). Frequently demonstrated aneuploidies include monosomy 13 and trisomies 3, 5, 6, 7, 9, 11, 15, 17 and 19 [60–63]. Common deletions are 13q14, 13q34, 17p13 and 11q [64]. Hyperdiploidy is seen in more than 50% of patients with the remainder showing hypodiploidy, pseudodiploidy and near tetraploidy [63]. In a very large series of patients (1064) the frequency of different abnormalities was: del(13), 48%; hyperdiploidy, 39%; t(11;14), 21%; t(4;14), 14%; translocations involving *MYC*, 13%; and del(17p), 11% [65]. In a study of IgM myeloma four of eight patients had del(13q) and five of eight had t(11;14) (with cyclin D1 expression) [24].

Deletions of 11q, 13q14 and 17p13 have been found to have a poor prognostic significance [64,66], with 13q14 abnormalities being very fairly consistently found to have a poor prognosis. Trisomy 8 has been associated with disease progression [59]. The t(4;14) translocation is associated with shorter survival [67]. Hyperdiploidy has been found to have a better prognosis than other abnormal karyotypes (pseudodiploidy, hypodiploidy and hypotetraploidy grouped together) [68] and hypodiploidy has been specifically related to a poor prognosis [66]. In univariate analysis of a very large series of patients, del(13), t(4;14) and del(17p) were adverse and hyperdiploidy was favourable [58]. In multivariate analysis t(4;14), del(17p), high β_2-microglobulin and a haemoglobin concentration less than 100 g/l were of adverse prognostic significance, but the prognostic significance of del(13) was found to be because of its association with the other two adverse rearrangements [58].

In one study expression of *CCND1* mRNA, detected by *in situ* hybridization, was found in 32% of patients, expression correlating with high grade and higher stage disease [53]. *MYC* is often involved in complex translocations. There may be loss of *TP53*, associated with disease progression. *NRAS* and *KRAS* mutations are also associated with disease progression.

Epigenetic events include hypermethylation of tumour suppressor genes, *DAPK*, *SOCS1*, *CDKN2B* (p15) and *CDKN2A* (p16).

Another technique applicable to the molecular genetic analysis of myeloma is microarray analysis of gene expression. Potential uses include: (i) detection of loss of 13q14; (ii) detection of overexpression of genes activated by proximity to the *IGH* locus, such as *MMSET* with t(4;14), *FGFR3* with t(4;14), *CCND1* with t(11;14), *CCND3* with t(6;14) and *MAF* with t(14;16); and (iii) prediction of response to therapy. Microarray analysis can distinguish cells of myeloma and MGUS from normal plasma cells but does not distinguish these two disorders from each other.

Problems and pitfalls

Problems can occur in distinguishing myeloma from reactive plasmacytosis and from other lymphoproliferative disorders with plasmacytic differentiation. The diagnosis must therefore be based on

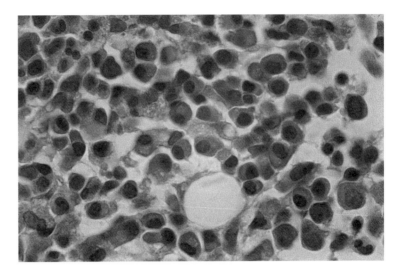

Fig. 7.22 Bone-marrow trephine biopsy section showing heavy reactive plasma cell infiltration in HIV infection. Paraffin-embedded, H&E ×100.

correlation of clinical, biochemical, radiological, cytological and histological features. Diagnosis is not always easy and sensitive biochemical tests may be needed, not only serum protein electrophoresis but also immunofixation of a concentrated urine sample to detect Bence–Jones protein. Measurement of the ratio of free κ to free λ light chains in the serum can also be useful, being abnormal in patients with Bence–Jones myeloma and even in the majority of those with non-secretory myeloma.

Increased numbers of bone marrow plasma cells can be seen as a reactive phenomenon in a wide range of conditions (see page 134). They can comprise more than 10% of cells (Fig. 7.22) and sometimes considerably more. Rarely, as many as 30–50% plasma cells are present as a reactive change; 30% were reported in a patient with Sjögren's syndrome [69], 50% in a patient with syphilis, 50% in an HIV-positive patient with tuberculosis [70] and at least 50% in a patient with relapsed AML [71]. A marked reactive plasmacytosis with 10–80% bone marrow plasma cells was reported during haemopoietic recovery in patients with myeloma treated with high dose melphalan and peripheral blood stem cell transplantation [72]; the reactive plasma cells were distinguishable from myeloma cells on the basis of genotype and phenotype. Since there is no cut-off point that reliably distinguishes myeloma from reactive conditions, cytological features (and other pathological and

clinical features) must be assessed as well as plasma cell number. The presence of plasmablasts and marked plasma cell dysplasia, e.g. giant forms, striking nuclear lobulation and prominent nucleoli, are strongly suggestive of myeloma.

Three trephine biopsy features have been reported to be specific for myeloma: (i) homogeneous nodules of plasma cells occupying at least half a high power field; (ii) monotypic plasma cell aggregates occupying the space between fat cells; and (iii) marked diffuse plasmacytosis with monotypic light chain expression [42].

Increased numbers of plasma cells are seen in MGUS (see below) and this condition therefore needs to be distinguished from myeloma [73,74]. In some cases of myeloma, the neoplastic cells have the features of lymphoplasmacytoid lymphocytes rather than of plasma cells; such cases need to be distinguished from lymphoplasmacytic lymphoma.

In rare cases of myeloma that show a very marked fibroblastic response it may be difficult to recognize distorted plasma cells (Fig. 7.23); immunohistochemistry is useful to confirm their presence.

In some patients with myeloma, the neoplastic cells are so immature or atypical that they are cytologically indistinguishable from the neoplastic cells of large cell lymphoma or other anaplastic tumours, including carcinoma, melanoma and AML. Plasmablastic myeloma and large cell lymphoma with cells having the features of immunoblasts are particularly likely to

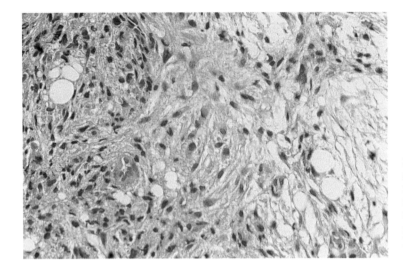

Fig. 7.23 BM trephine biopsy section, myeloma, showing a fibroblastic reaction to myelomatous infiltration. Immunohistochemistry is useful for identifying the distorted neoplastic cells in the fibrous tissue. Paraffin-embedded, H&E ×40. (By courtesy of Dr J. Jip, Bolton.)

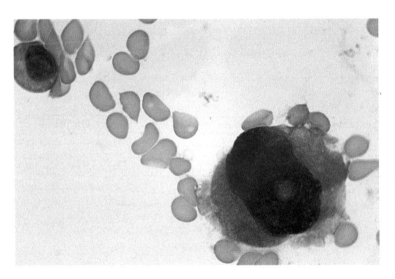

Fig. 7.24 BM aspirate, myeloma, showing a giant myeloma cell which could easily be confused with a megakaryocyte; the presence of an intranuclear inclusion (a Dutcher body) is a clue to the correct diagnosis. MGG ×100.

be confused. Myeloma cells sometimes also resemble carcinoma cells in forming cohesive masses [75]. Immunohistochemistry may add to the confusion if the possibility of a plasma cell neoplasm is not considered, since myeloma cells may be CD45 negative and epithelial membrane antigen positive. Giant, pleomorphic plasma cells may be confused with megakaryocytes (Figs 7.24 and 7.25). When there is diagnostic difficulty a careful search will usually show that even in anaplastic myeloma some cells show clear signs of plasmacytic differentiation.

A Giemsa stain can be very useful in highlighting plasma cell differentiation in an apparently anaplastic tumour but immunohistochemistry, using an appropriate panel of antibodies, is often crucial in making a correct diagnosis. Large cell lymphoma can be distinguished from myeloma immunohistochemically since lymphoma cells are usually positive for CD45, CD79a and CD20 and do not express cytoplasmic immunoglobulin. Myeloma cells are usually negative for CD45 and CD20, vary in their expression of CD79a and show strong cytoplasmic expression of monotypic immunoglobulin. AIDS-

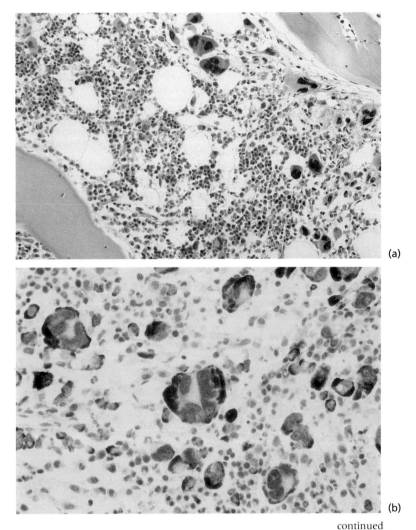

(a)

(b)

Fig. 7.25 BM trephine biopsy section (same patient as Fig. 7.24) showing giant myeloma cells which were confused with megakaryocytes. However, the giant cells were negative for CD61, positive for a plasma cell marker and showed light chain restriction. (a) Paraffin-embedded, H&E ×20. (b) Positive reaction with VS38c. Paraffin-embedded, immunoperoxidase ×40.

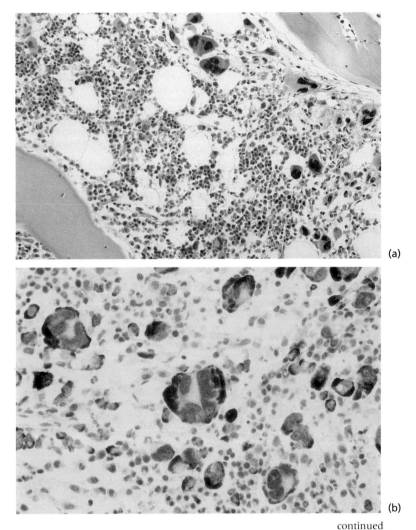

continued

related large cell lymphomas without any apparent plasmacytic differentiation may fail to express CD20 but usually express CD45. Anaplastic large cell lymphoma is among the large cell lymphomas which can be confused with anaplastic myeloma; both conditions are usually negative for B-cell markers and can lack CD45 expression but are positive for CD30 and may express epithelial membrane antigen. Staining for ALK1 can be useful for distinguishing ALK1-positive anaplastic large cell lymphoma from myeloma but not for distinguishing the ALK1-negative category. CD45RO, often

used as a T-cell marker, is expressed in some cases of myeloma [55]. The demonstration of light chain restriction using labelled oligonucleotide or peptide nucleic acid probes complementary to κ and λ light chain mRNA can be useful in distinguishing myeloma from large cell lymphoma and from other tumours.

Anaplastic carcinoma cells do not express CD45 or CD20 and usually express epithelial membrane antigen and high or low molecular weight cytokeratins. However, in this context, it should be noted that some myeloma cells also express epithe-

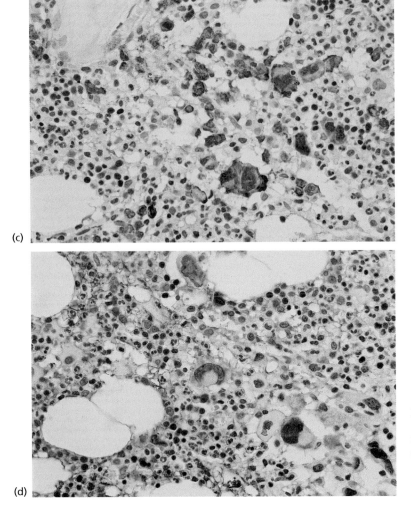

(c)

(d)

Fig. 7.25 (continued)
(c) Positive reaction with anti-κ.
Paraffin-embedded,
immunoperoxidase ×40.
(d) Negative reaction with anti-λ.
Paraffin-embedded,
immunoperoxidase ×40.

lial membrane antigen and, likewise, CD138 may be expressed by non-lymphoid tumours including some anaplastic carcinomas. It is usual practice to apply a broad panel of monoclonal antibodies in an attempt to determine the nature of anaplastic tumours. If reactions are all negative it is important to consider anaplastic myeloma and carry out immunostaining or *in situ* hybridization for κ and λ light chains. Immunostaining for CD138 and the antigen (p63) reactive with VS38c can also be useful in this context [46,47]. It should be noted that VS38c also reacts with endothelial cells,

lymphoma cells in lymphoplasmacytic lymphoma, lymphoma cells in a third of cases of diffuse large B-cell lymphoma, and neoplastic cells of some non-haemopoietic tumours [23]. MUM1/IRF4 can also be expressed in other neoplastic and normal plasma cells and in a proportion of normal post-germinal centre B cells and activated T cells.

Plasma cell leukaemia

The term plasma cell leukaemia may be used to designate a *de novo* leukaemia or the terminal phase of myeloma when neoplastic cells are present in the peripheral blood in large numbers. Plasma cell leukaemia has been defined by the presence in the circulating blood of at least 2 × 10⁹/l plasma cells, which also constitute at least 20% of circulating cells [76], but the WHO classification accepts either of these criteria as adequate [1]. Patients with *de novo* or primary plasma cell leukaemia show clinical features that are common in myeloma such as bone pain, lytic lesions, hypercalcaemia and renal failure but they have a higher incidence of extramedullary lesions and, in addition, often have hepatomegaly and splenomegaly. The disease is more aggressive than myeloma with a median survival of less than a year. Patients with established myeloma who develop a secondary plasma cell leukaemia have advanced disease which is usually refractory to treatment. Their prognosis is likewise poor.

Peripheral blood
The blood film shows large numbers of circulating neoplastic plasma cells (Fig. 7.26), the morphology of which varies between patients from cells resembling normal plasma cells to primitive, blastic cells showing only minimal evidence of plasma cell differentiation. Anaemia is almost invariable and neutropenia and thrombocytopenia are common. Increased rouleaux formation and increased background staining are usual; in patients with plasma cell leukaemia as the terminal phase of myeloma

these abnormalities are often striking since the paraprotein level is commonly high.

Bone marrow cytology
The bone marrow is heavily infiltrated with neoplastic cells showing the same morphological features as those in the peripheral blood. Normal haemopoietic elements are reduced.

Flow cytometric immunophenotyping
The immunophenotype is similar to that of myeloma but CD20 is more often expressed and CD56 less often [77]. Expression of CD38 is weaker [78].

Bone marrow histology
There is a diffuse infiltrate of plasma cells, which make up the majority of cells in the marrow [79,80]. In most cases, the cytological features are similar to those of myeloma; in a minority, the cells are very immature with little morphological evidence of plasma cell differentiation (Fig. 7.27).

Cytogenetic and molecular genetic analysis
Clonal cytogenetic abnormalities are common in plasma cell leukaemia. Although no consistent association is recognized, monosomy 13 is common [61,62] and there are often chromosomal rearrangements, such as the cryptic t(4;14)(p15;q32),

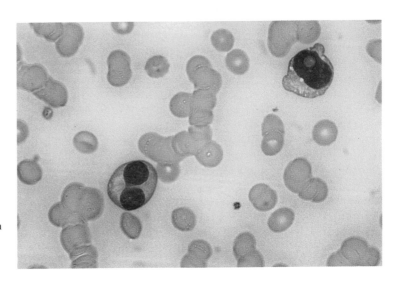

Fig. 7.26 Peripheral blood (PB) film, plasma cell leukaemia, showing marked rouleaux formation and two dysplastic plasma cells, one with an intranuclear inclusion (Dutcher body). MGG ×100.

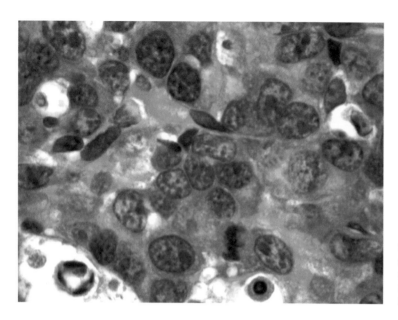

Fig. 7.27 BM trephine biopsy section from a patient with plasma cell leukaemia showing highly atypical plasmablasts. Paraffin-embedded, H&E ×100.

with a 14q32 breakpoint. Monosomy 13 and both t(11;14)(q13;q32) and t(14;16)(q32;q23) are more prevalent than in myeloma and, in contrast to myeloma, hypodiploidy is common whereas hyperdiploidy is not [61–63,81]. Deletion of *RB1* is common [61,62].

Monoclonal gammopathy of undetermined significance

Monoclonal gammopathy of undetermined significance (MGUS), previously known as 'benign monoclonal gammopathy', denotes a condition in which there is proliferation of a clone of plasma cells with production of a paraprotein but without the signs of disease that are characteristic of myeloma or B-cell lymphoma. The paraprotein is usually an immunoglobulin (either IgG, IgA or IgM) but is occasionally a Bence–Jones protein. The paraprotein concentration is relatively low (e.g. in the case of an IgG paraprotein <30 g/l, in the case of an IgA or IgM paraprotein <20 g/l or, if the International Myeloma Working Group criteria are adopted, <30 g/l, regardless of heavy chain type) and is usually stable. Since there are no features of disease, the diagnosis is necessarily made incidentally. MGUS is common. Paraproteins can be detected in about 3% of individuals over the age of 50 years, being as high as 5% in those aged 70 or

older and 7.5% in those aged 85 years or older [82]. The prevalence is higher in those with African ancestry than in Caucasians, being three times more frequent in Afro-Americans than in white Americans [83,84]. Immune paresis is not usually a feature but, in a population survey, 28% of tested subjects with MGUS had a reduction of normal immunoglobulins [82]. Most individuals with MGUS do not have urinary Bence–Jones protein but in the same population survey it was detected in 21.5% of those who were tested [82]. It is not always possible to make a distinction between myeloma and MGUS on the basis of any single feature. It is necessary to assess clinical and haematological features, bone marrow cytology and bone marrow histology in order to make the distinction. A period of observation may also be necessary to establish that the concentration of the paraprotein is stable and no disease features are appearing. It should be noted that although this condition may be clinically benign it does represent a neoplastic proliferation. If patients are followed for a prolonged period, a significant proportion eventually develop overt myeloma or a related condition. There is an increased incidence of skeletal fractures in patients in whom a diagnosis of MGUS has been made, as a result of reduced bone mineral density [85]. Patients with an IgG or IgA paraprotein tend to progress to myeloma or light chain-associated amyloidosis whereas those with an IgM paraprotein tend to progress to lymphoplasmacytic lymphoma, light chain-associated amyloidosis or chronic lymphocytic leukaemia. In a series of over 1300 patients followed for between 5 and 40 years the cumulative rate of progression was 12% at 10 years, 25% at 20 years and 35% at 25 years [86]. Progression is more likely in patients with a paraprotein concentration of more than 10 g/l [87]. Although the prevalence is greater in Afro-Americans, the rate of progression to myeloma is no greater than in white Americans [84]. It is because the likelihood of progression cannot be predicted for individual patients, that the designation 'monoclonal gammopathy of undetermined significance' is preferred to the previously used term 'benign monoclonal gammopathy'.

It should be noted that although definitions of MGUS include there being fewer than 10% plasma cells in the bone marrow and normal skeletal radiography, common sense should be applied when deciding whether individual patients with a paraprotein require further investigation. The incidental discovery of a paraprotein in an otherwise healthy, elderly person is not necessarily an indication for bone marrow examination.

Peripheral blood
The peripheral blood film may show increased rouleaux formation but this is generally less marked than in myeloma, anaemia does not occur and circulating plasma cells are not present.

Bone marrow cytology
The bone marrow may appear completely normal or there may be an increase of plasma cells. Plasma cells do not usually exceed 5% of nucleated cells but may comprise up to 10%. The presence of more than 2% plasma cells has been found predictive of later progression [87]. The plasma cells are usually morphologically fairly normal but minor dysplastic features may be noted. In one study the presence of nucleoli in more than 10% of plasma cells was found to be strongly predictive of myeloma rather than MGUS [88]. Crystal-laden macrophages, resembling Gaucher cells, are occasionally observed and may be much more conspicuous than the accompanying plasma cells [11].

Flow cytometric immunophenotyping
Often two populations of plasma cells are demonstrated – normal polyclonal plasma cells (CD19+, CD56−) and monoclonal plasma cells (often CD19− and either CD56+ or CD56−).

Bone marrow histology
Plasma cell infiltration is usually minimal with an interstitial increase and focal accumulation around capillaries that is often indistinguishable from a reactive plasmacytosis [26]. Crystal-laden macrophages are occasionally observed and may be much more conspicuous than the accompanying plasma cells [11].

Immunohistochemistry
CD138 and MUM1/IRF4 staining is important for highlighting the presence of increased numbers of plasma cells. CD56 is sometimes positive, whereas it is negative in reactive plasma cells. In situ hybridization for mRNA or, when technically adequate, immunohistochemical staining for κ and λ light chains shows κ:λ or λ:κ ratios of greater than four in approximately 65% of cases, the majority having ratios between four and 16. In comparison, almost all cases of overt myeloma have κ:λ or λ:κ ratios of greater than 16, the majority being greater than 100 [89]. Because it represents a reversal of the normal situation, an excess of λ over κ indicates the presence of monoclonal plasma cells reliably at lower ratios than when there is an excess of κ over λ.

Cytogenetic and molecular genetic analysis
Because the neoplastic cells make up a low proportion of bone marrow cells and have a low proliferative rate it is uncommon for cytogenetic analysis to demonstrate any clonal abnormality in patients with MGUS. Nevertheless, FISH techniques show that translocations with a 14q32 breakpoint, such as t(4;14)(p16;q32) and t(11;14)(q13;q32), occur with a similar frequency to that seen in myeloma [60]. Various aneuploidies have also been demonstrated (e.g. +3, +7, +9 +11) and 13q− is also found. Monosomy 13, however, has been found to be much less common than in myeloma and, when present, is likely to be predictive of disease progression [60].

Problems and pitfalls

It can be difficult to estimate κ:λ ratios when plasma cells constitute less than 5% of total cells [90] and in a significant minority of patients an abnormal κ:λ ratio cannot be demonstrated. However, it should been noted that this is not an essential investigation if it is known that the patient has a paraprotein. The major purpose of the trephine biopsy in this context is to distinguish between MGUS and myeloma using criteria such as the distribution and cytology of plasma cells as well as their number.

Waldenström macroglobulinaemia

The condition described by Waldenström as 'essential hyperglobulinaemia' is a disease characterized by a lymphoma, most often lymphoplasmacytic lymphoma, with secretion of large amounts of an IgM paraprotein leading to hyperviscosity, although the term is often used more loosely to include patients with a low concentration of IgM and no features of hyperviscosity. Most cases represent a variant of lymphoplasmacytic lymphoma (see page 327) and are distinguished from other cases of this lymphoma on the basis of clinical and biochemical features rather than by cytological or histological criteria. Less often, Waldenström macroglobulinaemia (IgM paraprotein of 3.2–8.8 g/l with clinical features of hyperviscosity) is a manifestation of extranodal marginal zone lymphoma of mucosa-associated lymphoid tissue (MALT lymphoma) [91]. Predominant signs and symptoms are either characteristic of a lymphoma or are caused by the hyperviscosity of blood consequent on the high concentration of IgM. Hepatomegaly, splenomegaly and lymphadenopathy are common; less often there is a lymphoma at an extranodal site such as the ocular adnexae or lung. Clinical features resulting from the high concentration of the paraprotein include anaemia (due to a greatly increased plasma volume), impaired vision, cerebral effects, cardiac failure and a bleeding tendency. In some patients the paraprotein has characteristics of a cold agglutinin or a cryoglobulin and in others it is amyloidogenic. Peripheral neuropathy is common and the paraprotein can sometimes be shown to have antibody activity against neural antigens. The incidence of Waldenström macroglobulinaemia is about a tenth that of myeloma.

Peripheral blood

There is usually a normocytic normochromic anaemia, increased rouleaux formation and increased background staining. Some patients have thrombocytopenia. When the paraprotein has the characteristics of a cold agglutinin or of a cryoglobulin, either red cell agglutinates or a cryoglobulin precipitate may be detected in the blood film. The lymphocyte count may be normal or elevated, with the neoplastic cells usually being mature small lymphocytes showing some features of differentiation to plasma cells.

Bone marrow cytology

The bone marrow is infiltrated by neoplastic cells which most often have the morphology of small lymphocytes, with a variable proportion of cells showing some plasmacytoid features (Figs 7.28 and 7.29). Plasma cells are usually increased and, in some patients, plasmacytic differentiation is prominent. Intranuclear or intracytoplasmic inclusions, which are usually PAS positive, are sometimes present. Macrophages and mast cells (Fig. 7.28) are often increased. Lymphoplasmacytoid cells may be clustered around macrophages.

Bone marrow histology

The bone marrow histology is not uniform [92–94]. In some patients, the infiltrating cells are predominantly lymphocytes, including plasmacytoid lymphocytes whereas, in others, there is prominent plasma cell differentiation. Some patients have an interstitial infiltrate or well-circumscribed nodules of lymphoid cells but in the majority there is either diffuse infiltration or a mixed nodular diffuse pattern. Paratrabecular infiltration can also occur, often accompanied by increased reticulin deposition. A variable proportion of cells show features of plasmacytic differentiation, including Russell bodies and Dutcher bodies (Fig. 7.30). Mature plasma cells are usually increased, as are macrophages, mast cells and, sometimes, eosinophils. Mast cells may be specifically associated with lymphoid infiltrates. Overall, about half of the cases show increased reticulin deposition. Trephine biopsy sections sometimes show infiltration when the bone marrow aspirate is normal. Rare observations in Waldenström macroglobulinaemia include the deposition of paraprotein in the bone marrow

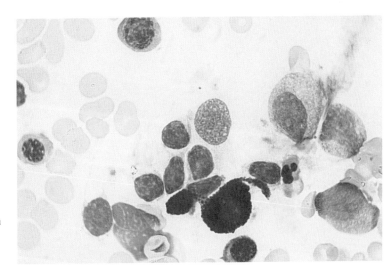

Fig. 7.28 BM aspirate, Waldenström macroglobulinaemia, showing a mast cell and mature small lymphocytes. MGG ×100.

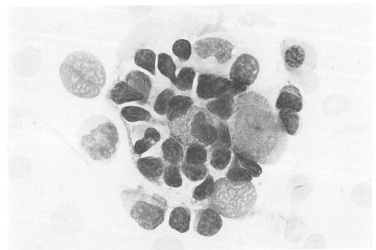

Fig. 7.29 BM aspirate, Waldenström macroglobulinaemia (same patient as Fig. 7.28), showing mature small lymphocytes and one plasmacytoid lymphocyte clustered around a macrophage. MGG ×100.

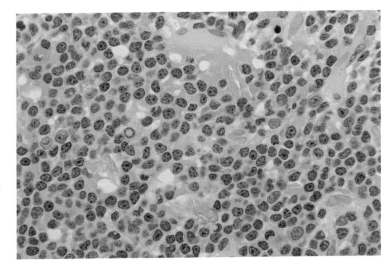

Fig. 7.30 BM trephine biopsy, Waldenström macroglobulinaemia, showing a diffuse infiltrate of small lymphoid cells, some of which show evidence of plasmacytoid differentiation (Dutcher bodies, 'clock-face' chromatin pattern and/ or a Golgi zone). Resin-embedded, H&E ×40.

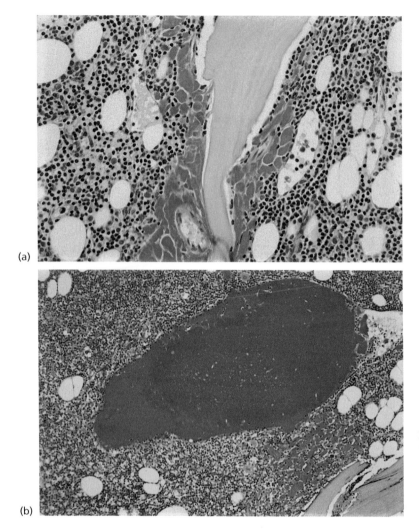

(a)

(b)

Fig. 7.31 Paraffin-embedded BM trephine biopsy sections, Waldenström macroglobulinaemia. (a) Interstitial deposition of IgM paraprotein adjacent to a trabecula. PAS stain ×20. (b) Intrasinusoidal paraprotein. PAS stain ×10.

interstitium and an abnormal staining pattern caused by intrasinusoidal paraprotein (Fig. 7.31).

Immunohistochemistry

Immunohistochemical features vary between and within cases, depending on the degree of plasma-cytic differentiation shown. There is usually strong expression of CD79a by most of the cells, while any neoplastic plasma cells show monotypic cytoplas-mic immunoglobulin (κ or λ) and react with VS38c, CD38, CD138 and MUM1/IRF4.

Other syndromes associated with secretion of a paraprotein

There are a number of other, relatively uncommon, syndromes associated with the secretion of a para-protein. In some of these the features of a lympho-proliferative disorder are prominent; in others the clinical and pathological features relate to the char-acteristics of the paraprotein and only detailed investigation reveals the presence of an abnormal clone of plasma cells, plasmacytoid lymphocytes or

Table 7.3 Monoclonal gammopathies (modified from reference [95]).

Plasma cell myeloma (including smouldering myeloma)

Solitary plasmacytoma (of bone or extramedullary)

Lymphoplasmacytic lymphoma including Waldenström macroglobulinaemia and other types of non-Hodgkin lymphoma with a serum or urinary paraprotein

Monoclonal gammopathy of undetermined significance including idiopathic Bence–Jones proteinuria

Light chain-associated amyloidosis

Light chain or other immunoglobulin deposition disease

Adult-acquired Fanconi syndrome (renal tubular deposition and excretion of monoclonal light chain)

Essential cryoglobulinaemia (type I and type II cryoglobulinaemia)

Chronic cold haemagglutinin disease

Alpha, gamma and mu (α, γ and μ) heavy chain disease

The POEMS syndrome

Acquired angio-oedema associated with monoclonal gammopathy

Monoclonal gammopathy with peripheral neuropathy

Scleromyxoedema (mucinous deposition in the skin plus serum paraprotein)

Systemic capillary leak syndrome with paraproteinaemia

Acquired C1 inhibitor deficiency with paraproteinaemia

lymphocytes. These conditions are summarized in Table 7.3 [95].

Light chain-associated amyloidosis

Light chain-associated amyloidosis (AL type of amyloidosis), in the 2008 WHO classification designated primary amyloidosis, is a disease resulting from a plasma cell neoplasm in which there is production of an amyloidogenic light chain [96–101]. The features of the disease are usually caused by the amyloidosis rather than by other features of the plasma cell proliferation. Heart failure and renal failure are common manifestations. In a minority of patients, light chain-associated amyloidosis is associated with overt myeloma or with Waldenström macroglobulinaemia or other forms of lymphoplasmacytic lymphoma [99]. However, in the majority of patients, the plasma cell neoplasm would be classified as MGUS if it were not for the amyloidogenic characteristics of the light chains. In a small minority of patients no paraprotein is detectable in the serum or urine but, in this group also, the disease results from a neoplastic proliferation of plasma cells, albeit occult. The term primary amyloidosis may be used to describe cases without evidence of myeloma or other overt plasma cell neoplasm. Amyloid can be formed from either κ or λ light chains but, in the majority of patients (70–80%), it is derived from λ light chains.

Peripheral blood

The peripheral blood may be normal or may show the features usually associated with myeloma or lymphoplasmacytic lymphoma. Occasionally, features of hyposplenism are present, indicating that the spleen is infiltrated by amyloid and has become hypofunctional. Thrombocytosis, observed in 9% of cases in one large series, may be indicative of hyposplenism [100]. Using sensitive immunophenotyping techniques, monoclonal plasma cells can be detected in the peripheral blood in a significant minority of patients, their presence being indicative of a worse prognosis [102].

Bone marrow cytology

The bone marrow aspirate varies from normal through increased numbers of plasma cells of normal morphology to overt myeloma or lymphoplasmacytic lymphoma. In a large series of patients, 40% had at least 10% bone marrow plasma cells [100]; the presence of increased numbers is indicative of a worse prognosis [102]. When the bone marrow aspirate is apparently normal, κ:λ imbalance may indicate the presence of an abnormal clone of cells, even though the total number of plasma cells is not increased. Very rarely, a bone marrow aspirate from a patient with amyloidosis contains either neutrophils that have ingested amyloid [103] or extracellular amyloid deposits (Fig. 7.32).

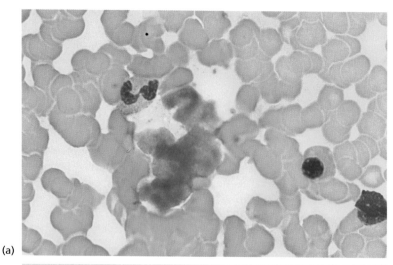

(a)

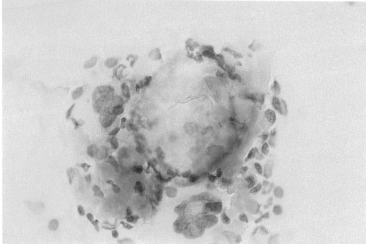

(b)

Fig. 7.32 BM aspirate showing amyloid. (a) MGG ×100. (b) Congo red ×50.

Bone marrow histology

Bone marrow biopsy sections may be normal or may show increased plasma cells. Patients with increased plasma cells may also have lymphoid aggregates and occasional patients have granulomas [101]. Sometimes, characteristic features of myeloma or lymphoplasmacytic lymphoma are present. In addition, amyloid may be detected either in the walls of small blood vessels (Figs 7.33 and 7.34) or in the interstitium (Fig. 7.35). Amyloid was detected in bone marrow sections in 56% of one large series of patients [103]. In another study

of 100 patients, amyloid was detected in bone marrow sections in 60%, in 39% in blood vessels and in 21% interstitially [101]. In the same series, a neoplastic plasma cell infiltrate was detected in 83% when histology was supplemented by immunohistochemistry [101]. In sections stained with H&E, amyloid is homogeneous and pink (Fig. 7.33a) whereas with a Giemsa stain it is blue (Fig. 7.34). It stains orange-red with Congo red (Fig. 7.33b) or Sirius red, and with both stains there is apple-green birefringence on examination with polarized light (Fig. 7.33c). Amyloid stains meta-

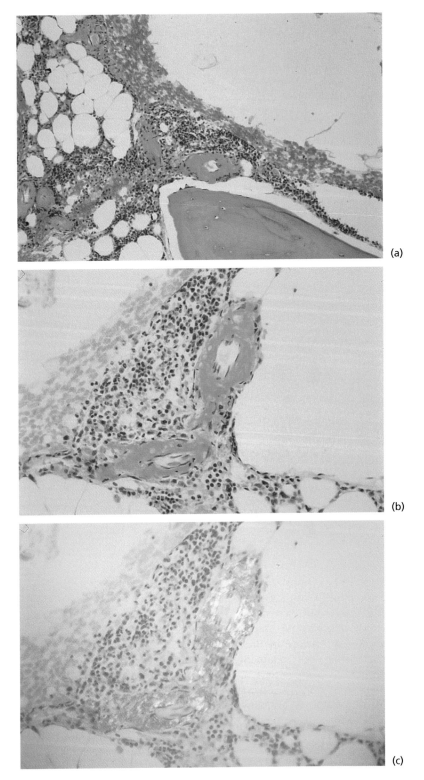

(a)

(b)

(c)

Fig. 7.33 BM trephine biopsy sections showing amyloid in the walls of small blood vessels. Paraffin-embedded: (a) H&E ×10; (b) Congo red stain ×40; (c) Congo red stain viewed under polarized light ×40.

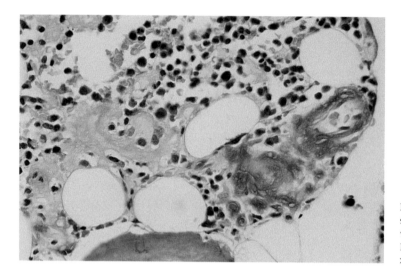

Fig. 7.34 BM trephine biopsy section showing amyloid in the walls of small blood vessels. Paraffin-embedded, Giemsa stain ×40.

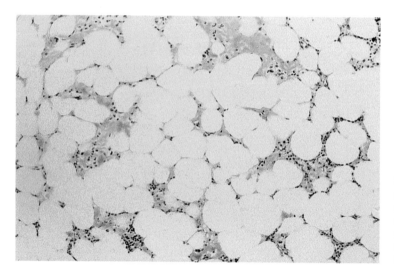

Fig. 7.35 BM trephine biopsy section, light chain-associated amyloidosis (AL type), showing deposition of amorphous eosinophilic material in the interstitium. Paraffin-embedded, H&E ×10.

chromatically with crystal violet and methyl violet and fluoresces after staining with thioflavine-T [104]. AL amyloid can be distinguished from amyloid of AA type by the abolition of Congo red staining by prior treatment with potassium permanganate in the latter type [104].

Trephine biopsy is important in the diagnosis of AL amyloidosis. In one series it was estimated that 96% of patients would have been detected by the combination of a bone marrow trephine biopsy and a biopsy of the abdominal fat pad [101].

Immunohistochemistry

Amyloid can be demonstrated using a monoclonal antibody that reacts with the P protein common to AL and other forms of amyloid. A positive identification of AL amyloid can sometimes be made with type-specific anti-light-chain sera; this was possible in fewer than 50% of patients in one series [105] and in 67% in another [101]. Neoplastic lymphocytes and plasma cells, when present in increased numbers, show the expected patterns of reactivity. Light chain restriction is demonstrable in the great majority of those with at least 6% of plasma cells and in two thirds of those with 5% or fewer [101].

Cytogenetic and molecular genetic analysis

Clonal chromosome abnormalities are common in AL amyloidosis but, because the neoplastic cells constitute a low percentage of bone marrow cells, demonstration of these abnormalities requires FISH techniques [106], preferably performed on purified plasma cells. Numerical abnormalities, both monosomies and trisomies, are common as are complex cytogenetic abnormalities. Both t(11;14) and del(13q) occur in a significant proportion of cases [107]. The pattern of abnormal findings is similar to that observed in MGUS and myeloma.

Problems and pitfalls

Since monoclonal gammopathy is quite common in older people it cannot be assumed that patients with amyloidosis and a paraprotein necessarily have AL amyloidosis. Some such patients have hereditary amyloidosis [105] and in other patients also the association may be coincidental. Misdiagnosis should be avoided since treatment directed at AL amyloidosis can have significant morbidity. Measurement of the ratio of free κ to free λ light chains in the serum can be useful in providing evidence of a plasma cell neoplasm in patients without a serum paraprotein but the same proviso applies, that this does not prove causality.

Light chain deposition disease

Light chain deposition disease [104,108–110] describes a syndrome of organ damage consequent on the systemic deposition of free light chains. There is an associated neoplastic proliferation of plasma cells, which may be occult or overt. About 70% of patients have relevant clinical features, most often of plasma cell myeloma but occasionally of solitary plasmacytoma, lymphoplasmacytic lymphoma or other non-Hodgkin lymphoma. The remaining patients either have features that would usually be interpreted as MGUS (about 15% of cases) or have no serum or urinary paraprotein detectable (also about 15% of cases) [104]. Those without a detectable paraprotein nevertheless have an occult plasma cell neoplasm, the neoplastic cells producing a light chain type that has a propensity

to deposit in and damage tissues. Cases with κ light chains are over-represented relative to cases with λ light chains. In occasional patients, a similar syndrome is associated with systemic deposition of heavy chains in addition to light chains (light and heavy chain deposition disease); the term 'monoclonal immunoglobulin deposition disease' has been suggested to include these cases [110,111] and is the preferred terminology in the WHO 2008 classification. The predominant organ damage is renal, with glomerular and tubular deposition causing the nephrotic syndrome, renal failure or both. Occasional patients have presented with clinical features of hepatic, cardiac or adrenal involvement.

Peripheral blood and bone marrow

There are no specific peripheral blood findings other than those usually associated with renal failure or with myeloma or other plasma cell neoplasm.

The bone marrow may appear normal or may show features usually associated with MGUS, myeloma or a related condition. Some patients who initially have no evidence of myeloma subsequently develop typical features of this disease. In those cases in which the bone marrow is apparently normal it may be possible to demonstrate a monoclonal population of plasma cells by flow cytometry. Rarely, light chains are deposited in the bone marrow, either in the interstitium or in the walls of blood vessels [104,109]. Light chain deposits are morphologically similar to amyloid deposits when stained with H&E but they do not stain with Congo red, or show birefringence with polarized light, and are negative or react weakly with thioflavine-T; they are PAS positive and stain blue with a Giemsa or Gomori trichrome stain. The nature of light chain deposits may be confirmed by immunohistochemistry with anti-κ or anti-λ antiserum but this is technically difficult because of background staining.

Measurement of the ratio of free κ to free λ light chains in the serum can be of use in diagnosis.

Essential and other paraprotein-associated cryoglobulinaemia

A plasma cell disorder may lead to cryoglobulinaemia, either when there is secretion of a paraprotein with the characteristics of a cryoglobulin (type I cryoglobulinaemia) or when a paraprotein has antibody activity against another immunoglobulin and the immune complex formed is a cryoglobulin (type II cryoglobulinaemia); in the latter type, the paraprotein is usually IgMκ with antibody activity against polyclonal IgG (i.e. it has rheumatoid factor activity). In about a quarter of patients, cryoglobulinaemia is a manifestation of myeloma or of Waldenström macroglobulinaemia. In the other three quarters of patients, in whom no overtly neoplastic proliferation of plasma cells is present, the term 'essential cryoglobulinaemia' has been used but this term is not appropriate if an underlying cause can be found. In these cases the clone of cells secreting the paraprotein is too small to produce any pathological manifestations other than those due to the characteristics of the cryoglobulin. The majority of cases of type II cryoglobulinaemia are secondary to hepatitis C infection, while some are associated with a lymphoproliferative disorder [112] or an autoimmune disease (e.g. Sjögren's syndrome) [112] and a small minority are associated with hepatitis B [113]. Some hepatitis C-associated cases have oligoclonal lymphoid infiltrates in the bone marrow while a smaller proportion of patients have overt low grade non-Hodgkin

lymphoma [113]. The clinical features of cryoglobulinaemia, e.g. purpura and peripheral cyanosis, may relate to precipitation of the immunoglobulin on chilling or, in the case of type II cryoglobulinaemia, to immune complex formation. Some patients with type II cryoglobulinaemia have polyarthralgia, peripheral neuropathy, sicca syndrome or renal impairment due to glomerulonephritis.

Peripheral blood

In the absence of overt myeloma or lymphoplasmacytic lymphoma, the peripheral blood film is often normal. In a minority of patients, a cryoglobulin precipitate is present, usually as weakly basophilic globular masses, less often as crystals or a fibrillar deposit. Occasionally cryoglobulin precipitates have been ingested by neutrophils or monocytes and are seen as globular, variably basophilic intracytoplasmic inclusions.

Bone marrow cytology and histology

In type I cryoglobulinaemia the bone marrow findings are either normal or are those of myeloma, a low grade non-Hodgkin lymphoma or MGUS. Occasionally there is deposition of cryoglobulin in marrow films (Fig. 7.36). In hepatitis C-associated type II cryoglobulinaemia the bone marrow may be

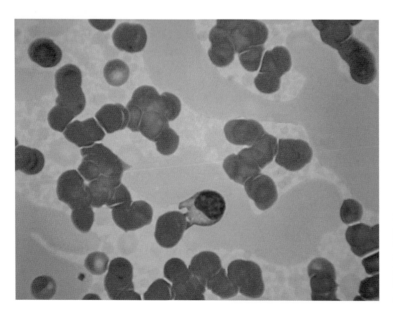

Fig. 7.36 BM aspirate from a patient with plasma cell myeloma and associated cryoglobulinaemia showing deposition of cryoglobulin in the bone marrow. A lymphoplasmacytoid cell is also apparent. MGG ×100.

normal, may show oligoclonal lymphoid infiltrates comprised of mature small lymphocytes, prolymphocytes and para-immunoblasts [113] or may show overt monoclonal low grade B-cell lymphoma.

Cytogenetic and molecular genetic analysis
IGH/BCL2 rearrangements and t(14;18) have been found to be common in mixed cryoglobulinaemia associated with hepatitis C infection [113,114].

Chronic cold haemagglutinin disease
Chronic cold haemagglutinin disease (CHAD) is a disease characterized by chronic, cold-induced haemolytic anaemia consequent on a lymphoplasmacytic neoplasm, which may be either occult or overt. In patients who do not have clinical or pathological features of a lymphoma at presentation, these may evolve subsequently.

Peripheral blood
Unless it has been prepared from warmed blood, the blood film shows red cell agglutinates. If there has been a recent episode of haemolysis a few spherocytes may be present together with polychromatic macrocytes. Some patients have lymphocytosis, with the cells either having the morphology of normal mature lymphocytes or showing some plasmacytic features.

Bone marrow cytology and histology
The bone marrow appearances vary from normal to those of an overt lymphoplasmacytic lymphoma. There is usually erythroid hyperplasia.

Alpha heavy chain disease
Alpha heavy chain disease is a variant of MALT lymphoma, also known as immunoproliferative small intestinal disease (IPSID) [50]. It usually affects predominantly the small bowel and is associated with the secretion of a truncated IgA heavy chain into the serum or into the bowel lumen. Some cases evolve into large cell lymphoma. This disease has been recognized particularly in relatively young persons living in poor socioeconomic conditions around the Mediterranean region, the Middle East, the Far East and Africa. In the early

stages a response to antibiotic therapy is often seen. Infection by *Campylobacter jejuni* is an aetiological factor [115]. Serum IgA may be increased or there may be free α chain in the serum.

Peripheral blood and bone marrow
The peripheral blood usually shows no specific abnormality. Rarely there are circulating plasmacytoid lymphocytes [115]. The bone marrow is usually normal but may be infiltrated by plasma cells.

Gamma heavy chain disease
Gamma heavy chain disease is a lymphoplasmacytic neoplasm characterized by lymphadenopathy, hepatomegaly, splenomegaly and involvement of Waldeyer's ring, together with the secretion of a defective IgG heavy chain. About a third of patients have associated autoimmune disease, most often rheumatoid arthritis [116]. Some patients have developed amyloidosis; rarely, amyloid (AH amyloid) can be derived from immunoglobulin heavy chains as well as light chains [117].

Peripheral blood
Anaemia, leucopenia and thrombocytopenia are common. Anaemia and thrombocytopenia may be autoimmune in nature [50,118]. In about half of cases there are atypical lymphoplasmacytoid cells and some plasma cells in the peripheral blood. Some patients have eosinophilia.

Bone marrow cytology and histology
The bone marrow is infiltrated by lymphocytes, lymphoplasmacytoid cells or plasma cells. Infiltration may be focal [116]. Admixed eosinophils and macrophages may create infiltrates that resemble those of angioimmunoblastic T-cell lymphoma.

Mu heavy chain disease
Mu heavy chain disease [119–122] is a lymphoproliferative disorder characterized by the secretion of a defective IgM heavy chain. Most patients described in the published literature have had the pathological features of chronic lymphocytic leukaemia although one case was associated

with Waldenström macroglobulinaemia [123]. Hepatomegaly and splenomegaly are usual; abdominal lymphadenopathy is more prominent than peripheral lymphadenopathy. Light chain secretion may also occur and may give rise to Bence–Jones proteinuria and amyloidosis.

Peripheral blood and bone marrow

The majority of patients show features indistinguishable from chronic lymphocytic leukaemia except that vacuolated plasma cells are often present [50].

The POEMS syndrome

The POEMS, or 'polyneuropathy, organomegaly, endocrinopathy, M protein, skin changes' syndrome [124–127] describes a curious constellation of pathological manifestations that have been associated with myeloma (particularly, but not exclusively, osteosclerotic myeloma), solitary plasmacytoma and lymphoplasmacytic lymphoma. In addition, POEMS has been described in patients with bone marrow appearances which, but for the many associated pathological features, would be designated MGUS. The syndrome is rare and occurs at a younger age than is usual in myeloma. The 'polyneuropathy' is both motor and sensory but motor neuropathy predominates. The 'organomegaly' refers to hepatomegaly, splenomegaly and lymphadenopathy. The pathological features of the enlarged lymph nodes approximate to those of the hyaline-vascular type of Castleman's disease; there is follicular hyperplasia, vascular proliferation and an interfollicular infiltrate of lymphocytes, plasma cells and immunoblasts. The 'endocrinopathy' may include primary gonadal failure, hypothyroidism, hypoparathyroidism, Addison's disease and diabetes mellitus. The 'monoclonal gammopathy', present in about three quarters of patients, is usually an IgGλ or IgAλ paraprotein. Fifteen per cent of cases are non-secretory [128]. Because the concentration of paraprotein is usually low, immunofixation should be used for detection. 'Skin' manifestations include skin thickening resembling that of scleroderma, oedema, hypertrichosis, hyperpigmentation and Raynaud's phenomenon. Other features of the syndrome include pleural effusion, ascites, papilloedema, pulmonary

hypertension, restrictive lung disease and finger clubbing.

Peripheral blood and bone marrow

There are no specific peripheral blood features. Anaemia is rare; erythrocytosis and thrombocytosis can occur [50]. The bone marrow findings range from normal to those of overt lymphoplasmacytic lymphoma or myeloma. In as many as a quarter of patients the bone marrow appears normal [128]; in the same large series of patients, 17% were considered to have the bone marrow features of myeloma while the remaining patients showed some increase in plasma cells. Osteosclerosis is usual but some patients have osteolytic lesions. The plasma cells are almost always λ restricted. Rarely Castleman's disease is detected in the trephine biopsy specimen (Fig. 7.37).

Acquired angio-oedema associated with plasma cell neoplasia

The majority of cases of acquired angio-oedema described have been associated with a neoplastic plasma cell proliferation or with other mature B-lineage neoplasms, with or without secretion of a paraprotein [129–131]. Associated conditions have included myeloma, lymphoplasmacytic lymphoma, splenic lymphoma with villous lymphocytes and other non-Hodgkin lymphomas, essential cryoglobulinaemia, MGUS and chronic lymphocytic leukaemia. The mechanism of the acquired angio-oedema is C1 inhibitor deficiency consequent on excessive consumption; it is likely that consumption of C1 inhibitor can be due to precipitation of a cryoglobulin, to an immunological reaction involving the paraprotein or to reaction of autoantibodies with neoplastic cells. Deficiency of C1 inhibitor may precede the development of overt lymphoproliferative disease by many years [132].

Peripheral blood and bone marrow

The peripheral blood and bone marrow findings are those usually associated with myeloma, lymphoplasmacytic lymphoma or other lymphoproliferative disease. In a minority of cases the bone marrow shows only a slight increase in plasma cells or is normal.

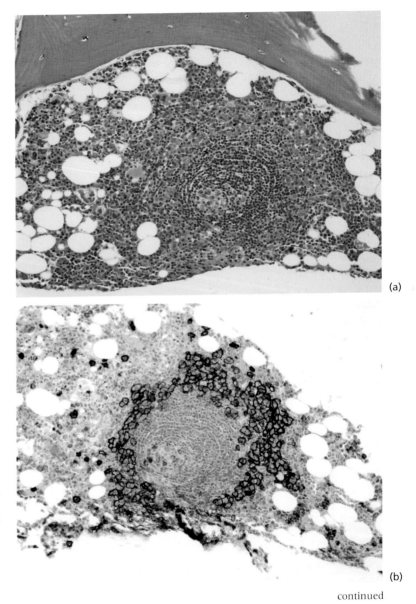

(a)

(b)

Fig. 7.37 BM trephine biopsy section from a patient with POEMS and Castleman's disease showing a lymphoid follicle surrounded by plasma cells. (a) Paraffin-embedded, H&E ×20. (b) Immunoperoxidase for CD138 showing that, in contrast to human herpesvirus 8 (HHV8)-associated Castleman's disease, these neoplastic plasma cells clearly surround the follicle. Paraffin-embedded, ×20.

continued

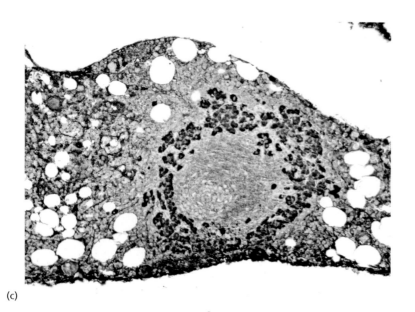

(c)

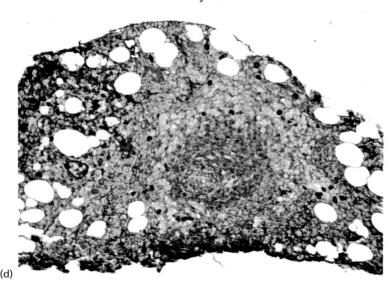

(d)

Fig. 7.37 (continued) (c) Immunoperoxidase for λ light chain and (d) immunoperoxidase for κ light chain showing that plasma cells are light chain restricted, expressing only λ light chain. Paraffin-embedded, ×20. (By courtesy of Dr Ahmet Dogan, Rochester, Minnesota.)

References

1 McKenna RW, Kyle RA, Kuehl WM, Grogan TM, Harris NL and Coupland RW (2008) Plasma cell neoplasms. In: Swerdlow SH, Campo E, Harris NL, Jaffe ES, Pileri SA, Stein H, Thiele J and Vardiman JW (eds) *World Health Organization Classification of Tumours of Haematopoietic and Lymphoid Tissues.* IARC Press, Lyon, pp. 200–213.

2 Smith A, Wisloff F, Samson D, the UK Myeloma Forum, Nordic Myeloma Study Group and British Committee for Standards in Haematology (2006)

Guidelines on the diagnosis and management of multiple myeloma 2005. *Br J Haematol*, **132**, 410–451.

3 Phekoo KJ, Schey SA, Richards MA, Bevan DH, Bell S, Gillett D and Moller H (2004) A population study to define the incidence and survival of multiple myeloma in a National Health Service Region in the UK. *Br J Haematol*, **127**, 299–304.

4 Morton LM, Wang SS, Devesa SS, Hartge P, Weisenburger DD and Linet MS (2006) Lymphoma incidence patterns by WHO subtype in the United States, 1992–2001. *Blood*, **107**, 265–276.

5 Ögmundsdóttir HM, Haraldsdóttir W, Jóhannesson GM, Bjarnadóttir G, Ólafsdóttir GK, Sigvaldason H and Tulinius H (2005) Familiality of benign and malignant paraproteinemias. A population-based cancer-registry study of multiple myeloma families. *Haematologica*, **90**, 66–71.

6 Österborg A and Mellstedt H (1996) Clinical features and staging. In: Gahrton G and Durie BGM (eds) *Multiple Myeloma*. Arnold, London.

7 The International Myeloma Working Group (2003) Criteria for the classification of monoclonal gammopathies, multiple myeloma and related disorders: a report of the International Myeloma Working Group. *Br J Haematol*, **121**, 749–757.

8 Ghevaert C, Fournier M, Bernardi F, Genevieve F, Pouyol F and Zandecki M (1997) Non-secretory multiple myeloma with multinucleated giant plasma cells. *Leuk Lymphoma*, **27**, 185–189.

9 Dimov ND, Zynger DL and Peterson LC (2006) Plasma cell satellitism in plasma cell myeloma. *J Clin Pathol*, **59**, 1003.

10 Vidulich K, Hanks D and Etzell JE (2006) Iron in neoplastic plasma cells of plasma cell myeloma. *Am J Hematol*, **81**, 216–217.

11 Lebeau A, Zeindl-Eberhart E, Müller E-C, Müller-Höcker J, Jungblut PR, Emmerich B and Löhrs U (2002) Generalized crystal-storing histiocytosis associated with monoclonal gammopathy: molecular analysis of a disorder with rapid clinical course and review of the literature. *Blood*, **100**, 1817–1827.

12 Brodie C, Agrawal S, Rahemtulla A, O'Shea D, Lampert I and Naresh KN (2007) Multiple myeloma with bone marrow extracellular crystal deposition. *J Clin Pathol*, **60**, 1064–1065.

13 Merlini G, Gobbi PG and Ascari E (1989) The Merlini, Waldenström, Jayakar staging system revisited. *Eur J Haematol*, **43** (Suppl. 51), 105–110.

14 Pasqualetti P, Casale R, Collacciani A, Abruzzo BP and Colantonio D (1990) Multiple myeloma: relationship between survival and cellular morphology. *Am J Hematol*, **33**, 145–147.

15 Finnish Leukaemia Group (1999) Long-term survival in multiple myeloma: a Finnish Leukaemia Group study. *Br J Haematol*, **105**, 942–947.

16 Greipp PR, Raymond NM, Kyle RA and O'Fallon WM (1985) Multiple myeloma: significance of plasmablastic morphological classification. *Blood*, **65**, 305–310.

17 Carter A, Hocherman I, Linn S, Cohen Y and Tatarsky I (1987) Prognostic significance of plasma cell morphology in multiple myeloma. *Cancer*, **60**, 1060–1065.

18 Goasguen JE, Zandecki M, Mathiot C, Scheiff JM, Bizet M, Ly-Sunnaram B *et al.* (1999) Mature plasma cells as indicator of better prognosis in multiple myeloma. New methodology for the assessment of plasma cell morphology. *Leuk Res*, **23**, 1133–1140.

19 Kyle RA, Remstein ED, Therneau TM, Dispenzieri A, Kurtin PJ, Hodnefield JM *et al.* (2007) Clinical course and prognosis of smoldering (asymptomatic) multiple myeloma. *N Engl J Med*, **356**, 2582–2590.

20 Almeida J, Orfao A, Ocqueteau M, Mateo G, Corral M, Caballero MD *et al.* (1999) High-sensitive immunophenotyping and DNA ploidy studies in the investigation of minimal residual disease in multiple myeloma. *Br J Haematol*, **107**, 121–131.

21 Ruiz-Arguelles GJ and San Miguel JF (1994) Cell surface markers in multiple myeloma. *Mayo Clin Proc*, **96**, 684–690.

22 Kraj M, Poglód R, Kopeć-Szlęzak J, Sokolowska U, Woźniak J and Kruk B (2004) C-kit receptor (CD117) expression on plasma cells in monoclonal gammopathies. *Leuk Lymphoma*, **45**, 2281–2289.

23 Wei A and Juneja S (2003) Bone marrow immunohistology of plasma cell neoplasms. *J Clin Pathol*, **56**, 406–441.

24 Feyler S, O'Connor SJ, Rawstron AC, Subash C, Ross FM, Pratt G *et al.* (2008) IgM myeloma: a rare entity characterized by a CD20-CD56-CD117- immunophenotype and the t(11;14). *Br J Haematol*, **140**, 547–551.

25 Owen RG and Rawstrom AC (2005) Minimal residual disease monitoring in multiple myeloma: flow cytometry is the method of choice. *Br J Haematol*, **128**, 732–733.

26 Bartl R, Frisch B, Diem H, Møndel M and Fateh-Moghadam A (1989) Bone marrow histology and serum β 2 microglobulin in multiple myeloma – a new prognostic strategy. *Eur J Haematol*, **43** (Suppl. 51), 88–98.

27 Pileri S, Poggi S, Baglioni P, Montanari M, Sabattini E, Galieni P *et al.* (1989) Histology and immunohistology of bone marrow biopsy in multiple myeloma. *Eur J Haematol*, **43** (Suppl. 51), 52–59.

28 Ribatti D, Vacca A, Nico B, Quondamatteo F, Ria R, Minischetti M *et al.* (1990) Bone marrow angiogenesis and mast cell density increase simultaneously with progression of human multiple myeloma. *Br J Cancer*, **79**, 451–455.

29 Vacca A, Ribatti D, Presta M, Minischetti M, Iurlaro M, Ria R *et al.* (1999) Bone marrow neovascularization, plasma cell angiogenic potential, and matrix metalloproteinase-2 secretion parallel progression of human multiple myeloma. *Blood*, **93**, 3064–3073.

30 Schreiber S, Ackermann J, Obermair A, Kaufmann H, Urbauer E, Aletaha K *et al.* (2000) Multiple myeloma with deletion of chromosome 13q is characterized by increased bone marrow neovascularization. *Br J Haematol*, **110**, 605–609.

31 Xu JL, Lai R, Kinoshita T, Nakashima B and Nagasaka T (2002) Proliferation, apoptosis, and intratumoral vascularity in multiple myeloma: correlation with clinical stage and cytological grade. *J Clin Pathol*, **55**, 530–534.

32 Foucar K (2001) *Bone Marrow Pathology*, 2nd edn. ASCP Press, Chicago.

33 Nakamura H, Sakamoto M, Wakasugi K and Toyama K (1991) IgD-lambda multiple myeloma associated with bone marrow fibrosis. *Rinsho Ketsueki*, **32**, 395–398.

34 Lam KY and Chan KW (1993) Unusual findings in a myeloma kidney: a light- and electron-microscopic study. *Nephron*, **65**, 133–136.

35 Abildgaard N, Bendix-Hansen K, Kristensen JE, Vejlgaard T, Risteli L, Nielsen JL and Heickendorff L (1997) Bone marrow fibrosis and disease activity in multiple myeloma monitored by the aminoterminal propeptide of procollagen III in serum. *Br J Haematol*, **99**, 641–648.

36 Desikan KR, Dhodapkar MV, Hough A, Waldron T, Jagannath S, Siegel D, Barlogie B and Tricot G (1997) Incidence and impact of light chain associated (AL) amyloidosis on the prognosis of patients with multiple myeloma treated with autologous transplantation. *Leuk Lymphoma*, **27**, 315–319.

37 Bartl R and Frisch B (1995) Diagnostic morphology in multiple myeloma. *Current Diagnostic Pathol*, **2**, 222–235.

38 Bains MA, Pardoe LE and Rudin CE (2007) Osteitis fibrosa cystica and secondary hyperparathyroidism in multiple myeloma. *Br J Haematol*, **136**, 179.

39 Pich A, Chiusa L, Marmont F and Navone R (1997) Risk groups of myeloma patients by histologic pattern and proliferative activity. *Am J Surg Pathol*, **21**, 339–347.

40 Strand WR, Banks PM and Kyle RA (1984) Anaplastic plasma cell myeloma and immunoblastic lymphoma: clinical, pathologic and immunologic comparison. *Am J Med*, **76**, 861–867.

41 Bartl R, Frisch B, Fateh-Moghadam A, Kettner G, Jaeger K and Sommerfeld W (1986) Histologic classification and staging of multiple myeloma. *Am J Clin Pathol*, **87**, 342–355.

42 Sukpanichnant S, Cousar JB, Leelasiri A, Graber SE, Greer JP, Collins RD (1994) Diagnostic criteria and histologic grading in multiple myeloma: histologic and immunohistologic analysis of 176 cases with clinical correlation. *Hum Pathol*, **25**, 308–318.

43 Bhatti SS, Kumar L, Dinda AK and Dawar R (2006) Prognostic value of bone marrow angiogenesis in multiple myeloma: use of light microscopy as well as computerized image analyzer in the assessment of microvessel density and total vascular area in multiple myeloma and its correlation with various clinical, histological, and laboratory parameters. *Am J Hematol*, **81**, 649–656.

44 Joshi R, Horncastle D, Elderfield K, Lampert I, Rahemtulla A and Naresh KN (2007) Bone marrow trephine combined with immunohistochemistry is superior to bone marrow aspirate in follow-up of myeloma patients. *J Clin Pathol*, **61**, 213–216.

45 Anderson KC, Bates MP, Slaughtenhoupt B, Schlossman SF and Nadler LM (1984) A monoclonal antibody with reactivity restricted to normal and neoplastic plasma cells. *J Immunol*, **132**, 3172–3177.

46 Dhodapkar MV, Abe E, Theus A, Lacy M, Langford JK, Barlogie B and Sanderson RD (1998) Syndecan-1 is a multifunctional regulator of myeloma pathobiology: control of tumour cell survival, growth and bone differentiation. *Blood*, **91**, 2679–2688.

47 Turley H, Jones M, Erber W, Mayne K, de Waele M and Gatter K (1994) VS38: a new monoclonal antibody for detecting plasma cell differentiation in routine sections. *J Clin Pathol*, **47**, 418–422.

48 Vallario A, Chilosi M, Adami F, Montagna L, Deaglio S, Malavasi F and Calgaris-Cappio F (1999) Human myeloma cells express the CD38 ligand CD31. *Br J Haematol*, **105**, 441–444.

49 Robillard N, Avet-Loiseau H, Garand R, Moreau P, Pineau D, Rapp M-J *et al.* (2003) CD20 is associated with a small mature plasma cell morphology and t(11;14) in multiple myeloma. *Blood*, **102**, 1070–1071.

50 Grogan TM, van Camp B, Kyle RA, Müller-Hermelink HK and Harris NL (2001) Plasma cell neoplasms. In: Jaffe ES, Harris NL, Stein H and Vardiman JW (eds) *World Health Organization Classification of Tumours: Pathology and Genetics of Tumours of Haematopoietic and Lymphoid Tissues*. IARC Press, Lyon, pp. 142–156.

51 Petruch UR, Horny H-P and Kaiserling E (1992) Frequent expression of haemopoietic and non-haemopoietic antigens by neoplastic plasma cells: an immunohistochemical study using formalin-fixed, paraffin-embedded tissue. *Histopathol*, **20**, 35–40.

52 Hoyer JD, Hanson CA, Fonseca R, Greipp PR, Dewald GW and Kurtin PJ (2000) The t(11;14)(q13;q32) translocation in multiple myeloma: a morphologic and immunohistochemical study. *Am J Clin Pathol*, **113**, 831–837.

53 Athanasiou E, Kaloutsi V, Kotoula V, Hytiroglou P, Kostopoulos I, Zervas *et al.* (2001) Cyclin D1 over-

expression in multiple myeloma. *Am J Clin Pathol*, **116**, 535–542.

54 Chang H, Stewart AK, Qi XY, Li ZH, Yi QL and Trudel S (2005) Immunohistochemistry accurately predicts FGFR3 aberrant expression and t(4;14) in multiple myeloma. *Blood*, **106**, 353–355.

55 Menke DM, Horny HP, Griesser H, Atkinson EJ, Kaiserling E and Kyle RA (1998) Immunophenotypic and genotypic characterisation of multiple myelomas with adverse prognosis characterised by immunohistological expression of the T cell related antigen CD45RO (UCHL-1). *J Clin Pathol*, **51**, 432–437.

56 Boersma-Vreugdenhil GR, Peeters T and Bast BJEG (2003) Translocation of the IgH locus is nearly ubiquitous in multiple myeloma as detected by immuno-FISH. *Blood*, **101**, 1653.

57 Fonseca R, Blood EA, Oken MM, Kyle RA, Dewald GW, Bailey RJ *et al.* (2002) Myeloma and the t(11;14) (q13;q32); evidence for a biologically defined unique subset of patients. *Blood*, **99**, 3735–3741.

58 Avet-Loiseau H, Garand R, Lodé L, Harousseau J-L and Bataille R for the Intergroupe Francophone du Myélome (2003) Translocation t(11;14)(q13;q32) is the hallmark of IgM, IgE, and nonsecretory multiple myeloma variants. *Blood*, **101**, 1570–1571.

59 Gozzetti A and Le Beau M (2000) Fluorescence in situ hybridization: uses and limitations. *Semin Hematol*, **37**, 320–333.

60 Avet-Loiseau H, Li J-Y, Morineau N, Facon T, Brigaudeau C, Harousseau J-L *et al.* on behalf of the Intergroupe Francophone du Myélome (1999) Monosomy 13 is associated with the transition of monoclonal gammopathy of undetermined significance to multiple myeloma. *Blood*, **94**, 2583–2589.

61 García-Sanz R, Orfão A, González M, Tabernero MD, Bladé J, Moro MJ *et al.* (1999) Primary plasma cell leukemia: clinical, immunophenotypic, DNA ploidy and cytogenetic characteristics. *Blood*, **93**, 1032–1037.

62 García-Sanz R, Orfão A and San Miguel JF (1999b) Primary plasma cell leukemia and multiple myeloma: one or two disease according to the methodology – response. *Blood*, **94**, 3608–3609.

63 Smadja NV, Bastard C and Brigaudeau C (1999) Primary plasma cell leukemia and multiple myeloma: one or two disease according to the methodology. *Blood*, **94**, 3607.

64 Konigsberg R, Zojer N, Ackermann J, Kromer E, Kittler H, Fritz E *et al.* (2000) Predictive role of interphase cytogenetics for survival of patients with multiple myeloma. *J Clin Oncol*, **18**, 804–812.

65 Avet-Loiseau H, Attal M, Moreau P, Charbonnel C, Garban F, Hulin C *et al.* (2007) Genetic abnormalities and survival in multiple myeloma: the experience of the Intergroupe Francophone du Myélome. *Blood*, **109**, 3489–3495.

66 Fassas AB-T, Spencer T, Sawyer J, Zangari M, Lee C-K, Anaissie E *et al.* (2002) Both hypodiploidy and deletion of chromosome 13 independently confer poor prognosis in multiple myeloma. *Br J Haematol*, **118**, 1041–1047.

67 Winkler JM, Greiff PR and Fonseca R (2003) t(4;14) (p16.3)(q32) is strongly associated with a shorter survival in myeloma patients. *Br J Haematol*, **120**, 166–171.

68 Smadja NV, Bastard C, Brigaudeau B, Leroux D and Fruchart C on behalf of the Groupe Français de Cytogénétique Hématologique (2001) Hypodiploidy is a major prognostic factor in multiple myeloma. *Blood*, **98**, 2229–2238.

69 Tanvetyanon T and Leighton JC (2002) Severe anemia and marrow plasmacytosis as presentation of Sjögren's syndrome. *Am J Hematol*, **69**, 233.

70 Bayley J, Pavlû J and Thompson M (2008) Striking bone marrow plasmacytosis in a patient with sickle cell anaemia. *Br J Haematol*, **144**, 457.

71 Torlakovic EE, Naresh KN and Brunning RD (2008) *Bone Marrow Immunohistochemistry*. ASCP Press, Chicago, p. 134.

72 Jego G, Avet-Loiseau H, Robillard N, Moreau P, Amiot M, Harousseau J *et al.* (2000) Reactive plasmacytoses in multiple myeloma during hematopoietic recovery with G- or GM-CSF. *Leuk Res*, **24**, 627–630.

73 Riccardi A, Ucci G, Luoni R, Castello A, Coci A, Magrini U and Ascari E (1990) Bone marrow biopsy in monoclonal gammopathies: correlations between pathological findings and clinical data. *J Clin Pathol*, **43**, 469–475.

74 Thiry A, Delvenne P, Fontaine MA and Boniver J (1993) Comparison of bone marrow sections, smears and immunohistological staining for immunoglobulin light chains in the diagnosis of benign and malignant plasma cell proliferations. *Histopathology*, **22**, 423–428.

75 Gatter K and Brown D (1997) *An Illustrated Guide to Bone Marrow Diagnosis*. Blackwell Science, Oxford.

76 Kyle RA, Maldonado JE and Bayrd ED (1974) Plasma cell leukemia. Report on 17 cases. *Arch Intern Med*, **133**, 813–818.

77 Garcia-Sanz R, Orfao A, Gonzales M, Tabernero MD, Blade J, Moro MJ *et al.* (1999) Primary plasma cell leukemia: clinical, immunophenotypic, DNA ploidy, and cytogenetic characteristics. *Blood*, **93**, 1032–1037.

78 Perez-Andres M, Almeida J, Martin-Ayuso M, Moro MJ, Martin-Nunez G, Galende J *et al.* (2005) Clonal plasma cells from monoclonal gammopathy of undetermined significance, multiple myeloma and plasma cell leukemia show different expression profiles of molecules involved in the interaction with the

immunological bone marrow microenvironment. *Leukemia*, **19**, 449–455.

79 Kosmo MA and Gale RP (1987) Plasma cell leukemia. *Semin Hematol*, **24**, 202–208.

80 Bernasconi G, Castelli G, Pagnucco G and Brusamolino E (1989) Plasma cell leukemia: a report on 15 patients. *Eur J Haematol*, **43** (Suppl. 51), 76–83.

81 Avet-Loiseau H, Daviet A, Brigaudeau C, Callet-Bauchu E, Terré C, Lafage-Pochitaloff M *et al.* (2001) Cytogenetic, interphase, and multicolour fluorescence in situ hybridization analyses in primary plasma cell leukemia: a study of 40 patients at diagnosis, on behalf of the Intergroupe Francophone du Myélome and the Groupe Français de Cytogénetique Hématologique. *Blood*, **97**, 822–835.

82 Kyle RA, Therneau TM, Rajkumar SV, Larson DR, Plevak MF, Offord JR *et al.* (2006) Prevalence of monoclonal gammopathy of undetermined significance. *N Engl J Med*, **354**, 1362–1369.

83 Cohen HJ, Crawford J, Rao MK, Pieper CF and Currie MS (1998) Racial differences in the prevalence of monoclonal gammopathy in a community-based sample of the elderly. *Am J Med*, **104**, 439–444.

84 Landgren O, Gridley G, Turesson I, Caporaso NE, Goldin LR, Baris D *et al.* (2006) Risk of monoclonal gammopathy of undetermined significance (MGUS) and subsequent multiple myeloma among African American and white veterans in the United States. *Blood*, **107**, 904–906.

85 Pepe J, Petrucci MT, Nofroni I, Fassino V, Diacinti D, Romagnoli E and Minisola S (2006) Lumbar bone mineral density as the major factor determining increased prevalence of vertebral fractures in monoclonal gammopathy of undetermined significance. *Br J Haematol*, **134**, 485–490.

86 Kyle RA, Therneau TM, Rajkumar SV, Offord JR, Larson DR, Plevak MF and Melton LJ (2002) A long term study of prognosis in monoclonal gammopathy of undetermined significance. *N Engl J Med*, **346**, 564–569.

87 van den Donk N, de Weerdt O, Eurelings M, Bloem A and Lokhorst H (2001) Malignant transformation of monoclonal gammopathy of undetermined significance: cumulative incidence and prognostic factors. *Leuk Lymphoma*, **42**, 609–618.

88 Millá F, Oriol A, Aguilar J, Aventín A, Ayats R, Alonso E *et al.* (2001) Usefulness and reproducibility of cytomorphologic evaluations to differentiate myeloma from monoclonal gammopathies of unknown significance. *Am J Clin Pathol*, **115**, 127–135.

89 Peterson LC, Brown BA, Crosson JT and Mladenovic J (1985) Application of the immunoperoxidase technique to bone marrow trephine biopsies in the classification of patients with monoclonal gammopathies. *Am J Clin Pathol*, **85**, 688–693.

90 Menke DM, Greipp PR, Colon Otero G, Solberg LA Jr, Cockerill KJ, Hook CC and Witzig TE (1994) Bone marrow aspirate immunofluorescent and bone marrow biopsy immunoperoxidase staining of plasma cells in histologically occult plasma cell proliferative marrow disorders. *Arch Pathol Lab Med*, **118**, 811–814.

91 Valdez R, Finn WG, Ross CW, Singleton TP, Tworek JA and Schnitzer B (2001) Waldenström's macroglobulinemia caused by extranodal marginal zone B-cell lymphoma. *Am J Clin Pathol*, **116**, 683–690.

92 Rywlin AM, Civantos F, Ortega, RS and Dominguez CJ (1975) Bone marrow histology in monoclonal macroglobulinemia. *Am J Clin Pathol*, **63**, 769–777.

93 Chalazzi G, Bettini R and Pinotti G (1979) Bone marrow patterns and survival in Waldenström's macroglobulinaemia. *Lancet*, **ii**, 965–966.

94 Pangalis GA and Kittas C (1988) Bone marrow involvement in chronic lymphocytic leukaemia, small lymphocytic (well differentiated) and lymphoplasmacytic (macroglobulinaemia of Waldenström) non-Hodgkin's lymphoma. In: Polliack A and Catovsky D (eds) *Chronic Lymphocytic Leukaemia*. Harwood Academic Publishers, Chur.

95 Griepp PR and Lust JA (1996) Monoclonal gammopathies of undetermined significance: their relationship to multiple myeloma. In: Gahrton G and Durie BGM (eds) *Multiple Myeloma*. Arnold, London.

96 Sezer O, Eucker J, Jakob C and Possinger K (2000) Diagnosis and treatment of AL amyloidosis. *Clin Nephrol*, **53**, 417–423.

97 Perfetti V, Ubbiali P, Vignarelli MC, Diegoli M, Fasani R, Stoppini M *et al.* (1998) Evidence that amyloidogenic light chains undergo antigen-driven selection. *Blood*, **91**, 2948–2954.

98 Perfetti V, Vignarelli MC, Anesi E, Garini P, Quaglini S, Ascari E and Merlini G (1999) The degrees of plasma cell clonality and marrow infiltration adversely influence the prognosis of AL amyloidosis patients. *Haematologica*, **84**, 218–221.

99 Gertz MA, Kyle RA and Noel P (1993). Primary systemic amyloidosis: a rare complication of immunoglobulin M monoclonal gammopathies and Waldenstrom's macroglobulinemia. *J Clin Oncol*, **11**, 914–920.

100 Kyle RA and Gertz MA (1995) Primary systemic amyloidosis: clinical and laboratory features in 474 cases. *Semin Hematol*, **32**, 45–59.

101 Swan N, Skinner M and O'Hara CT (2003) Bone marrow core biopsy specimens in AL (primary) amyloidosis. *Am J Clin Pathol*, **120**, 610–616.

102 Pardanani A, Witzig TE, Schroeder G, McElroy EA, Fonseca R, Dispenzieri A *et al.* (2003) Circulating peripheral blood plasma cells as a prognostic indica-

tor in patients with primary systemic amyloidosis. *Blood*, **101**, 827–830.

103 Park YK, Trubowitz S and Davis S (1982) Plasma cells in the bone marrow. In: Trubowitz S and Davis S (eds) *The Human Bone Marrow: Anatomy, physiology and pathophysiology*, vol. 2. CRC Press, Boca Raton.

104 Feiner HD (1988) Pathology of dysproteinemia: light chain amyloidosis, non-amyloid immunoglobulin deposition disease, cryoglobulinemia syndromes and macroglobulinemia of Waldenström. *Hum Pathol*, **11**, 1255–1272.

105 Lachmann HJ, Booth DR, Booth SE, Bybee A, Gilbertson JA, Gillmore JD *et al.* (2002) Misdiagnosis of hereditary amyloidosis as AL (primary) amyloidosis. *New Engl J Med*, **346**, 1786–1791.

106 Fonseca R, Ahmann GJ, Jalal SM, Dewald GW, Larson DR, Therneau TM *et al.* (1998) Chromosomal abnormalities in systemic amyloidosis. *Br J Haematol*, **103**, 704–710.

107 Harrison CJ, Mazzullo H, Ross FM, Cheung KL, Gerrard G, Harewood L *et al.* (2002) Translocations of 14q32 and deletions of 13q14 are common chromosomal abnormalities in systemic amyloidosis. *Br J Haematol*, **117**, 427–435.

108 Tubbs RR, Gephardt GN, McMahon JT, Hall PM, Valenzuela R and Vidt DG (1981) Light chain nephropathy. *Am J Med*, **71**, 263–269.

109 Silver MM, Hearn SA, Ritchie S, Slinger RP, Sholdice JA, Cordy PS and Hodsman AB (1986) Renal and systemic light chain deposits and their plasma cell origin identified by immunoelectron microscopy. *Am J Pathol*, **122**, 17–27.

110 Gallo G, Picken M, Buxbaum J and Frangione B (1989) The spectrum of monoclonal immunoglobulin deposition disease associated with immunocytic dyscrasias. *Semin Hematol*, **26**, 234–243.

111 Buxbaum JN, Chuba JV, Hellman GC, Solomon A and Gallo GR (1990) Monoclonal immunoglobulin deposition disease: light chain and light and heavy chain deposition diseases and their relation to light chain amyloidosis. Clinical features, immunopathology, and molecular analysis. *Ann Intern Med*, **112**, 455–464.

112 Bryce AH, Kyle RA, Dispenzieri A and Gertz MA (2006) Natural history and therapy of 66 patients with mixed cryoglobulinaemia. *Am J Hematol*, **81**, 511–518.

113 Ferri C, Zignego AL and Pileri SA (2002) Cryoglobulins. *J Clin Pathol*, **55**, 4–13.

114 Kitay-Cohen Y, Amiel A, Hilzenrat N, Buskila D, Ashur Y, Fejgin M *et al.* (2000) Bcl-2 rearrangement in patients with chronic hepatitis C associated with essential mixed cryoglobulinemia type II. *Blood*, **96**, 2910–2912.

115 Lecuit M, Abachin E, Martin A, Poyart C, Pochart P, Suarez F *et al.* (2004) Immunoproliferative small intestinal disease associated with *Campylobacter jejuni*. *N Engl J Med*, **350**, 239–248.

116 Munshi NC, Digunarthy S and Rahemtulla A (2008) Case records of the Massachusetts General Hospital. Case 13-2008. A 46-year-old man with rheumatoid arthritis and lymphadenopathy. *N Engl J Med*, **358**, 1838–1848.

117 Yazaki M, Fushimi T, Tohuda T, Kametani F, Yamamoto K, Matsuda M *et al.* (2004) A patient with severe renal amyloidosis associated with an immunoglobulin gamma-heavy chain fragment. *Am J Kidney Dis*, **43**, e23–28.

118 Berger F, Isaacson PG, Piris MA, Harris NL, Müller-Hermelink HK, Nathwani BN and Swerdlow SH (2001) Lymphoplasmacytic lymphoma/Waldenström macroglobulinaemia. In: Jaffe ES, Harris NL, Stein H and Vardiman JW (eds) *World Health Organization Classification of Tumours: Pathology and genetics of tumours of haematopoietic and lymphoid tissues*. IARC Press, Lyon, pp. 132–134.

119 Fermand JP, Brouet JC, Danon F and Seligmann M (1989) Gamma heavy chain 'diseases': heterogeneity of the clinicopathologic features. Report of 16 cases and review of the literature. *Medicine*, **68**, 321–335.

120 Husby G (2000) Is there a pathogenic link between gamma heavy chain disease and chronic arthritis? *Curr Opin Rheumatol*, **12**, 65–70.

121 Katz A, Zent R and Bargman JM (1994) IgG heavy-chain deposition disease. *Mod Pathol*, **7**, 874–878.

122 Khamlichi AA, Aucouturier P, Preud'Homme JL and Cogne M (1995) Structure of abnormal heavy chains in human heavy-chain-deposition disease. *Eur J Biochem*, **229**, 54–60.

123 Iwasaki T, Hamano T, Kobayashi K and Kakishita E (1997) A case of mu-heavy chain disease: combined features of mu-chain disease and macroglobulinemia. *Int J Hematol*, **66**, 359–365.

124 Bardwick PA, Zvaifler NJ, Gill GN, Newman D, Greenway GD and Resnick DC (1980) Plasma cell dyscrasia with polyneuropathy, organomegaly, endocrinopathy, M-protein, and skin changes: the POEMS syndrome. *Medicine*, **59**, 311–322.

125 Moya-Mir MS, Martin-Martin F, Barbadillo R, Cuervas-Mons V, Martin-Jimenez T and Sanchez-Miro I (1980) Plasma cell dyscrasia with polyneuritis and dermato-endocrine alterations. Report of a new case outside Japan. *Postgrad Med J*, **56**, 427–430.

126 Solomons REB and Gibbs DD (1982) Plasma cell dyscrasia with polyneuropathy, organomegaly, endocrinopathy, monoclonal gammopathy and skin changes. *J Roy Soc Med*, **75**, 553–555.

127 Pareyson D, Marazzi R, Confalonieri P, Mancardi GL, Schenone A and Sghirlanzoni A (1994) The POEMS syndrome: report of six cases. *Ital J Neurol Sci*, **15**, 353–358.

128 Dispenzieri A, Gertz MA, Lacy MQ, Fonseca R, Rajkumar SV, Greipp PR *et al.* (1999) POEMS syndrome: review of 93 cases. *Blood*, **94** (Suppl. 1), 538a.

129 Bain BJ, Catovsky D and Ewan PW (1993) Acquired angioedema as the presenting feature of lymphoproliferative disorders of mature B-lymphocytes. *Cancer*, **72**, 3318–3322.

130 Mathur R, Toghill PJ and Johnston IDA (1993). Acquired C1 inhibitor deficiency with lymphoma causing recurrent angioedema. *Postgrad Med J*, **69**, 646–648.

131 Gordon MM, Lucic N and Porter D (2000) Acquired C1q deficiency caused by monoclonal paraproteinaemia. *Lupus*, **9**, 68–71.

132 Qaseem T, Paterson WD, Jardine GWH, Wild G, Milford Ward A and Large DM (1991) Acquired C1-inhibitor deficiency preceding malignant lymphoma by 7 years. *J R Soc Med*, **84**, 628.

EIGHT

DISORDERS OF ERYTHROPOIESIS, GRANULOPOIESIS AND THROMBOPOIESIS

In this chapter we shall discuss non-neoplastic hae-matological disorders, both congenital and acquired, which affect predominantly a single lineage – either erythroid, granulocytic or megakaryocytic. For a more detailed discussion of the peripheral blood features the reader is referred to reference 1 [1]. In the majority of these conditions diagnosis is based on peripheral blood and bone marrow aspirate fea-tures and on supplementary tests. In general a tre-phine biopsy is of little importance and is not often performed. The changes consequent on infection have been discussed in Chapter 3 and will therefore not be dealt with further here.

Iron deficiency anaemia

Iron deficiency anaemia results from inadequate iron intake, increased loss of iron from the body or a combination of the two. Peripheral blood fea-tures, supplemented by biochemical assays, are often sufficient for a definitive diagnosis. In more complicated cases bone marrow aspiration permits a definitive diagnosis. Trephine biopsy is of little importance and, if iron is leached out during decal-cification, histological sections can be misleading.

Useful biochemical tests in the diagnosis of iron deficiency include estimations of serum ferritin and serum iron concentration, the latter only if com-bined with an estimate of either transferrin concen-tration or serum total iron binding capacity. Serum ferritin and serum iron concentrations are reduced whereas serum transferrin concentration and total iron binding capacity are increased. The concentra-tion of soluble serum transferrin receptors is also

Bone Marrow Pathology. By Barbara Bain, David Clark and Bridget Wilkins. © 2010, Blackwell Publishing.

increased but this test is not very specific for iron deficiency since concentration is also increased if there is increased erythropoiesis.

Peripheral blood

The peripheral blood shows initially a normocytic normochromic anaemia and later, when the defi-ciency is more severe, a hypochromic microcytic anaemia. Red cells also show anisocytosis, aniso-chromasia and poikilocytosis, particularly the presence of elliptocytes. Some patients show thrombocytosis, thrombocytopenia or the presence of occasional hypersegmented neutrophils.

Bone marrow cytology

Bone marrow cellularity is mildly increased as a result of a moderate degree of erythroid hyper-plasia. Erythropoiesis is micronormoblastic with erythroblasts being smaller than normal with scanty or ragged cytoplasm or with cytoplasmic vacuolation (Fig. 8.1). There is a minor degree of dyserythropoiesis. An iron stain shows siderotic granules to be severely reduced or absent and there is a complete or virtual absence of the iron within macrophages, which usually contain the body's iron stores (see Fig. 2.2). Since iron is irregularly distributed in the marrow, a number of bone marrow fragments must be available for assessment with an iron stain before it can be concluded that storage iron is lacking. In iron deficiency, the bone marrow sometimes shows occasional giant meta-myelocytes but granulopoiesis and thrombopoiesis are otherwise usually normal. Individuals whose bone marrows lack storage iron but in whom erythropoiesis is normal should be regarded as iron depleted rather than as iron deficient; a significant proportion of healthy women fall into this group.

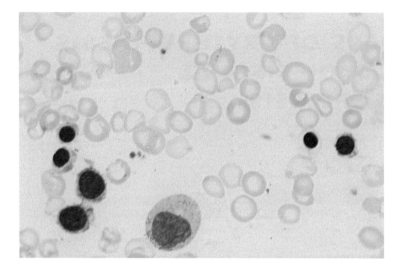

Fig. 8.1 Bone marrow (BM) aspirate film, iron deficiency anaemia, showing erythroblasts with poorly haemoglobinized vacuolated cytoplasm. May–Grünwald–Giemsa (MGG) ×100.

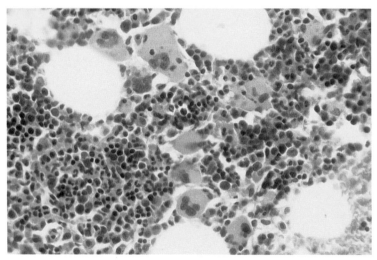

Fig. 8.2 BM trephine biopsy section, iron deficiency anaemia. Paraffin-embedded, haematoxylin and eosin (H&E) ×40.

Bone marrow histology

Trephine biopsy sections show mild hypercellularity, erythroid hyperplasia and absent iron stores. Megakaryocytes are sometimes increased (Fig. 8.2).

Problems and pitfalls

An iron stain performed on a resin-embedded, non-decalcified trephine biopsy section permits reliable assessment of iron stores. However, it should be noted that the decalcification needed for paraffin-embedded biopsy specimens leads to leaching out of some or all of the iron. It is therefore possible to exclude a diagnosis of iron deficiency if stainable iron is present but it is not possible to state reliably that iron stores are absent or reduced. A diagnosis of iron deficiency therefore cannot be made from a biopsy specimen that has been decalcified.

Sideroblastic anaemia

Sideroblastic anaemia as a feature of myelodysplastic syndromes (MDS), e.g. refractory anaemia with ring sideroblasts or refractory cytopenia with multilineage dysplasia, has been discussed in Chapter 4. Sideroblastic anaemia may also be inherited [2–5] (Table 8.1) or be secondary to exogenous agents such as lead, alcohol and drugs, including chloramphenicol, isoniazid, fusidic acid and linezolid [6,7].

Table 8.1 Causes of congenital sideroblastic anaemia.

Condition	Gene	Inheritance
Mitochondrial disorders [2]		
Pearson's syndrome	Mitochondrial	
Kearns–Sayre syndrome	Mitochondrial	
Sideroblastic anaemia with cerebellar ataxia	Mutation in *ABCB7* encoding a mitochondrial protein [3]	Autosomal recessive
Mitochondrial myopathy, lactic acidosis and sideroblastic anaemia	Mutation in *PUS1* gene encoding pseudo-uridine synthase	Autosomal recessive
Mitochondrial depletion syndrome	Mutation of one of a number of autosomal genes that leads to depletion of mitochondrial DNA	Autosomal recessive
Other		
X-linked sideroblastic anaemia	*ALAS2* encoding ALA synthase	X-linked recessive
Thiamine-responsive sideroblastic anaemia	*SLC19A2* encoding a thiamine transporter protein	Autosomal recessive
Erythropoietic porphyria (rarely) [4]	*UROS* gene encoding uroporphyrinogen III synthase	Autosomal recessive
Autosomal recessive sideroblastic anaemia [5] (one patient)	Homozygous mutation of *GLRX5* encoding glutaredoxin	Autosomal recessive

Copper deficiency, sometimes as a result of zinc excess, can cause acquired sideroblastic erythropoiesis [8]. Sideroblastic anaemia is most readily diagnosed from a bone marrow aspirate but diagnosis is also possible from sections of resin-embedded trephine biopsy specimens.

Peripheral blood

Congenital and secondary sideroblastic anaemias are associated with microcytosis and hypochromia (Fig. 8.3), in contrast to the macrocytosis which is usual when sideroblastic erythropoiesis is a feature of MDS. In some patients the peripheral blood film is dimorphic with a mixture of hypochromic microcytes and normochromic normocytes. In congenital cases, the anaemia varies from moderate to severe; in secondary cases it varies from mild to moderately severe. In families in which males have sideroblastic anaemia, female heterozygotes can show a small population of hypochromic microcytes.

Bone marrow cytology

The bone marrow shows mild hypercellularity and mild erythroid hyperplasia. A proportion of the erythroblasts show micronormoblastic maturation and defective haemoglobinization with ragged or vacuolated cytoplasm (Fig. 8.4). An iron stain shows the presence of abnormal sideroblasts including frequent ring sideroblasts (Fig. 8.5). Iron stores are usually increased. Plasma cells may contain haemosiderin (see Fig. 2.4). Heterozygous carriers of a mutated *ABC7* gene, causing sideroblastic anaemia with ataxia in hemizygous males, may have some ring sideroblasts [3].

Bone marrow histology

Trephine biopsy sections show some degree of erythroid hyperplasia. Increased storage iron and ring sideroblasts are detectable in resin-embedded sections but abnormal sideroblasts are not detectable in sections of decalcified paraffin-embedded biopsy specimens and although increased storage iron may be recognizable it cannot be quantified reliably. Plasma cells may contain haemosiderin (see Fig. 2.8). A trephine biopsy is not indicated in the investigation of suspected congenital sideroblastic anaemia but is useful if acquired sideroblastic

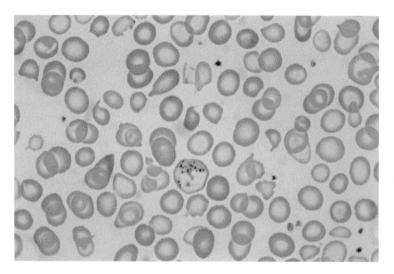

Fig. 8.3 Peripheral blood (PB) film from a boy with congenital sideroblastic anaemia showing many hypochromic and microcytic cells; there is moderate poikilocytosis and one cell containing multiple Pappenheimer bodies. MGG ×100.

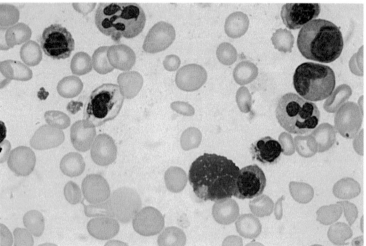

Fig. 8.4 BM aspirate film from a boy with congenital sideroblastic anaemia (same patient as Fig. 8.3) showing granulocyte precursors and five erythroblasts, one of which has a very severe defect in haemoglobinization. MGG ×100.

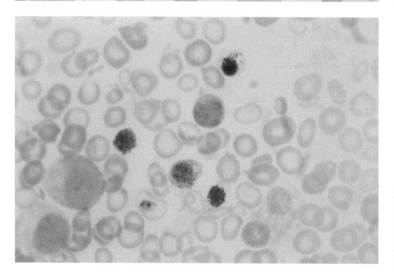

Fig. 8.5 BM aspirate film from a boy with congenital sideroblastic anaemia (same patient as Fig. 8.3) showing abnormal sideroblasts, including one ring sideroblast. Perls' stain ×100.

anaemia, particularly as a feature of MDS, is suspected.

Problems and pitfalls

Making a distinction between congenital and acquired sideroblastic anaemias and between primary and secondary sideroblastic anaemias is not always possible from the peripheral blood and bone marrow features alone. In some cases a family history, drug history and supplementary tests are needed.

A diagnosis of sideroblastic anaemia cannot be made from acid-decalcified trephine biopsy specimens.

Thalassaemia trait and thalassaemia intermedia

The various thalassaemic disorders, including thalassaemia trait, are most readily diagnosed from peripheral blood features but it is necessary for haematologists and pathologists to be aware of the bone marrow features to avoid misdiagnosis as other conditions. Bone marrow aspiration and trephine biopsy are not of any importance in the diagnosis.

Thalassaemia trait (also known as thalassaemia minor) is the term used to describe an asymptomatic condition usually consequent on dysfunction of one of the two β genes or lack of one or two of the four α genes. The term thalassaemia intermedia denotes a symptomatic condition, more severe than thalassaemia trait, but in which blood transfusion is not generally necessary; the genetic basis is diverse.

Diagnosis of β thalassaemia trait is based on a typical blood count and blood film together with demonstration of an elevated percentage of haemoglobin A_2. There may or may not be an elevated percentage of haemoglobin F. The diagnosis of β thalassaemia intermedia is made on the basis of clinical and haematological features, haemoglobin electrophoresis and DNA analysis. A presumptive diagnosis of α thalassaemia trait is made when there is microcytosis that is not explained by other more readily diagnosable conditions such as iron deficiency anaemia or β thalassaemia trait. A definitive diagnosis of α thalassaemia trait requires DNA analysis, most cases being caused by deletion of one or more of the α genes.

Peripheral blood

In β thalassaemia trait, and in cases of α thalassaemia trait in which two of the four α genes are lacking, the peripheral blood shows microcytosis and sometimes a degree of hypochromia. Some, but not all, cases of β thalassaemia trait also have basophilic stippling and moderate poikilocytosis, including the presence of target cells. In cases of α thalassaemia trait in which only one of the four α genes is lacking, the haematological abnormalities are much less and the diagnosis may not be suspected. In β thalassaemia intermedia the haematological features are intermediate between those of thalassaemia trait and thalassaemia major.

Bone marrow cytology

In thalassaemia trait, the bone marrow aspirate shows moderate erythroid hyperplasia. Erythropoiesis is micronormoblastic and there is moderate dyserythropoiesis including nuclear lobulation and nuclei of irregular shape (Fig. 8.6). An iron stain shows increased siderotic granulation and occasional ring sideroblasts. Storage iron is commonly increased. In thalassaemia intermedia, erythroid hyperplasia and dyserythropoiesis are marked and storage iron is increased.

Bone marrow histology

Trephine biopsy sections show erythroid hyperplasia and dyserythropoiesis.

Problems and pitfalls

Misdiagnosis of β thalassaemia intermedia as MDS can occur if the possibility of thalassaemia is not considered and if it is not appreciated that dysplastic features are confined to the erythroid lineage.

Thalassaemia major

Thalassaemia major indicates a transfusion-dependent thalassaemic condition, usually consequent on homozygosity or compound heterozygosity for β thalassaemia.

Peripheral blood

The peripheral blood shows striking hypochromia, microcytosis, anisocytosis and poikilocytosis. Basophilic stippling, Pappenheimer bodies and dysplastic circulating erythroblasts are also present. If the patient has been transfused, the blood film is dimorphic.

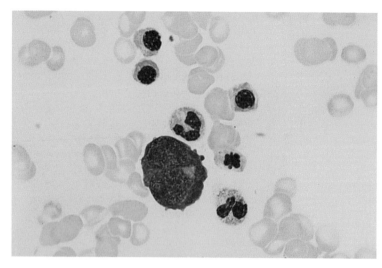

Fig. 8.6 BM aspirate film, β thalassaemia trait, showing erythroid hyperplasia and dyserythropoiesis. There is a binucleated early erythroblast and the late erythroblasts are small and have irregular or lobulated nuclei. MGG ×100.

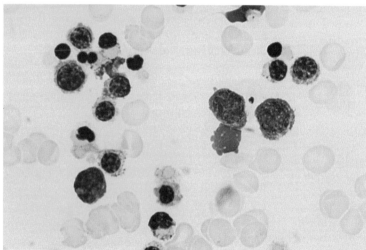

Fig. 8.7 BM aspirate film, β thalassaemia major, showing erythroid hyperplasia and dyserythropoiesis. Several cells contain cytoplasmic inclusions, composed of precipitated α chains. MGG ×100.

Bone marrow cytology

The bone marrow shows very marked erythroid hyperplasia, severe erythroid dysplasia and poor haemoglobinization (Fig. 8.7). Some erythroblasts contain cytoplasmic inclusions, seen with difficulty in May–Grünwald–Giemsa (MGG)-stained films, which represent precipitated α chains. There is an increase in macrophages, which contain degenerating erythroblasts, cellular debris and haemosiderin. In some patients the increased cell turnover leads to the formation of pseudo-Gaucher cells and sea-blue histiocytes (see pages 531 and 535). An iron stain shows numerous abnormal sideroblasts and small numbers of ring sideroblasts. Storage iron is considerably increased. Plasma cells may contain haemosiderin.

Bone marrow histology

Bone marrow sections show marked erythroid hyperplasia with disappearance of fat spaces. Dyserythropoiesis is also very marked and iron stores are increased. Pseudo-Gaucher cells and sea-blue histiocytes may be present. Plasma cells and the endothelial cells lining sinusoids may contain haemosiderin.

Haemoglobin H disease

Haemoglobin H disease is a thalassaemic condition resulting from the lack of three of the four α genes

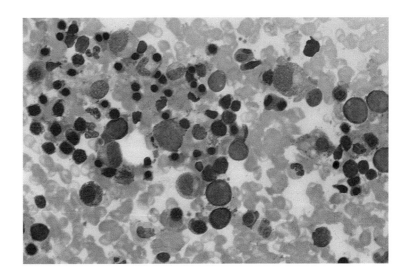

Fig. 8.8 BM aspirate film, haemoglobin H disease, showing marked erythroid hyperplasia with micronormoblastic maturation. MGG ×40.

or a functionally similar defect. There is also a decreased red cell life span. Diagnosis rests on peripheral blood features and the results of haemoglobin electrophoresis; bone marrow examination contributes little. Haemoglobin electrophoresis shows a small percentage of haemoglobin H and haemoglobin H inclusions are seen within red cells that have been exposed to a suitable supravital dye. Occasionally haemoglobin H disease is an acquired condition, occurring as a feature of MDS.

Peripheral blood
The peripheral blood shows marked hypochromia, microcytosis, anisocytosis and poikilocytosis. Because of the haemolytic component, there is also polychromasia and the reticulocyte count is elevated.

Bone marrow cytology
The bone marrow is hypercellular with marked erythroid hyperplasia, defective haemoglobinization and some dyserythropoietic features (Fig. 8.8).

Bone marrow histology
Bone marrow sections show hypercellularity due to erythroid hyperplasia.

Problems and pitfalls
It is important to distinguish acquired haemoglobin H disease from the much more common inherited

condition. This is possible by examination of cells of other haemopoietic lineages.

Haemolytic anaemias
Haemolytic anaemia may be inherited or acquired. Aetiological factors, pathogenetic mechanisms and morphological features are very varied [1]. Examination of the peripheral blood is of great importance in the diagnosis but examination of the bone marrow adds little, except in detecting complicating megaloblastic anaemia or pure red cell aplasia or, occasionally, an associated lymphoma.

Peripheral blood
Haemolytic anaemias have in common polychromasia and an increased reticulocyte count. Macrocytosis is usual in those patients in whom haemolysis is chronic and severe. Other morphological features are very variable, depending on the precise nature of the condition [1].

Bone marrow cytology
The bone marrow is hypercellular as a consequence of erythroid hyperplasia (Fig. 8.9). The degree of hyperplasia reflects the extent to which the red cell life span is shortened. In some patients, fat cells are totally lost. Haemopoiesis is often macronormoblastic, i.e. the erythroblasts are increased in size but have nuclear and cytoplasmic characteristics similar to those of normoblasts. Some cases of haemolytic

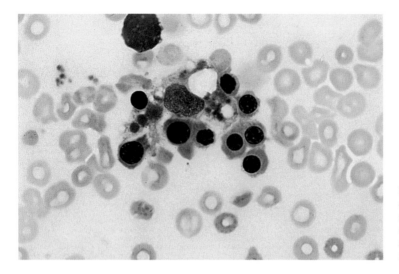

Fig. 8.9 BM aspirate film, autoimmune haemolytic anaemia, showing an erythroid island composed of erythroblasts clustered around a debris-laden macrophage. MGG ×100.

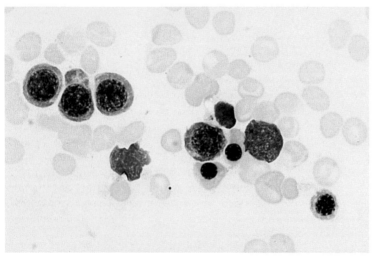

Fig. 8.10 BM aspirate film, haemoglobin C disease, showing erythroid hyperplasia and an irregular nuclear outline which is characteristic of this condition. MGG ×100.

anaemia have quite marked dyserythropoiesis. This may occur transiently in autoimmune haemolytic anaemia [9] and has also been observed in haemolytic anaemia associated with the familial autoimmune lymphoproliferative disorder caused by *FAS* gene mutations [10]. Dyserythropoiesis is often very striking when severe haemolytic anaemia occurs in a neonate, e.g. in haemolytic disease of the newborn. A specific dyserythropoietic feature is associated with haemolytic anaemia due to haemoglobin C disease; normoblasts have irregular nuclear membranes (Fig. 8.10). Macronormoblastic erythropoiesis should be distinguished from mildly megaloblastic erythropoiesis which may occur in

the haemolytic anaemias when there is complicating folic acid deficiency. When haemolysis is extravascular, bone marrow macrophages are increased and contain cellular debris. Iron stores are commonly increased, except when there is severe intravascular haemolysis with consequent loss of iron from the body. Siderotic granulation is somewhat increased.

Bone marrow histology
The bone marrow is hypercellular with erythroid hyperplasia (Fig. 8.11) and a variable degree of dyserythropoiesis. The number of erythroid islands is increased and the central macrophage is large

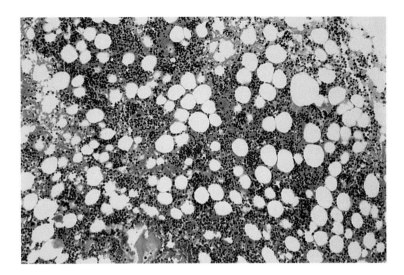

Fig. 8.11 BM trephine biopsy section, autoimmune haemolytic anaemia, showing erythroid hyperplasia. Paraffin-embedded, H&E ×10.

and prominent, often staining a dirty green colour with a Giemsa stain because of the presence of increased haemosiderin. A Perls' stain confirms increased storage iron.

Problems and pitfalls

Misinterpretation of erythroid hyperplasia with a variable degree of dyserythropoiesis, which is a consequence of haemolytic anaemia, is possible if a peripheral blood film is not examined as part of the assessment of a bone marrow aspirate and trephine biopsy. This may result in failure to consider haemolysis as a diagnostic possibility.

Congenital dyserythropoietic anaemia

The congenital dyserythropoietic anaemias (CDAs) are a diverse group of inherited conditions [11,12], all of which are characterized by anaemia resulting from dysplastic and ineffective erythropoiesis. Splenomegaly and expansion of the bone marrow cavity are common, as are jaundice (reflecting both ineffective erythropoiesis and shortened red cell life span) and gallstones. Three major types of CDA have been recognized but a considerable number of cases not conforming to these categories have also been described. Both peripheral blood and bone marrow aspirate features are important in making the diagnosis. In type II CDA, demonstration of a positive acidified serum lysis test, using a number of normal sera to exclude false-negative

results, is required for confirmation. Trephine biopsy is not important in diagnosis. Complicating parvovirus B19-induced pure red cell aplasia has been reported in several patients with CDA type II [13].

Peripheral blood

Specific morphological features vary, depending on the category of CDA (Table 8.2). All are characterized by anisocytosis and poikilocytosis (Figs 8.12 and 8.13), which often includes the presence of fragments and irregularly contracted cells. Basophilic stippling is common. In all categories, the reticulocyte count is not elevated appropriately for the degree of anaemia.

Bone marrow cytology

Bone marrow features characteristic of the different categories of CDA are summarized in Table 8.2 and illustrated in Figs 8.14–8.16. In all types there is erythroid hyperplasia and dyserythropoiesis. In type II CDA the increase in cell turnover is such that pseudo-Gaucher cells may be present (Fig. 8.17). Iron stores are commonly increased. Ultrastructural examination of bone marrow cells is diagnostically useful, showing a 'Swiss cheese' appearance of the nucleus in CDA type I, a double membrane, representing endoplasmic reticulum, parallel to the cell membrane in CDA type II and a variety of defects in CDA type III [12].

Table 8.2 Genetic, peripheral blood and bone marrow features of the congenital dyserythropoietic anaemias; features of most diagnostic importance are shown in bold.

	Type I	Type II (HEMPAS)	Type III
Inheritance	Autosomal recessive	Autosomal recessive	Autosomal dominant (in two families)
Peripheral blood	Mild to moderate anaemia, **macrocytosis**, marked anisocytosis and poikilocytosis including teardrop poikilocytes, basophilic stippling	Mild to severe anaemia, **normocytic red cells**, moderate anisocytosis and poikilocytosis including teardrop poikilocytes, variable anisochromasia, irregularly contracted cells, basophilic stippling	Mild anaemia, **macrocytosis (with some particularly large macrocytes)**, marked anisocytosis and poikilocytosis, basophilic stippling
Bone marrow	Hyperplastic, mildly megaloblastic, moderate binuclearity and **internuclear chromatin bridges**, nuclear budding, increased Howell–Jolly bodies and karyorrhexis, basophilic stippling	Hyperplastic, normoblastic, **marked binuclearity and multinuclearity**, basophilic stippling, karyorrhexis	Hyperplastic, some cells megaloblastic, **giant erythroblasts with single nuclei or marked multinuclearity – up to a dozen nuclei per cell**, basophilic stippling, nuclear lobulation, karyorrhexis

HEMPAS, hereditary erythroid multinuclearity with positive acidified serum test.

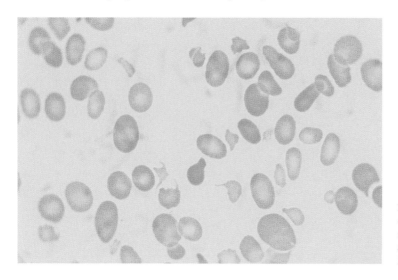

Fig. 8.12 PB film, congenital dyserythropoietic anaemia type I, showing macrocytosis, marked anisocytosis and poikilocytosis. MGG ×100.

Bone marrow histology

Examination of trephine biopsy or bone marrow clot sections confirms erythroid hyperplasia and dyserythropoiesis (Fig. 8.18).

Problems and pitfalls

Delay in diagnosis is common in CDA. The presence of anaemia and jaundice has led to misdiagnosis as hereditary spherocytosis in cases presenting in infancy, but the reticulocyte count is not elevated. Other cases of CDA present quite late in life. Misdiagnosis as MDS may occur if the possibility of CDA is not considered and if due consideration is not given to the fact that the abnormalities are essentially confined to the erythroid lineage. CDA may be confused with the many other causes of

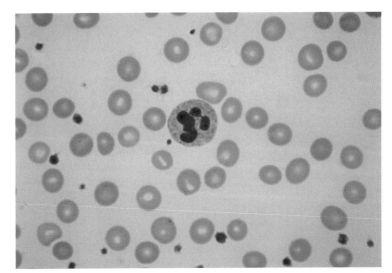

Fig. 8.13 PB film, congenital dyserythropoietic anaemia type II (herditary erythroid multinuclearity with positive acidified serum lysis test (HEMPAS)), showing mild anisocytosis. MGG ×100.

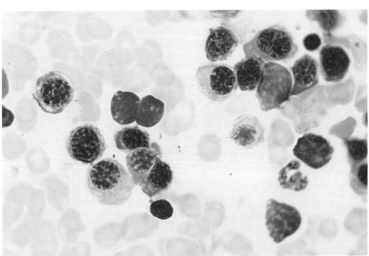

Fig. 8.14 BM aspirate film, congenital dyserythropoietic anaemia type I, showing erythroid hyperplasia and dyserythropoietic features including two pairs of erythroblasts joined by cytoplasmic and nuclear bridges respectively. The cell (top right) with two nuclei joined together over a considerable distance is typical of this type of CDA. MGG ×100.

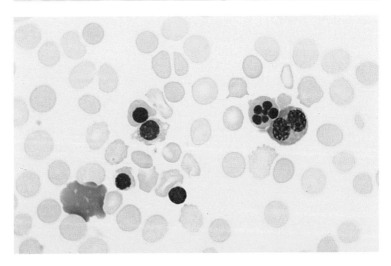

Fig. 8.15 BM aspirate film, congenital dyserythropoietic anaemia type II, showing one binucleate erythroblast and one erythroblast with a multilobulated nucleus. MGG ×100.

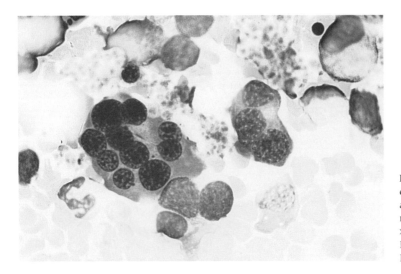

Fig. 8.16 BM aspirate film, congenital dyserythropoietic anaemia type III, showing giant, multinucleated erythroblasts. MGG ×100. (By courtesy of the late Professor S. N. Wickramasinghe, London.)

dyserythropoiesis. Dyserythropoiesis without anaemia has been described in a single patient with Ellis–van Creveld syndrome (a rare autosomal recessive disorder characterized by chondrodysplasia, ectodermal dysplasia, polydactyly and congenital heart disease) [14].

Megaloblastic anaemia

Megaloblastic anaemia is usually consequent on deficiency of vitamin B_{12} or folic acid. Less often, it is attributable to administration of a drug that interferes with DNA synthesis or, rarely, to a congenital metabolic defect. Some patients with acute myeloid leukaemia (AML) or MDS also have megaloblastic erythropoiesis. The presence of megaloblastic anaemia can usually be suspected from examination of the peripheral blood and, if features are totally typical, bone marrow aspiration is often not done. The ready availability of accurate assays for vitamin B_{12} and folic acid has lessened the importance of bone marrow examination. However, if typical peripheral blood features of megaloblastic erythropoiesis are lacking or if atypical features are present, bone marrow aspiration should be performed. Further tests indicated in patients with megaloblastic anaemia are assays of serum vitamin B_{12} and red cell folate followed, when appropriate, by tests for autoantibodies and a Schilling test. If pernicious anaemia is suspected, tests for parietal cell and intrinsic factor antibodies are indicated; the former is more sensitive but less specific than the

latter. If coeliac disease is suspected as a cause of malabsorption of folic acid or vitamin B_{12}, tests indicated include those for relevant autoantibodies (anti-reticulin and anti-endomysium antibodies), anti-gliadin antibodies and a small bowel biopsy.

In young infants the possible causes of megaloblastic anaemia are rather different from the causes later in life. In the first 2 years of life, causes include transcobalamin deficiency, congenital absence of intrinsic factor, congenital vitamin B_{12} malabsorption, congenital folic acid malabsorption, goat's milk anaemia and maternal vitamin B_{12} deficiency (including pernicious anaemia and maternal veganism) [15].

Peripheral blood

In most cases there is a macrocytic anaemia, with oval macrocytes being particularly characteristic. The mildest cases have macrocytosis without anaemia. Some degree of anisocytosis and poikilocytosis is usual and, when anaemia is severe, there are striking morphological abnormalities including the presence of teardrop poikilocytes, fragments, basophilic stippling and occasional Howell–Jolly bodies and circulating megaloblasts. Hypersegmented neutrophils are usually present; they are highly suggestive of megaloblastic erythropoiesis although not pathognomonic. They persist for a week or more after commencement of vitamin B_{12} or folic acid therapy. There may also be increased numbers of macropolycytes (tetraploid

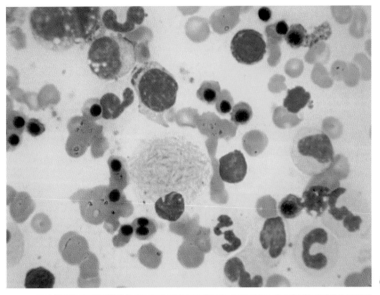

(a)

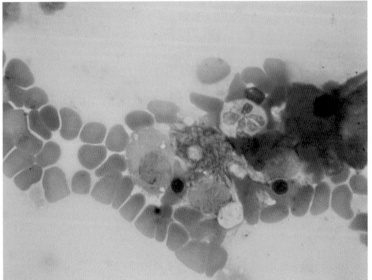

(b)

Fig. 8.17 BM aspirate film, congenital dyserythropoietic anaemia type II, showing pseudo-Gaucher cells. (a) MGG ×100. (b) Perls' stain ×100.

neutrophils) but this feature is less strongly associated with megaloblastic erythropoiesis. In severe megaloblastic anaemia, leucopenia and thrombocytopenia also occur.

Bone marrow cytology

The bone marrow is hypercellular, often markedly so. Erythropoiesis is hyperplastic and is character-ized by the presence of megaloblasts (Fig. 8.19). These are large cells with a chromatin pattern more primitive than is appropriate for the degree of maturation of the cytoplasm. Late megaloblasts may be fully haemoglobinized and lack any cytoplasmic basophilia. They may therefore be described as orthochromatic, a term that is not really appropriate in describing normal erythropoiesis, in which

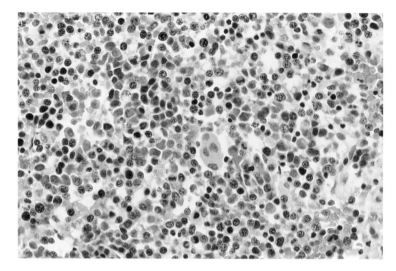

Fig. 8.18 BM clot section, congenital dyserythropoietic anaemia type I, showing marked erythroid hyperplasia with large numbers of immature erythroid precursors and marked dyserythropoiesis. The chromatin pattern is very abnormal. Paraffin-embedded, H&E ×40.

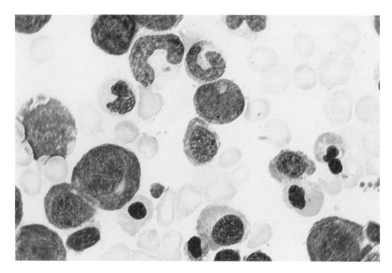

Fig. 8.19 BM aspirate film, megaloblastic anaemia, showing hyperplastic megaloblastic erythropoiesis and a giant metamyelocyte. MGG ×100.

the most mature erythroblasts are polychromatic. Erythropoiesis is ineffective so that early erythroid cells are over-represented in comparison with mature cells; macrophages are increased and contain defective red cell precursors and cellular debris. An iron stain shows abnormally prominent siderotic granules and sometimes occasional ring sideroblasts. Storage iron is usually increased. Plasma cells may contain iron. The mitotic count is increased and examination of cells in metaphase may show that chromosomes are unusually long.

Granulopoiesis is also hyperplastic although less so than erythropoiesis. Giant metamyelocytes are usually present (Fig. 8.19). They are twice to three times the size of a normal metamyelocyte and often have nuclei of unusual shapes, e.g. E- or Z-shaped rather than U-shaped. Myelocytes and promyelocytes are also increased in size but this abnormality is less obvious and less distinctive than the abnormality of metamyelocytes. When megaloblastic features in erythroblasts are partly or largely masked by coexisting iron deficiency, the detection of giant metamyelocytes is diagnostically important.

Megakaryocytes are hyperlobated and have more finely stippled chromatin than normal megakaryocytes.

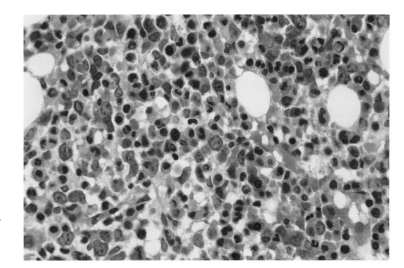

Fig. 8.20 BM trephine biopsy section, megaloblastic anaemia, showing marked erythroid hyperplasia with numerous early, intermediate and late megaloblasts. Giant metamyelocytes are also present. Paraffin-embedded, H&E ×40.

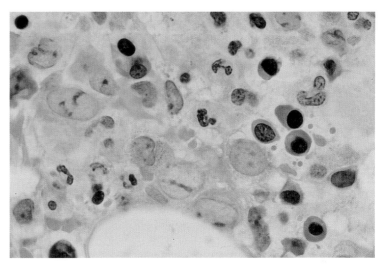

Fig. 8.21 BM trephine biopsy section, megaloblastic anaemia, showing several early megaloblasts with prominent, often elongated nucleoli which frequently abut on the nuclear membrane. Numerous late megaloblasts are also seen. Resin-embedded, H&E ×100.

Bone marrow histology

There is variable hypercellularity with loss of fat cells. In some cases this can be so severe that it may resemble the 'packed marrow' appearance seen in acute leukaemia on examination at low power. There is erythroid hyperplasia with predominance of immature precursors (Figs 8.20 and 8.21). The early erythroid cells have large, round-to-oval nuclei with one or more basophilic nucleoli, which often appear to have rather irregular margins and often abut on the nuclear membrane (Fig. 8.21); there is usually a moderate amount of intensely basophilic cytoplasm. Small Golgi zones may be seen. The later erythroid cells show asynchrony of nuclear and cytoplasmic maturation with cells having immature nuclei but haemoglobinized cytoplasm. Granulocytic precursors are increased but may appear relatively inconspicuous in the presence of profound erythroid hyperplasia. Giant metamyelocytes are usually easily seen (Fig. 8.20). Megakaryocyte numbers may be normal or decreased.

Problems and pitfalls

It is critically important that a bone marrow aspirate in severe megaloblastic anaemia is not misinterpreted as AML. The likelihood of these errors has probably increased in recent years as haematolo-

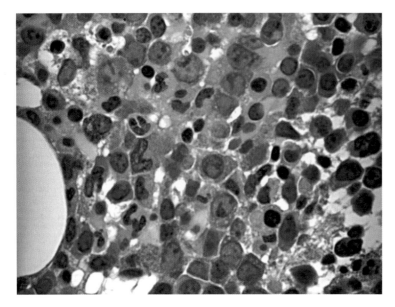

Fig. 8.22 BM trephine biopsy section, megaloblastic anaemia due to vitamin B_{12} deficiency. There are numerous early megaloblasts; late megaloblasts and phagocytic macrophages are also present. Noting the presence of giant metamyelocytes (one in field shown) should avoid misdiagnosis as erythroleukaemia. Paraffin-embedded, H&E ×60.

gists have had less experience in interpreting bone marrows from patients with straightforward megaloblastic anaemia. An appearance of 'maturation arrest' and gross dyserythropoiesis may suggest acute leukaemia but these are also features of severe megaloblastosis. Confusion with FAB M6 AML should not occur since the bone marrow in megaloblastic anaemia does not have any increase in myeloblasts. However, confusion may occur with 'M6 variant' AML in which the primitive cells present are all erythroid. It is important that the diagnosis of megaloblastic anaemia is always considered in such patients. Hypersegmented neutrophils and giant metamyelocytes should be sought since they are not a feature of AML. If there is any real doubt as to the correct diagnosis, a trial of vitamin B_{12} and folic acid therapy should be given.

Examination of a trephine biopsy specimen is rarely useful in the diagnosis of megaloblastic anaemia but it is important for pathologists to be able to recognize the typical histological features so that misdiagnosis, particularly as acute leukaemia, does not occur (Fig. 8.22). Megaloblastic change in biopsy sections may be mistaken for acute leukaemia if the histology is reported without referring to the blood film and marrow aspirate findings and if the possibility of megaloblastic anaemia is not con-

sidered. Less often, there may have been failure to obtain an aspirate or the presence of immature cells in the peripheral blood in a patient with complicating infection may have given rise to the clinical suspicion of leukaemia; in these circumstances misdiagnosis of leukaemia is more likely [16].

Erythroid islands composed of early megaloblasts are also sometimes mistaken for clusters of carcinoma cells or for 'abnormal localization of immature precursors' in MDS (see Fig. 4.78). If there is any real doubt as to their nature, immunohistochemistry can be used.

Anaemia of chronic disease

Anaemia of chronic disease is characterized by a normocytic normochromic anaemia or, when more severe, by a hypochromic microcytic anaemia. Such anaemia is secondary to infection, inflammation or malignancy. Diagnosis is usually based on peripheral blood features and biochemical assays. Serum iron and transferrin are reduced whereas serum ferritin is normal or increased. Serum transferrin receptor concentration tends to be normal. A bone marrow aspirate is sometimes necessary to confirm or exclude coexisting iron deficiency in a patient who has features of anaemia of chronic disease. A bone marrow trephine biopsy does not usually give diagnostically useful information.

Peripheral blood

In addition to the possible occurrence of hypochromia and microcytosis, the peripheral blood usually shows increased rouleaux formation and sometimes increased background staining due to a reactive increase in various serum proteins (reflected also in a raised erythrocyte sedimentation rate).

Bone marrow cytology

The bone marrow is usually of normal cellularity. Erythropoiesis may show no specific abnormality or may be micronormoblastic with defective haemoglobinization. An iron stain shows storage iron to be increased, often markedly so when the condition is very chronic. Erythroblasts show reduced or absent siderotic granulation. The bone marrow often shows non-specific inflammatory changes including increased plasma cells, mast cells and macrophages.

Bone marrow histology

Sections of bone marrow trephine biopsy cores usually show normal cellularity. There may be increased lymphoid nodules, plasma cells, mast cells and macrophages. A Perls' stain shows increased storage iron.

Problems and pitfalls

An iron stain may be falsely negative, if a trephine biopsy specimen has been decalcified, leading to a mistaken assumption that the patient has iron deficiency anaemia.

Sickle cell disease

The term 'sickle cell disease' encompasses sickle cell anaemia and compound heterozygous states that also lead to tissue damage from sickle cell formation. Sickle cell anaemia refers specifically to homozygosity for the β^S gene. Other forms of sickle cell disease include the compound heterozygous states, sickle cell/haemoglobin C disease and sickle cell/β thalassaemia. Diagnosis of sickle cell anaemia is dependent on peripheral blood features and haemoglobin electrophoresis or an equivalent technique. Haemoglobin S comprises almost all the total haemoglobin, haemoglobin A being absent. Bone marrow aspiration is usually only indicated to detect suspected complications such as megaloblastic anaemia, pure red cell aplasia or bone marrow necrosis. Trephine biopsy is not often indicated.

Peripheral blood

The peripheral blood shows anaemia, usually with a haemoglobin concentration of 60–100 g/l. There are variable numbers of sickle cells and, in addition, target cells and polychromasia; nucleated red blood cells may be present. Beyond the age of 6 months, features of hyposplenism start to appear, particularly Howell–Jolly bodies and Pappenheimer bodies. The neutrophil count may be increased, particularly during episodes of sickling. The blood film in compound heterozygous states is often similar to that of sickle cell anaemia although patients with sickle cell/haemoglobin C disease may have occasional cells containing haemoglobin C crystals and those with sickle cell/β thalassaemia have microcytosis.

Bone marrow cytology

The bone marrow aspirate shows hypercellularity due to erythroid hyperplasia. Iron stores are often increased and sickle cells are usually present. Sometimes they are much more elongated than is usual for sickle cells in the circulating blood. When there are complicating conditions such as megaloblastic anaemia, pure red cell aplasia or bone marrow necrosis, the appropriate morphological features are superimposed on those of the underlying disease. Bone marrow macrophages may contain occasional or numerous sickle cells (Fig. 8.23). Macrophages and various storage cells are sometimes increased (Figs 8.23 and 8.24) as a consequence of increased cell turnover and episodes of bone marrow infarction. Occasionally, during a sickle cell crisis, there is sufficient macrophage activation for clinical and pathological features to resemble those of a haemophagocytic syndrome [17]. In sickle cell/β thalassaemia, erythropoiesis is hyperplastic and micronormoblastic (Fig. 8.25).

Bone marrow histology

Trephine biopsy sections show hypercellularity due to erythroid hyperplasia. Sickle cells may be seen within bone marrow sinusoids (Fig. 8.26). Blood vessels may be distended by sickle cells and perivascular fibrosis is common [18]. As for bone marrow aspirate films, bone marrow sections may show

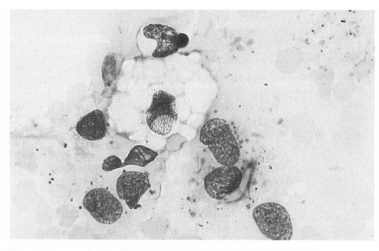

Fig. 8.23 BM aspirate film, sickle cell anaemia, showing a foamy macrophage and a macrophage containing a sickled cell. MGG ×100. (By courtesy of Professor Sally Davies, London.)

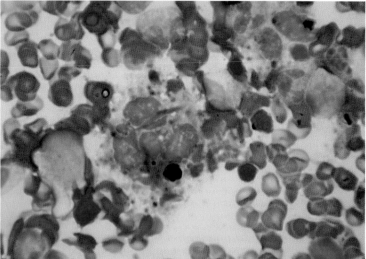

Fig. 8.24 BM aspirate, sickle cell anaemia, showing a sea-blue histiocyte which has ingested a sickled cell. MGG ×100.

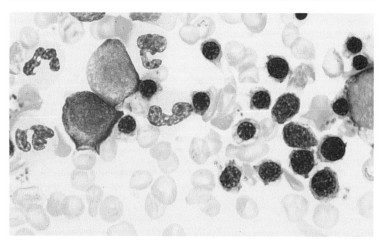

Fig. 8.25 BM aspirate, sickle cell/β^0 thalassaemia compound heterozygosity, showing erythroid hyperplasia and erythroblasts with scanty cytoplasm and defective haemoglobinization; several sickle cells are present. MGG ×100.

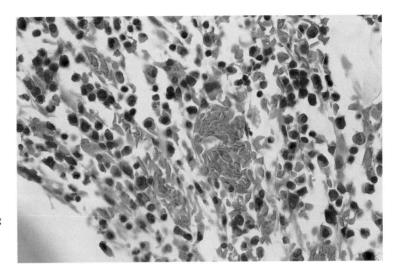

Fig. 8.26 BM trephine biopsy section, sickle cell anaemia, showing sinusoids distended by irreversibly sickled erythrocytes. Paraffin-embedded, H&E ×40.

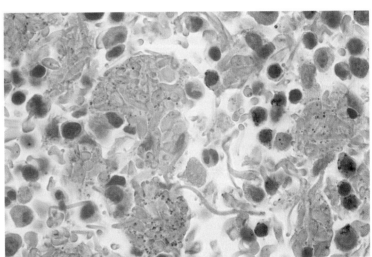

Fig. 8.27 Section of clotted BM aspirate showing macrophages stuffed with sickle cells and several extremely long sickled cells. Paraffin-embedded, H&E ×100.

sickle cells that are much more elongated than the typical cells seen in blood films (Fig. 8.27). Infarcted bone and bone marrow may be present in patients who have recently experienced a sickling crisis. Foamy macrophages and small fibrotic scars may mark the sites of previous bone marrow infarction. Thin and irregular bone trabeculae have been reported [18].

Problems and pitfalls

It should be noted that in the bone marrow at autopsy, sickle cells may be present not only in patients with sickle cell disease but also in those with sickle cell trait. The presence of sickled cells

therefore does not necessarily indicate that the patient has sickle cell disease, nor that a sickle cell crisis has occurred in a patient with sickle cell disease.

Pure red cell aplasia (including Blackfan–Diamond syndrome)

Pure red cell aplasia has been defined as severe anaemia with the reticulocyte count being less than 1% and mature erythroblasts in a normocellular bone marrow being less than 0.5% [19]. Pure red cell aplasia may be either constitutional or acquired and either acute or chronic.

Constitutional pure red cell aplasia, also known as the Blackfan–Diamond syndrome, is a chronic condition which usually becomes manifest during the first year of life. It appears to be a trilineage disorder, consequent on an inherited stem cell defect, rather than a purely erythroid disorder. It shows some responsiveness to corticosteroids. Inheritance is usually autosomal dominant, with variable penetrance, but some cases are autosomal recessive. Many cases appear to be sporadic. A significant proportion of cases are due to a mutation in the gene encoding ribosomal protein S19 at 19q13 (*RPS19*) [20]; others are linked to 8p23.3-23.1 [21]. Sometimes the red cell aplasia is transient [22]. Red cell adenosine deaminase is elevated in the great majority of patients with Diamond–Blackfan anaemia and in some family members this may be the only sign of the underlying genetic abnormality [22]. A small percentage of patients subsequently develop bone marrow aplasia [23], MDS [23] or AML.

Infants, usually but not always over 1 year in age, may also suffer from acute pure red cell aplasia designated transient erythroblastopenia of childhood [24,25]; in this condition the aplasia, which usually results from infection by human herpesvirus 6 [26], lasts only a matter of months and does not require specific treatment. Occasional cases result from infection by other viruses, e.g. Epstein–Barr virus [27] or parvovirus B19 [28]. Transient erythroblastopenia has been described as a feature of Kawasaki's syndrome [29]. It can also occur as the presenting feature of childhood coeliac disease, an aetiological relationship being suspected [30].

In older children and adults, the most commonly recognized cause of acute aplasia is parvovirus infection; the aplasia is usually of brief duration and therefore causes symptomatic anaemia only in subjects with a pre-existing intrinsic red cell defect or with an extrinsic cause of shortened red cell life span (i.e. with haemolytic anaemia or compensated haemolysis). However, in certain circumstances, parvovirus B19 infection is persistent and thus leads to chronic pure red cell aplasia. This occurs particularly, but not exclusively, in patients with evident causes of immune deficiency, either congenital or acquired. Congenital causes include severe combined immune deficiency, hyperimmunoglobulinaemia M syndrome, Nezelof's syndrome and hypogammaglobulinaemia. Acquired immune deficiency states that have been reported in association with chronic parvovirus infection include common variable immune deficiency [31], HIV infection and the prior administration of immunosuppressive drugs or monoclonal antibodies directed at lymphocytes, such as rituximab [32,33] and alemtuzumab [34]. Cases have occurred following renal and bone marrow transplantation, following chemotherapy for solid tumours [35] and Waldenström macroglobulinaemia [36] and during maintenance treatment for acute lymphoblastic leukaemia (ALL). Occasionally parvovirus-induced chronic pure red cell aplasia is seen in patients with no apparent defect in immune responses [37].

In adults, chronic red cell aplasia is commonly immunological in origin (T-cell, natural killer (NK) cell or antibody mediated) and may be associated with a thymoma, Hodgkin or non-Hodgkin lymphoma, chronic lymphocytic leukaemia, carcinoma, rheumatoid arthritis and systemic lupus erythematosus. Rare cases are associated with pregnancy [38]. Pure red cell aplasia is a relatively common complication of T-cell large granular lymphocytic leukaemia [39]; the lymphoproliferative disorder may be occult. In one series, almost 20% of cases of pure red cell aplasia were attributed to large granular lymphocyte leukaemia [40]. Marked erythroid hypoplasia may also be a feature of protein-calorie deprivation (kwashiorkor), be induced by hypothermia [41], occur as part of a hypersensitivity reaction to a drug or be the dominant feature of MDS [42]. Stem cell transplantation across an ABO barrier may lead to red cell aplasia.

Peripheral blood

The peripheral blood shows no specific abnormality. There is a complete absence of polychromatic cells and the reticulocyte count is zero or virtually zero. Associated features differ according to the cause of the red cell aplasia. Macrocytosis is usual in the Blackfan–Diamond syndrome and the red cells have some characteristics similar to those of fetal red cells; occasionally there is mild neutropenia and the platelet count may be somewhat elevated [24]. In transient erythroblastopenia of childhood the red cells are of normal size and lack fetal characteristics. Neutropenia, which may be moderately severe, occurs in about a quarter of cases and thrombocytosis in about a third [24,25]. There may be lymphocytosis with atypical reactive lymphocytes [26]. Since symptomatic anaemia following parvovirus-induced aplasia is largely confined to patients with an underlying red cell defect, the blood film shows features of the associated disease, most often hereditary spherocytosis or sickle cell anaemia. In such cases the absence of polychromasia, despite marked anaemia, is diagnostically important and should lead to a reticulocyte count being performed. Neutrophil and platelet counts are only occasionally reduced in patients with parvovirus-induced red cell aplasia. Patients with red cell aplasia associated with thymoma or with autoimmune disease sometimes also have neutropenia or thrombocytopenia. In patients with red cell aplasia as the dominant feature of MDS it is sometimes possible to detect dysplastic features in cells of other lineages. In patients with an underlying lymphoproliferative disorder, neoplastic cells may be present.

Bone marrow cytology

Bone marrow cellularity is usually somewhat reduced. There is a striking reduction of maturing erythroid cells. Proerythroblasts are usually present in normal numbers but are sometimes increased (Fig. 8.28). Other lineages are usually normal. In Blackfan–Diamond syndrome (Fig. 8.29) there are scattered proerythroblasts and sometimes minimal evidence of maturation. Haematogones and mature lymphocytes may be increased [43]; the haematogones show variable expression of CD10 and terminal deoxynucleotidyl transferase [25,26]. In transient erythroblastopenia of childhood, granulopoiesis may be left shifted, and in patients with neutropenia there may be apparent arrest of maturation at the myelocyte stage [26]. In parvovirus-induced aplasia, giant proerythroblasts with prominent nucleoli are often noted (Fig. 8.30). Iron stores are commonly increased since the iron normally in erythroid cells has been deposited in the stores.

Bone marrow histology

The overall bone marrow cellularity is somewhat reduced. There is a striking lack of erythroid islands and of maturing erythroblasts (Figs 8.31 and 8.32). Large proerythroblasts with strongly basophilic cytoplasm are readily apparent. Occasionally there is a striking increase in proerythroblasts (Fig. 8.33). There may be non-specific inflammatory changes including increased lymphocytes (including haematogones), plasma cells, macrophages (which may be iron-laden) and mast cells [44]. In parvovirus infection, the giant proerythroblasts, which may be many times the size of normal proerythroblasts, may show intranuclear eosinophilic virus inclusions, with peripheral condensation of chromatin (Fig. 8.34). In immunocompetent patients, the bone marrow is hypercellular and megakaryocytes are increased [43]. Immunohistochemistry

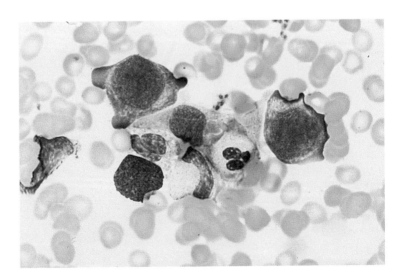

Fig. 8.28 BM aspirate, chronic idiopathic pure red cell aplasia, showing increased proerythroblasts and a lack of maturing erythroblasts. MGG ×100.

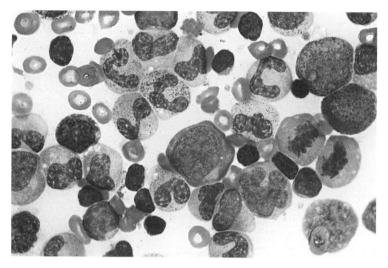

Fig. 8.29 BM aspirate, Blackfan–Diamond syndrome, showing a single intermediate erythroblast but no maturing cells. MGG ×100. (By courtesy of Dr R. Brunning, Minneapolis.)

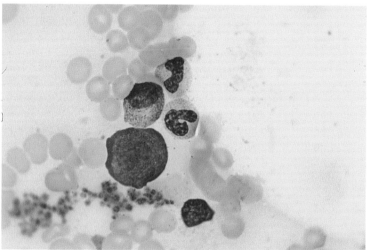

Fig. 8.30 BM aspirate, chronic pure red cell aplasia caused by parvovirus B19 infection in an HIV-positive child. MGG ×100.

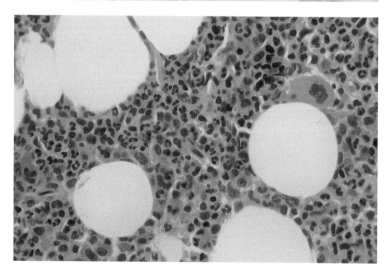

Fig. 8.31 BM trephine biopsy section, pure red cell aplasia, showing absence of erythroblastic islands and late erythroblasts; only occasional early and intermediate erythroblasts are present. Paraffin-embedded, H&E ×40.

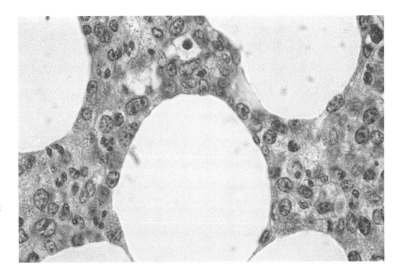

Fig. 8.32 BM trephine biopsy section, Blackfan–Diamond syndrome, showing prominent proerythroblasts and early erythroblasts but very few maturing erythroid cells (same patient as Fig. 8.29). Paraffin-embedded, H&E ×100. (By courtesy of Dr R. Brunning, Minneapolis.)

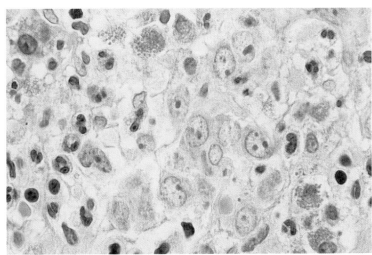

Fig. 8.33 BM trephine biopsy section, chronic pure red cell aplasia, probably autoimmune in nature, showing a striking increase of proerythroblasts. Paraffin-embedded, H&E ×100. (By courtesy of Dr Haley, Vancouver.)

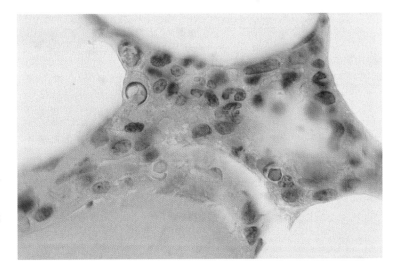

Fig. 8.34 BM trephine biopsy section, chronic parvovirus B19-induced pure red cell aplasia in an HIV-positive child (same patient as Fig. 8.30), showing several apoptotic cells and a proerythroblast with an eosinophilic intranuclear inclusion. Paraffin-embedded, H&E ×100.

can be used to show parvovirus antigens. In transient erythroblastopenia of childhood, there are large proerythroblasts, which may have small cytoplasmic vacuoles but lack the intranuclear viral inclusions discernible in parvovirus infection [26].

Problems and pitfalls

Occasionally patients with pure red cell aplasia show a striking increase of proerythroblasts (see Fig. 8.33) which can cause diagnostic confusion with a haematological neoplasm. A lack of maturing erythroblasts should alert the observer to the true nature of these cells, which can be confirmed by immunohistochemistry.

Increased numbers of haematogones can raise the suspicion of ALL in children with Blackfan–Diamond anaemia or transient erythroblastopenia of childhood.

Since red cell aplasia may be the major manifestation of MDS, it is important to examine other lineages carefully for dysplastic features.

It should be noted that, in patients with immune deficiency, seronegativity does not exclude parvovirus B19 as a cause of red cell aplasia; immunohistochemistry on a biopsy section or DNA analysis of peripheral blood is required.

Congenital neutropenia

Severe congenital neutropenia is a heterogeneous group of disorders with either autosomal dominant, autosomal recessive or X-linked recessive inheritance. The term Kostmann syndrome should probably be reserved for cases showing autosomal recessive inheritance, as was present in the family reported by Kostmann. Severe congenital neutropenia is mainly autosomal dominant and may result from a mutation in ELA2, the gene encoding neutrophil elastase [45]. Less often, severe congenital neutropenia results from mutation in GFI1, CSF3R (the gene encoding granulocyte colony-stimulating factor (G-CSF) receptor) [46], WAS [47], HAX1 (Kostmann's family), G6PC3 or AP3B1. Isolated congenital neutropenia may also be mild with a benign clinical course. Congenital neutropenia can be cyclical with variation, over a period of 3 weeks or more, from very low to normal or above normal levels. There is phenotypic overlap between severe congenital neutropenia and cyclical neutropenia since both can show autosomal domi-

nant inheritance and result from mutations in ELA2. Patients can show cycling at some times and not at others and, in addition, some family members can have cyclical neutropenia while others with the same mutation do not exhibit cycling [45]. In these conditions, neutrophils are either cytologically normal or show toxic changes, whereas myelokathexis, an autosomal dominant condition attributable to accelerated apoptosis in neutrophil precursors, is characterized by neutropenia with specific cytological abnormalities in neutrophils [48,49]. Congenital neutropenia also occurs as a feature of other congenital syndromes. For example, Shwachman–Diamond syndrome, which results from homozygosity or compound heterozygosity for mutations in the SBDS gene, is characterized by neutropenia plus exocrine pancreatic dysfunction, growth retardation and skeletal abnormalities; it may progress to aplastic anaemia. Severe congenital neutropenia can occur in the X-linked Barth syndrome (cardiomyopathy with abnormal mitochondria), which results from a mutation in the TAZ (G4.5) gene at Xq28.

Myelodysplastic syndromes and AML frequently develop during the course of Shwachman–Diamond syndrome. There is also a significant incidence of these complications in severe congenital neutropenia if early death is prevented by therapy with G-CSF. The occurrence of a mutation in CSF3R makes the development of MDS and AML more likely but this is not the only pathway of leukaemogenesis [50,51]. Evolution to MDS or AML is not a feature of cyclical neutropenia.

Peripheral blood

In severe congenital neutropenia the peripheral blood shows severe neutropenia and often monocytosis, eosinophilia, thrombocytosis and the effects of chronic or recurrent infection such as anaemia and increased rouleaux formation. In neutropenia resulting from a WAS mutation there may be monocytopenia, lymphopenia and a borderline low platelet count [47,50]. In neutropenia resulting from a G6PC3 mutation there may be intermittent thrombocytopenia [52]. In Shwachman–Diamond syndrome the neutropenia can be intermittent [53]. In myelokathexis the neutrophils are hypersegmented with pronounced chromatin condensation and long filaments separating nuclear lobes

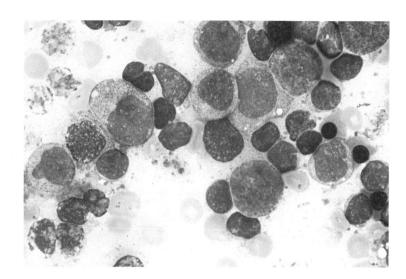

Fig. 8.35 BM aspirate film, severe congenital neutropenia, showing neutrophil maturation apparently arrested at the promyelocyte stage; cells of eosinophil lineage are increased. MGG ×100.

[48]; in some families there is also neutrophil vacuolation.

Bone marrow cytology and histology

Most cases of severe congenital neutropenia show an arrest at the promyelocyte stage of differentiation (Fig. 8.35). Large promyelocytes, often binucleated, may be common [54]. Haematogones may be increased. Some cases show a severe reduction of all granulopoietic cells with residual cells sometimes being morphologically atypical. The latter pattern may predict failure to respond to G-CSF therapy [55]. An association between severe congenital neutropenia and osteoporosis has been observed [56]. In Barth syndrome, apparent maturation arrest at the myelocyte stage has been described. Trilineage myelodysplasia can occur in association with *WAS* mutations [47,50,51]. Congenital neutropenia associated with hyperimmunoglobulin M syndrome is characterized by maturation arrest and vacuolated promyelocytes [50].

In the Shwachman–Diamond syndrome, the bone marrow may show granulocytic hypoplasia, left shift or apparent maturation arrest [57,58]; with disease progression, generalized bone marrow hypoplasia develops [58]. In myelokathexis the bone marrow is hypercellular with marked granulocyte hyperplasia; the neutrophils show the same abnormalities as those in the blood [48] (Fig. 8.36).

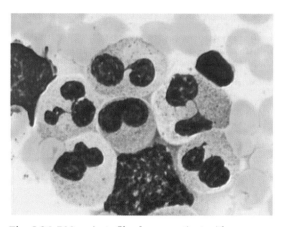

Fig. 8.36 BM aspirate film from a patient with myelokathexis as part of the WHIM (warts, hypogammaglobulinaemia, infections and myelokathexis) syndrome, showing the characteristic long filaments between nuclear lobes. MGG ×100. (Courtesy of Dr Véronique Latger-Cannard, Nancy and the *British Journal of Haematology*).

Table 8.3 Drugs most often implicated in agranulocytosis.

Class of drug	Example
Venotonic	Calcium dobesilate
Anti-thyroid	Carbimazole, methimazole, propylthiouracil
Analgesic	Dipyrone
Diuretic	Spironolactone
Anti-epileptic	Carbamazepine
Antibacterial and related	Sulphonamides including co-trimoxazole and dapsone and sulfasalazine, β-lactam antibiotics (penicillins and cephalosporins)
Non-steroidal anti-inflammatory	Diclofenac, phenylbutazone
Anti-psychotic	Clozapine
Anti-arrhythmic	Procainamide
Iron-chelating	Deferiprone

In cyclical neutropenia there is myeloid hypoplasia with lack of maturation beyond the myelocyte stage during the neutropenic phase but, when the neutrophil count is normal, the bone marrow appears normal or shows granulocytic hyperplasia. In neutropenia associated with Cohen's syndrome, bone marrow examination shows left-shifted granulopoiesis [59].

Cytogenetic analysis

Shwachman–Diamond syndrome can be associated with an acquired isochromosome of the long arm of chromosome 7, i(7)(q10), which is not predictive of disease progression [60]. Monosomy 7 and del(20q) may also be observed; the cytogenetic abnormalities may be transient [53].

Agranulocytosis

Agranulocytosis is an acute, severe, reversible lack of circulating neutrophils consequent on an idiosyncratic reaction to a drug or chemical. Incidence varies greatly between countries, e.g. from 1.1 to 4.9 per 10 million per year in one study [61]. Drugs commonly implicated also vary between countries, the more important being shown in Table 8.3 [62]. At least some cases result from the development of antibodies against the causative drug with destruction of neutrophils being caused by the interaction of the antibody and the drug. However, some cases may result from abnormal metabolism of a drug so

that toxic levels develop when normal doses are administered. Persistent parvovirus infection is a very rare cause of recurrent agranulocytosis [63]. Clinical features of agranulocytosis result from neutropenia-related sepsis.

Peripheral blood

The neutrophil count is greatly reduced, usually to less than $0.5 \times 10^9/1$. Residual neutrophils may be morphologically normal but often they show toxic changes consequent on superimposed sepsis. During recovery there is a transient outpouring of immature granulocytes into the peripheral blood, constituting a leukaemoid reaction.

Bone marrow cytology

The bone marrow aspirate shows a marked reduction in mature neutrophils. Sometimes myelocytes are also greatly reduced. The degree of granulocyte compartment depletion is predictive of speed of recovery; if promyelocytes and myelocytes are present, recovery usually occurs in 4–7 days, without administration of growth factors, whereas if promyelocytes and myelocytes are absent recovery takes 14 days or more [64]. In severe cases with superimposed sepsis, the majority of cells of granulocytic lineage may be promyelocytes with very heavy granulation. This appearance has been confused with hypergranular promyelocytic leukaemia. Useful points allowing differentiation of the

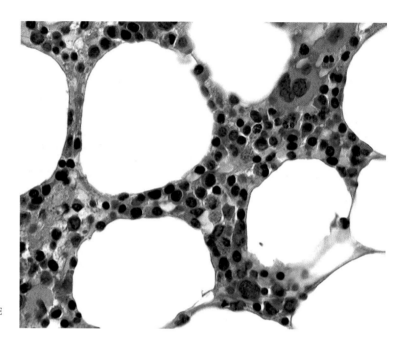

Fig. 8.37 BM trephine biopsy section from a patient with agranulocytosis. There is a striking absence of neutrophil granulocyte precursors. Paraffin-embedded, H&E ×40.

two conditions are the prominent Golgi zone in the promyelocytes of agranulocytosis and the absence of Auer rods and giant granules.

Bone marrow histology

Bone marrow sections show a lack of mature granulocytes and, often, superimposed changes due to infection (Fig. 8.37). Stromal changes, including oedema and red cell extravasation, result from damage to small vessels [44].

Other drug-induced neutropenia

Many cytotoxic agents lead to neutropenia, which is transient but often severe if the drugs are used in high dose intermittent schedules. Other drugs can cause a dose-related neutropenia: they include phenothiazines, anti-thyroid drugs, clozapine, zidovudine and azathioprine. Rituximab can cause late-onset prolonged neutropenia with reduced granulocyte precursors in the bone marrow [65]; apparent arrest of granulopoiesis at the promyelocyte stage has been observed [66].

Autoimmune neutropenia

Autoimmune neutropenia may occur as an isolated phenomenon or be one manifestation of an autoimmune disease such as systemic lupus erythematosus. It may also occur in association with thymoma and as a complication of T-cell large granular lymphocytic leukaemia (with or without associated rheumatoid arthritis). Neutropenia associated with T-cell large granular lymphocytic leukaemia may be cyclical [40].

Peripheral blood

There is a reduction in neutrophils but those present are cytologically normal.

Bone marrow cytology

Granulopoiesis appears normal or hyperplastic with a reduced proportion of mature neutrophils. An uncommon observation is phagocytosis of neutrophils by bone marrow macrophages [67] (Fig. 8.38). In agranulocytosis associated with thymoma, the bone marrow may show either apparent arrest at the promyelocytic stage or a total absence of myelopoiesis [68].

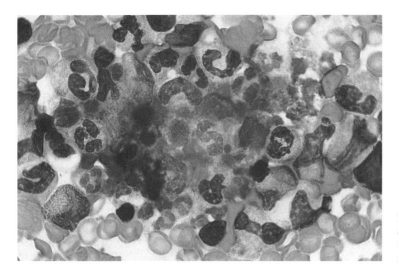

Fig. 8.38 BM aspirate film, autoimmune neutropenia, showing neutrophil shadows within macrophages. MGG ×100.

Idiopathic hypereosinophilic syndrome

The idiopathic hypereosinophilic syndrome is a condition of unknown aetiology and nature characterized by sustained hypereosinophilia and damage to tissues, usually including the heart and central nervous system, by eosinophil products. The clinical features are due to this tissue damage. The idiopathic hypereosinophilic syndrome has been arbitrarily defined as requiring the eosinophil count to be at least $1.5 \times 10^9/l$ for more than 6 months and for tissue damage to have occurred [69]. The number of diagnoses of idiopathic hypereosinophilic syndrome has been considerably reduced since the discovery that many cases were actually chronic eosinophilic leukaemia with a *FIP1L1-PDGFRA* fusion gene [70]. When such cases are excluded the male predominance that was once described is absent or less marked [71,72].

Diagnosis of the idiopathic hypereosinophilic syndrome is mainly dependent on peripheral blood and clinical features and on the exclusion of other diagnoses. The diagnosis cannot be made without cytogenetic and molecular genetic analysis to exclude cases of eosinophilic leukaemia (Table 8.4). A bone marrow aspirate and trephine biopsy are of importance in excluding eosinophilic leukaemia and lymphoma, the latter being an important cause of reactive eosinophilia. Some cases of idiopathic hypereosinophilic syndrome represent a myeloproliferative disorder and subsequently transform to AML despite initially displaying no specific evidence of the nature of the underlying disorder. Some cases of otherwise unexplained eosinophilia result from cytokine secretion by aberrant, sometimes monoclonal, T cells [73].

Peripheral blood

The eosinophil count is considerably elevated and eosinophils usually show some degree of hypogranularity and cytoplasmic vacuolation; completely agranular eosinophils are sometimes present. Eosinophil nuclei may be non-segmented, hypersegmented or, occasionally, ring shaped. Neutrophils may show heavy granulation. In contrast to eosinophilic leukaemia, there are usually only occasional if any granulocyte precursors in the peripheral blood. There may be a mild anaemia and thrombocytopenia with red cells showing anisocytosis and poikilocytosis. Nucleated red cells are sometimes present.

Bone marrow cytology

The bone marrow shows an increase of eosinophils and their precursors (Fig. 8.39). Some eosinophil myelocytes have granules with basophilic staining characteristics but this feature is much less striking than in AML of M4Eo type (see page 178). There

Table 8.4 Diagnostic criteria for idiopathic hypereosinophilic syndrome.

- Eosinophil count at least $1.5 \times 10^9/l$ for more than 6 months with tissue damage
- No cause of eosinophilia found from clinical history, physical examination and supplementary investigations (e.g. stool examination and serology for parasites, bone marrow trephine biopsy for systemic mastocytosis or lymphoma)
- Normal bone marrow cytogenetic analysis
- *FIP1L1-PDGFRA* fusion gene not detected by FISH or nested PCR
- No aberrant T-cell population

FISH, fluorescence *in situ* hybridization; PCR, polymerase chain reaction.

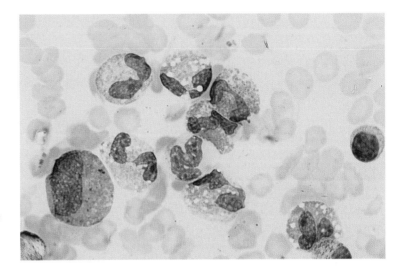

Fig. 8.39 BM aspirate film, idiopathic hypereosinophilic syndrome, showing eosinophil hyperplasia; note partial degranulation of the eosinophils. This patient was investigated before analysis for the *FIP1L1-PDGFRA* fusion gene was available. MGG ×100.

is no increase in blast cells. Macrophages may contain Charcot–Leyden crystals [74].

Bone marrow histology

Cellularity may be normal or increased. Eosinophils and their precursors are increased (Fig. 8.40). A third of patients are reported to show increased bone marrow mast cells with aberrant CD2 and CD25 expression [75]. Reticulin may be increased. It is important to exclude marrow infiltration by lymphoma since this may be easily overlooked. However, it should be noted that reactive lymphoid aggregates have been reported in the idiopathic hypereosinophilic syndrome [76].

Problems and pitfalls

The idiopathic hypereosinophilic syndrome is a diagnosis of exclusion. The bone marrow aspirate should be examined for any increase of blast cells, indicating a diagnosis of eosinophilic leukaemia. Bone marrow aspirate films and trephine biopsy sections should be examined carefully for features of systemic mastocytosis, which occasionally presents with striking eosinophilia. Bone marrow cytogenetic analysis and peripheral blood molecular genetic analysis for *FIP1L1-PDGFRA* are essential since demonstration of a clonal abnormality means that the condition is not 'idiopathic' but represents a chronic eosinophilic leukaemia [70,77,78]. Immunophenotyping of peripheral blood lymphocytes is indicated and, when an aberrant population is found, a diagnosis of idiopathic hypereosinophilic syndrome is not made. T-cell receptor gene analysis can be used to determine whether such a population is monoclonal.

Despite thorough investigation some patients with apparently idiopathic hypereosinophilic syndrome can be recognized as having chronic eosinophilic leukaemia only in retrospect when they

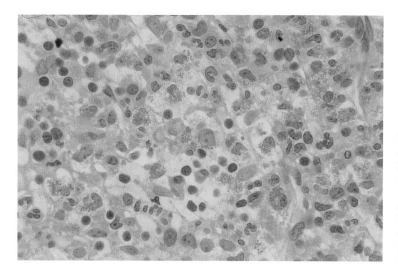

Fig. 8.40 BM trephine biopsy specimen, idiopathic hypereosinophilic syndrome, showing marked granulocytic hyperplasia and increased numbers of eosinophil precursors. This patient was investigated before analysis for the *FIP1L1-PDGFRA* fusion gene was available. Resin-embedded, H&E ×40.

subsequently develop a granulocytic sarcoma or AML.

Chédiak–Higashi syndrome

Chédiak–Higashi syndrome is a fatal inherited condition characterized by a defect in the formation of lysosomes in multiple cell lineages. Patients suffer from albinism, neurological abnormalities and recurrent infections. Haematological abnormalities are most apparent in the granulocyte series although anaemia and thrombocytopenia also occur.

Peripheral blood

All granulocyte lineages show striking abnormalities. Granules are very large and also have abnormal staining characteristics. Lymphocytes and monocytes may also have abnormally prominent granules. With disease progression, there is development of anaemia, neutropenia and thrombocytopenia.

Bone marrow cytology

Granulocyte precursors as well as mature granulocytes show giant granules with unusual staining characteristics (Fig. 8.41a, b). Sometimes there is also vacuolation. A secondary haemophagocytic syndrome may occur; it is likely to be consequent on immune deficiency and superimposed infection.

Bone marrow histology

Giant granules may be apparent in granulocyte precursors (Fig. 8.41c, d) but, in general, detection is easier in bone marrow aspirate films. Marked haemophagocytosis may be seen during the terminal phase.

Congenital thrombocytopenia

Congenital thrombocytopenia may be inherited or may be secondary to intra-uterine infection, mutagen exposure or platelet destruction by maternal anti-platelet antibodies.

Peripheral blood

Morphological features are dependent on which specific defect is responsible for thrombocytopenia [1]. In inherited thrombocytopenia, the platelets may be of normal size, increased in size as in Bernard–Soulier syndrome and *GATA1* mutations [79] or decreased in size as in the Wiskott–Aldrich syndrome. In the grey platelet syndrome they are increased in size and lack normal azurophilic granules. Platelets may also be hypogranular in patients with a *GATA1* mutation [80]. In the May–Hegglin anomaly, and in several other rare inherited defects, thrombocytopenia and giant platelets are associated with weakly basophilic cytoplasmic inclusions, resembling Döhle bodies, in neutrophils. When thrombocytopenia is secondary to intra-uterine platelet destruction or damage to megakaryocytes,

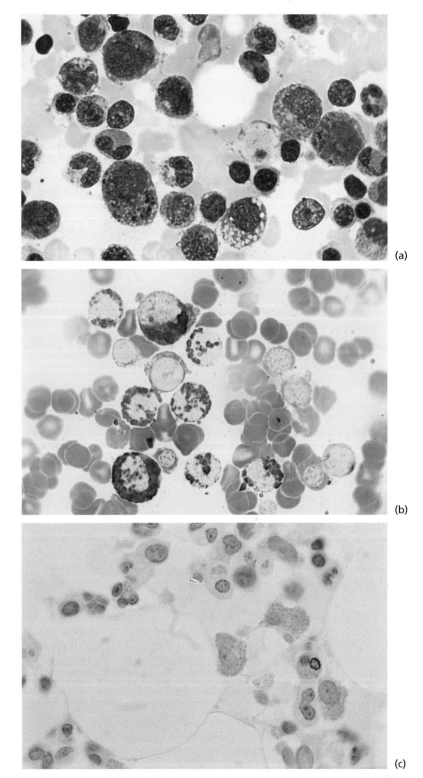

Fig. 8.41 Chédiak–Higashi syndrome. (a, b) BM aspirate, showing giant granules and vacuolation of granulocyte precursors. (a) MGG ×100. (b) Sudan black B ×100. (c, d) BM trephine biopsy section. (c) H&E stain showing giant granules. Paraffin-embedded ×100.

continued

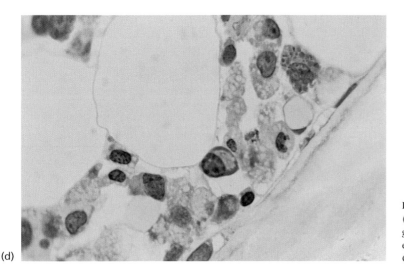

(d)

Fig. 8.41 (continued)
(d) Dominicini stain showing giant granules and vacuolation. Paraffin-embedded ×100. (By courtesy of Dr C. J. McCallum, Kirkaldy.)

the platelets are usually normal in size and morphology.

Other lineages are generally normal, but infants with the thrombocytopenia-absent radii (TAR) syndrome have been noted to be prone to leukaemoid reactions and some patients with amegakaryocytic thrombocytopenia resulting from mutation of the *MPL* or the *HOXA11* gene progress to pancytopenia [79,81]. Patients with Fanconi anaemia or dyskeratosis congenita may also initially present with an isolated thrombocytopenia with later progression to aplastic anaemia.

Bone marrow cytology

In inherited thrombocytopenia, megakaryocytes may be present in normal numbers, as in Bernard–Soulier syndrome, or may be severely reduced in number, as in constitutional amegakaryocytic thrombocytopenia. In the TAR syndrome megakaryocytes are greatly reduced in number and are small with poorly lobulated nuclei; eosinophilia is common. In the Wiskott–Aldrich syndrome megakaryocyte size and cytoplasmic mass are normal and numbers may be somewhat increased, although platelet production is about a third of normal [82]. In the Jacobsen syndrome (Paris–Trousseau thrombocytopenia), associated with a heterozygous constitutional deletion of the long arm of chromosome 11, there are some normal megakaryocytes and some small immature megakaryocytes [83,84]. In

the May–Hegglin anomaly the bone marrow may show inclusions in neutrophils and budding of large platelets (Fig. 8.42). The bone marrow in one patient with probable Epstein syndrome (thrombocytopenia, sensorineural deafness and nephritis) showed increased megakaryocyte ploidy [85]. In one family with autosomal dominant thrombocytopenia with normal platelet size, the megakaryocytes tended to be reduced in number and small with low ploidy [79]. In autosomal recessive dysmegakaryopoietic thrombocytopenia, the megakaryocytes are normal or increased in number but small and dysmorphic [86]. In thrombocytopenia with macrothrombocytes resulting from a *GATA1* mutation there is usually a hypercellular marrow with dysmegakaryopoiesis; there may be either apparently normal erythropoiesis or dyserythropoiesis with or without anaemia or associated β thalassaemia [87,88]. In thrombocytopenia with normal-sized platelets linked to 10p11-12, there are small hypolobated megakaryocytes [88]. Megakaryocytes also tend to be relatively small, with reduced ploidy, in *GATA1* mutation and in familial platelet disorder with propensity to AML associated with a *RUNX1* (*AML1*) mutation [80]. In other rare syndromes characterized by familial thrombocytopenia, megakaryocyte numbers are variously increased, normal or decreased and megakaryocyte size may likewise be increased, normal or decreased [89].

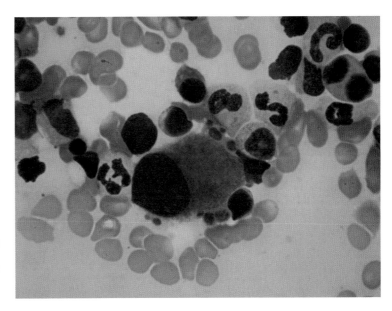

Fig. 8.42 BM aspirate film, May–Hegglin anomaly, showing two neutrophils with cytoplasmic inclusions and a megakaryocyte that is budding off large platelets. MGG ×100.

When thrombocytopenia results from intra-uterine damage to megakaryocytes these cells are usually reduced in number. When platelets have been destroyed by exposure to maternal anti-platelet antibodies, megakaryocytes are present in normal or increased numbers.

Bone marrow histology
A bone marrow biopsy is not often needed in determining the cause of congenital thrombocytopenia but it can be useful in permitting an accurate assessment of megakaryocyte numbers and morphology. In the grey platelet syndrome there may be associated myelofibrosis, probably resulting from intramedullary release by megakaryocytes of granular contents capable of stimulating fibroblasts.

Acquired thrombocytopenias
Isolated acquired thrombocytopenia is commonly due to peripheral destruction of platelets, caused by anti-platelet antibodies, drug-dependent antibodies or immune complexes; the latter may attach to platelets both in autoimmune diseases and during or after viral infections, including infection by HIV. Thrombocytopenia may also result from platelet consumption, as in thrombotic thrombocytopenic purpura or disseminated intravascular coagulation.

Less often, acquired thrombocytopenia results from megakaryocytic hypoplasia, such as that induced by thiazide diuretics, or a failure of megakaryocytes to produce platelets, as in some patients with MDS who present with isolated thrombocytopenia. Antibody-mediated amegakaryocytic thrombocytopenia is a rare cause [90]. Autoimmune thrombocytopenia and, rarely, amegakaryocytic thrombocytopenic purpura may be associated with large granular lymphocyte leukaemia [40].

Peripheral blood
When thrombocytopenia is caused by a sustained increase in peripheral destruction or consumption of platelets there is usually an increase in platelet size with some giant platelets being present. When thrombocytopenia is due to failure of production, as in sepsis or during chemotherapy, the platelets are small. When thrombocytopenia is consequent on MDS, platelets often show increased variation in size and hypogranular or agranular forms may be present.

Bone marrow cytology
If thrombocytopenia resulting from peripheral destruction or consumption of platelets has developed acutely, the bone marrow may show no relevant abnormality, megakaryocytes being present

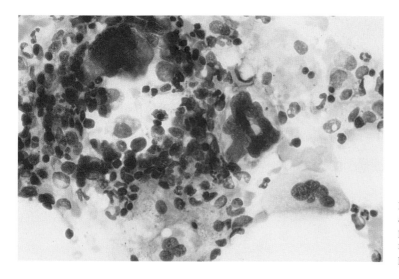

Fig. 8.43 BM aspirate film, autoimmune thrombocytopenic purpura, showing five megakaryocytes of varying size and ploidy levels. MGG ×40.

in normal numbers. With sustained thrombocytopenia, there is an increase in megakaryocyte numbers (Fig. 8.43) and a reduction in average size. There is often very little morphological evidence of platelet production despite the increased platelet turnover that can be demonstrated by isotopic studies. Bone marrow examination is not necessary in adults or children who appear to have uncomplicated autoimmune ('idiopathic') thrombocytopenic purpura. It is, however, advised in adults who (i) have atypical features; (ii) are aged above 60 years; (iii) have relapsed; or (iv) require splenectomy [91]. It is similarly advised in children who (i) have atypical features; (ii) relapse; or (iii) require corticosteroid therapy [91].

When thrombocytopenia results from ineffective thrombopoiesis, for example in MDS, megakaryocytes may be present in normal or increased numbers and may show dysplastic features. In acquired megakaryocytic hypoplasia, for example as an adverse drug effect, megakaryocytes are usually morphologically normal although reduced in number. Antibody-mediated amegakaryocytic thrombocytopenia may be cyclical. In these cases, megakaryocyte numbers are reduced and megakaryocytes are small when the platelet count is falling. When the count is rising, they are normal or increased in number and cytologically normal [90]. Cyclical amegakaryocytic thrombocytopenic purpura can occur as a stem cell as well as an autoimmune disorder; in these cases also there is variation in megakaryocyte numbers in synchrony with the platelet count [92]. Thrombocytopenia, resulting from development of anti-thrombopoietin antibodies, can develop in subjects to whom pegylated recombinant human thrombopoietin is administered; the bone marrow shows reduced numbers of megakaryocytes, which are small and have hypolobated nuclei and scanty cytoplasm [93].

Bone marrow histology

Trephine biopsy is not usually necessary in the investigation of suspected immune thrombocytopenia but is useful in confirming megakaryocytic hypoplasia and in investigating suspected MDS, e.g. in elderly patients. Because of the possibility of underlying carcinoma, bone marrow aspiration and trephine biopsy should be considered in middle-aged and elderly patients with suspected autoimmune thrombocytopenic purpura.

In autoimmune thrombocytopenia the bone marrow is normocellular with increased numbers of megakaryocytes (Fig. 8.44). Mean megakaryocyte diameter is decreased. There is increased variation in size so that, although small megakaryocytes predominate, there are also increased numbers of large forms. There is no abnormal localization of megakaryocytes and clusters are not usually seen [94]. In cyclical, antibody-mediated amegakaryocytic thrombocytopenia, megakaryocyte numbers are reduced when the platelet count is falling and normal when it is rising [90].

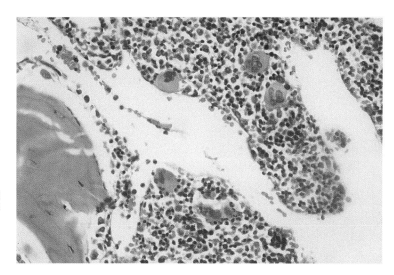

Fig. 8.44 BM trephine biopsy specimen, autoimmune thrombocytopenic purpura, showing increased megakaryocytes which are not clustered and are normally sited; two are adjacent to sinusoids. Paraffin-embedded, H&E ×40. (By courtesy of Dr S. Wright, London.)

Problems and pitfalls

The differential diagnosis of isolated thrombocytopenia in children includes ALL. Leukaemia is unlikely if the haemoglobin concentration and white cell count are normal. However, a small but significant proportion of children in whom a presumptive diagnosis of autoimmune or post-viral thrombocytopenia is made turn out to have ALL. This has led to controversy as to whether a bone marrow aspirate is required in children with isolated thrombocytopenia [95]. There is concern that administration of corticosteroids without a pretreatment bone marrow examination may lead to inadvertent suboptimal treatment of undiagnosed ALL. For this reason, UK guidelines suggest that bone marrow aspiration should be performed before corticosteroid therapy is given, whereas this is not considered essential prior to high dose immunoglobulin therapy or if no treatment is required. USA guidelines, however, do not regard a bone marrow examination as necessary if there are no atypical clinical or haematological features.

Frequent apparently bare megakaryocyte nuclei and reactive stromal changes may indicate unsuspected HIV infection as a cause of thrombocytopenia.

Familial thrombocytosis

Familial thrombocytosis has been reported in at least 17 individuals in eight families [96]. In most families inheritance appears to be autosomal dominant. In one Arab family inheritance was recessive, probably X-linked recessive [97]. In some, but not all, families the cause is a mutation in the thrombopoietin gene (*THPO*). A minority of individuals have had splenomegaly.

Peripheral blood

The blood film and count show thrombocytosis as an isolated abnormality. Platelet morphology has sometimes been reported as abnormal [96].

Bone marrow cytology and histology

Megakaryocytes are increased in number and have sometimes been considered to be cytologically abnormal [96]. In the Arab family with recessively inherited thrombocytosis the megakaryocytes were cytologically normal but increased in number and clustered [97]. Bone marrow cellularity is sometimes increased.

Problems and pitfalls

Use of the term 'essential thrombocythaemia' to describe familial thrombocytosis is not recommended since the condition clearly differs from the myeloproliferative neoplasm (MPN) that is usually intended by this term. This MPN is rare in children, with a significant proportion of cases of primary thrombocythaemia being found to be familial. Investigation of parents and siblings is therefore indicated when persistent unexplained thrombocytosis is found in a child or adolescent.

Reactive thrombocytosis

The platelet count may increase in response to infection, inflammation and malignant disease. In reactive thrombocytosis it is uncommon for the platelet count to exceed 1000×10^9/l.

Peripheral blood

In contrast to MPN, there is no increase in platelet size when thrombocytosis is reactive. The blood film may show other reactive changes including leucocytosis and neutrophilia but the presence of basophilia suggests an MPN.

Bone marrow cytology

The bone marrow aspirate shows increased numbers of megakaryocytes of normal morphology.

Bone marrow histology

Megakaryocyte numbers are increased. The average megakaryocyte diameter is increased in comparison with normal and there is increased variation in size. There is no clustering or abnormality of distribution [94].

Problems and pitfalls

The differential diagnosis of reactive thrombocytosis includes hyposplenism and essential thrombocythaemia. Changes of hyposplenism should therefore be sought in the blood film. An increased basophil count, increased reticulin deposition in the bone marrow and clustering of megakaryocytes favours a diagnosis of an MPN.

References

1 Bain BJ (2006) *Blood Cells: A practical guide*, 4th edn. Blackwell Publishing, Oxford.

2 Finisterer J (2007) Hematological manifestations of primary mitochondrial disorders. *Acta Haematol*, **118**, 88–98.

3 Maguire A, Hellier K, Hammans S and May A (2001) X-linked cerebellar ataxia and sideroblastic anaemia associated with a missense mutation in the *ABC7* gene predicting V411L. *Br J Haematol*, **315**, 910–917.

4 Morrell R, O'Marcaigh A, May A, Connolly K and Crotty G (2004) Severe sideroblastic anaemia with raised erythrocyte protopophyrins – a variant of erythropoietic protoporphyria (EPP). *Br J Haematol*, **125** (Suppl. 1), 27–28.

5 Camaschella C, Campanella A, De Falco L, Boschetto L, Merlini R, Silvestri L *et al.* (2007) The human counterpart of zebrafish shiraz shows sideroblastic-like microcytic anemia and iron overload. *Blood*, **110**, 1353–1358.

6 Vial T, Grignon M, Daumont M, Guy C, Zenut M, Germain ML *et al.* (2004) Sideroblastic anaemia during fusidic acid treatment. *Eur J Haematol*, **72**, 358–360.

7 Dawson MA, Davis A, Elliott P and Cole-Sinclair M. (2005) Linezolid-induced dyserythropoiesis: chloramphenicol toxicity revisited. *Intern Med J*, **35**, 626–628.

8 Miyoshi I, Saito T and Iwahara Y (2004) Copper deficiency anaemia. *Br J Haematol*, **125**, 106.

9 Bodnar A, Rosenthal NS and Yomtovian R (1996) Severe hemolytic anemia with marrow dyserythropoiesis. *Am J Clin Pathol*, **105**, 509.

10 Bader-Meunier B, Rieux-Laucat F, Croisille L, Yvart J, Mielot F, Dommergues JP *et al.* (2000) Dyserythropoiesis associated with a Fas-deficient condition in childhood. *Br J Haematol*, **108**, 300–304.

11 Wickramasinghe SNW (1997) Dyserythropoiesis and congenital dyserythropoietic anaemias. *Br J Haematol*, **98**, 785–797.

12 Wickramasinghe SN (1998) Congenital dyserythropoietic anaemia: clinical features, haematological morphology and new biochemical data. *Blood Rev*, **12**, 178–200.

13 Heimpel H, Wilts H, Hirschmann WD, Hofman WK, Siciliano RD, Steinke B and Weschler JG (2007) Aplastic crisis as a complication of congenital dyserythropoietic anemia type II. *Acta Haematol*, **117**, 115–118.

14 Scurlock D, Ostler D, Nguyen A and Wahed A (2005) Ellis–van Creveld syndrome and dyserythropoiesis. *Arch Path Lab Med*, **129**, 680–682.

15 Chanarin I (1983) Management of megaloblastic anaemia in the very young. *Br J Haematol*, **53**, 1–3.

16 Dokal IS, Cox TC and Galton DAG (1990) Vitamin B_{12} and folate deficiency presenting as leukaemia. *BMJ*, **300**, 1263–1264.

17 Kio E, Onitilo A, Lazarchick J, Hanna M, Brunson C and Chaudhary U (2004) Sickle cell crisis associated with hemophagocytic lymphohistiocytosis. *Am J Hematol*, **77**, 229–232.

18 Manci EA, Culberson DE, Gardner JM, Brogdon BG, Shah AK, Holladay JE *et al.* (2004) Perivascular fibrosis in the bone marrow in sickle cell disease. *Arch Path Lab Med*, **128**, 634–639.

19 Maung ZT, Norden J, Middleton PG, Jack FR and Chandler JE (1994) Pure red cell aplasia: further evidence of a T cell clonal disorder. *Br J Haematol*, **87**, 189–192.

20 Ramenghi U, Garelli E, Valtolina S, Campagnoli MF, Timeuus F, Crescenzio N et al. (1999) Diamond–Blackfan anaemia in the Italian population. *Br J Haematol*, **104**, 841–848.

21 Freedman MH (2000) Diamond–Blackfan anaemia. *Bailliere's Clin Haematol*, **13**, 391–406.

22 Orfali KA, Ohene-Abuakwa Y and Ball SE (2004) Diamond Blackfan anaemia in the UK: clinical and genetic heterogeneity. *Br J Haematol*, **125**, 243–252.

23 Giri N, Kang E, Tisdale JF, Follman D, Rivera M, Schwartz GN et al. (2000) Clinical and laboratory evidence for a trilineage haematopoietic defect in patients with refractory Diamond–Blackfan anaemia. *Br J Haematol*, **108**, 167–175.

24 Glader BE (1987) Diagnosis and management of red cell aplasia in children. *Hematol Oncol Clin North Am*, **1**, 431–447.

25 Foot ABM, Potter MN, Ropner JE, Wallington TB and Oakhill A (1990) Transient erythroblastopenia of childhood with CD10, TdT, and cytoplasmic μ lymphocyte positivity in bone marrow. *J Clin Pathol*, **43**, 857–859.

26 Penchansky L and Jordan JA (1997) Transient erythroblastopenia of childhood associated with human herpesvirus type 6, variant B. *Am J Clin Pathol*, **108**, 127–132.

27 Skeppner G, Kreuger A and Elinder G (2002) Transient erythroblastopenia of childhood: prospective study of 10 patients with special reference to viral infections. *J Pediatr Hematol Oncol*, **24**, 294–298.

28 Nagai K, Morohoshi T, Kudoh T, Yoto Y, Suzuki N and Matsunaga Y (1992) Transient erythroblastopenia of childhood with megakaryocytopenia associated with human parvovirus B19 infection. *Br J Haematol*, **80**, 131–132.

29 Frank GR, Cherrick I, Karayalcin G, Valderrama E and Lanzkowsky P (1994) Transient erythroblastopenia in a child with Kawasaki syndrome: a case report. *Am J Pediatr Hematol Oncol*, **16**, 271–274.

30 Guariso G, Messina C, Gazzola MV and Chiarelli S (2001) Transient erythroblastopenia in coeliac disease. *Haematologica*, **86**, E23.

31 Chuhjo T, Nakao S and Matsuda T (1999) Successful treatment of persistent erythroid aplasia caused by parvovirus B19 infection in a patient with common variable immunodeficiency with low-dose immunoglobulin. *Am J Hematol*, **60**, 222–224.

32 Frickhofen N, Chen ZJ, Young NS, Cohen BJ, Heimpel H and Abkowitz JL (1994) Parvovirus B19 as a cause of acquired chronic pure red cell aplasia. *Br J Haematol*, **87**, 818–824.

33 Sharma VR, Fleming DR and Slone SP (2000) Pure red cell aplasia due to parvovirus B19 in a patient treated with rituximab. *Blood*, **96**, 1184–1186.

34 Herbert KE, Prince HM and Westerman DA (2003) Pure red-cell aplasia due to parvovirus B19 infection in a patient treated with alemtuzumab. *Blood*, **101**, 1654.

35 Shaw PJ, Eden T and Cohen BJ (1993) Parvovirus as a cause of chronic anemia in rhabdomyosarcoma. *Cancer*, **72**, 945–949.

36 Karmochkine M, Oksenhendler E, Leruez-Ville M, Jaccard A, Morinet F and Herson S (1995) Persistent parvovirus B19 infection and pure red cell aplasia in Waldenström's macroglobulinemia: successful treatment with high dose intravenous immunoglobulin. *Am J Hematol*, **50**, 227–228.

37 Lugassy G (2002) Chronic pure red cell aplasia associated with parvovirus B19 infection in an immunocompetent patient. *Am J Hematol*, **71**, 238–239.

38 Fleming AF (1999) Pregnancy and aplastic anaemia. *Br J Haematol*, **105**, 313–320.

39 Kwong YL and Wong KF (1998) Association of pure red cell aplasia with large granular lymphocyte leukaemia. *J Clin Pathol*, **51**, 672–675.

40 Lamy T and Loughran TP (1999) Current concepts: large granular lymphocyte leukemia. *Blood Rev*, **13**, 230–240.

41 O'Brien H, Amess JAL and Mollin DL (1982) Recurrent thrombocytopenia, erythroid hypoplasia and sideroblastic anaemia associated with hypothermia. *Br J Haematol*, **51**, 451–456.

42 Uprichard J and Bain BJ (2008) Case 39: an elderly man with red cell aplasia. *Leuk Lymphoma*, **49**, 1810–1812.

43 Koduri PR (1998) Novel cytomorphology of the giant proerythroblasts of parvovirus B19 infection. *Am J Hematol*, **58**, 95–99.

44 Frisch B and Bartl R (1999) *Biopsy Interpretation of Bone and Bone Marrow: Histology and immunohistology in paraffin and plastic*, 2nd edn. Arnold, London.

45 Dale DC, Person RE, Bolyard AA, Aprikyan AG, Bos C, Bonilla MA et al. (2000) Mutation in the gene encoding neutrophil elastase in congenital and cyclical neutropenia. *Blood*, **96**, 2317–2322.

46 Sinha S, Watkins S and Corey SJ (2001) Genetic and biochemical characterization of a deletional mutation of the extra-cellular domain of the human G-CSF receptor in a child with severe congenital neutropenia unresponsive to Neupogen. *Blood*, **98**, 440a.

47 Ancliff PJ, Blundell MP, Gale RE, Liesner R, Hann IM, Thrasher AJ and Linch DC (2001) Activating mutations in the Wiskott Aldrich syndrome protein may define a subgroup of severe congenital neutropenia (SCN) with specific and unusual laboratory features. *Blood*, **98**, 439a.

48 Aprikyan AAG, Liles WC, Park JR, Jonas M, Chi EY and Dale DC (2000) Myelokathexis, a congenital disorder of severe neutropenia characterized by accelerated apoptosis and defective expression of bcl-x in neutrophil precursors. *Blood*, **95**, 320–327.

49 Latger-Cannard V, Bensoussan D and Bordigoni P (2006) The WHIM syndrome shows a peculiar dysgranulopoiesis: myelokathexis. *Br J Haematol*, **132**, 669.

50 Ancliff PJ (2003) Congenital neutropenia. *Blood Rev*, **17**, 209–216.

51 Ancliff PJ, Gale RE, Liesner R, Hann I and Linch DC (2003) Long-term follow-up of granulocyte colony-stimulating factor receptor mutations in patients with severe congenital neutropenia: implications for leukaemogenesis and therapy. *Br J Haematol*, **120**, 685–690.

52 Boztug K, Appaswamy G, Ashikov A, Schäffer AA, Salzer U, Diestelhorst J et al. (2009) A syndrome with congenital neutropenia and mutations in *G6PC3*. *N Engl J Med*, **360**, 32–43.

53 Kuijpers TW, Alders M, Tool AT, Mellink C, Roos D and Hennekam RC (2005) Hematologic abnormalities in Shwachman Diamond syndrome: lack of genotype–phenotype relationship. *Blood*, **106**, 356–361.

54 Foucar K (2001) Bone Marrow Pathology, 2nd edn. ASCP Press, Chicago.

55 Ryan M, Will AM, Testa N, Hayworth C and Darbyshire PJ (1995) Severe congenital neutropenia unresponsive to G-CSF. *Br J Haematol*, **91**, 43–45.

56 Simon M, Lengfelder E, Reiter S and Hehlmann R (1996) Osteoporosis in severe congenital neutropenia: inherent in the disease or a sequel of G-CSF treatment? *Am J Hematol*, **52**, 127.

57 Van den Tweel JG (1997) Preleukaemic disorders in children: hereditary disorders and myelodysplastic syndrome. *Curr Diagn Pathol*, **4**, 45–50.

58 Dror Y and Freedman MH (2002) Shwachman–Diamond syndrome. *Br J Haematol*, **118**, 701–713.

59 Kivitie-Kallio S, Rajantie J, Juvonen E and Norio R (1997) Granulocytopenia in Cohen syndrome. *Br J Haematol*, **98**, 308–311.

60 Cunningham J, Sales M, Pearce A, Howard J, Stallings R, Telford N et al. (2002) Does isochromosome 7q mandate bone marrow transplant in children with the Shwachman–Diamond syndrome? *Br J Haematol*, **119**, 1062–1069.

61 Kaufman DW, Kelly JP, Issaragrisil S, Laporte J-R, Anderson T, Levy M et al. (2006) Relative incidence of agranulocytosis and aplastic anemia. *Am J Hematol*, **81**, 65–67.

62 Ibáñez L, Vidal X, Ballarín E and Laporte JR (2005) Population-based drug-induced agranulocytosis. *Arch Intern Med*, **165**, 869–874.

63 Post J, Puchhammer-Stöckl E, Chott A, Popow-Kraupp T, Kienzer H, Postner G and Honetz N (1992) Recurrent granulocytic aplasia as clinical presentation of a persistent parvovirus B19 infection. *Br J Haematol*, **80**, 160–165.

64 Patton WN (1993) Use of colony stimulating factors for the treatment of drug-induced agranulocytosis. *Br J Haematol*, **84**, 182–186.

65 Chaiwatanatorn K, Lee N, Frigg A, Filsgie R and Firkin F (2003) Delayed-onset neutropenia associated with rituximab therapy. *Br J Haematol*, **121**, 913–918.

66 Tesfa D, Gelius T, Sander B, Kimby E, Fadeel B, Palmblad J and Hägglund H (2008) Late-onset neutropenia associated with rituximab therapy: evidence for a maturation arrest at the (pro)myelocyte stage of granulopoiesis. *Med Oncol*, **25**, 374–379.

67 Shimizu H, Sawada K, Katano N, Sasaki K, Kawai S and Fujimoto T (1990) Intramedullary neutrophil phagocytosis by histiocytes in autoimmune neutropenia of infancy. *Acta Haematol*, **84**, 201–203.

68 Yip D, Rasko JEJ, Lee C, Kronenberg H and O'Neill B (1996) Thymoma and agranulocytosis: two case reports and literature review. *Br J Haematol*, **95**, 52–56.

69 Chusid MJ, Dale DC, West BC and Wolff SM (1975) The hypereosinophilic syndrome. *Medicine*, **54**, 1–27.

70 Cools J, DeAngelo DJ, Gotlib J, Stover EH, Legare RD, Cortes J et al. (2003) A tyrosine kinase created by the fusion of the PDGFRA and FIP1L1 genes as a therapeutic target of imatinib in idiopathic hypereosinophilic syndrome. *N Engl J Med*, **348**, 1201–1214.

71 Brito-Babapulle F and Cross NCP (2007) Redefinition of hypereosinophilic disorders based on analysis of 28 cases of FIP1L1-PDGFRA negative persistent unexplained eosinophilia (PUE) with eosinophil end-organ damage. *Blood*, **110**, 972A.

72 Baccarani M, Cilloni D, Rondoni M, Ottaviani F, Messa F, Merante S et al. (2007) The efficacy of imatinib mesylate in patients with FIP1L1-PDGFRα-positive hypereosinophilic syndrome. Results of a multicenter study. *Haematologica*, **92**, 1173–1179.

73 Simon HU, Plötz SG, Dummer R and Blaser K (1999) Abnormal clones of interleukin-5-producing T cells in idiopathic eosinophilia. *N Engl J Med*, **341**, 1112–1120.

74 Brunning RD and McKenna RW (1993) *Atlas of Tumor Pathology, 3rd series, fascicle 9, Tumors of the Bone Marrow*. Armed Forces Institute of Pathology, Washington.

75 Metzgeroth G, Walz C, Erben P, Popp H, Schmitt-Graeff A, Haferlach C et al. (2008) Safety and efficacy of imatinib in chronic eosinophilic leukaemia and hypereosinophilic syndrome – a phase-II study. *Br J Haematol*, **143**, 707–715.

76 Metz J, McGrath KM, Savoia HF, Begley CG and Chetty R (1993) T cell lymphoid aggregates in bone marrow in idiopathic hypereosinophilic syndrome. *J Clin Pathol*, **46**, 955–958.

77 Bain BJ (1996) Eosinophilic leukaemias and the idiopathic hypereosinophilic syndrome. *Br J Haematol*, **95**, 2–9.

78 Bain BJ (1999) Eosinophilia – idiopathic or not? *N Engl J Med*, **341**, 1141–1143.

79 Drachman JG, Jarvik GP and Mehaffey M (2000) Inherited thrombocytopenia in two kindreds. *Acta Haematol*, **103** (Suppl. 1), 18.

80 Geddis AE (2005) Congenital cytopenias. The molecular basis of congenital; thrombocytopenias: insights into megakaryopoiesis. *Hematology*, **10** (Suppl. 1), 299–305.

81 Ihara K, Ishii I, Eguchi M, Takada H, Suminoe A, Good RA and Hara T (1999) Identification of mutations in the c-mpl gene in congenital amegakaryocytic thrombocytopenia. *Proc Natl Acad Sci USA*, **96**, 3132–3136.

82 Ochs HD, Slichter SJ, Harker LA, Von Behrens WE, Clark RA and Wedgwood RJ (1980) The Wiskott–Aldrich syndrome: studies of lymphocytes, granulocytes, and platelets. *Blood*, **55**, 243–252.

83 Gangarossa S, Schiliró G, Mattina T, Scardilli S, Mollica F and Cavallari V (1996) Dysmegakaryopoietic thrombocytopenia in patients with distal chromosome 11q deletion. *Blood*, **87**, 4915–4916.

84 Raslova H, Favier R, Albagli O and Vainchenker W (2004) Une haplo-insuffisance de Fli1 à l'origine de la thrombopénie Paris-Trousseau. *Med Sci (Paris)*, **20**, 962–964.

85 Cahill MR and Newland AC (1997) Is it refractory idiopathic thrombocytopenic purpura. *Lancet*, **349**, 1066.

86 van den Oudenrijn S, Bruin M, Folman CC, Bussel J, de Haas M and von dem Borne AEGKr (2002) Three parameters, plasma thrombopoietin levels, plasma glycocalicin levels and megakaryocyte culture, distinguish between different causes of congenital thrombocytopenia. *Br J Haematol*, **117**, 390–398.

87 Mehaffey MG, Newton AL, Gandhi MJ, Crossley M and Drachman JG (2001) X-linked thrombocytopenia caused by a novel mutation of *GATA-1*. *Blood*, **98**, 2681–2688.

88 Drachman JG (2004) Inherited thrombocytopenia: when a low platelet count does not mean ITP. *Blood*, **103**, 390–398.

89 Bellucci S (1997) Megakaryocytes and inherited thrombocytopenias. *Bailliere's Clin Haematol*, **10**, 149–162.

90 Zent CS, Ratajczak J, Ratajczak MZ, Anastasi J, Hoffman PC and Gewirtz AM (1999) Relationship between megakaryocyte mass and serum thrombopoietin levels as revealed by a case of cyclic amegakaryocytic thrombocytopenic purpura. *Br J Haematol*, **105**, 452–458.

91 British Committee for Standards in Haematology, General Haematology Task Force (2003) Guidelines for the investigation and management of idiopathic thrombocytopenic purpura in adults, children and in pregnancy. *Br J Haematol*, **120**, 574–596.

92 Kashyap R, Chouddry VP and Pati HP (1999) Danazol therapy in cyclic acquired amegakaryocytic thrombocytopenic purpura: a case report. *Am J Hematol*, **60**, 225–228.

93 Li J, Yang C, Xia Y, Bertino A, Glaspy J, Roberts M and Kuter DJ (2001) Thrombocytopenia caused by the development of antibodies to thrombopoietin. *Blood*, **98**, 3241–3248.

94 Thiele J and Fischer R (1991) Megakaryocytopoiesis in haematological disorders: diagnostic features of bone marrow biopsies. *Virchows Archiv A Pathol Anat Histopathol*, **418**, 87–97.

95 Bolton-Maggs PHB (1998) The management of acute childhood immune thrombocytopenic purpura – a controversy revisited. *CME Bull Haematol*, **1**, 79–81.

96 Dror Y and Blanchette VS (1999) Essential thrombocythaemia in children. *Br J Haematol*, **107**, 691–698.

97 Sturhmann M, Bashawri L, Ahmed MA, Al-Awamy BH, Kühnau W, Schmidtke J and El-Harith EA (2001) Familial thrombocytosis as a recessive, possibly X-linked trait in an Arab family. *Br J Haematol*, **112**, 616–620.

NINE

MISCELLANEOUS DISORDERS

Non-metastatic effects of cancer

Patients with cancer but without bone marrow metastases may have a variety of haematological abnormalities.

Peripheral blood

Anaemia is common. Red cells may be normocytic and normochromic or microcytic and hypochromic. Rouleaux formation is often increased. Some patients have neutrophil leucocytosis, eosinophilia, monocytosis or thrombocytosis.

Bone marrow cytology

Erythropoiesis often shows the features of anaemia of chronic disease. There may also be dyserythropoiesis. Granulopoiesis (neutrophil and/or eosinophil) may be increased and there may also be hypogranularity or some cells showing the acquired Pelger–Huët anomaly [1]. Megakaryocytes are often increased, as are macrophages, plasma cells and sometimes mast cells. Bone marrow necrosis may occur. It has been suggested that this may be mediated by tumour necrosis factor [2].

Bone marrow histology

There may be suppression of erythropoiesis, granulocytic hyperplasia and increased megakaryocytes (Fig. 9.1). Dyserythropoiesis, abnormal localization of immature granulocytes and dysplastic megakaryocytes are sometimes noted [1]. Macrophages, plasma cells and mast cells are sometimes increased. Stromal changes can include paratrabecular fibrosis, sinusoidal congestion, oedema and bone remodelling [1]. In patients with advanced disease there may be gelatinous transformation, which is sometimes extensive. Patients with parathyroid hormone-secreting tumours may show changes of hyperparathyroidism. Iron stores may be increased.

Bone marrow dysplasia with polyclonal haemopoiesis

Bone marrow dysplasia can be primary – inherited disorders or the myelodysplastic syndromes (MDS) – or secondary. It is important to distinguish MDS from other primary myelodysplasia and from secondary dysplasia. Myelodysplastic syndromes are characterized by dysplastic and ineffective clonal haemopoiesis. They are neoplastic conditions, which are potentially preleukaemic. Secondary myelodysplasia is neither neoplastic nor preleukaemic and, if the underlying cause can be removed, it is reversible. In secondary myelodysplasia and when dysplasia is the result of an inherited condition, haemopoiesis is polyclonal.

Dysplasia as a feature of an inherited condition

Dyserythropoiesis as a feature of an inherited condition is seen not only in the congenital dyserythropoietic anaemias and thalassaemias but also in other uncommon or rare defects including congenital dyserythropoietic porphyria [3], the mitochondrial cytopathies, hereditary sideroblastic anaemia [4], homozygosity for haemoglobin C [4], heterozygosity for some unstable haemoglobins [4], homozygosity for pyruvate kinase deficiency [4] and in some cases of thiamine-responsive anaemia with diabetes and deafness [4]. Dyserythropoiesis is a feature of 'stress erythropoiesis', e.g. in severe haemolytic anaemia. Dysgranulopoiesis can also be a feature of inherited abnormalities, e.g. the mitochondrial cytopathies and myelokathexis. Rather non-specific

Bone Marrow Pathology. By Barbara Bain, David Clark and Bridget Wilkins. © 2010, Blackwell Publishing.

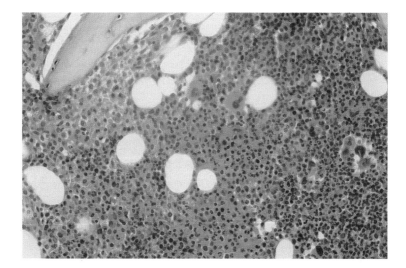

Fig. 9.1 Bone marrow (BM) trephine biopsy section from a patient with cancer showing granulocytic and megakaryocytic hyperplasia and an increase of granulocyte precursors in a paratrabecular position. The haemoglobin concentration was 97 g/l. The white cell count and platelet count were normal. Paraffin-embedded, haematoxylin and eosin (H&E) ×25.

dyserythropoiesis and dysgranulopoiesis, including an increased frequency of macropolycytes, have been described in patients with diGeorge syndrome, associated with microdeletion of 22q11.2 [5]. Familial *GATA1* mutations can cause anaemia and neutropenia with a hypocellular bone marrow and trilineage dysplasia; there may be macrocytosis and pseudo-Pelger–Huët neutrophils [6]. Inherited thrombocytopenias can have dysplastic megakaryocytes.

Secondary myelodysplasia

Dysplasia can be secondary to illness, exposure to drugs or toxins (see pages 505 and 510) or a deficiency state. The commonest causative illnesses are infections (for example, HIV infection, tuberculosis, malaria (*Plasmodium falciparum* and *P. vivax*) and leishmaniasis), critical illness (often with multiorgan failure) [7], liver disease and autoimmune diseases (see below). Dyserythropoiesis, possibly with an autoimmune basis, has been reported in the autoimmune lymphoproliferative syndrome associated with Fas or Fas ligand deficiency [8]. Equally rare is an unusual type of dyserythropoiesis in patients with a lymphoproliferative disorder, designated erythroblastic synartesis and mediated by a monoclonal immunoglobulin [9,10]. Parvovirus B19 infection can cause sufficient dyserythropoiesis to be confused with congenital dyserythropoietic anaemia [11]. Dysplastic changes have been reported following liver and other solid organ transplantation [12]. Macrocytosis and trilineage myelodysplasia are seen in a significant minority of patients with large granular lymphocyte leukaemia. Other lymphomas can have associated dysplasia. Anaemia with sideroblastic erythropoiesis has been observed in hypothermia [13].

When vitamin B_{12} and folate deficiency lead to severe megaloblastic anaemia, the dysplastic features are very prominent and there is associated pancytopenia; this combination has led to misdiagnosis as MDS or erythroleukaemia. Copper deficiency can cause microcytic, normocytic or macrocytic anaemia, neutropenia, vacuolation of haemopoietic cells, dyserythropoiesis (megaloblastic or sideroblastic erythropoiesis), increased macrophage iron, haemosiderin in plasma cells and bone marrow hypocellularity [14,15] (Fig. 9.2, see also Figs 9.15 and 9.16); again, misdiagnosis as MDS has occurred. Protein-calorie malnutrition also causes dysplasia.

The characteristic haematological effects of autoimmune diseases (see page 504), HIV infection (see page 144), anti-cancer and immunosuppressive chemotherapy (see page 505), other drugs and toxins (see page 510), excess alcohol intake (see page 513) and protein-calorie malnutrition (see page 529) are dealt with in detail elsewhere. The general features of secondary bone marrow dysplasia will be described here.

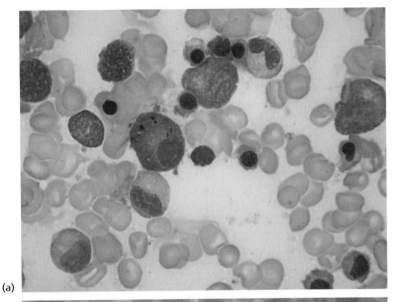

(a)

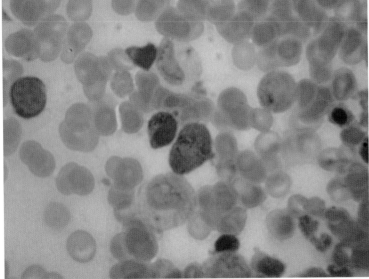

(b)

Fig. 9.2 BM aspirate film from a patient with copper deficiency showing haemosiderin in plasma cells. (a) May–Grünwald–Giemsa (MGG) ×100. (b) Perls' stain ×100.

Peripheral blood

Anaemia is usual and thrombocytopenia is common. Some patients have leucopenia or pancytopenia. Red cells may show anisocytosis, macrocytosis or poikilocytosis. The reticulocyte count is likely to be reduced. Neutrophils may show nonspecific abnormalities such as cytoplasmic vacuolation, variable granulation, abnormalities of nuclear shape, binuclearity and detached nuclear fragments. Agranular neutrophils and the acquired Pelger–Huët anomaly are uncommon but do occur.

Bone marrow cytology

Dyserythropoiesis is common (Figs 9.3 and 9.4). Abnormalities seen include increased cytoplasmic bridging, abnormal nuclear lobulation, binuclearity

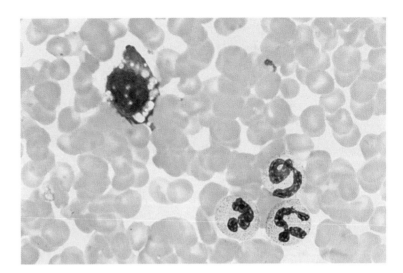

Fig. 9.3 BM aspirate from an intensive care ward patient with multiorgan failure showing a heavily vacuolated dysplastic proerythroblast. MGG ×100.

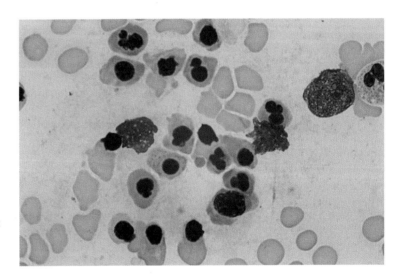

Fig. 9.4 BM aspirate from a patient with tuberculosis showing quite marked dyserythropoiesis. MGG ×100.

and vacuolation. Erythropoiesis is sometimes megaloblastic [7]. Ring sideroblasts may be present although they are usually less frequent than in MDS. Granulocytic cells may show abnormal chromatin clumping, hypolobation, left shift, vacuolation, hypogranularity or variable granulation and the presence of giant metamyelocytes. Erythroid and granulocyte precursors are sometimes vacuolated. Multinucleated or non-lobulated megakaryocytes may be present. In contrast to MDS, very small mononuclear or binuclear megakaryocytes are uncommon in secondary dysplasia. The

specific type of dyserythropoiesis designated erythroblastic synartesis is characterized by clumps of closely apposed erythroblasts with a clear non-basophilic zone of cytoplasm at the cell junctions [9,10] (Fig. 9.5). The diagnosis is confirmed by ultrastructural examination, which shows interdigitating cell membranes.

Bone marrow histology
The bone marrow may be hypercellular, normocellular or hypocellular. There is often a discrepancy

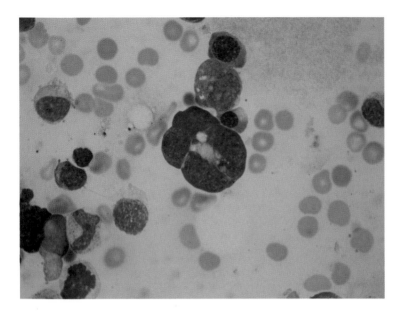

Fig. 9.5 BM aspirate film from a patient with small lymphocytic lymphoma showing synartesis, a phenomenon of closely linked erythroblasts joined by interdigitating cell processes; this is a rare form of autoimmune dyserythropoiesis. MGG ×100. (By courtesy of Dr John Apostolidis, Athens.)

between a hypercellular or normocellular marrow and peripheral cytopenia. Erythropoiesis is often decreased. Dyserythropoiesis is usually present with disorganization of erythroblastic islands and sometimes megaloblastosis. Megakaryocyte atypia, clustering and 'bare' nuclei can be present but micromegakaryocytes are not a feature. Reactive changes (e.g. increased macrophages with haemophagocytosis, increased lymphocytes or increased plasma cells) are often present and some patients show gelatinous transformation or stromal oedema. Marrow architecture may be disturbed and reticulin may be increased.

Problems and pitfalls

It is important not to over-interpret dysplastic features in the bone marrows of patients with severe illness. The diagnosis of MDS requires assessment of clinical, haematological, histological and genetic features rather than just the observation of dysplasia. It is also important to distinguish dysplastic features that are a direct effect of chemotherapeutic agents from therapy-induced MDS. The former disappear following cessation of the causative agent whereas the latter do not.

Leishmaniasis may be missed on bone marrow examination of patients in whom this is the cause

of myelodysplasia [16]. Bone marrow dysplasia has been reported in association with blastic plasmacytoid dendritic cell neoplasm but several of these patients had a prior diagnosis of MDS. It is not yet clear whether such patients have polyclonal haemopoiesis or whether they have myeloid and plasmacytoid dendritic cell neoplasms with a common clonal origin [17].

The bone marrow in connective tissue and autoimmune disorders

There are few specific abnormalities in connective tissue disorders but non-specific abnormalities are common.

Peripheral blood

In systemic lupus erythematosus there may be haemolytic anaemia, thrombocytopenia or neutropenia with an autoimmune basis. In rheumatoid arthritis the features of anaemia of chronic disease (normocytic normochromic or microcytic hypochromic anaemia with increased background staining and rouleaux formation) are usual. There is also a relationship between rheumatoid arthritis and T-lineage large granular lymphocytic leukaemia (see page 367). Felty's syndrome, splenomegaly with pancytopenia occurring in rheumatoid arthritis, may be a feature of this type of leukaemia.

Bone marrow aspirate

There may be dysplasia with polyclonal haemopoiesis (see above), increased lymphocytes and plasma cells and the features of anaemia of chronic disease. Autoimmune cytopenias (thrombocytopenia, haemolytic anaemia) may be reflected in the bone marrow by an increase in megakaryocytes or erythroid precursors, respectively. Other autoimmune processes – pure red cell aplasia and aplastic anaemia – affect the bone marrow more directly. Systemic lupus erythematosus has been associated with reversible dyserythropoiesis, including sideroblastic erythropoiesis, which appears to have an autoimmune basis [18,19]. Rheumatoid arthritis has also been associated with autoimmune dyserythropoiesis. Rarely, if a bone marrow aspirate is anti-coagulated and there is delay in spreading films, specific LE (lupus erythematosus) cells are seen [20,21] (Fig. 9.6). These are neutrophils containing a rounded mass of amorphous purple material that represents degraded nuclear material.

Bone marrow trephine biopsy

Trephine biopsy sections show the same features as described for the bone marrow aspirate. In addition, there is an increased prevalence of lymphoid aggregates. Aplastic anaemia in both systemic lupus erythematosus and rheumatoid arthritis can show an associated increased in lymphoid aggregates [22]. Abnormal localization of immature precursors (ALIP) and erythroid cells and megakaryocytes in a paratrabecular position have been described as common features in systemic lupus erythematosus [23]; haemophagocytosis and bone marrow necrosis can also occur. A very rare finding in this condition is that of LE cells in bone marrow biopsy sections [24]. A marked increase in reticulin deposition can also be a feature. Amyloid deposition has been seen in the bone marrow in rheumatoid arthritis and haemophagocytosis in juvenile-onset rheumatoid arthritis.

Problems and pitfalls

Reactive changes in autoimmune disorders, particularly systemic lupus erythematosus, may closely resemble those seen in association with HIV infection.

The haematological effects of anti-cancer and immunosuppressive chemotherapy

The majority of anti-cancer and immunosuppressive chemotherapeutic agents are damaging to the bone marrow. Most cause hypoplasia, some cause megaloblastosis and some have other, more specific effects. The nature of the bone marrow damage depends on dose and duration of therapy. A drug

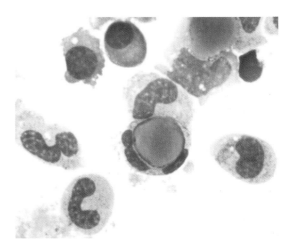

Fig. 9.6 BM aspirate film from a patient with previously undiagnosed systemic lupus erythematosus showing an LE cell. MGG ×100. (Courtesy of Dr Anne Angellilo-Scherrer, Lausanne and www.bloodmed.com.)

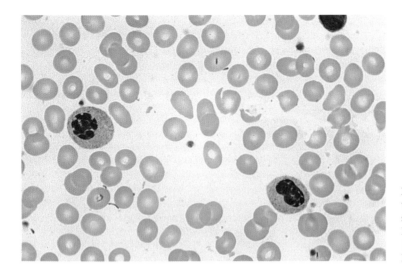

Fig. 9.7 PB film from a patient taking mycophenolate mofetil showing a reversible, acquired Pelger–Huët anomaly. MGG ×100. (By courtesy of Dr Ozay Halil, London.)

may, for example, cause erythroid hyperplasia and megaloblastic erythropoiesis at a low dose and severe hypoplasia at a higher dose.

Some anti-cancer drugs can also induce MDS, acute myeloid leukaemia (AML) and, rarely, acute lymphoblastic leukaemia (ALL) (see page 190) with an interval of some years between their administration and the onset of the haematological neoplasm. It is possible that immunosuppressive drugs such as azathioprine also increase the incidence of AML and MDS. Alemtuzumab (anti-CD52) is likewise suspected of inducing MDS [25].

Early reversible bone marrow damage with dysplasia must be distinguished from therapy-related MDS.

Peripheral blood

The most prominent effect of anti-cancer chemotherapy is pancytopenia. This is usual with all of the commonly employed agents, exceptions being vincristine and bleomycin. Neutropenia and thrombocytopenia are apparent well in advance of anaemia. Some degree of anisocytosis and poikilocytosis, together with basophilic stippling and Howell–Jolly bodies, occur as a consequence of the dyserythropoiesis induced by chemotherapeutic agents. When megaloblastic change is induced, formation of Howell–Jolly bodies is more marked and

macrocytosis is common. Dysplastic changes, including abnormalities of nuclear shape and presence of nuclear inclusions within the cytoplasm, may also be apparent in neutrophils. A reversible acquired Pelger–Huët anomaly has been observed with a number of drugs including chlorambucil, tacrolimus and mycophenolate mofetil (Fig. 9.7). Imatinib often causes anaemia and neutropenia and can cause pancytopenia [26].

Platelets are small but do not show any specific morphological abnormality. Vincristine is unusual in occasionally causing thrombocytosis, although not when it is given in combination with other drugs that are highly toxic to the bone marrow.

Occasionally chemotherapy is followed by the development of microangiopathic haemolytic anaemia. This appears to be a particular feature of mitomycin C therapy.

Alemtuzumab can cause anaemia, neutropenia, lymphopenia and thrombocytopenia [25].

Bone marrow cytology

The bone marrow aspirate shows a variable degree of hypoplasia. If bone marrow aspiration is performed after an episode of severe hypoplasia, early regeneration can produce appearances misinterpreted as 'maturation arrest' (Fig. 9.8). Erythropoiesis is dysplastic, often strikingly so. Drugs that cause

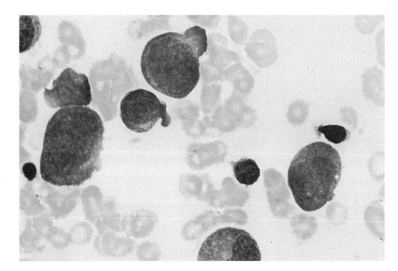

Fig. 9.8 BM aspirate from a patient with severe methotrexate toxicity showing 'maturation arrest'; two promyelocytes and one proerythroblast are seen but maturing cells are severely diminished. MGG ×100.

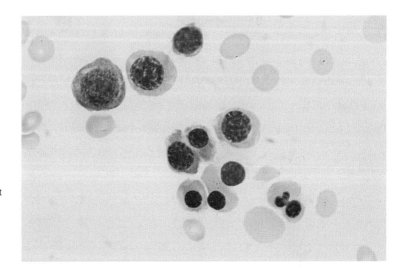

Fig. 9.9 BM aspirate from a patient taking hydroxycarbamide for psoriasis showing erythroid hyperplasia, mild megaloblastosis and one dyserythropoietic cell. MGG ×100.

megaloblastosis include methotrexate, cyclophosphamide, daunorubicin, doxorubicin, cytarabine, hydroxycarbamide (previously known as hydroxyurea), azathioprine and zidovudine. The megaloblastosis induced by anti-cancer chemotherapeutic agents, with the exception of folate antagonists, differs from that due to vitamin B_{12} or folate deficiency in that dyserythropoiesis is very striking and hypersegmented neutrophils and giant metamyelocytes are either not a feature or are less marked. Depending on drug dose, megaloblastosis may be associated with erythroid hyperplasia (Fig. 9.9) or

hypoplasia. Other drugs cause dysplastic features without megaloblastosis. Erythroid dysplasia may be striking, both with megaloblastic and with normoblastic erythropoiesis. Vincristine and other spindle poisons cause mitotic arrest in quite a high proportion of erythroblasts; this is detected if a bone marrow aspirate is performed 1–2 days after the administration of one of these drugs (Fig. 9.10). Bone marrow aspirates taken shortly after the administration of chemotherapeutic agents may show increased apoptosis and increased numbers of macrophages containing cellular debris.

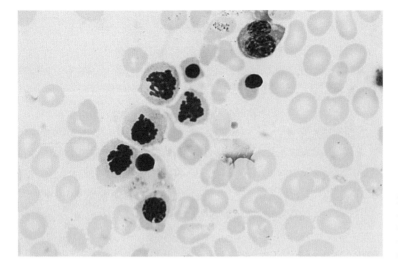

Fig. 9.10 BM aspirate, performed about 24 hours after administration of vincristine, showing a binucleate erythroblast and four erythroblasts arrested in mitosis. MGG ×940.

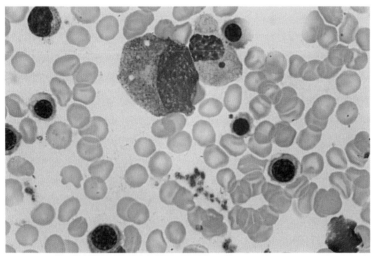

Fig. 9.11 BM aspirate from a patient taking mycophenolate mofetil showing a myelocyte with abnormal chromatin clumping and a detached nuclear fragment (same patient as Fig. 9.7). MGG ×100. (By courtesy of Dr Ozay Halil.)

When mycophenolate mofetil causes the acquired Pelger–Huët anomaly, abnormal chromatin clumping and detached nuclear fragments can be seen in granulocyte precursors in the bone marrow as well as in peripheral blood cells (Fig. 9.11). Alemtuzumab can be associated with dysplastic features, bone marrow hypoplasia and an increased incidence of parvovirus infection, cytomegalovirus reactivation and Epstein–Barr virus (EBV)-related haemophagocytic syndrome [25].

Bone marrow histology

Cells exposed to chemotherapeutic agents show apoptosis. Dead cells degenerate to granular eosino-philic debris. With intensive chemotherapy, depletion of haemopoietic cells is severe and stromal elements become prominent. There are dilated sinusoids containing red cells and fibrin [27], and sometimes residual lymphocytes and plasma cells, the latter particularly along small blood vessels. Red cells may be extravasated from dilated and disrupted sinusoids. Macrophages are prominent. In the acute phase of bone marrow damage there may be interstitial oedema; at this stage stains for stromal mucin are negative. Subsequently, typical features of gelatinous transformation may develop.

In the majority of patients treated with intensive chemotherapy for acute leukaemia [27,28], the

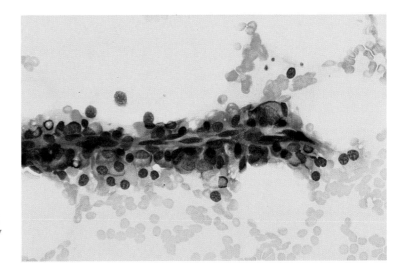

Fig. 9.12 BM aspirate, post-chemotherapy (for AML), showing plasma cells surrounding a capillary in a severely hypoplastic bone marrow. MGG ×40.

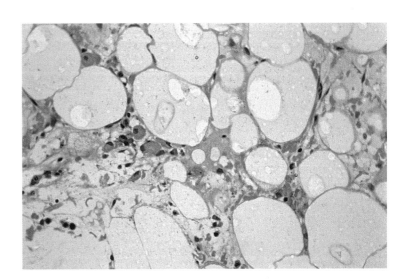

Fig. 9.13 BM trephine biopsy section, regeneration post-chemotherapy, showing decreased cellularity, oedema and a cluster of immature regenerating megakaryocytes. Resin-embedded, H&E ×20.

marrow is almost completely emptied of haemopoietic cells, particularly when therapy is of the type used in AML. Varying degrees of stromal damage occur, including stromal necrosis. Viable osteocytes are decreased [29]. Prominent residual plasma cells (Fig. 9.12) are more a feature of AML than of ALL [28]. Cellular depletion persists for 3–4 weeks, to be followed by regeneration of fat cells, which are initially multivesicular, then by regeneration of haemopoietic cells. Erythroid and megakaryocytic regeneration often occurs before granulocytic regeneration, but this is variable. In the early stages of regeneration, clusters of haemopoietic precursors made up of cells from a single lineage (Fig. 9.13) are often seen. Topography may be abnormal with erythroid islands adjacent to trabeculae, ALIP and megakaryocyte clustering. Reticulin fibres are increased. There may be collagen deposition, increased osteoblastic activity and focal appositional or intertrabecular bone formation [27]. Extensive osteoid seams, resembling those in osteomalacia, may be seen [29] and bone remodelling may be prominent. These bone changes are likely to indicate prior necrosis and central areas of dead bone with empty osteocyte lacunae within trabeculae are often still present.

Imatinib can cause bone marrow aplasia [26].

Problems and pitfalls

Megakaryocyte clustering and ALIP are common features during recovery from intensive chemotherapy and may persist for many months. In this context these abnormalities should not be interpreted as evidence of MDS. It is important to know if chemotherapeutic regimens include growth factors such as granulocyte colony-stimulating factor (G-CSF), since this will complicate the interpretation of increased numbers of myeloblasts and promyelocytes. Following cessation of chemotherapy, particularly in children, there may be a rebound increase in immature lymphoid cells (haematogones). This should not be confused with relapse of leukaemia.

The haematological effects of other drugs and chemicals

Anti-cancer and related drugs have predictable haematological toxicity. Other drugs more often cause idiosyncratic reactions with an immunological mechanism such as agranulocytosis (see page 486), immune haemolytic anaemia and aplastic anaemia (see page 515). There is also a small group of other drugs with predictable toxicity. Oxidant drugs and chemicals can cause haemolytic anaemia. Chloramphenicol, as well as causing severe idiosyncratic reactions, regularly causes mild bone marrow suppression with ring sideroblasts and vacuolation of erythroid and granulocyte precursors. A number of drugs including isoniazid can cause sideroblastic anaemia. The antimicrobial agent, linezolid, can cause both vacuolation of erythroid precursors and ring sideroblasts, associated with anaemia or pancytopenia [30]. Drugs other than those used for anti-cancer treatment can cause megaloblastosis by interfering with vitamin B_{12} or folate metabolism. Nitrous oxide (an inactivator of hydroxocobalamin) can cause megaloblastosis and a single case of megaloblastic anaemia apparently resulting from pentamidine therapy has been reported [31]. Megaloblastic erythropoiesis is particularly common in intensive care ward patients who have been exposed to nitrous oxide [7]. Antimonial therapy (sodium stibogluconate) for leishmaniasis has been associated with severe anaemia and striking karyorrhexis of bone marrow erythroblasts [32].

The haematological effects of recombinant human growth factors, which include myelodysplasia, are dealt with on page 526.

Lead poisoning can cause basophilic stippling of erythrocytes, hypochromic microcytic anaemia, haemolytic anaemia and sideroblastic erythropoiesis; reported sources include 'herbal' or other alternative medications, lead-glazed pottery, cosmetics and contaminated marihuana. Arsenic can cause leucopenia, anaemia, thrombocytopenia and pancytopenia with dysplastic or megaloblastic erythropoiesis [33–36] (Fig. 9.14); reported causes of arsenic toxicity include use of 'herbal' and other alternative medical remedies and attempted homicide. Erythrocytes may be normocytic or macrocytic. Dyserythropoiesis can be very prominent, with basophilic stippling, binuclearity, multinuclearity, nuclear lobulation, internuclear bridges, karyorrhexis and the presence of ring sideroblasts [33–36]. Aplastic anaemia has also been reported [35]. Zinc toxicity can lead to copper deficiency with consequent anaemia, neutropenia, sideroblastic erythropoiesis and vacuolation of erythroid and myeloid precursors [37]. Similar features are seen with copper-depleting drugs such as penicillamine, trientine and ammonium tetrathiomolybdate used in the treatment of Wilson's disease [38] (Figs 9.15 and 9.16). Hypervitaminosis A has been associated with anaemia and thrombocytopenia with reduced erythroid precursors and megakaryocytes [39].

Mustard gas can produce effects similar to those of alkylating agents; delayed neutropenia, thrombocytopenia and bone marrow hypoplasia were reported following exposure during the Iran–Iraq war [40].

The effect of irradiation on the bone marrow

Irradiation of a significant proportion of the bone marrow causes a fall in neutrophil and platelet counts. Extensive irradiation causes pancytopenia. Monitoring of blood counts is therefore carried out during radiotherapy.

Peripheral blood

The blood film may show neutropenia, thrombocytopenia and the features of anaemia.

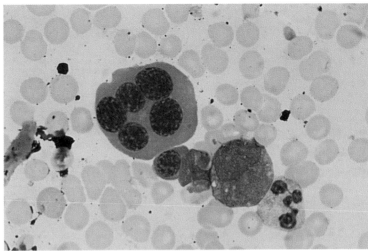

Fig. 9.14 BM aspirate showing dyserythropoiesis induced by arsenic. MGG ×100. (By courtesy of Professor A. Newlands, London.)

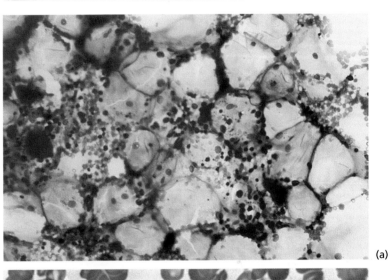

(a)

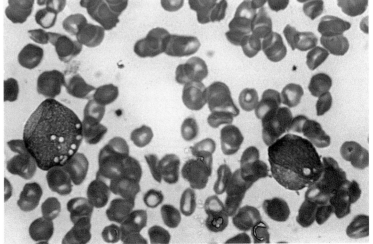

(b)

Fig. 9.15 BM aspirate from a patient with copper deficiency caused by chelation therapy for Wilson's disease. (a) Hypocellularity. MGG ×20. (b) Vacuolation of granulocyte precursors. MGG ×100. (By courtesy of Dr A. Grigg, Melbourne.)

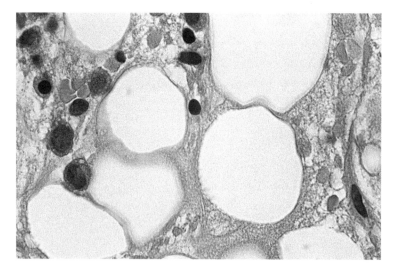

Fig. 9.16 BM trephine biopsy section from a patient with copper deficiency caused by chelation therapy for Wilson's disease (same patient as Fig. 9.15) showing hypocellularity and vacuolation of granulocyte precursors. H&E ×100. (By courtesy of Dr A. Grigg, Melbourne.)

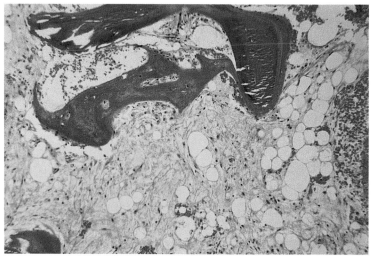

Fig. 9.17 BM trephine biopsy section showing stromal damage and radiation-induced osteodysplasia. H&E ×10. (By courtesy of Dr Ruth Langholm, Oslo.)

Bone marrow cytology

The initial change in irradiated bone marrow is pyknosis and karyorrhexis of haemopoietic cells followed by disappearance of haemopoietic and fat cells and replacement by areas of gelatinous transformation. Subsequently, at the site of irradiation, hypoplastic marrow is found, with haemopoietic cells being replaced by fat. Extensive high dose irradiation of the bone marrow is followed by aplastic anaemia.

Bone marrow histology

Initially, there may be necrosis of the bone marrow within the field that has received high dose radia-

tion. Cell loss is initially greatest adjacent to trabeculae as more mature post-proliferative cells in the central marrow space are more radio resistant. There is endothelial cell swelling, sinusoidal dilation, interstitial haemorrhage and sometimes stromal necrosis. Haemosiderin-laden macrophages appear on a background of eosinophilic debris. Subsequently, gelatinous transformation may occur. Bone necrosis may also occur during the acute phase and may be followed by bone remodelling and radiation-induced osteodysplasia (Fig. 9.17). Later, there is permanent replacement of haemopoietic marrow by fat or, less often, fibrous tissue.

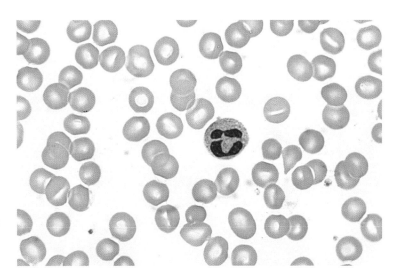

Fig. 9.18 Peripheral blood (PB) film showing macrocytosis with some stomatocytes, consequent on excess alcohol intake. MGG ×100.

The haematological effects of alcohol

Excess intake of ethanol is often complicated by dietary deficiency and liver disease. However, ethanol itself has well-defined haematological toxicity.

Peripheral blood

There is a normocytic or macrocytic anaemia with red cells being normochromic. Macrocytes differ from those of megaloblastic anaemia in that they are usually round rather than oval (Fig. 9.18). Stomatocytes are common and target cells are sometimes present. A dimorphic blood film has been reported but is not common. Heavy alcohol intake and acute alcoholic liver disease have been associated with haemolytic anaemia and hyperlipidaemia, with the blood film showing spherocytes or irregularly contracted cells; this is designated Zieve's syndrome. The neutrophil count is usually normal but the capacity of the bone marrow to mount a neutrophil response to infection is reduced and infection may lead to neutropenia. Neutrophils may be vacuolated. The lymphocyte count may be reduced. Thrombocytopenia is common. If alcohol intake is suddenly stopped a rebound thrombocytosis can occur.

Bone marrow cytology

Erythropoiesis is normoblastic, macronormoblastic or mildly megaloblastic. Siderotic granules are prominent and there may be ring sideroblasts; sometimes these are numerous. There are other dyserythropoietic features such as erythroid multinuclearity. Erythroid and granulocyte precursors are sometimes vacuolated (Fig. 9.19). Iron stores may be increased; sometimes haemosiderin inclusions are present in plasma cells [41]. In Zieve's syndrome there may be an excess of iron-laden foamy macrophages (Fig. 9.20). Megakaryocytes are often increased [42] but a marked decrease has also been reported [43]. Alcohol-induced reversible bone marrow hypoplasia has been reported [44].

Bone marrow histology

Trephine biopsy sections show dyserythropoiesis. There may be increased iron in macrophages and iron in plasma cells [41] and endothelial cells [42]. The latter phenomenon may be noted in the absence of any increase in macrophage iron [42]. Megakaryocytes may be increased [42] or markedly decreased [43].

Problems and pitfalls

It is important to be aware of the likelihood of excess alcohol intake in interpreting cytopenias and dysplastic features. Otherwise there may be a misdiagnosis of MDS.

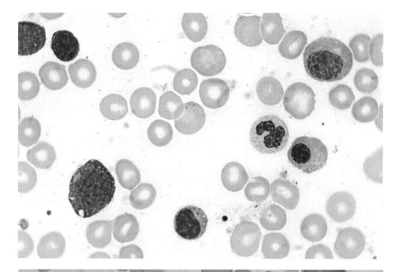

Fig. 9.19 BM aspirate showing macronormoblastic erythropoiesis and erythroblast vacuolation caused by excess alcohol intake (same patient as Fig. 9.18). MGG ×100.

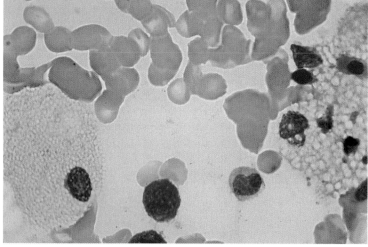

(a)

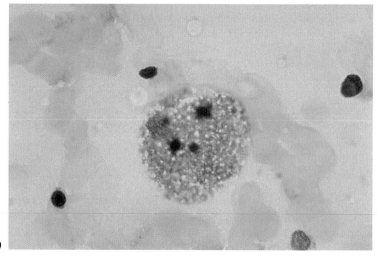

(b)

Fig. 9.20 BM aspirate from a patient with Zieve's syndrome. (a) Foamy macrophages. MGG ×100. (b) An iron-laden foamy macrophage. Perls' stain ×100. (By courtesy of Dr Sue Fairhead, London.)

Table 9.1 Causes of aplastic anaemia.

Inherited
Fanconi anaemia
Dyskeratosis congenita
Diamond–Blackfan syndrome (disease evolution)
Shwachman–Diamond syndrome (disease evolution)
Amegakaryocytic thrombocytopenia (disease
    evolution)
Dubowitz syndrome
Seckel syndrome
Ataxia-pancytopenia syndrome

Acquired
Drugs (e.g. chloramphenicol, phenylbutazone,
    carbamazepine, phenytoin, felbamate,
    acetazolamide, indomethacin, piroxicam, gold)
Chemicals (e.g. benzene, organophosphates,
    chlorinated hydrocarbons)
Irradiation
Autoimmune (including association with large
    granular lymphocytic leukaemia and, rarely,
    thymoma, and with autoimmune diseases such as
    systemic lupus erythematosus, autoimmune
    thyroid disease and eosinophilic fasciiitis and
    possibly with pregnancy)
Graft-versus-host disease
Unknown

Aplastic anaemia

Aplastic anaemia is a heterogeneous disorder characterized by pancytopenia and a hypocellular marrow without any apparent underlying neoplastic process. It may be inherited or acquired. The name, although well established, is somewhat misleading since all haemopoietic lineages are involved. The causes are summarized in Table 9.1. Aplastic anaemia is rare. The reported incidence varies considerably between countries, e.g. from 0.7 to 4.1 per 10 million per year in one study [45]. Incidence is lower in Europe and North America than in various other parts of the world, e.g. Asia; an incidence of 4.1 per 10 million per year having been reported in Thailand and of 11 per 10 million per year in Japan. Although some cases of aplastic anaemia result from an inherited disorder and

develop in infancy or childhood, the incidence, in general, increases with age.

The commonest inherited form of aplastic anaemia is Fanconi anaemia. This is an autosomal recessive condition in which sufferers have defective DNA repair mechanisms. The pancytopenia usually develops between the ages of 5 and 10 years. Without bone marrow transplantation many patients die from infection or bleeding, but approximately 20% develop AML [46]. Fanconi anaemia is heterogeneous, there being at least 11 different genetic loci where mutations can give rise to this phenotype. Spontaneous improvement of blood counts can occur as a result of a second acquired mutation that corrects or compensates for the inherited mutation [47].

Other inherited disorders that may progress to aplastic anaemia include dyskeratosis congenita (a heterogeneous disorder with either X-linked recessive inheritance, resulting from mutation in the *DKC1* gene, or autosomal dominant inheritance resulting from mutation in either the *TERC* gene or the *TERT* gene), Hoyeraal–Hreidarsson syndrome (a severe variant of dyskeratosis congenita) [48], Shwachman–Diamond syndrome and amegakaryocytic thrombocytopenia without physical defects [49]. In Shwachman–Diamond syndrome, neutropenia often develops first, with pancytopenia – resulting from aplastic anaemia – following.

Known causes of acquired aplastic anaemia include radiation exposure, autoimmune disease, orthodox and recreational drugs (such as chloramphenicol and 3,4-methylenedioxymethamphetamine ('ecstasy'), respectively[50]) and chemicals (such as benzene). Aplastic anaemia can follow hepatitis that clinically resembles viral hepatitis but evidence of a viral aetiology has not been found. Aplastic anaemia can be the initial presentation of systemic lupus erythematosus [51]. Pregnancy appears to be a rare cause of aplastic anaemia [52]. In many cases the cause is not apparent and the designation 'idiopathic aplastic anaemia' is then used. An autoimmune origin is likely in many 'idiopathic' cases. Mutation of either the *TERC* gene or the *TERT* gene can predispose to apparently idiopathic acquired aplastic anaemia without the stigmata of dyskeratosis congenita [53]; it is probable that these mutations make stem cells vulnerable to injury [53].

The diagnosis of aplastic anaemia may be suspected from peripheral blood and bone marrow aspirate findings but trephine biopsy is essential for diagnosis. This is because of the frequent difficulty in obtaining an adequate aspirate and the variable degree of hypoplasia in different areas of the marrow. If bone marrow examination does not confirm a strong clinical suspicion of aplastic anaemia, repeat examination at another site is indicated since the bone marrow may be affected in an uneven manner.

Prior to the development of stem cell transplantation and immunosuppressive therapy, the prognosis of aplastic anaemia was poor with severe cases having a median survival of less than a year. With immunosuppressive therapy (antilymphocyte globulin plus ciclosporin) or stem cell transplantation from a histocompatible sibling, 5-year survivals of the order of 50–70% can be anticipated. Bone marrow or other stem cell transplantation may cure aplastic anaemia whereas, following immunosuppressive therapy, defective stem cells persist giving the possibility of evolution into paroxysmal nocturnal haemoglobinuria, MDS or AML.

Aplastic anaemia has been categorized, on the basis of peripheral blood and bone marrow features as severe, very severe or non-severe. Aplastic anaemia is classified as severe if at least two of three peripheral blood criteria are met – reticulocyte count less than 1% or less than $60 \times 10^9/l$, neutrophil count less than $0.5 \times 10^9/l$ and platelet count less than $20 \times 10^9/l$; in addition, bone marrow cellularity must be less than 25% [22]. Patients with very severe aplastic anaemia have a granulocyte count less than $0.2 \times 10^9/l$. Other cases are categorized as non-severe.

Peripheral blood

Severe cases are characterized by pancytopenia and a low reticulocyte count. The lymphocyte count is also low. The anaemia may be normocytic or macrocytic, polychromasia is absent and poikilocytes may be present; sometimes poikilocytosis is marked. Neutrophils often have dark red granules and high alkaline phosphatase activity, even in the absence of any apparent infection. Platelets are of normal size, in contrast to the large platelets that are common when thrombocytopenia is the result of increased platelet destruction. Macrocytosis and borderline cytopenias may persist following remission induced by immunosuppressive therapy.

Bone marrow cytology

Bone marrow may be difficult to aspirate with the result being a 'dry tap' or 'blood tap', but more often aspiration of fragments is possible [22]. In the majority of patients a hypocellular aspirate is obtained with the fragments being composed largely of fat (Fig. 9.21). The cell trails are also hypocellular. Different lineages are affected to a variable extent so that the myeloid:erythroid ratio may be increased, normal or decreased. Dyserythropoiesis may be seen and is often marked. Ring sideroblasts are not usually a feature but otherwise the changes seen can be similar to those observed in MDS [54,55]. Dysplastic changes in granulocytes are less common and pseudo-Pelger neutrophils are not a feature. There is no disproportionate increase in immature granulocyte precursors. Megakaryocytes are often so infrequent in the aspirate that it is difficult to assess their morphology but dysplasia is not a feature.

In a minority of patients the aspirate is normocellular or even hypercellular [54,55]. Examination of trephine biopsy specimens from such patients shows that such 'hot spots' coexist with extensive areas of hypoplastic marrow.

The bone marrow aspirate shows at least a relative increase in lymphocytes and sometimes an absolute increase. There may also be increased numbers of plasma cells, macrophages and mast cells. Foamy macrophages are sometimes present and macrophage iron is increased. Early after disease onset, haemophagocytosis may be marked [22].

Bone marrow histology

Trephine biopsy is crucial in the diagnosis of aplastic anaemia. The bone marrow is usually hypocellular with a marked reduction of haemopoietic cells (Figs 9.22–9.24). Myeloid cells are mainly replaced by fat but there is a variable inflammatory infiltrate composed of lymphocytes, plasma cells, macrophages, mast cells and sometimes eosinophils [56] (Fig. 9.23). As in the aspirate, in the early stages of the disease there may be prominent haemophagocytosis [22]. Lymphocytes, which are CD3 positive

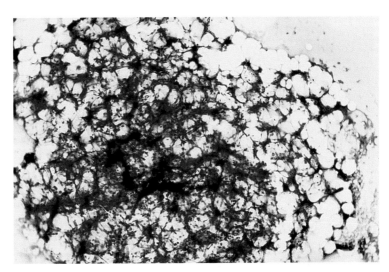

Fig. 9.21 BM aspirate, aplastic anaemia, showing a severely hypoplastic fragment. MGG ×10.

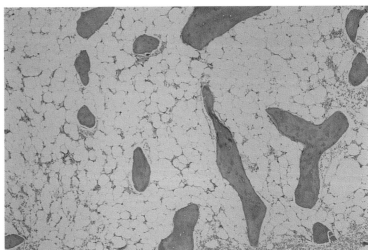

Fig. 9.22 BM trephine biopsy section, aplastic anaemia, showing marked hypocellularity. Resin-embedded, H&E ×4.

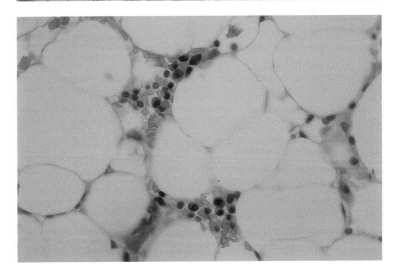

Fig. 9.23 BM trephine biopsy section, aplastic anaemia, showing a marked reduction in haemopoietic precursors; many of the remaining cells are plasma cells. Resin-embedded, H&E ×40.

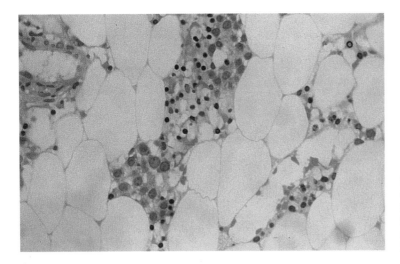

Fig. 9.24 BM trephine biopsy section, Fanconi anaemia, showing large, poorly formed erythroblastic islands containing increased numbers of early erythroblasts. Resin-embedded, H&E ×20.

and either CD4 or CD8 positive, are preferentially increased in areas of residual haemopoiesis [57]. Reactive lymphoid aggregates are also increased, particularly early in the disease course and in patients in whom aplastic anaemia develops in the setting of rheumatoid arthritis or systemic lupus erythematosus [22]. Necrotic cells and cellular debris may be present. Walls of sinusoids may be disrupted and there may be oedema and haemorrhage. In some patients the inflammatory infiltrate is so heavy that the marked reduction of haemopoietic cells is not immediately apparent. Sinusoids are reduced but arterioles and capillaries are normal or increased [58] Residual erythroid cells show dysplastic features [56]. Macrophage iron is increased. A distinctive appearance has been observed in aplastic anaemia induced by acetazolamide. In many of these patients there is depletion of haemopoietic cells leaving abnormal stroma, lymphocytes and plasma cells but without replacement by fat.

A minority of cases have some areas of normal or increased cellularity. Such cellular areas are commonly adjacent to sinusoids [58] and are composed of erythroid cells, all at the same stage of development and showing dysplastic features [55]. This finding is more common in Fanconi anaemia (Fig. 9.24). In this condition the marrow is initially normocellular but becomes hypocellular. Megakaryocytes are often the first lineage to show reduction, followed by granulo-

cytes and then erythroid cells. *In situ* techniques for the detection of apoptosis show a marked increase in apoptotic cells [59].

There is usually little if any increase in reticulin fibres. Various abnormalities of bone have been reported. Some studies have found osteoporosis and others increased osteoblastic and osteoclastic activity with irregular remodelling of bone [56]. Osteoporosis is said to be characteristic of long-standing aplastic anaemia [29].

When aplastic anaemia remits, for example following therapy with anti-thymocyte or anti-lymphocyte globulin, dysplastic features are very evident [60,61] and the inflammatory infiltrate often persists [61].

The presence of trilineage dysplasia and increased reticulin deposition is indicative of a worse prognosis (see below). Otherwise there is little relationship between histological features and prognosis. Assessment of cellularity has not been found particularly useful in this regard. Prior to the development of modern treatment, an intense inflammatory infiltrate was shown to correlate with a worse prognosis [56,62] but this was not so in three large series of patients treated either with anti-thymocyte globulin or by bone marrow transplantation [61,63].

Trephine biopsy for assessing bone marrow cellularity is essential to establish if the criteria for severe aplastic anaemia are met.

Cytogenetic and molecular genetic analysis

At presentation, a significant proportion of patients with acquired aplastic anaemia are found to have a clonal cytogenetic abnormality, most often trisomy 6 or 8 or anomalies of chromosomes 5 or 7. Although this indicates the presence of a neoplastic clone it does not necessarily predict progression to MDS or AML [64], this being dependent on the specific abnormality detected. Abnormalities of chromosome 7 and complex cytogenetic abnormalities have been found predictive of leukaemic transformation [65] whereas del(13)(q12q14) and trisomies are not indicative of a poor prognosis [66,67]. Overall, the prognosis is no worse in patients with a clonal cytogenetic abnormality [67]. An abnormal clone may disappear following immunosuppressive therapy [64]. In Fanconi anaemia, gains of 3q26q29 have been found to have an adverse prognostic significance [68].

Clonal cytogenetic abnormalities that appear following a response to immunosuppressive therapy are of more significance. They are often present at the time of evolution to MDS or AML. Abnormalities observed have included monosomy 6 and monosomy or deletion of chromosome 7.

The molecular genetic abnormalities underlying many types of inherited aplastic anaemia have been defined. Fanconi anaemia is associated with chromosomal fragility and cytogenetic analysis following exposure to clastogenic agents, such as diepoxybutane, is diagnostically important. More than 100 specific mutations in 11 different genes have been identified in different families with Fanconi anaemia.

Problems and pitfalls

A diagnosis of aplastic anaemia should not be based on a bone marrow aspirate alone. Trephine biopsy is essential in order both to assess cellularity of an adequate sample of marrow and to assess the cytological features of residual cells. Trephine biopsy is particularly important in distinguishing aplastic anaemia from hypoplastic MDS and AML and from conditions in which bone marrow fibrosis leads to a hypocellular uninformative aspirate. Abnormal cells such as blast cells or hairy cells may be present in trephine biopsy sections although not detectable in a hypocellular aspirate.

An adequate clinical history is important in order to avoid performing a bone marrow biopsy at the site of previous radiotherapy; the bone marrow at such sites is hypocellular and histological features may be indistinguishable from those of aplastic anaemia (Fig. 9.25). It should be noted that subcortical bone marrow is hypocellular (Fig. 9.26) so that a diagnosis of aplastic anaemia should never be based on an inadequate biopsy composed mainly of cortical bone and subcortical bone marrow.

The relationship of aplastic anaemia to hypocellular MDS is problematical since neoplastic clones

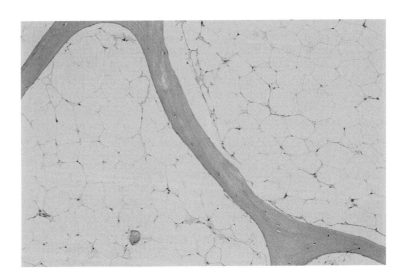

Fig. 9.25 BM trephine biopsy section inadvertently taken from the site of previous radiotherapy, showing marked hypocellularity. Paraffin-embedded, H&E ×10.

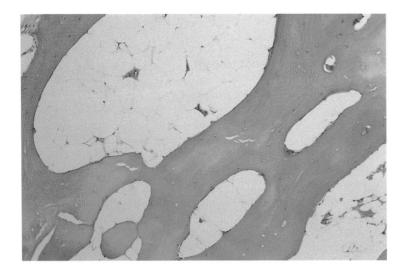

Fig. 9.26 BM trephine section from a patient with essential thrombocythaemia showing very hypocellular subcortical bone marrow; elsewhere marrow was of normal cellularity with increased megakaryocytes. Paraffin-embedded, H&E ×10.

arise in some cases of aplastic anaemia and may be predictive of subsequent MDS and AML. However, it should be noted that although the detection of a clonal cytogenetic abnormality in a hypoplastic bone marrow indicates a neoplastic clone it is not necessarily predictive of disease progression. Such clones sometimes disappear spontaneously. It may be that hypocellular MDS represents an intermediate stage of evolution of typical aplastic anaemia to MDS [49] or to AML. Aplastic anaemia can also progress through typical hypercellular MDS to AML [69]. Of long-term survivors of aplastic anaemia, the number developing MDS and AML may be as high as 10% [70]. In the differential diagnosis of hypoplastic MDS and aplastic anaemia the most important feature is the presence of clusters of blasts, which are indicative of the former diagnosis. Other features which have been found, to some extent, to be predictive of progression to AML and which can therefore be considered to favour a diagnosis of hypocellular MDS are: (i) trilineage atypia, particularly megakaryocyte atypia; (ii) increased numbers or clustering of megakaryocytes; and (iii) reticulin fibrosis [69]. In Fanconi anaemia the development of trilineage dysplasia and reticulin fibrosis may herald transformation to AML.

The relationship of aplastic anaemia to paroxysmal nocturnal haemoglobinuria is discussed below.

It should be noted that, in children, apparent aplastic anaemia may represent an aplastic presentation of ALL. Spontaneous recovery of haemopoiesis occurs, to be followed within a few months by frank ALL; increased reticulin is common in pre-ALL aplasia and a proportion of patients also have prominent bone marrow lymphocytes [71]. DNA analysis has shown that leukaemic cells are present in significant numbers in the hypoplastic stage [72].

Careful examination of bone marrow sections should avoid the pitfall of confusing hairy cell leukaemia with aplastic anaemia but, if there is doubt, immunohistochemistry will resolve the problem.

Other causes of bone marrow aplasia and hypoplasia

Reversible aplasia follows intensive cytotoxic chemotherapy. In subjects unable to mount a normal immune response to EBV, primary infection by the virus may cause bone marrow aplasia. Hypoplasia can also be a feature of cytomegalovirus (CMV) infection and, rarely, brucellosis [73]. Advanced HIV infection is associated with bone marrow hypoplasia with reticulin fibrosis. Other infections, including toxoplasmosis, sometimes cause bone marrow aplasia [74]. Bone marrow aplasia is also one of the features of graft-versus-host disease (see below).

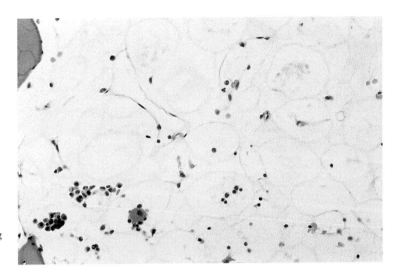

Fig. 9.27 BM trephine biopsy section in anorexia nervosa showing marked hypocellularity. Paraffin-embedded, H&E ×20.

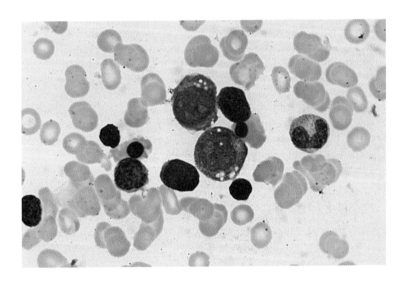

Fig. 9.28 BM aspirate from a patient with probable Pearson's syndrome showing vacuolation of haemopoietic precursors. MGG ×100. (By courtesy of Dr S. Jan, Pakistan.)

Other causes of bone marrow hypoplasia include starvation, anorexia nervosa (Fig. 9.27), severe hypothyroidism, hypopituitarism [75], copper deficiency (see Fig. 9.16) and arsenic toxicity.

Pearson's syndrome and other mitochondrial cytopathies

Several congenital syndromes with mitochondrial inheritance cause anaemia and cytopenia with an onset during childhood [76]. There may be associated pancreatic dysfunction, metabolic disorder or developmental delay.

Peripheral blood
Normocytic normochromic or macrocytic anaemia, neutropenia and thrombocytopenia occur in variable combinations. The anaemia may be severe enough to render the child transfusion dependent [77].

Bone marrow cytology
In classical Pearson's syndrome there is dyserythropoiesis with numerous ring sideroblasts and vacuolation of erythroid and granulocytic precursors (Fig. 9.28). However, mitochondrial cytopathies

are heterogeneous and these features have not been described in all cases [77].

Other constitutional abnormalities associated with abnormal haemopoiesis

Down's syndrome may be associated, in the neonatal period, with otherwise unexplained polycythaemia or with transient abnormal myelopoiesis, which represents transient leukaemia [78]. Subsequently there may be trilineage myelodysplasia. The incidence of AML, specifically acute megakaryoblastic leukaemia, is greatly increased.

Griscelli syndrome is a rare fatal disorder with abnormal pigmentation and variable cellular immune deficiency [79]. Pancytopenia is characteristic. The bone marrow may appear normal or there may be lymphohistiocytic infiltration with haemophagocytosis.

Thiamine-responsive anaemia is an autosomal recessive condition that can cause not only megaloblastic anaemia but also pancytopenia with trilineage myelodysplasia. Features include small and hypolobated megakaryocytes, multinucleated megakaryocytes and hypolobated neutrophils [80].

Many inborn errors of metabolism lead to haematological abnormalities but the bone marrow features have often not been described. Isovaleric acidaemia can cause neutropenia, thrombocytopenia and pancytopenia; the bone marrow may show apparent arrest of granulopoiesis at the promyelocyte stage [81].

Paroxysmal nocturnal haemoglobinuria

Paroxysmal nocturnal haemoglobinuria (PNH) is a heterogeneous disease, the essential feature of which is abnormal complement sensitivity of red cells. PNH is a clonal disorder resulting from a somatic mutation in a multipotent myeloid stem cell. In the majority of cases, cells of the abnormal clone coexist with normal polyclonal haemopoietic cells; in a minority the PNH clone constitutes virtually all haemopoietic tissue [82]. The causative mutation occurs in an X-chromosome gene, *PIGA*, which encodes a protein essential for the biosynthesis of glycosyl phosphatidylinositol (GPI). This protein is an important component of the red cell membrane, providing an anchor for many proteins. GPI-anchored proteins include CD55 (a complement-regulatory protein) and CD59. The resulting defect in the red cell membrane leads, *in vitro*, to lysis of cells when serum is acidified and, *in vivo*, to intravascular haemolysis, which is often nocturnal.

Approximately one quarter of cases of PNH evolve to aplastic anaemia [49]. Conversely, 5–10% of patients with aplastic anaemia acquire a PNH clone during the course of their illness, often with associated clinical improvement [49,82]. In a small percentage of cases of PNH there is evolution to AML. The specific PNH defect of red cells leading to a positive acid lysis test has also been observed, occasionally, in patients with other clonal haemopoietic disorders including MDS (refractory anaemia with ring sideroblasts and refractory anaemia with excess of blasts) and myeloproliferative neoplasms (myelofibrosis and unclassified myeloproliferative neoplasm). It is not uncommon for clonal cytogenetic abnormalities to occur in PNH [83]; however, they do not always persist and are not generally predictive of progression to MDS or AML. Recovery of PNH can occur with the abnormal clone disappearing and being replaced by normal polyclonal haemopoietic cells.

The diagnosis of PNH is confirmed by an acid lysis (Ham) test or sugar-water test showing complement sensitivity of red cells. Alternatively, the diagnosis can be confirmed by flow cytometry, using monoclonal antibodies to demonstrate a deficiency of GPI-linked proteins such as CD59.

Peripheral blood

Paroxysmal nocturnal haemoglobinuria is characterized by varying degrees of chronic haemolysis with episodes of more severe haemolysis. Red cells do not show any morphological abnormalities other than polychromasia associated with an elevated reticulocyte count. Some patients have neutropenia, thrombocytopenia or both. Neutrophil alkaline phosphatase activity is typically low or absent.

Bone marrow cytology

The most characteristic bone marrow abnormality is hypercellularity due, at least in part, to erythroid hyperplasia (Fig. 9.29); there is often also granulocytic and megakaryocytic hyperplasia. However, in some patients the specific red cell abnormality of PNH occurs when there is bone marrow hypopla-

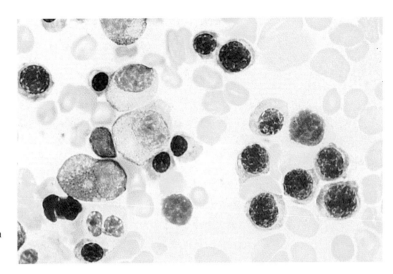

Fig. 9.29 BM aspirate, paroxysmal nocturnal haemoglobinuria, showing erythroid hyperplasia and a somewhat abnormal chromatin pattern. MGG ×100.

sia. Haemopoietic cells may be cytologically normal or may show dysplastic features; if present, dysplasia is usually milder than in MDS but there is some overlap [83]. Mast cells may be increased.

Bone marrow histology

Trephine biopsy sections may show erythroid hyperplasia or generalized hypoplasia.

Bone marrow and other haemopoietic stem cell transplantation

Allogeneic haemopoietic stem cells suitable for transplantation may be obtained by bone marrow aspiration from volunteer donors. Alternatively, they may be obtained from cord blood or may be harvested from peripheral blood, following stimulation by growth factors such as G-CSF. Since stem cell transplantation necessitates prior immunosuppression, and often also ablative chemotherapy, the haematological features of bone marrow aplasia precede the signs of stem cell engraftment. Stem cell transplantation may be complicated by a variety of pathological processes [84] including sepsis, rejection and graft-versus-host disease. ABO-incompatible transplantation can be followed by pure red cell aplasia (Fig. 9.30). Infection with CMV [85] and human herpesvirus 6 [86] post-transplant can cause bone marrow hypoplasia leading to pancytopenia. EBV-induced lymphoproliferative disease (see page 399) occurs but is

uncommon in comparison with the incidence following solid organ transplantation; it occurs in about 1% of stem cell transplant recipients. Chronic parvovirus B19-induced red cell aplasia may develop as a consequence of post-transplant immune deficiency. In the early post-transplant period there is hyposplenism. Post-transplant there is also an increased incidence of autoimmune thrombocytopenic purpura (often associated with chronic graft-versus-host disease), autoimmune neutropenia, autoimmune haemolytic anaemia and Evans syndrome [87]. Microangiopathic haemolytic anaemia is also observed in some patients, occurring as a result of endothelial damage caused by ciclosporin or other agents.

Autologous stem cell transplantation may lead to some of the same pathological processes that follow allogeneic stem cell transplantation, since there is a period of bone marrow aplasia and immune deficiency, but graft-versus-host disease does not occur.

Post-transplantation, a bone marrow trephine biopsy is generally more informative than the peripheral blood film or bone marrow aspirate.

Peripheral blood

Initially there is a period of 2–3 weeks of severe pancytopenia, followed by a gradual rise of white cell and platelet counts as engraftment occurs. If there is failure of engraftment or if rejection occurs there is a failure of counts to rise or a subsequent

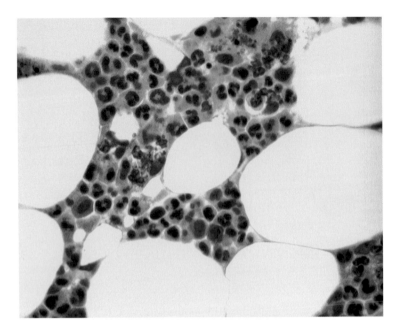

Fig. 9.30 BM trephine biopsy section from patient with red cell aplasia following an ABO incompatible allogeneic bone marrow transplant. There is a striking absence of erythroid precursors and large numbers of apoptotic cells within the macrophages. Paraffin-embedded, H&E ×40.

fall. Features of hyposplenism may be present. Those who develop autoimmune complications or microangiopathic haemolytic anaemia show the expected peripheral blood features. If patients develop EBV-induced lymphoproliferative disease following transplantation the peripheral blood film may be leucoerythroblastic and show atypical lymphoid cells.

Bone marrow cytology

The bone marrow aspirate is initially severely hypoplastic. Subsequently, haemopoietic cells gradually reappear. Dysplastic features, particularly dyserythropoiesis, may be present [88]. In the months following transplantation an appreciable increase may occur in haematogones, lymphoid cells which morphologically and immuno-phenotypically resemble lymphoblasts of French–American–British (FAB) L1 ALL [89]; with prolonged follow-up these are no longer apparent. If rejection occurs the abnormalities noted include lymphocytosis, plasmacytosis, increased macrophages and increased iron stores [84]. If chronic parvovirus infection occurs, the bone marrow aspirate shows a lack of erythroid cells beyond the proerythroblast stage. EBV-induced lymphoproliferative disease is associated with bone marrow infiltration by highly atypical lymphoid cells including bizarre plasmacytoid lymphocytes. Patients with failure to engraft, particularly but not exclusively those treated with granulocyte–macrophage colony-stimulating factor (GM-CSF), may have an increase of foamy histiocytes in a hypocellular marrow [90]. When autoimmune complications occur, the expected erythroid or megakaryocytic hyperplasia may be seen but this is dependent on adequate haemopoietic reconstitution.

Bone marrow histology [84,91–93]

The speed of haemopoietic regeneration depends on the type of transplantation; engraftment is much more rapid after transplantation of autologous peripheral blood stem cells, least rapid after allografting from unrelated donors and intermediate with allografts from related donors. In general, during the first 2 weeks cellularity is very low. Thereafter, clusters of proliferating cells appear at a variable rate. In the early stages of engraftment, foci of regenerating cells commonly contain cells of only one lineage and cells may be all at the same stage of development. The topography may be abnormal, with foci of granulocyte precursors present in the intertrabecular area rather than in a paratrabecular position. Megakaryocytes are often

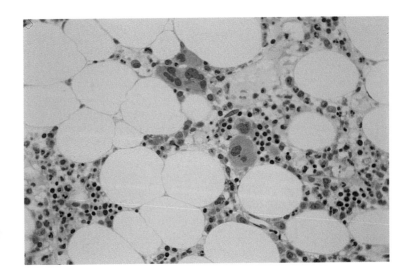

Fig. 9.31 BM trephine biopsy section showing regeneration following bone marrow transplantation; note the cluster of megakaryocytes. Resin-embedded, H&E ×20.

clustered (Fig. 9.31). Haemopoietic cells may be dysplastic. Often there are stromal changes such as oedema, the presence of foamy macrophages, formation of small granulomas, sinusoidal ectasia and extravasation of red cells into the interstitium; these abnormalities are probably a result of damage caused by the ablative therapy employed prior to grafting and are more marked in patients transplanted for leukaemia. There may also be lymphoid foci, sometimes with associated eosinophils. Plasma cells may be increased in patients who have had a stem cell transplant for acute leukaemia. In patients with increased reticulin or collagen, there is gradual stromal remodelling with a return to normal or near normal appearances. If rejection occurs, the trephine biopsy sections may show oedema and fat necrosis, in addition to the features apparent in the aspirate that have been mentioned above. There may be small foci of lymphoblast-like cells. A hypoplastic bone marrow biopsy specimen post-transplant may result from failure of engraftment, infection by herpesviruses or stromal damage resulting from graft-versus-host disease. Selective loss of maturing red cells is seen in parvovirus B19-induced chronic pure red cell aplasia.

Problems and pitfalls
Patients who have had an autologous stem cell transplant show an increased incidence of MDS as a result of damage to stem cells by preceding chem-

otherapy. However, the diagnosis of MDS should be made with circumspection since disturbed architecture and dysplastic features are common in the early post-transplant period. Cytogenetic and molecular genetic analysis can be useful in making the distinction.

In patients transplanted for ALL, a post-transplant excess of haematogones must be distinguished from relapse. Immunophenotyping and cytogenetic and molecular genetic analysis can be useful in making the distinction.

In patients transplanted for multiple myeloma (plasma cell myeloma), increased monoclonal plasma cells are often present in the first 1–2 months after transplantation. These represent residual myeloma cells rather than relapse and are not predictive of disease progression [94].

Graft-versus-host disease (including the effects of donor-lymphocyte infusion)
Graft-versus-host disease (GVHD) occurs not only in the setting of stem cell transplantation but also when viable, immunocompetent, histo-incompatible lymphocytes have been transferred to an immuno-incompetent host. This may occur *in utero*, when there is transfer of maternal lymphocytes to a fetus with severe combined immune deficiency. Following birth, it can occur following blood transfusion in congenital and certain acquired

immune deficiency states. It has been recognized in patients being treated for Hodgkin lymphoma and in patients with low grade lymphoproliferative disorders who have received treatment with nucleoside analogues such as fludarabine.

Graft-versus-host disease can also occur when blood for transfusion was derived from a donor who was homozygous for a human leucocyte antigen (HLA) haplotype identical to one of the host's haplotypes; the host is then unable to recognize the recipient's lymphocytes as foreign and so cannot destroy them, whereas the transfused lymphocytes are capable of recognizing and attacking host tissues. GVHD in immunologically normal hosts has most often resulted from transfusions from closely related family members.

Donor-lymphocyte transfusion, increasingly practised for post-transplant relapse of chronic granulocytic leukaemia or other haemopoietic neoplasms, can also be complicated by GVHD. Inadvertent transfer of donor lymphocytes following solid organ transplantation has also led to GVHD [95].

The bone marrow features of GVHD differ depending on whether bone marrow has been transplanted or not. When viable lymphocytes only have been transferred the host's bone marrow will be among the tissues that come under immunological attack and bone marrow aplasia results. In patients who have received donor bone marrow containing viable lymphocytes other tissues are attacked but since the bone marrow is donor in origin it will not be recognized as foreign by donor lymphocytes. The haemopoietic marrow may, however, be indirectly damaged by the immunological reaction between donor cells and host cells, including those of the bone marrow stroma. This damage may be severe with necrosis of haemopoietic cells and stroma, oedema and haemorrhage [29].

It was previously suggested that Omenn syndrome, a condition of infants characterized by combined immunodeficiency and signs suggestive of GVHD, might represent GVHD consequent on transplacental passage of lymphocytes [96]. However, this condition is now known to be an inherited disorder resulting from a mutation in one of the recombination activating genes, *RAG1* and *RAG2* [97].

Peripheral blood

In patients who have received histo-incompatible donor lymphocytes the consequent bone marrow hypoplasia is reflected in peripheral blood pancytopenia. In bone marrow transplant recipients there are no specific peripheral blood features that indicate the occurrence of GVHD but there is a delay in the appearance of signs of engraftment.

Bone marrow cytology

The bone marrow aspirate is usually hypocellular. In patients who have received a stem cell transplant, bone marrow eosinophils of more than 7% have been found predictive of acute GVHD [98].

Bone marrow histology

When donor lymphocytes have been transferred without donor bone marrow, histological sections of trephine biopsies show aplasia. In GVHD in the setting of bone marrow transplantation, histological abnormalities include a decrease in haemopoietic cells, increased macrophages, erythrophagocytosis, oedema and perivenous lymphoid infiltrates [91].

Effects of haemopoietic growth factors and other cytokines

An increasing number of haemopoietic growth factors and other cytokines are being administered to patients. Haematological effects are often profound.

Peripheral blood

Administration of G-CSF and GM-CSF causes neutrophilia and monocytosis with a marked left shift, 'toxic' granulation, neutrophil vacuolation and a variety of dysplastic changes in neutrophils including abnormal neutrophil lobulation and the presence of macropolycytes. Blast cells may appear in the blood following G-CSF therapy [99]. GM-CSF causes more marked monocytosis than G-CSF and can also cause eosinophilia. In patients with MDS, the administration of G-CSF can be associated with the appearance of significant numbers of myeloblasts in the peripheral blood [100]. Neutrophilia is induced by various interleukins (IL1, IL2, IL3 and IL6) and by stem cell factor [101]. Eosinophilia is induced by IL2, IL3 and IL5. Lymphocytosis is induced by IL2, IL3, IL6, IL11 and thrombopoietin

[102]. Thrombocytosis is induced by IL1, IL3, IL6 and thrombopoietin. Thrombopoietin administration may also cause megakaryocytes to appear in the peripheral blood [103]. The administration of IL2 leads to anaemia and thrombocytopenia and IL6 and IL11 [104] also cause anaemia. Erythropoietin administration raises the haemoglobin concentration as a result of erythroid hyperplasia.

Bone marrow cytology

Administration of G-CSF and GM-CSF causes a marked left shift of granulopoiesis. This is particularly prominent when these cytokines are administered to patients with suppressed bone marrow function. Myeloblasts may reach 20–40% and promyelocytes 12–60% leading to possible confusion with FAB M2 and M3 categories of AML [105]. In haematologically normal subjects, G-CSF causes a marked increase in cellularity and an increase of all cells of neutrophil lineage [106]; the greatest increase is in promyelocytes and myelocytes. Morphological alterations include increased granularity, particularly of early cells, and an increased prevalence of ring neutrophils [106]. GM-CSF can cause a marked increase in macrophage numbers and its administration has been associated with the development of a haemophagocytic syndrome [107]. The administration of IL5 causes an increase in bone marrow eosinophils. Stem cell factor causes some increase in cellularity with increased promyelocytes and, in some cases, increased basophils and mast cells [101]. Administration of thrombopoietin (in the form of pegylated recombinant human thrombopoietin, now withdrawn) led to increased numbers of large megakaryocytes with increased nuclear lobation and abundant cytoplasm [102].

Bone marrow histology

The bone marrow following administration of G-CSF and GM-CSF may be hypocellular, normocellular or hypercellular, depending on the underlying disease and prior therapy. There is granulocytic hyperplasia, left-shifted granulopoiesis and expansion of the paratrabecular zone of neutrophil precursors (Fig. 9.32). There may be aggregates of granulocyte precursors [105] resembling ALIP seen in MDS. Administration of thrombopoietin increases megakaryocyte numbers, size and nuclear lobation [102] and leads to megakaryocyte clustering with increased reticulin deposition (Fig. 9.33). In another study, administration of thrombopoietin was found to be associated with atypical megakaryocytes including small hypolobated forms and cells with hyperchromatic nuclei, as well as large hyperlobated forms [103]. In addition, in some patients, administration of thrombopoietin was associated

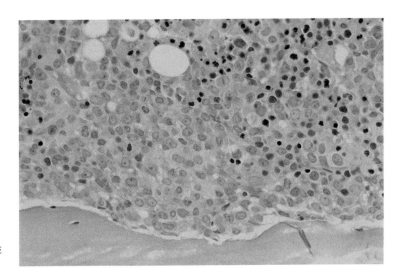

Fig. 9.32 BM trephine biopsy specimen from a patient receiving G-CSF showing an expanded paratrabecular seam of neutrophil precursors. Paraffin-embedded, H&E ×40.

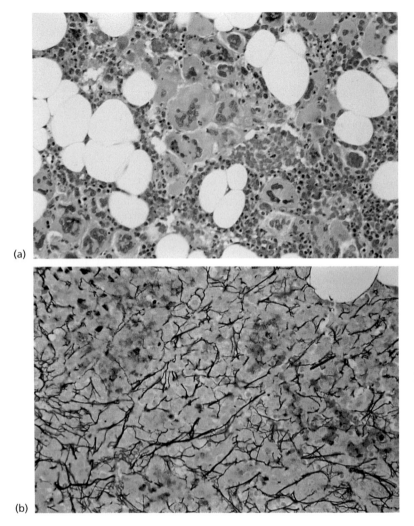

(a)

(b)

Fig. 9.33 BM trephine biopsy specimen from a patient receiving thrombopoietin showing: (a) a marked increase in megakaryocytes which are pleomorphic and forming clusters; (b) increased reticulin deposition. Both abnormalities reversed on cessation of therapy. (a) Paraffin-embedded, H&E ×20. (b) Paraffin-embedded, reticulin stain ×20.

with increased mitoses in megakaryocytes, increased emperipolesis, intrasinusoidal megakaryocytes and new bone formation [103].

Problems and pitfalls

When blast cells appear in the peripheral blood in response to G-CSF therapy there are usually other granulocyte precursors present and maturing cells show 'toxic' changes such as heavy granulation. These blast cells also show some immunophenotypic differences from leukaemic myeloblasts [99]. They express CD34 but not terminal deoxynu-

cleotidyl transferase, coexpress CD19 and express CD13 and CD33 weakly [99].

In patients receiving G-CSF following induction therapy for AML, an increased blast cell percentage may be misinterpreted as persisting leukaemia [108]. G-CSF can also increase the blast cell percentage in MDS so that AML is simulated [100,109].

An adequate clinical history should prevent ALIP resulting from G-CSF therapy leading to a misdiagnosis of MDS and, similarly, should prevent the changes induced by thrombopoietin from being misinterpreted as a myeloproliferative neoplasm.

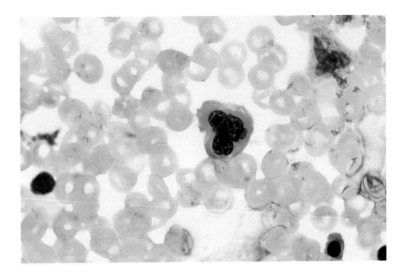

Fig. 9.34 BM aspirate showing dyserythropoiesis in protein-calorie malnutrition. MGG ×100. (By courtesy of the late Professor S. N. Wickramasinghe, London.)

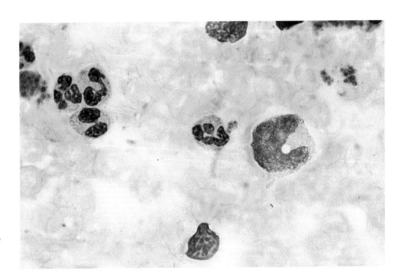

Fig. 9.35 BM aspirate showing a giant metamyelocyte in a patient with protein-calorie malnutrition. MGG ×100. (By courtesy of the late Professor S. N. Wickramasinghe, London.)

Protein-calorie malnutrition and calorie deficiency

Peripheral blood

Protein-calorie malnutrition (kwashiorkor or marasmus) is not usually associated with deficiency of specific haematinics such as iron, vitamin B_{12} or folate but, nevertheless, anaemia occurs. Red cells are normocytic and normochromic. The white cell and platelet counts may also be reduced. Severely reduced calorie intake, as in anorexia nervosa, is associated with mild anaemia, lymphopenia, neutropenia and thrombocytopenia; the blood film may show small numbers of acanthocytes.

Bone marrow cytology

The bone marrow in protein-calorie malnutrition usually shows reduced cellularity with normoblastic but dyserythropoietic haemopoiesis (Fig. 9.34). Giant metamyelocytes (Fig. 9.35) are common, even in the majority of cases which have normoblastic erythropoiesis. There is vacuolation of erythroid and granulocyte precursors. Dysmegakaryopoiesis is uncommon. Iron stores are normal or increased. There may be abnormal sideroblasts including ring sideroblasts. In anorexia nervosa, the bone marrow is hypocellular and may show gelatinous transformation.

Storage diseases and storage cells in the bone marrow [110–114]

In various inherited diseases the deficiency of an enzyme leads to accumulation of a metabolite in body cells, often in macrophages. The morphologically abnormal bone marrow macrophages, containing an excess of the relevant metabolite, are referred to as storage cells. Storage cells may also result from an abnormal load of a metabolite such that the enzymes of normal cells are unable to cope. Both bone marrow aspiration and trephine biopsy are useful in the detection of storage diseases. Peripheral blood cells may show related abnormalities [110,115].

Gaucher's disease
Gaucher's disease (hereditary glucosyl ceramide lipidosis) is an inherited condition in which glucocerebrosides accumulate in macrophages including those in the liver, spleen and bone marrow. Although Gaucher's disease can be readily diagnosed by bone marrow aspiration and by trephine

biopsy it has been pointed out that this is unnecessary when assays for the relevant enzyme, β-glucocerebrosidase, are available [116]. Gaucher's disease can be transferred to graft recipients by bone marrow transplantation [117].

Peripheral blood
There are usually no specific peripheral blood features although very occasionally Gaucher's cells may be seen in the peripheral blood, particularly after splenectomy. Pancytopenia develops slowly, as a consequence of hypersplenism. The monocytes of patients with Gaucher's disease are positive for tartrate-resistant acid phosphatase (TRAP) activity, whereas normal monocytes are not [114].

Bone marrow cytology
Gaucher cells are large, round or oval cells with a small, usually eccentric nucleus and voluminous weakly basophilic cytoplasm with a wrinkled or fibrillar pattern (Fig. 9.36). The fibrillar or striated appearance is the result of elongation of lysosomes. Gaucher cells may show extensive erythrophagocytosis [118]. These cells stain with Sudan black B (SBB) and periodic acid–Schiff (PAS). They are non-specific esterase and TRAP positive and may be positive for iron, particularly in older children and adults. Patients with Gaucher's disease may also have an increase in foamy macrophages and

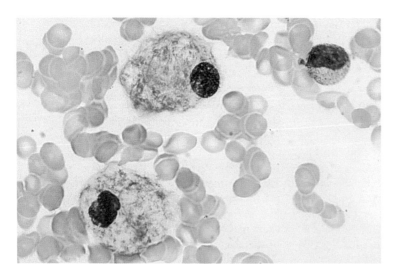

Fig. 9.36 BM aspirate, Gaucher's disease, showing two Gaucher cells. MGG ×100.

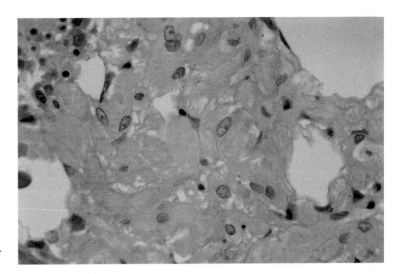

Fig. 9.37 BM trephine biopsy section, Gaucher's disease, showing a sheet of large macrophages with characteristic 'watered silk' texture to their cytoplasm. Resin-embedded, H&E ×40.

in cells that resemble typical Gaucher cells but have more strongly basophilic granules.

Bone marrow histology

Gaucher cells may be isolated or appear in clumps or sheets, sometimes replacing large areas of the marrow (Fig. 9.37). The cells have abundant pale-staining cytoplasm with a texture that has been likened to watered silk or crumpled tissue paper. The fibrillar pattern is accentuated by PAS staining. A Perls' stain is often positive, even in decalcified specimens. There may be an increase in reticulin and collagen deposition [114]. In advanced disease, osteolytic lesions occur [119]. Gaucher cells are strongly positive with an immunohistochemical stain for TRAP [119] but it is usually sufficient to confirm their macrophage origin by staining for CD68R.

Treatment with glucocerebrosidase leads to reduction in the number of Gaucher cells and improvement of haemopoiesis but in one study was associated with an unexpected increase in osteopenia [120].

Pseudo-Gaucher cells

Cells resembling Gaucher cells, but not identical to them on ultrastructural examination [111], are seen in the bone marrow in a variety of haematological conditions [112,113] in which they result from an abnormal load of glucocerebroside

presented to macrophages. In contrast to Gaucher cells, which are often positive for iron, pseudo-Gaucher cells are negative [121]. They are seen in chronic granulocytic leukaemia (Fig. 9.38), chronic neutrophilic leukaemia [122], acute leukaemia, occasional cases of MDS [123], thalassaemia major and congenital dyserythropoietic anaemia (particularly type II). They have also been recognized in occasional patients with Hodgkin lymphoma, non-Hodgkin lymphoma and a variety of other conditions [112,124]. They have been reported as a consequence of repeated platelet transfusions [125].

Problems and pitfalls

If there is any difficulty distinguishing pseudo-Gaucher cells from Gaucher cells it is possible to assay β-glucosidase in peripheral blood leucocytes.

Cells resembling Gaucher cells have been seen in multiple myeloma and in lymphoplasmacytic or immunoblastic lymphoma but the macrophages in these cases contain material derived from immunoglobulin rather than glucocerebroside and are better regarded as crystal-storing histiocytosis [124,126]. Cells considered to resemble Gaucher cells have also been reported in the bone marrow of a patient with atypical mycobacterial infection complicating AIDS [127]; in this case it appears that the abnormal morphology was consequent on large numbers of mycobacteria packing the macrophage

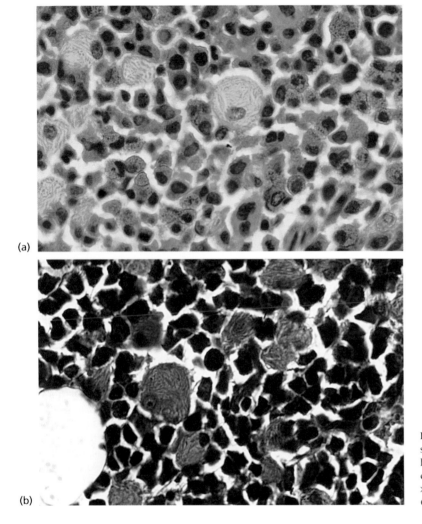

(a)

(b)

Fig. 9.38 BM trephine biopsy section in chronic granulocytic leukaemia showing pseudo-Gaucher cells. (a) Paraffin-embedded, H&E ×100. (b) Paraffin-embedded, Giemsa stain ×100.

cytoplasm rather than on storage of a metabolic breakdown product. Similar appearances have been reported in an immunosuppressed patient who had received a renal transplant [128]. The distinction is easily made with a stain for acid-fast bacilli.

Crystal-storing histiocytosis
Macrophages containing immunoglobulin crystals in the lysosomal compartment can be observed in patients with lymphoplasmacytic lymphoma, myeloma and other conditions associated with the presence of a paraprotein [124,126]. On light microscopy they can resemble Gaucher cells. There appears to be a strong association with κ light chains [129]; there is no specific heavy chain association although immunoglobulin M has been observed most often.

Niemann–Pick disease
Niemann–Pick disease is an inherited condition (sphingomyelin lipidosis) caused by reduced sphingomyelinase activity (type I), or a related ill-defined defect of cholesterol esterification (type II). It is

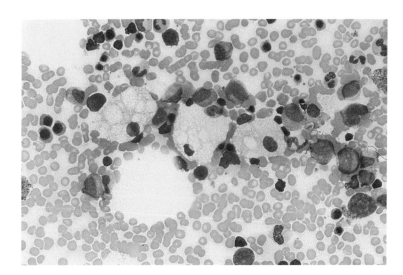

Fig. 9.39 BM aspirate, Niemann–Pick disease, showing foamy macrophages. MGG ×40. (By courtesy of Dr S. G. Davis, Birmingham.)

characterized by the presence of foamy lipid-containing macrophages in the bone marrow and other tissues.

Peripheral blood

Lipid-containing monocytes and lymphocytes may be present in the peripheral blood. Anaemia and various cytopenias may occur as a consequence of hypersplenism.

Bone marrow cytology

The foamy macrophages of Niemann–Pick disease are large cells (exceeding 50 µm in diameter) with a nucleus that is usually central. They stain pale blue with Romanowsky stains (Fig. 9.39) and variably with PAS and lipid stains. They may contain lamellated cytoplasmic inclusions [130]. There are also increased numbers of sea-blue histiocytes (see below), possibly reflecting slow conversion of sphingomyelin to ceroid [112].

Bone marrow histology

Foamy macrophages may appear bluish when stained with Giemsa and are light brown or pink in haematoxylin and eosin (H&E)-stained sections (Fig. 9.40); they are PAS positive and may be positive for iron [114]. Inclusion bodies are demonstrated within foamy macrophages; on ultrastructural examination they are osmiophilic electron-dense structures [130].

Other causes of foamy macrophages

Other metabolic defects that can lead to the presence of increased numbers of foamy macrophages in the bone marrow [113] include familial hypercholesterolaemia [131], hyperchylomicronaemia, Wolman's disease (Fig. 9.41), late-onset cholesteryl ester storage disease, Fabry's disease, neuronal lipofucsinosis (Batten's disease), Tangier disease and acquired hypercholesterolaemia, e.g. Zieve's syndrome (see Fig. 9.20). In Fabry's disease the storage cells have small globular inclusions which are weakly basophilic with a Romanowsky stain and lightly eosinophilic with H&E; they are PAS and SBB positive [132].

Foam cells are also increased as a result of damage to fat cells (Fig. 9.42) from, for example, trauma, fat necrosis, bone marrow infarction, infection, pancreatitis and recent performance of a bone marrow biopsy at the same site [133]. Acquired diseases that have been associated with an increase of foamy macrophages include Langerhans cell histiocytosis (Hand–Schüller–Christian disease, Letterer–Siwe disease and eosinophilic granuloma), bone marrow metastases (Fig. 9.43), sickle cell disease (see Fig. 8.23) and a variety of other conditions [112]. Foamy cells have been noted in subjects who have, in the past, received polyvinyl pyrrolidine as a plasma expander; they contain amorphous grey-blue material and are PAS, mucicarmine and Congo red positive [133–136]. In

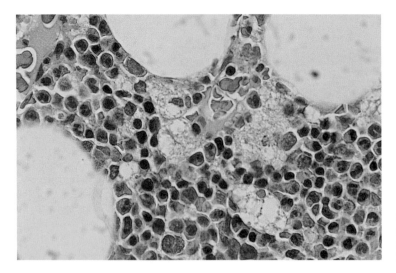

Fig. 9.40 BM trephine biopsy section, Niemann–Pick disease, showing foamy macrophages. Paraffin-embedded, H&E ×50.

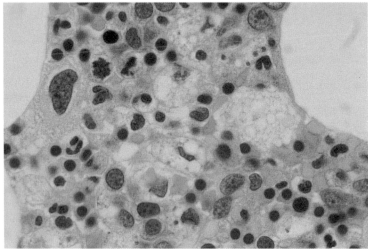

Fig. 9.41 BM trephine biopsy section, Wolman's disease showing foamy macrophages. Paraffin-embedded, H&E ×100.

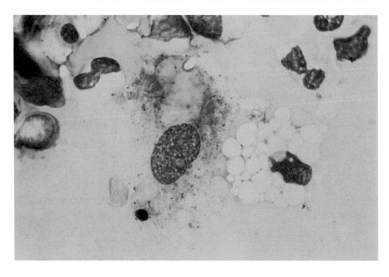

Fig. 9.42 BM aspirate, sickle cell anaemia, showing a foamy macrophage and a sea-blue histiocyte containing a clump of red cells. MGG ×100.

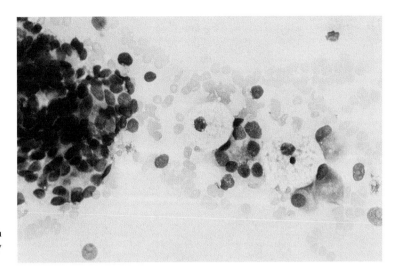

Fig. 9.43 BM aspirate, carcinoma of prostate, showing a clump of carcinoma cells, dispersed carcinoma cells, two osteoblasts and two foamy macrophages. MGG ×40.

trephine biopsy sections, reticulin is increased [136]. Occasionally the foamy cell infiltration is so heavy that bone marrow failure occurs [136]. Foamy ceroid-containing macrophages (see below) are seen in patients on prolonged intravenous nutrition with lipid emulsions [137].

Macrophages containing cholesterol crystals

Bone marrow macrophages may contain cholesterol crystals in various hyperlipidaemic conditions, both congenital and acquired. Such conditions include α-lipoprotein deficiency, hyperbetalipoproteinaemia, poorly controlled diabetes mellitus and hypothyroidism [29]. The cholesterol crystals are soluble and thus give rise to unstained needle-like clefts within the macrophages.

Sea-blue histiocytosis

The terms 'sea-blue histiocytosis' [138] and 'ceroid lipofucsinosis' [139] encompass an inherited group of conditions characterized by the presence of 'sea-blue histiocytes' – distinctive macrophages containing ceroid or lipofucsin – in the bone marrow, liver, spleen and other organs. The designation of the disease derives from the staining characteristics of the storage cells with Romanowsky stains. In unstained films, ceroid is brown. The inherited conditions causing increased numbers of sea-blue histiocytes include the Hermansky–Pudlak syndrome (oculo-cutaneous albinism with a bleeding

diathesis) and Niemann–Pick syndrome (in addition to the more typical storage cells).

Bone marrow cytology

Sea-blue histiocytes stain blue or blue-green with Romanowsky stains. They are SBB, PAS and oil red O positive and are sometimes positive for iron. With ultraviolet illumination they exhibit yellow-green autofluorescence.

Bone marrow histology

Sea-blue histiocytes are brownish yellow with H&E and blue with a Giemsa stain. They are PAS positive and positive for iron. Their cytoplasmic contents are acid fast and exhibit autofluorescence.

Other causes of sea-blue histiocytes

Increased numbers of sea-blue histiocytes are seen in the bone marrow in a great variety of conditions [138], including many of the same disorders in which pseudo-Gaucher cells are present or foamy macrophages are increased (Figs 9.42, 9.44 and 9.45). Most of these conditions are characterized by an increased turnover of bone marrow cells (e.g. myeloproliferative neoplasms, autoimmune thrombocytopenic purpura). There is also an association with hyperlipidaemia. Less often there is an exogenous cause, as in prolonged intravenous nutrition with fat emulsions [137] or sodium valproate administration [140].

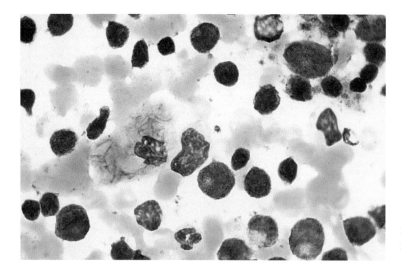

Fig. 9.44 BM aspirate from a patient with AML showing a sea-blue histiocyte. MGG ×100.

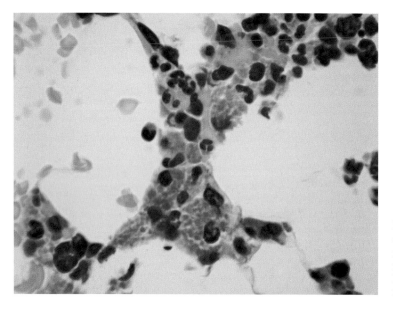

Fig. 9.45 BM trephine biopsy section from a patient with polycythaemia vera showing numerous sea-blue histiocytes. Paraffin-embedded, Giemsa stain ×50.

Cystinosis

Peripheral blood

There are no specific abnormalities in the peripheral blood. Progressive pancytopenia can occur [141].

Bone marrow cytology

Bone marrow macrophages are packed with almost colourless, refractile crystals of various shapes.

They are best seen under polarized light when they are birefringent but are also readily apparent with normal illumination (Fig. 9.46). Bone marrow aspiration has sometimes confirmed a provisional diagnosis of cystinosis when other diagnostic measures were negative [142].

Bone marrow histology

Crystals are colourless and in histological sections appear as a negative image (Figs 9.47 and 9.48).

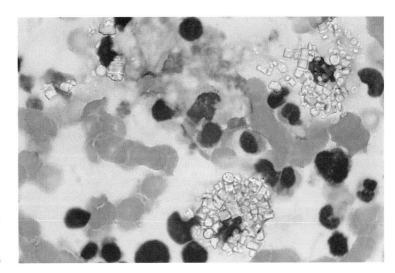

Fig. 9.46 BM aspirate from a patient with cystinosis showing two macrophages containing colourless cystine crystals. MGG ×100. (Courtesy of Dr J. Yin, Manchester.)

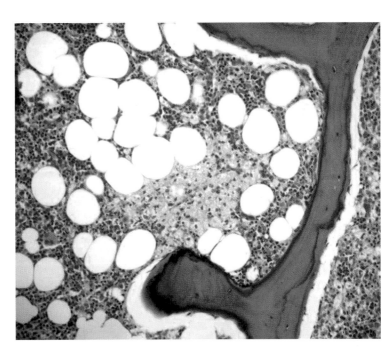

Fig. 9.47 BM trephine biopsy section from a patient with cystinosis showing an aggregate of macrophages containing cystine crystals. Paraffin-embedded, H&E ×20. (Courtesy of Dr Venetia Bigley, Middlesbrough.)

They are birefringent under polarized light [143].

Hyperoxaluria

Hyperoxaluria or oxalosis [144–146] is a metabolic disorder in which oxalate is deposited in various tissues including the bone, bone marrow, liver, spleen and kidneys. Renal deposition leads to renal failure. The introduction of haemodialysis has prolonged life in these patients and has permitted advanced bone marrow lesions to become apparent.

Peripheral blood

There is anaemia as a consequence of renal failure. Hypersplenism also contributes to anaemia and

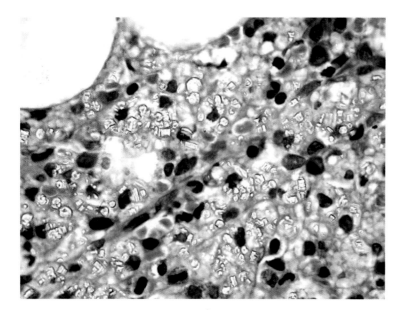

Fig. 9.48 BM trephine biopsy section from a patient with cystinosis showing an aggregate of macrophages containing cystine crystals, which are birefringent under polarized light. Paraffin-embedded, H&E ×100. (Courtesy of Dr Venetia Bigley, Middlesbrough and the *British Journal of Haematology*.)

may cause pancytopenia. Deposition of oxalate in the bone marrow further aggravates anaemia and other cytopenias and causes a leucoerythroblastic blood film.

Bone marrow biopsy

Intertrabecular bone marrow is extensively replaced by needle-like crystals arranged in a radial pattern (Fig. 9.49). There are variable numbers of epithelioid and multinucleated macrophages, including foreign body giant cells, at the periphery of the crystalline deposits and engulfing crystals. The surrounding bone marrow shows mild fibrosis.

Mucopolysaccharidoses

The mucopolysaccharidoses are inherited diseases characterized by the storage of various mucopolysaccharides [110]. They are consequent on a deficiency of one of the lysosomal enzymes needed to degrade mucopolysaccharide.

Peripheral blood

Peripheral blood neutrophils may show the Alder–Reilly anomaly (prominent granules) [110,115]. Lymphocytes may either be vacuolated or contain abnormal granules which stain metachromatically with toluidine blue.

Bone marrow cytology

Bone marrow granulocytes may contain inclusions similar to those observed in the peripheral blood. Similar inclusions have been observed in plasma cells. Bone marrow macrophages also contain abnormal metachromatic granules [110] (Fig. 9.50). Inclusions within vacuoles have been observed in osteoblasts in type VII mucopolysaccharidosis (β-glucuronidase deficiency) [147].

Bone marrow histology

In histological preparations, macrophages appear foamy since mucopolysaccharides are water soluble. Abnormal macrophages may be scattered between haemopoietic cells or in small clusters.

Glycogen storage disease

Periodic acid–Schiff-positive inclusions have been observed in osteoblasts in Pompe's disease (type II glycogen storage disease, acid maltase deficiency) [148].

Sinus histiocytosis with massive lymphadenopathy (Rosai–Dorfman disease)

Sinus histiocytosis with massive lymphadenopathy is a rare condition of unknown aetiology characterized by lymphophagocytic macrophages.

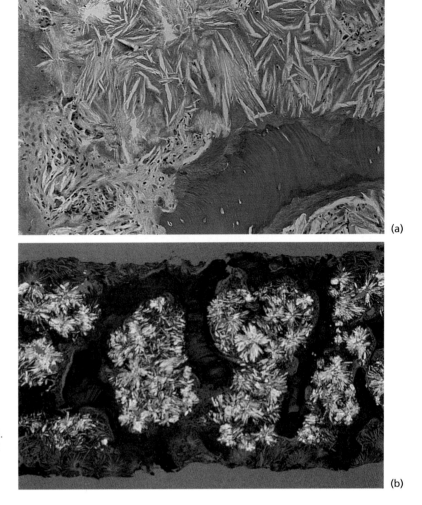

(a)

(b)

Fig. 9.49 BM trephine biopsy sections in oxalosis. (a) Paraffin-embedded, H&E ×10. (b) Paraffin-embedded, with polarized light ×2.5. (By courtesy of Dr M. J. Walter and Dr C. V. Dang, Johns Hopkins University School of Medicine, Baltimore.)

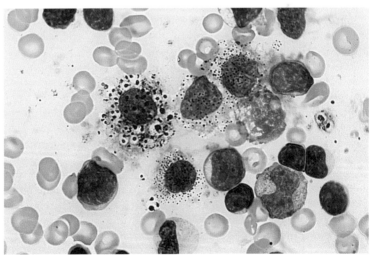

Fig. 9.50 BM aspirate, Sanfilippo syndrome, showing cells containing abnormal granules. MGG ×100. (By courtesy of Dr. R. Brunning, Minneapolis.)

Involvement of the bone marrow is very uncommon. There is a hypercellular marrow with plasmacytosis and large aggregates of S100-positive macrophages containing lymphocytes, neutrophils, erythrocytes and occasional plasma cells [149].

Deposition of foreign substances

Foreign substances may be deposited in the bone marrow, principally in bone marrow macrophages. Such substances may be apparent in bone marrow aspirates and in trephine biopsy sections. There are not usually any associated peripheral blood abnormalities.

In anthracosis there is widespread deposition of carbon pigment in body macrophages, including those of the bone marrow. Large aggregates of dense black particles are apparent [150]. Silica and anthracotic pigment are often co-deposited. Silica crystals are detected by their birefringence. There may be resultant granuloma formation.

Occasional patients are still seen who have, in the past, been exposed to Thorotrast as a radiographic medium. Thorotrast within macrophages appears as pale grey refractile material (see Fig. 10.30). Bone marrow abnormalities associated with the presence of Thorotrast include hypoplasia, hyperplasia, fibrosis and the development of MDS, acute leukaemia and haemangioendothelioma [151]. The peripheral blood film may be bizarre because of the combined effects of bone marrow fibrosis and Thorotrast-induced splenic atrophy.

Vascular and intravascular lesions [113,152]

The bone marrow vasculature may be altered as a consequence of bone marrow diseases but, in addition, blood vessels within the marrow, particularly arterioles and capillaries, may be involved in a variety of generalized diseases. The peripheral blood film may show related abnormalities but in general a bone marrow aspirate does not give relevant information and a trephine biopsy is necessary.

Peripheral blood

The peripheral blood shows red cell fragments in patients with thrombotic thrombocytopenic purpura or with microangiopathic haemolytic anaemia as a consequence of disseminated malignancy. Eosinophilia may be a feature of some types

of vasculitis and also of cholesterol embolism, which may involve the marrow as well as other tissues. Leucocytosis and an elevated erythrocyte sedimentation rate have also been associated with cholesterol embolism. The peripheral blood film may show pancytopenia and leucoerythroblastic features in patients with bone marrow necrosis as a consequence of vascular occlusion.

Bone marrow cytology

There are no specific abnormalities in the bone marrow aspirate in patients with vascular lesions.

Bone marrow histology

In patients with generalized arteriosclerosis, the bone marrow arterioles may show arteriosclerotic changes. In people with atherosclerosis, embolism of atheromatous material to bone marrow vessels may occur; the embolus may be acellular or composed of hyaline material or cholesterol crystals [153,154] (Fig. 9.51). Emboli are found in the bone marrow at autopsy in about 10% of patients with generalized cholesterol embolism [153]. Vessels are partly or totally occluded by this material and by the granulomatous tissue that develops as a reaction to it. Any cholesterol crystals appear as empty clefts. There may be foreign body giant cells in addition to macrophages, together with fibrosis and new bone formation simulating bone marrow metastases [155]. Vasculitic lesions can be seen in polyarteritis nodosa, with fibrinoid necrosis being a feature. Lesions of giant cell arteritis may show not only epithelioid macrophages but also foreign body giant cells in the inflamed vessels [156]. In patients with hypersensitivity reactions to drugs, a granulomatous vasculitis may occur. Patients with vasculitis may show granulocytic hyperplasia with both neutrophils and eosinophils being increased. Intravascular and subendothelial hyaline deposits may be seen in bone marrow capillaries in thrombotic thrombocytopenic purpura and there may be associated platelet thrombi. In patients with microangiopathic haemolytic anaemia as a consequence of disseminated carcinoma, the bone marrow capillaries, like other capillaries, may contain tumour thrombi. Thrombi may also be seen in patients with thrombophilia, e.g. in patients with anti-cardiolipin antibodies (Fig. 9.52). In patients with sickle cell disease, sickle cells are usually present in sinusoids.

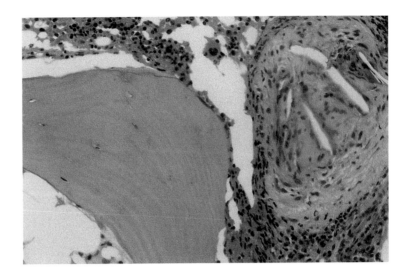

Fig. 9.51 BM trephine biopsy section showing a cholesterol embolus; cholesterol crystals are seen as negative images. Paraffin-embedded, H&E ×20.

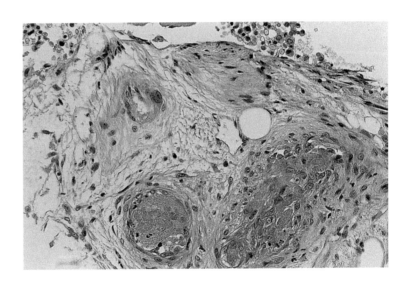

Fig. 9.52 BM trephine biopsy section from a patient with an anti-cardiolipin antibody showing thrombi in bone marrow vessels. Paraffin-embedded, H&E ×20.

During sickling crises there may also be thrombotic lesions and associated areas of bone marrow necrosis. Sickle cells may also be present in autopsy specimens from patients with sickle cell trait; their presence does not have any particular significance. Thrombi may also be noted in vessels in other patients with bone marrow necrosis. In amyloidosis, there may be deposition of amyloid in bone marrow vessels (see Fig. 7.33). In hyperparathyroidism, vessel walls may be calcified [29]. Abnormal vessels encircled by mast cells may be seen in systemic mastocytosis (see Fig. 5.42). Rarely the bone marrow has been affected by peliosis [157]. Equally rarely involvement has been reported in hereditary haemorrhagic telangiectasia [158] (Fig. 9.53).

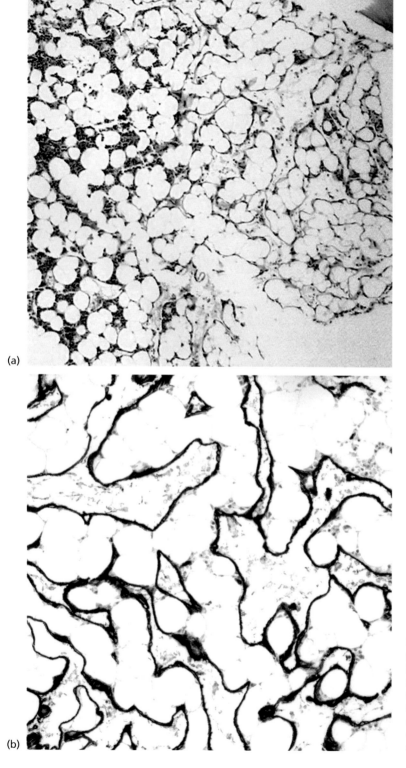

(a)

(b)

Fig. 9.53 BM trephine biopsy section from a patient with hereditary haemorrhagic telangiectasia showing replacement of a considerable part of the bone marrow by abnormal vascular channels. (a) H&E ×10. (b) Immunoperoxidase for CD34 × 20.

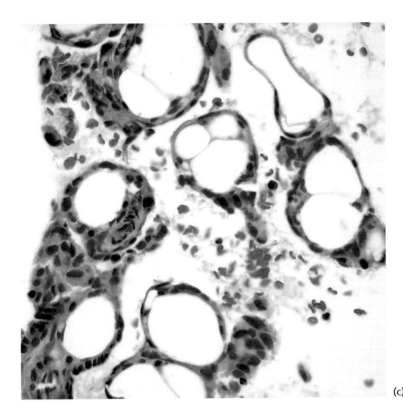

Fig. 9.53 (continued)
(c) H&E ×40. (Courtesy of Dr
Weina Chen, Dallas, Texas and the
British Journal of Haematology.)

(c)

References

1 Castello A, Coci A and Magrini U (1992) Paraneoplastic marrow alterations in patients with cancer. *Haematologica*, **77**, 392–397.

2 Knupp C, Pekala PH and Cornelius P (1988) Extensive bone marrow necrosis in patients with cancer and tumor necrosis factor in plasma. *Am J Hematol*, **29**, 215–221.

3 Kushner JP, Pimstone NR, Kjeldsberg CR, Pryor MA and Huntley A (1982) Congenital erythropoietic porphyria, diminished activity of uroporphyrinogen decarboxylase and dyserythropoiesis. *Blood*, **58**, 725–737.

4 Wickramasinghe SN and Wood WG (2005) Advances in the understanding of the congenital dyserythropoietic anaemias. *Br J Haematol*, **131**, 431–436.

5 Özbek N, Derbent M, Olcay L, Yilmaz Z and Tokel K (2004) Dysplastic changes in the peripheral blood in children with microdeletion 22q11.2. *Am J Hematol*, **77**, 126–131.

6 Hollanda LM, Lima CSP, Cunha AF, Albuquerque DM, Ozelo MC, De Souza CA *et al.* (2004) Inherited mutation in exon 2 of *GATA-1* is associated with a clinical and laboratory picture similar to familial hypocellular myelodysplastic syndrome (MDS). *Blood*, **104**, 936a.

7 Amos RJ, Deane M, Ferguson G, Jeffries G, Hinds CJ and Amess JAL (1990) Observations of the haemopoietic response to critical illness. *J Clin Pathol*, **43**, 850–856.

8 Bader-Meunier B, Rieux-Laucat F, Croisille L, Yvart J, Mielot F, Dommergues JP *et al.* (2000) Dyserythropoiesis associated with a Fas-deficient condition in childhood, *Br J Haematol*, **108**, 300–304.

9 Cramer EM, Garcia I, Massé J-M, Zini J-M, Lambin P, Oksenhendler E *et al.* (1999) Erythroblastic synartesis: an auto-immune dyserythropoiesis. *Blood*, **94**, 3683–3693.

10 Liapis K, Bakiri M and Apostolidis J (2008) Erythroblastic synartesis in a patient with small lymphocytic lymphoma. *Br J Haematol*, **142**, 2.

11 Carpenter SL, Zimmerman SA and Ware RE (2004) Acute parvovirus B19 infection mimicking congenital dyserythropoietic anemia. *J Pediatr Hematol Oncol*, **26**, 133–135.

12 Clatch RJ, Krigman HR, Peters MG and Zutter MM (1994) Dysplastic haemopoiesis following orthoptic liver transplantation: comparison with similar changes in HIV infection and primary myelodysplasia. *Br J Haematol*, **88**, 685–692.

13 O'Brien H, Amess JAL and Mollin DL (1982) Recurrent thrombocytopenia, erythroid hypoplasia and sideroblastic anaemia associated with hypothermia. *Br J Haematol*, **51**, 451–456.

14 Gregg KT, Reddy V and Prchal JT (2002) Copper deficiency masquerading as myelodysplastic syndrome. *Blood*, **100**, 1493–1495.

15 Huff JD, Keung YK, Thakuri M, Beaty MW, Hurd DD, Owen J and Molnar I (2007) Copper deficiency causes reversible myelodysplasia. *Am J Hematol*, **82**, 625–630.

16 Kopterides P, Halikias S and Tsavaris N (2003) Visceral leishmaniasis masquerading as myelodysplasia. *Am J Hematol*, **74**, 198–199.

17 Feuillard J, Jacob M-C, Valensi F, Maynadié M, Gressin R, Chaperot L *et al.* (2002) Clinical and biological features of CD4⁺CD56⁺ malignancies. *Blood*, **99**, 1556–1563.

18 Jiminez-Balderas FJ, Morales-Polanco MR and Guttierez L (1994) Acute sideroblastic anemia in active systemic lupus erythematosus. *Lupus*, **3**, 157–159.

19 Kettaneh A, Hayem G, Palazzo E, Debandt M, Lebail-Darné JL, Roux S *et al.* (1998) Une observation de remission post partum d'une dyserythropoiese acquise, une cause rare d'anémie au cours du lupus érythémateux disséminé. *Rev Méd Intern*, **19**, 571–574.

20 Ghevaert C, Oscier D and Hopkinson N (2003) History revisited. ... *Br J Haematol*, **123**, 756.

21 Ferrario C, Quaroz S and Angelillo-Scherrer A (2008) Diagnosis of systemic lupus erythematosus by bone marrow cytology. http://www.bloodmed.com/home/allslideatlas.asp.

22 Marsh JCW, Ball SE, Darbyshire P, Gordon-Smith EC, Keidan AJ, Martin A *et al.* on behalf of the British Committee for Standards in Haematology (BCSH) General Haematology Task Force (2003) Guidelines for the diagnosis and management of acquired aplastic anaemia. *Br J Haematol*, **123**, 782–801.

23 Voulgarelis M, Giannouli S, Tasidou A, Anagnostou D, Ziakis PD and Tzioufas AG (2006) Bone marrow histological findings in systemic lupus erythematosus with hematologic abnormalities: a clinicopathological study. *Am J Hematol*, **81**, 590–597.

24 Schleicher E (1973) *Bone Marrow Morphology and Mechanics of Biopsy*. Charles C. Thomas, Springfield.

25 Gibbs SDJ, Westerman DA, McCormack C, Seymour JF and Prince M (2005) Severe and prolonged myeloid haematopoietic toxicity with myelodysplastic features following alemtuzumab therapy in patients with peripheral T-cell lymphoproliferative disorders. *Br J Haematol*, **130**, 87–91.

26 Srinivas U, Pillai LS, Kumar R, Pati HP and Saxena R (2007) Bone marrow aplasia – a rare complication of imatinib therapy in CML patients. *Am J Hematol*, **82**, 314–316.

27 Wittels B (1980) Bone marrow biopsy changes following chemotherapy for acute leukemia. *Am J Surg Pathol*, **4**, 135–142.

28 Brody JP, Krause JR and Penchansky L (1985) Bone marrow response to chemotherapy in acute lymphocytic and acute non-lymphocytic leukaemia. *Scand J Haematol*, **35**, 240–245.

29 Frisch B and Bartl R (1999) *Biopsy Interpretation of Bone and Bone Marrow: Histology and immunohistology in paraffin and plastic*, 2nd edn. Arnold, London.

30 Dawson MA, Davis A, Elliott P and Cole-Sinclair M (2005) Linezolid-induced dyserythropoiesis: chloramphenicol toxicity revisited. *Int Med J*, **35**, 626–628.

31 Au WY, Ma ESK and Kwong YL (2002) Intravenous pentamidine induced megaloblastic anemia. *Haematologica*, **87**, ECRO6.

32 Hernandez JA, Navarro JT and Force L (2001) The irreplaceable image: acute toxicity in erythroid bone marrow progenitors after antimonial therapy. *Haematologica*, **86**, 1319.

33 Resuke WN, Anderson C, Pastuszak WT, Conway SR and Firshein SI (1991) Arsenic intoxication presenting as a myelodysplastic syndrome. *Am J Hematol*, **36**, 291–293.

34 Pye A, Kelsey SM, House IM and Newland AC (1992) Severe dyserythropoiesis and autoimmune thrombocytopenia associated with ingestion of kelp supplements. *Lancet*, **339**, 1540.

35 Westhoff DD, Samaha RJ and Barnes A (1975) Arsenic intoxication as a cause of megaloblastic anemia. *Blood*, **45**, 241–246.

36 Feussner JR, Shelburne JD, Bredhoeft S and Cohen HJ (1978) Arsenic-induced bone marrow toxicity: ultrastructural and electron-probe analysis. *Blood*, **53**, 820–827.

37 Phatak PD, Janas J-AS, Kouides PA, Sham RL and Marder VJ (1997) Unusual anemias. *Am J Hematol*, **54**, 249–252.

38 Karunajeewa H, Wall A, Metz J and Grigg A (1998) Cytopenias secondary to copper depletion complicating ammonium tetrathomolybdate therapy for Wilson's disease. *Aust NZ J Med*, **28**, 215–216.

39 Perrotta S, Nobili B, Rossi F, Criscuolo M, Iolascon A, Di Pinto D *et al.* (2002) Infant hypervitaminosis A causes severe anemia and thrombocytopenia: evidence of a retinol-dependent bone marrow growth inhibition. *Blood*, **99**, 2017–2022.

40 Abelman W and Virchis A (2005) An unusual cause of thrombocytopenia. *Clin Lab Haematol*, **27**, 215–216.

41 Michot F and Gut J (1987) Alcohol-induced bone marrow damage. A bone marrow study in alcohol dependent individuals. *Acta Haematol*, **78**, 252–257.

42 Wulfhekel U and Düllmann J (1999) Storage of iron in bone marrow plasma cells: ultrastructural characterization, mobilization, and diagnostic significance. *Acta Haematol*, **101**, 7–15.

43 Gewirtz AM and Hoffman R (1986) Transitory hypomegakaryocytic thrombocytopenia: aetiological association with ethanol abuse and implications regarding regulation of human megakaryocytopoiesis. *Br J Haematol*, **62**, 333–344.

44 Ballard HS (1980) Alcohol-associated pancytopenia with hypocellular bone marrow. *Am J Clin Pathol*, **73**, 830–834.

45 Kaufman DW, Kelly JP, Issaragrisil S, Laporte J-R, Anderson T, Levy M *et al.* (2006) Relative incidence of agranulocytosis and aplastic anemia. *Am J Hematol*, **81**, 65–67.

46 Gordon-Smith EC and Rutherford T (1989) Fanconi's anaemia – constitutional, familial aplastic anaemia. *Baillière's Clin Haematol*, **2**, 139–152.

47 Gross M, Hanenberg H, Lobitz S, Friedl R, Herterich S, Dietrich R *et al.* (2002) Reverse mosaicism in Fanconi anemia: natural gene therapy via molecular self-correction. *Cytogenet Genome Res*, **98**, 126–135.

48 Knight S, Heiss N, Vuillamy T, Aalfs C, McMahon C, Jones A *et al.* (1999) Hoyeraal–Hreidarsson syndrome of progressive pancytopenia, immunodeficiency, growth retardation, and cerebellar hypoplasia is due to mutations in the dyskeratosis congenita gene. *Br J Haematol*, **105** (Suppl. 1), 66.

49 Marsh JCW and Geary CG (1991) Is aplastic anaemia a pre-leukaemic disorder? *Br J Haematol*, **77**, 447–452.

50 Marsh JC, Abboudi ZH, Gibson FM, Scopes J, Daly S, O'Shaunnessy DF *et al.* (1994) Aplastic anaemia following exposure to 3,4-methylenedioxymethamphetamine ('Ecstasy'). *Br J Haematol*, **88**, 281–285.

51 Chute JP, Hofmeister K, Cotelingam J, Davis TA, Frame JN and Jamieson T (1996) Aplastic anaemia as the sole presentation of systemic lupus erythematosus. *Am J Haematol*, **51**, 237–239.

52 Fleming AF (1999) Pregnancy and aplastic anaemia. *Br J Haematol*, **105**, 313–320.

53 Yamaguchi H, Calado RT, Ly H, Kajigaya S, Baerlocher GM, Chanock SJ *et al.* (2005) Mutations in TERT, the gene for telomerase reverse transcriptase, in aplastic anemia. *N Engl J Med*, **352**, 1413–1424.

54 Frisch B and Lewis SM (1974) The bone marrow in aplastic anaemia: diagnostic and prognostic features. *J Clin Pathol*, **27**, 231–241.

55 Kansu E and Erslev AJ (1976) Aplastic anaemia with 'hot pockets'. *Scand J Haematol*, **17**, 326–334.

56 te Velde J and Haak HL (1977) Aplastic anaemia: histological investigation of methacrylate embedded bone marrow biopsy specimens: correlation with survival after conventional treatment in 15 adult patients. *Br J Haematol*, **35**, 61–69.

57 Melenhorst JJ, van Krieken JHM, Dreef E, Landegent JE, Willemze R and Fibbe WE (1997) T cells selectively infiltrate bone marrow areas with residual haemopoiesis of patients with acquired aplastic anaemia. *Br J Haematol*, **99**, 517–519.

58 Burkhardt R, Frisch B and Bartl B (1982) Bone biopsy in haematological disorders. *J Clin Pathol*, **35**, 257–284.

59 Tripathy VNK and Nityanand S (2002) Massive apoptosis of bone marrow cells in aplastic anaemia. *Br J Haematol*, **117**, 993–994.

60 Tichelli A, Gratwohl A, Würsh A, Nissen C and Speck B (1988) Late haematological complications in severe aplastic anaemia. *Br J Haematol*, **69**, 413–418.

61 de Planque MM, Van Krieken JHJM, Kluin-Nelemans HC, Colla LPJM, van der Burgh F, Brand A and Kluin PM (1989) Bone marrow histopathology of patients with severe aplastic anaemia before treatment and at follow-up. *Br J Haematol*, **72**, 439–444.

62 Heimpel H (2000) Aplastic anemia before bone marrow transplantation and antilymphocyte globulin. *Acta Haematol*, **103**, 11–15.

63 Sale GE, Rajantie J, Doney K, Appelbaum FR, Storb R and Thomas ED (1987) Does histologic grading of inflammation in bone marrow predict the response of aplastic anaemia patients to antithymocyte globulin therapy? *Br J Haematol*, **67**, 261–266.

64 Geary CG, Harrison CJ, Philpott NJ, Hows JM, Gordon-Smith EC and Marsh JC (1999) Abnormal cytogenetic clones in patients with aplastic anaemia: response to immunosuppressive therapy. *Br J Haematol*, **104**, 271–274.

65 Maciejewski JP, Risitano A, Sloand EM, Nunez O and Young NS (2002) Distinct clinical outcomes for cytogenetic abnormalities evolving from aplastic anemia. *Blood*, **99**, 3129–3135.

66 Ishiyama K, Karasawa M, Miyawaki S, Ueda Y, Noda M, Wakita A *et al.* (2002) Aplastic anaemia with 13q–: a benign subset of bone marrow failure responsive to immunosuppressive therapy. *Br J Haematol*, **117**, 747–750.

67 Gupta V, Brooker C, Tooze JA, Yi OL, Sage D, Turner D *et al.* (2006) Clinical relevance of cytogenetic abnormalities at diagnosis of acquired aplastic anaemia in adults. *Br J Haematol*, **134**, 95–99.

68 Tönnies H, Huber S, Kühl J-S, Gerlach A, Ebell W and Neitzel H (2003) Clonal chromosomal aberrations in bone marrow cells of Fanconi anemia patients: gains of the chromosomal segment 3q26q29 as an adverse risk factor. *Blood*, **101**, 3872–3874.

69 Fohlmeister I, Fischer R, Mödder B, Rister M and Schaefer H-E (1985) Aplastic anaemia and the hypocellular myelodysplastic syndrome: histomorphological, diagnostic, and prognostic features. *J Clin Pathol*, **38**, 1218–1224.

70 de Planque MM, Kluin-Nelemans HC, Van Krieken HJM, Kluin PM, Brand A, Beverstock GC, Willemze R and van Rood JJ (1988) Evolution of acquired severe aplastic anaemia to myelodysplasia and subsequent leukaemia. *Br J Haematol*, **70**, 55–62.

71 Reid MM and Summerfield GP (1992) Distinction between aleukaemic prodrome of childhood acute lymphoblastic leukaemia and aplastic anaemia. *J Clin Pathol*, **45**, 697–700.

72 Morley AA, Brisco MJ, Rice M, Snell L, Peng L-M, Hughes E, Neoh D-H and Sykes PJ (1997) Leukaemia presenting as marrow hypoplasia: molecular detection of the leukaemic clone. *Br J Haematol*, **98**, 940–944.

73 Yildirmak Y, Palanduz A, Telhan L, Arapoglu M and Kayaalp N (2003) Bone marrow hypoplasia during Brucella infection. *J Pediatr Hematol Oncol*, **25**, 63–64.

74 Beyan C, Ural AU, Çetin T, Omay SB, Doğanci L and Yalçin A (1997) Uncommon cause of severe pancytopenia: toxoplasmosis. *Am J Hematol*, **55**, 164.

75 Ferrari E, Ascari E, Bossolo PA and Barosi G (1976) Sheehan's syndrome with complete bone marrow aplasia: long-term results of substitution therapy with hormones. *Br J Haematol*, **33**, 575–582.

76 Pearson HA, Lobel JS, Kocoshis SA, Naiman JL, Windmiller J, Lammi A, Hoffman R and Marsh JC (1979) A new syndrome of refractory sideroblastic anemia with vacuolation of bone marrow precursors and exocrine pancreatic dysfunction. *J Pediat*, **95**, 976–984.

77 Lacbawan F, Tifft CJ, Luban NLC, Schmandt SM, Guerrera M, Weinstein S *et al.* (2000) Clinical heterogeneity in mitochondrial DNA deletion disorders: a diagnostic challenge of Pearson syndrome. *Am J Med Genet*, **95**, 266–268.

78 Bain BJ (1994) Transient leukaemia in newborn infants with Down's syndrome, *Leuk Res*, **18**, 723–724.

79 Çetin M, Hicsönmez G and Göğüs S (1998) Myelodysplastic syndrome associated with the Griscelli syndrome. *Leuk Res*, **22**, 859–862.

80 Bazarbachi A, Muakkit S, Ayas M, Taher A, Salem Z, Solh H and Haidar JH (1998) Thiamine-responsive myelodysplasia. *Br J Haematol*, **102**, 1098–1100.

81 Elfenbein DS, Barness EG, Pomerance HH and Barness LA (2000) Newborn infant with lethargy, poor feeding, dehydration, hypothermia, hyperammonemia, neutropenia, and thrombocytopenia. *Am J Med Genet*, **94**, 332–337.

82 Rotoli B and Luzzatto L (1989) Paroxysmal nocturnal haemoglobinuria. *Semin Haematol*, **26**, 201–207.

83 Araten DJ, Swirsky D, Karadimitris A, Notaro R, Nafa K and Bessler M (2001) Cytogenetic and morphological abnormalities in paroxysmal nocturnal haemoglobinuria. *Br J Haematol*, **115**, 360–368.

84 Sale GE and Buckner CD (1988) Pathology of bone marrow in transplant recipients. *Hematol Oncol Clin North Am*, **2**, 735–756.

85 Bilgrami S, Almeida GD, Quinn JJ, Tuck D, Bergstrom S, Dainiak N, Poliquin C and Ascensao JL (1994) Pancytopenia in allogeneic marrow transplant recipients: role of cytomegalovirus. *Br J Haematol*, **87**, 357–362.

86 Carrigan DR and Knox KK (1994) Human herpesvirus 6 (HHV-6) isolation from bone marrow: HHV-6-associated bone marrow suppression in bone marrow transplant patients. *Blood*, **84**, 3307–3310.

87 Rocha V, Devergie A, Socié G, Ribaud P, Espérou H, Parquet N and Gluckman E (1998) Unusual complications after bone marrow transplantation for dyskeratosis congenita. *Br J Haematol*, **103**, 243–248.

88 Rozman C, Feliu E, Granēna A, Brugues R, Woessner S and Vives Corrons JL (1982) Transient dyserythropoiesis in repopulated human bone marrow following transplantation: an ultrastructural study. *Br J Haematol*, **50**, 63–73.

89 Kobayashi SD, Seki K, Suwa N, Koama C, Yamamoto T, Aiba K *et al.* (1991) The transient appearance of small blastoid cells in the marrow after bone marrow transplantation. *Am J Clin Pathol*, **96**, 191–195.

90 Rosenthal NS and Fahri DC (1994) Failure to engraft after bone marrow transplantation: bone marrow morphologic findings. *Am J Clin Pathol*, **102**, 821–824.

91 Müller-Hermelink HK and Sale GE (1984) Pathological findings in human bone marrow transplantation. In: Lennert K and Hübner K (eds) *Pathology of the Bone Marrow*. Gustav Fischer Verlag, Stuttgart.

92 van den Berg H, Kluin PM, Zwaan FE and Vossen JM (1989) Histopathology of bone marrow reconstitution after bone marrow transplantation. *Histopathology*, **15**, 363–375.

93 van den Berg H, Kluin PM and Vossen JM (1990) Early reconstitution of haematopoiesis after allogeneic bone marrow transplantation: a prospective histopathologic study of bone marrow biopsy specimens. *J Clin Pathol*, **43**, 335–369.

94 Maia DM, Kell DL, Goates J and Warnke RA (1997) The significance of light chain-restricted bone marrow plasma cells after peripheral blood stem cell transplantation for multiple myeloma. *Am J Clin Pathol*, **107**, 643–652.

95 Au MY and Kwong YL (1999) Haemophagocytosis in the peripheral blood. *Br J Haematol*, **105**, 321.

96 Jouan H, Deist F Le and Nezelof C (1987) Omenn's syndrome – pathologic arguments in favour of a graft versus host pathogenesis: a report of nine cases. *Hum Pathol*, **18**, 1011–1108.

97 Wada T, Takei K, Kudo M, Shimura S, Kasahara Y, Koizumi S *et al.* (2000) Characterization of immune function and analysis of RAG gene mutations in Omenn syndrome and related disorders. *Clin Exp Immunol*, **119**, 148–155.

98 Basara N, Kiehl MG and Fauser AA (2002) Eosinophilia indicates the evolution of acute graft-versus-host disease. *Blood*, **100**, 3055.

99 Asplund SL, Miller ML and Kalacyio ME (1999) Immunophenotypic characterization of granulocyte colony-stimulating factor-induced blast cells in peripheral blood. *Am J Clin Pathol*, **112**, 558.

100 Meyerson HJ, Farhi DC and Rosenthal NC (1998) Transient increase in blasts mimicking acute leukemia and progressing myelodysplasia in patients receiving growth factor. *Am J Clin Pathol*, **109**, 675–681.

101 Orazi A, Gordon MS, John K, Sledge G, Neiman RS and Hoffman R (1995) *In vivo* effects of recombinant human stem cell factor treatment: a morphologic and immunohistochemical study of bone marrow biopsies. *Am J Clin Pathol*, **103**, 177–184.

102 Rasko JEJ, Basser RL, Boyd J, Mansfield R, O'Malley CJ, Hussein S *et al.* (1997) Multilineage mobilization of peripheral blood progenitor cells in humans following administration of PEG-rHu MGDF. *Br J Haematol*, **97**, 871–880.

103 Douglas VK, Tallman MS, Cripe LD and Peterson L-AC (2002) Thrombopoietin administered during induction chemotherapy to patients with acute myeloid leukemia induces transient morphologic changes that may resemble chronic myeloproliferative disorders. *Am J Clin Pathol*, **117**, 844–850.

104 Du X and Williams DA (1997) Interleukin-11: review of molecular, cell biology, and clinical use. *Blood*, **89**, 3897–3905.

105 Harris AC, Todd WM, Hackney MH and Ben-Ezra J (1994) Bone marrow changes associated with recombinant granulocyte–macrophage and granulocyte colony-stimulating factors. *Arch Pathol Lab Med*, **118**, 624–629.

106 Tegg EM, Tuck DM, Lowenthal RM and Marsden KA (1999) The effect of G-CSF on the composition of human bone marrow. *Clin Lab Haematol*, **21**, 265–270.

107 Urabe AU (1994) Colony stimulating factor and macrophage proliferation. *Am J Clin Pathol*, **101**, 116.

108 Kaddar A, Edinger M, Wirth K, Schaefer HE, Lubbert M and Lindemann A (1997) Increased numbers of bone marrow blasts in acute myeloid leukaemia patients treated with G-CSF after chemotherapy. *Br J Haematol*, **98**, 492–493.

109 Cummings GH (1998) The effect of growth factor therapy on blast percentages. *Am J Clin Pathol*, **111**, 709.

110 Brunning RD (1970) Morphological alterations in nucleated blood and marrow cells in genetic disorders. *Hum Pathol*, **1**, 99–124.

111 Hayhoe FGT, Flemans RJ and Cowling DC (1979) Acquired lipidosis of marrow macrophages. *J Clin Pathol*, **32**, 420–428.

112 Savage RA (1984) Specific and not-so-specific histiocytes in bone marrow. *Lab Med*, **15**, 467–471.

113 Bain BJ and Wickramasinghe SN (1986) Pathology of the bone marrow: general considerations. In: Wickramasinghe SN (ed), Symmers WStC (series ed) *Systemic Pathology*, vol. 2, *Blood and Bone Marrow*. Churchill Livingstone, Edinburgh.

114 Lee RE (1988) Histiocytic diseases of the bone marrow. *Hematol Oncol Clin North Am*, **2**, 657–667.

115 Bain BJ (2006) *Blood Cells: A practical guide*, 4th edn. Blackwell Publishing, Oxford.

116 Beutler E and Saven A (1990) Misuse of marrow examination in the diagnosis of Gaucher's disease. *Blood*, **76**, 646–648.

117 Beutler E (1988) Gaucher disease. *Blood Rev*, **2**, 59–70.

118 Bitton A, Etzell J, Grenert JP and Wang E (2004) Erythrophagocytosis in Gaucher cells. *Arch Path Lab Med*, **128**, 1191–1192.

119 Hoyer JD, Li C-Y, Yam LT, Hanson CA and Kurtin PJ (1997) Immunohistochemical demonstration of acid phosphatase isoenzyme 5 (tartrate-resistant) in paraffin sections of hairy cell leukemia and other hematologic disorders. *Am J Clin Pathol*, **108**, 308–315.

120 Rudski Z, Okon K, Machaczka M, Rucinska M, Papla B and Skotnicki AB (2002) Bone marrow histology in Gaucher disease treated with imuglucerase. *J Clin Pathol*, **55** (Suppl. 1), A8.

121 Weisberger J, Emmon F and Gorczyca W (2004) Cytochemical diagnosis of Gaucher's disease by iron stain. *Br J Haematol*, **124**, 696.

122 Tang DJ, Yu ZF, Song JZ, Chen MC and Wang ZW (1987) Gaucher-like cells in chronic neutrophilic leukemia. A case report. *Chin Med J (Engl)*, **100**, 988–989.

123 Stewart AJ and Jones RDG (1999) Pseudo-Gaucher cells in myelodysplasia. *J Clin Pathol*, **52**, 917–918.

124 Papadimitriou JC, Chakravarthy A and Heyman MR (1988) Pseudo-Gaucher cells preceding the appearance of immunoblastic lymphoma. *Am J Clin Pathol*, **90**, 454–458.

125 Yamauchi K and Shimamura K (1995) Mild thrombocytopenia induced by phagocytosis of marrow pseudo-Gaucher cells in a patient with chronic myelogenous leukaemia. *Eur J Haematol*, **54**, 55–56.

126 Scullin DC, Shelburne JD and Cohen HJ (1979) Pseudo-Gaucher cells in multiple myeloma. *Am J Med*, **67**, 347–352.

127 Solis OG, Belmonte AH, Ramaswamy G and Tchertkoff V (1986) Pseudogaucher cells in *Mycobacterium avium intracellulare* infections in acquired immune deficiency syndrome (AIDS). *Am J Clin Pathol*, **85**, 233–235.

128 Agiris A, Maun N and Berliner N (1999) Mycobacterium avium complex inclusions mimicking Gaucher's cells. *New Engl J Med*, **340**, 1372.

129 Schaefer HE (1996) Gammopathy-related crystal-storing histiocytosis, pseudo- and pseudo-pseudo-Gaucher cells. Critical commentary and mini-review. *Pathol Res Pract*, **192**, 1152–1162.

130 Cobcroft R, Marlston P, Silburn P, Walsh M and Boyle R (2000) Type C Niemann–Pick disease. *Br J Haematol*, **111**, 718.

131 Nam MH, Grande JP, Li CY, Kottke BA, Pineda AA and Weiland LH (1988) Familial hypercholesterolemia with unusual foamy histiocytes. Report of a case with myelophthisic anemia and xanthoma of the maxillary sinus. *Am J Clin Pathol*, **89**, 556–561.

132 Brunning RD (1989) Bone marrow. In: Rosai J (ed) *Ackerman's Surgical Pathology*, 7th edn, vol. 2. C. V. Mosby, St Louis.

133 Wong KF and Chan JKC (1989) Foamy histiocytes in repeat marrow aspirates. *Pathology*, **21**, 153–154.

134 Hyun BH, Gulati GL and Ashton JK (1986) *Color Atlas of Clinical Hematology*. Igaku-Shoin, New York.

135 Kuo TT and Hsueh S (1984) Mucicarminophilic histiocytosis in polyvinylpyrrolidine (PVP) storage disease simulating signet ring carcinoma. *Am J Surg Pathol*, **8**, 419–428.

136 Dunn P, Kuo T-t, Shi L-Y, Wang P-N, Sun C-F and Chang MJW (1998) Bone marrow failure and myelofibrosis in a case of PVP storage disease. *Am J Hematol*, **57**, 68–71.

137 Bigorne C, Le Torneau A, Messing B, Rio B, Giraud V, Molina T, Adouin J and Diebold J (1996) Sea-blue histiocyte syndrome in bone marrow secondary to total parenteral nutrition including fat-emulsion sources: a clinicopathologic study of seven cases. *Br J Haematol*, **95**, 258–262.

138 Varela-Duran J, Roholt PC and Ratliff NB (1980) Sea-blue histiocyte syndrome: a secondary degenerative process of macrophages? *Arch Pathol Lab Med*, **104**, 30–34.

139 Armstrong D, Gadoth N and Harvey J (1985) Sea-blue histiocytes in canine ceroid-lipofuscinosis. *Blood Cells*, **11**, 151–155.

140 Abramson N (2007) Beyond the wide blue sea. *Blood*, **109**, 1799.

141 Emadi A, Burns KH, Confer B and Borowitz MJ (2008) Hematological manifestations of nephropathic cystinosis. *Acta Haematol*, **19**, 169–172.

142 Varan A and Tuncer AM (1991) The importance of the bone marrow examination in cystinosis. *Pediatr Hematol Oncol*, **8**, 373–374.

143 Bigley V, Bhartia S and Wood A (2007) Nephropathic cystinosis with bone marrow involvement. *Br J Haematol*, **136**, 180.

144 Mathews M, Stauffer M, Cameron EC, Maloney N and Sherrard DJ (1979) Bone biopsy to diagnose hyperoxaluria in patients with renal failure. *Ann Intern Med*, **90**, 777–779.

145 Hricik DE and Hussain R (1984) Pancytopenia and hepatosplenomegaly in oxalosis. *Arch Intern Med*, **184**, 167–168.

146 Walter MJ and Dang CV (1998) Pancytopenia secondary to oxalosis in a 23-year-old woman. *Blood*, **91**, 4394.

147 Peterson L, Parkin J and Nelson A (1982) Mucopolysaccharidosis type VII. A morphologic, cytochemical, and ultrastructural study of the blood and bone marrow. *Am J Clin Pathol*, **78**, 544–548.

148 Foucar K (2001) *Bone Marrow Pathology*, 2nd edn. ASCP Press, Chicago.

149 Huang O, Chang KL and Weiss LM (2006) Extranodal Rosai–Dorfman disease involving the bone marrow: a case report. *Am J Surg Pathol*, **30**, 1189–1192.

150 Miller D (1959) Observations in a case of probable bone marrow anthracosis. *Blood*, **14**, 1350–1353.

151 Jennings RC and Priestley SE (1978) Haemangioendothelioma (Kupffer cell angiosarcoma), myelofibrosis, splenic atrophy, and myeloma paraproteinaemia after parenteral Thorotrast administration. *J Clin Pathol*, **31**, 1125–1132.

152 Rywlin AM (1976) *Histopathology of the Bone Marrow*. Little Brown, Boston.

153 Pierce JR, Wren MV and Cousar JB (1978) Cholesterol embolism: diagnosis antemortem by bone marrow biopsy. *Ann Intern Med*, **89**, 937–938.

154 Retan JW and Miller RE (1966) Microembolic complications of atherosclerosis. *Arch Intern Med*, **118**, 534–543.

155 Muretto P, Carnevali A and Ansini AL (1991) Cholesterol embolism of bone marrow clinically masquerading as systemic or metastatic tumor. *Haematologica*, **76**, 248–250.

156 Cahalin PA and Pawade J (2002) Giant cell arteritis detected by bone marrow trephine. *Br J Haematol*, **118**, 687.

157 Tsokos M and Erbersdobler A (2005) Pathology of peliosis. *Forensic Sci Int*, **149**, 25–33.

158 Willis J, Mayo MJ, Rogers TE and Chen W (2009) Hereditary haemorrhagic telangiectasia involving the bone marrow and liver. *Br J Haematol*, **145**, 150.

TEN

METASTATIC TUMOURS

The bone marrow is one of the more common organs to be involved by tumours that metastasize via the bloodstream. In adults the tumours most often seen are carcinomas of the prostate gland, breast and lung, although any tumour that gives rise to blood-borne metastases may infiltrate the marrow [1,2]. In children, neuroblastoma, rhabdomyosarcoma, Ewing's sarcoma, other primitive neuroectodermal tumours (PNET) and retinoblastoma account for the majority of metastases [3,4]. Bone marrow metastases from squamous cell carcinoma, other than that of the lung, and from soft tissue tumours of adults are uncommon [1]. Intracranial tumours rarely metastasize outside the cranial vault. Of those cases reported with bone marrow involvement, glioblastoma multiforme has been the most frequent [5]; examples of metastatic medulloblastoma [6] and oligodendroglioma [7] have also been recorded.

Infiltration of the marrow may be suspected on the basis of: (i) bone pain; (ii) pathological fractures, lytic lesions or sclerotic lesions demonstrated radiologically; (iii) unexplained 'hot spots' on isotopic bone scans or positron emission tomography (PET) scanning; (iv) an abnormal magnetic resonance imaging scan; (v) hypercalcaemia or elevated serum alkaline phosphatase activity; or (vi) unexplained haematological abnormalities. The haematological abnormality most suggestive of marrow infiltration, though not specific for it, is leucoerythroblastic anaemia (see below). Metastases are also demonstrated occasionally when bone marrow examination is carried out for staging purposes in the absence of any features suggestive of infiltra-

tion. Overall, the presence of leucoerythroblastic anaemia is a relatively insensitive indication of infiltration since it is observed in less than half of patients in whom bone marrow metastases can be demonstrated by biopsy [8–10]. Aspirates and trephine biopsies are occasionally positive even when skeletal radiology and isotopic bone scans [8,11] are normal.

Considering the small volume of tissue sampled, both bone marrow aspiration and trephine biopsy are relatively sensitive techniques for detecting bone marrow infiltration by metastatic tumours. In two autopsy studies which simulated biopsy procedures it was estimated that, when osseous metastases were present, a bone marrow aspirate would give positive results in 28% of cases [12] and a single trephine biopsy in 35–45% [13]. Trephine biopsy is more sensitive than bone marrow aspiration and sensitivity is increased by performing bilateral biopsies or by obtaining a single large biopsy specimen. The sensitivity of aspiration is increased if large numbers of films are examined and if a clot section is also assessed. It is common for tumour cells to be detectable in trephine biopsy sections when none are demonstrable in films of an aspirate [8,14]. Overall, about three quarters of metastases detected by a trephine biopsy are also detected by simultaneous bone marrow aspiration. Discrepancy between biopsy and aspirate findings usually results from a desmoplastic stromal reaction to the tumour that renders neoplastic cells more difficult to aspirate than residual haemopoietic cells. It is also, to some degree, a consequence of the different volumes of tissue sampled. Because of its greater sensitivity, a trephine biopsy should always be performed when metastatic malignancy is suspected. However, tumour cells are seen occasionally in aspirate films when trephine biopsy sec-

Bone Marrow Pathology. By Barbara Bain, David Clark and Bridget Wilkins. © 2010, Blackwell Publishing.

tions appear normal [2,8,14] and the two procedures should therefore be regarded as complementary.

Increasingly, bone marrow aspiration and trephine biopsy are being performed as staging procedures at the time of diagnosis in a number of solid tumours, principally neuroblastoma, PNET and rhabdomyosarcoma in children and carcinomas of the breast and lung in adults. Such investigations are indicated when there is a significant probability of bone marrow metastases and when knowledge of their presence would affect the choice of primary treatment. Biopsy may be indicated, for example, when radical surgery or radiotherapy with curative intent is to be undertaken or when intensive chemotherapy with autologous bone marrow transplantation is being considered.

It can be important to suggest the likely primary site of metastatic lesions detected in the bone marrow. This is particularly so in the case of adenocarcinoma since, although many such tumours are relatively resistant to therapy, those originating in the breast and prostate gland may respond to hormonal therapy or other targeted therapies (e.g. monoclonal antibody therapy directed at the *ERBB2* product, HER2, in some breast cancers). Identification of metastatic thyroid carcinoma is likewise important although, in practice, this tumour is rarely found unexpectedly in bone marrow biopsy samples since malignant thyroid tumours generally manifest themselves clearly at their primary site. Investigation for an unknown primary tumour is therefore rarely necessary in this context and radio-isotope imaging is the preferred staging technique for known thyroid malignancies.

The main areas of difficulty in the diagnosis of metastatic tumour in bone marrow are:
1 Distinguishing metastatic tumour cells from tumours of haemopoietic cells – for example, marrow involvement by high grade non-Hodgkin lymphoma or acute myeloid leukaemia with fibrosis (as in the World Health Organization (WHO) categories of acute megakaryocytic leukaemia and acute panmyelosis).
2 Determining the site of origin of metastatic tumour when the primary is unknown.
3 Detecting small foci of metastatic tumour in biopsies performed as part of tumour staging.
4 Identifying scanty metastatic malignant cells in severely sclerotic deposits.

Immunohistochemistry is very useful for the identification of metastatic tumours in the bone marrow [15–19] (Tables 10.1 and 10.2).

Peripheral blood

Normocytic normochromic anaemia is commonly present when there is infiltration of the bone marrow by malignant cells; other cytopenias are less common. In a third to a half of patients with bone marrow infiltration there are nucleated red cells and neutrophil precursors in the blood – designated leucoerythroblastic anaemia when the patient is also anaemic. The presence of a leuco-erythroblastic anaemia correlates with the degree of reactive bone marrow fibrosis rather than with the extent of malignant infiltration [9]; it is most commonly seen in association with carcinoma of the breast, stomach, prostate gland and lung. Sometimes bone marrow infiltration is identified in the absence of anaemia or any other abnormality in the peripheral blood.

Significant numbers of circulating malignant cells are rare but may occur in the small cell tumours of childhood, particularly neuroblastoma, rhabdomyosarcoma and medulloblastoma. Circulating neoplastic cells may also be seen in adult patients with carcinoma but this is a very rare occurrence.

Patients with metastatic malignant cells in the bone marrow may show peripheral blood abnormalities which are caused by the underlying malignant disease but are not directly due to bone marrow infiltration. Such abnormalities can include iron deficiency anaemia, the anaemia of chronic disease, microangiopathic haemolytic anaemia, neutrophilia, eosinophilia, thrombocytopenia, thrombocytosis and increased rouleaux formation.

Bone marrow cytology

When bone marrow infiltration has led to reactive myelofibrosis attempts at aspiration may result in a 'dry tap' or a 'blood tap', or a small amount of marrow containing haemopoietic cells, tumour cells or both may be aspirated with difficulty. When there is an associated increase in bone turnover the aspirate may contain a mixture of tumour cells, osteoblasts and osteoclasts (Fig. 10.1). Sometimes the aspirate is wholly or partly necrotic and this

Table 10.1 Antigens expressed by non-haemopoietic cells, useful for the demonstration of metastatic tumours by immunohistochemistry in fixed, decalcified bone marrow trephine biopsy specimens.

Antigen	Antibody	Specificity	Comments
Broad spectrum of cytokeratins (low molecular weights)*	CAM5.2, AE1, MNF116, 5D3	Epithelial cells (cytoplasmic expression)	Cells in occasional cases of anaplastic large cell lymphoma and plasma cell neoplasms are also positive; leukaemic myeloblasts may be positive
Broad spectrum of cytokeratins (high molecular weights)*	AE3, LP34, C-11, 34βE12	Epithelial cells (cytoplasmic expression)	Cells in occasional cases of anaplastic large cell lymphoma and plasma cell neoplasms are also positive; leukaemic myeloblasts may be positive
Cytokeratin 7 (CK7)	RN7, LP5K	See Table 10.2	
Cytokeratin 20 (CK20)	PW31, CK205, Ks20.8	See Table 10.2	
Cytokeratin 8 (CK8)	TS1, 5D3 (8 and 18)	Epithelial cells	Usually coexpressed with CK18
Cytokeratin 18 (CK18)	DC-10, 5D3 (8 and 18)	Epithelial cells	Usually coexpressed with CK8
Cytokeratins 5 and 6	D5/16 B4 (5 and 6)	Epithelial cells with squamous differentiation	
Thyroid transcription factor 1 (TTF1)	SPT24, 8G7G3/1	Thyroid follicular epithelial cells and some other glandular epithelia (nuclear staining)	Among adenocarcinomas has specificity for thyroid and lung origin; expressed in small cell carcinomas (including those of non-pulmonary origin)
CD10	56C6	Subsets of B cells, renal tubular epithelial cells	Renal cell carcinoma usually positive; hepatocellular carcinomas often express CD10, but rarely metastasize to bone marrow; expressed in common and pre-B-ALL, Burkitt lymphoma and follicular lymphoma; also expressed by a subset of marrow stromal cells and some neutrophils
Uncharacterized renal cell-associated antigen	66.4.C2, SPM314	Renal tubular epithelial cells	
Epithelial cell adhesion molecule (Ep-CAM)	BerEP4, 17-1A	Epithelial cells (membrane expression)	
Epithelial membrane antigen	E29, GP1.4	Epithelial cells (membrane expression)	Anaplastic large cell lymphomas, non-neoplastic and some neoplastic plasma cells also positive; early erythroid cells may be positive
Carcino-embryonic antigen (epitopes include CD66)	Polyclonal antisera and 85A12, 12-140-10, II-7	Epithelial cells (membrane expression, often apical or periluminal distribution)	Metamyelocytes and mature neutrophils are also positive
Prostate-specific antigen	ER-PR8, PSA 28/A4, 35H9	Prostatic epithelial cells (cytoplasmic expression)	Fairly specific for prostatic adenocarcinoma, but staining may be patchy

continued

Table 10.1 (continued)

Antigen	Antibody	Specificity	Comments
Prostate-specific acid phosphatase	PASE/4LJ	Prostatic epithelial cells (preferential apical/periluminal distribution)	
Thyroglobulin	DAK-Tg6, 1D4	Thyroid epithelial cells (cytoplasmic expression)	
Calcitonin	Polyclonal antisera and CAL-3-F5	Thyroid medullary C cells (cytoplasmic expression)	
Oestrogen receptor	1D5, 6F11	Oestrogen-sensitive cells, including those of breast, ovary and endometrium (nuclear expression)	Of limited diagnostic value in metastases from an unknown primary source but valuable in determining whether metastatic breast carcinoma is likely to respond to anti-oestrogen therapy
Progesterone receptor	1A6, 16, PgR 636	Oestrogen-sensitive cells, including those of breast, ovary and endometrium (nuclear expression)	May be helpful in determining whether ER-negative metastatic breast carcinoma is likely to respond to anti-oestrogen therapy
HER2 (c-erbB-2) (CD340)	5A2, CB11, CBE1, PN2A	Overexpressed HER2 protein; main use is in breast carcinoma to help predict responsiveness to anti-CD340 (trastuzumab) immunotherapy	Many other carcinomas are positive, including many of female genital tract, urothelial, prostatic and pancreatic origin, non-small cell cancers of the lung, and squamous cell carcinomas of diverse tissue origins
S100 protein	Polyclonal antisera	Malignant melanoma (nuclear and cytoplasmic expression)	Perineural cells, a subset of macrophages, cells of Langerhans cell histiocytosis and 20% of breast cancers are positive
Melanosome matrix protein gp100-cl	HMB-45	Malignant melanoma (cytoplasmic expression)	Varying proportions of cells are negative in many melanomas
Melanoma-associated MART-1 gene product (melan A)	A103	Malignant melanoma (cytoplasmic expression)	
CD56	1B6, CD565, 123C3	Neuroendocrine tumours (small cell carcinoma of the lung and other sites, carcinoid tumour, medullary carcinoma of the thyroid, other neuroendocrine carcinomas)	Also expressed by NK cells, some T cells, neoplastic plasma cells, cells of myelomonocytic lineage including some AML, and plasmacytoid dendritic cells
Chromogranin A	5H7, DAK-A3	Neuroendocrine tumours (as above)	
Synaptophysin	27G12, SY38	Neuroendocrine tumours (as above)	

Table 10.1 (continued)

Antigen	Antibody	Specificity	Comments
Neurofilament protein	2F11, DA2, N52.1.7	Neuroendocrine tumours (as above); expressed in some neuroblastomas with neuroglial differentiation (may be present *de novo* or develop in patients undergoing treatment)	
Protein gene product 9.5 (PGP9.5) – ubiquitin related	Polyclonal antisera, 10A1	Neuroectodermal tumours including PNET (especially neuroblastoma) and neuroendocrine tumours (as above) (nuclear and cytoplasmic staining)	Newly produced reticulin, chondrocytes and late granulocyte precursors may be positive
Uncharacterized	NB84	PNET, especially neuroblastoma (cytoplasmic expression), but less sensitive than PGP95	Extensive background nuclear staining occurs with some fixation protocols; endothelial cells and some adult malignant epithelial tumours may also be positive
Uncharacterised	NeuN	PNET, especially neuroblastoma (cytoplasmic expression)	
Glial fibrillary acidic protein	6F2, GA5	Cells with glial differentiation	Useful after treatment of neuroblastoma, when neuroglial differentiation may occur and maturing tumour may mimic scar tissue
CD99 (MIC2)	12E7, HO36-1.1	PNET, especially Ewing's sarcoma (membrane expression)	Some normal T lymphocytes and cells in most cases of B- and T-lineage ALL are also positive
FLI-1	GI146-222 Alternative polyclonal antisera give high background staining	PNET, especially Ewing's sarcoma with t(11;22) and *EWS–FLI1* fusion (nuclear expression)	Some melanomas and Merckel cell tumours are also positive; neutrophils and megakaryocytes are variably positive, which may mimic low levels of metastatic involvement
Desmin	D33, DE-R-11	Rhabdomyosarcoma (cytoplasmic expression)	
MyoD1	5.8A	Rhabdomyosarcoma (nuclear expression)	Cytoplasmic staining is found in most neuroblastomas and occasional cases of Ewing's sarcoma/PNET; consistent good performance with the currently available McAb is difficult to achieve in fixed tissue
Myogenin	F5D	Rhabdomyosarcoma (nuclear expression)	

continued

Table 10.1 (continued)

Antigen	Antibody	Specificity	Comments
Myoglobin	MG-1, MYO18 and polyclonal antisera	Rhabdomyosarcoma (cytoplasmic expression)	
von Willebrand factor (previously known as factor VIII-related antigen)	F8/86, 36B11 and polyclonal antisera	Endothelium, tumours of endothelial origin and megakaryocytes	
CD34	QBEnd10	Endothelium, tumours of endothelial origin and primitive haemopoietic cells	Some non-endothelial spindle cell tumours
CD31	JC70a, 1A10	Endothelium and tumours of endothelial origin; monocytes, macrophages, osteoclasts, megakaryocytes and plasma cells	
p53	DO1, D07, PAb1801	Tumours of diverse origins with excessive wild-type p53 or mutant p53 (nuclear expression)	
p21 (WAF1)	4D10, SX118	Used in combination with p53 detection to aid distinction of wild type from mutant p53 expression	

ALL, acute lymphoblastic leukaemia; AML, acute myeloid leukaemia; ER, oestrogen receptor; HER2, human epidermal growth factor receptor 2; McAb, monoclonal antibody; NK, natural killer; PNET, primitive neuroectodermal tumours.
*Cytokeratins (epithelial cytoskeletal intermediate filaments) are classified according to size. Different epithelial cell types are characterized by the expression of particular combinations of cytokeratin filaments; few cells express more than a limited range of the full repertoire. Many commercially available monoclonal anti-cytokeratin bodies react with epitopes shared by filaments of more than one size and hence represent useful broad-spectrum reagents to separate epithelial from non-epithelial cells. Some are further combined into cocktails (e.g. AE1/AE3) to extend their coverage. However, antibodies reactive with epitopes restricted to single cytokeratin types (e.g. CK7 or CK20) are useful because they react more specifically with epithelial cells showing distinct patterns of differentiation (e.g. breast ductal differentiation).

observation should lead to the suspicion of malignant infiltration. When a satisfactory aspirate is obtained it may contain large numbers of tumour cells mixed with a variable number of residual haemopoietic cells, or tumour cells may be scanty and found only after a prolonged search. Examination of the tail and edges of the film and examination of many films is important if scanty tumour cells are to be detected. The detection of scattered neoplastic cells in films of bone marrow aspirates is enhanced by the use of appropriate monoclonal antibodies such as those reactive with cytokeratins, carcino-embryonic antigen and epithelial membrane antigen (EMA) [20,21]. Positive reactions with such antibodies allow single neoplastic cells to be identified with more confidence.

Malignant cells are usually considerably larger than any haemopoietic cells other than megakaryocytes. However, in the small cell tumours of childhood, malignant cells may be similar in size to blast

Table 10.2 Expression of cytokeratin 7 (CK7), cytokeratin 20 (CK20) and other markers in some common carcinomas that may metastasize to the bone marrow [15–19].

	CK7+ CK20+	CK7+ CK20–	CK7– CK20+	CK7– CK20–	Other markers
Breast – ductal carcinoma	0–16%	82–95%	0–3%	0–5%	ER (70–80% positive), HER2 (overexpression in approximately 15%)
Breast – lobular carcinoma	0–9%	91–100%	0%	0%	ER (92% positive), HER2 overexpression uncommon
Colon or rectum – adenocarcinoma	5–10%	0%	75–95%	0–15%	
Lung – adenocarcinoma	10%	90%	0%	0%	TTF1
Lung – squamous cell carcinoma	0%	0–47%	0–8%	53–89%	CK5/6 usually positive
Lung – small cell carcinoma	0%	18–43%	0%	57–82%	CD56, TTF1 (non-pulmonary small cell carcinoma may also express TTF1)
Kidney – renal cell carcinoma	0%	11–24%	0–6%	71–81%	CD10 positive
Prostate – adenocarcinoma	0–8%	0–8%	0–23%	62–100%	PSA, PSAP
Stomach – adenocarcinoma	13–38%	17–25%	35–37%	10–25%	
Thyroid – follicular, papillary carcinoma	0%	98%	0%	2%	Thyroglobulin, TTF1
Thyroid – medullary carcinoma	0%	0%	0%	2%	Calcitonin, CEA, TTF1

CEA, carcino-embryonic antigen; ER, oestrogen receptor; HER2, human epidermal growth factor receptor 2; PSA, prostate-specific antigen; PSAP, prostate-specific acid phosphatase; TTF1, thyroid transcription factor 1.

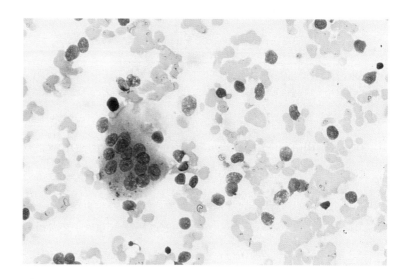

Fig. 10.1 Bone marrow (BM) aspirate, carcinoma of prostate, showing carcinoma cells and an osteoclast. May–Grünwald–Giemsa (MGG) ×40.

cells and acute leukaemia then enters into the differential diagnosis. Malignant cells are commonly cohesive and therefore occur as tight clumps with or without dispersed cells. Sometimes only irregu- larly distributed, dispersed cells are present. Neoplastic cells are usually pleomorphic with regard to size, shape and nuclear characteristics. Cell outlines may be indistinct or cells may appear

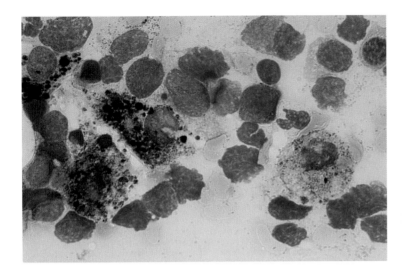

Fig. 10.2 BM aspirate, malignant melanoma, showing melanoma cells containing melanin. MGG ×100. (By courtesy of Dr J. Luckit, London.)

smudged. Some cells are multinucleated. The nuclei are often hyperchromatic and may contain nucleoli. Mitotic figures may be numerous. Carcinoma cells usually have moderately abundant cytoplasm, which shows a variable degree of basophilia and may contain vacuoles; they are sometimes phagocytic. In the small cell tumours of childhood, cytoplasm may be scanty, thus increasing the resemblance to leukaemic blast cells, and sometimes, because of their marked fragility, the cells are represented only by single or clustered bare nuclei. It should also be noted that neuroblastoma cells are positive for α-naphthyl acetate esterase activity [22]. However, they do not resemble cells of the monocyte lineage cytologically and they lack α-naphthyl butyrate esterase activity. Occasionally tumour cells in the bone marrow appear to be phagocytic. This has been reported for carcinoma of the breast and lung [23–25], medulloblastoma [26], rhabdomyosarcoma [27], Ewing's sarcoma [27] and haemangio-endothelioma. In the case of medulloblastoma, there was autophagocytosis of tumour cells [26].

It is not usually possible to predict the tissue of origin from the cytological features of neoplastic cells in films of bone marrow aspirates. In view of this, it is important also to examine histological sections of marrow particles, particularly if a trephine biopsy has not been performed. Sections may show features, such as gland formation, which are helpful in suggesting the tissue of origin. In a small percentage of cases, cytological features in aspirate films may suggest the tissue of origin. Melanoma cells may be recognized by the presence of pigment (Fig. 10.2), the nature of which can be confirmed by specific stains (see below). Such stains may be positive even when no pigment is detected in routinely stained films but otherwise the cells of amelanotic melanoma cannot be distinguished from other neoplastic cells. Melanin may also be present in macrophages (Fig. 10.3). Clear cell carcinomas are distinctive and suggest a renal primary; the cells have a relatively small nucleus and abundant, very weakly basophilic cytoplasm (Fig. 10.4). Cells of metastatic carcinoid tumour also have a relatively small nucleus and moderately abundant cytoplasm (Fig. 10.5). In children, neuroblastoma (Fig. 10.6) may sometimes be identified by the presence of extracellular blue-grey fibrillar material or by the presence of cells with irregular 'tails'; rosettes of tumour cells are distinctive and are found in up to two thirds of patients [28]. Rosettes are uncommon in other small cell tumours of childhood but small numbers may be seen in Ewing's sarcoma [28] and other PNET. In metastatic rhabdomyosarcoma there may be multinucleated giant cells or spindle-shaped binucleated rhabdomyoblasts [4]. The cytoplasm is often vacuolated and large vacuoles may coalesce to form lakes [29] (Fig. 10.7). Such cells are periodic acid–Schiff (PAS) positive. In some cases some of the tumour cells are phagocytic [27]. Less specific changes, such as

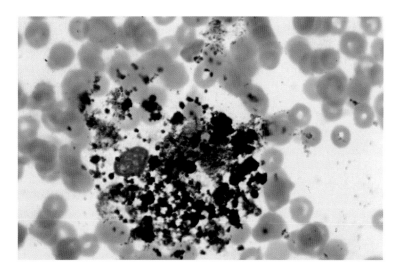

Fig. 10.3 BM aspirate from a patient with metastatic malignant melanoma showing a macrophage containing melanin. MGG ×100.

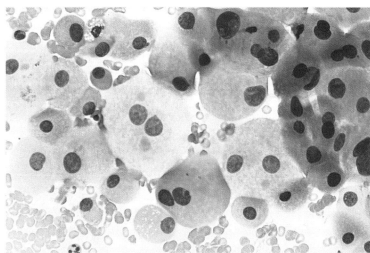

Fig. 10.4 BM aspirate, carcinoma of kidney, showing 'clear cells' with voluminous pale cytoplasm. MGG ×40. (By courtesy of Dr D. Gill, Brisbane.)

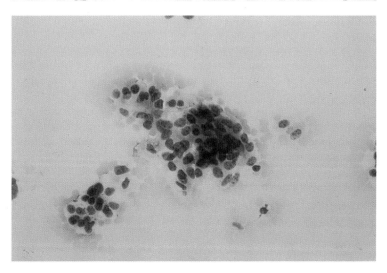

Fig. 10.5 BM aspirate, carcinoid tumour, showing cells with relatively small nuclei and a variable amount of cytoplasm. MGG ×40.

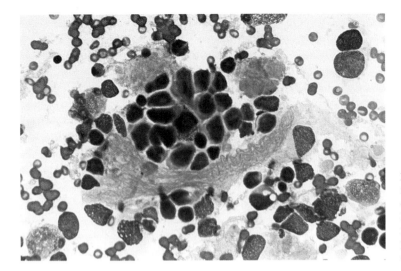

Fig. 10.6 BM aspirate, neuroblastoma, showing neoplastic cells which are relatively small and have a high nucleo-cytoplasmic ratio and a diffuse chromatin pattern. Neurofibrillary bundles are apparent. MGG ×40.

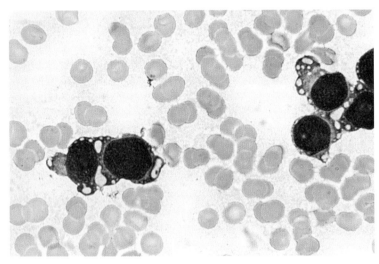

Fig. 10.7 BM aspirate, rhabdomyosarcoma, showing coalescing vacuoles. MGG ×100.

foamy or vacuolated cytoplasm or displacement of nuclei by cytoplasmic mucin, may be noted in metastatic adenocarcinoma originating from various primary sites (Fig. 10.8). In squamous cell carcinoma, metastatic tumour cells have sometimes been noted, on Romanowsky stains, to have a reddish cytoplasmic margin with the cytoplasm adjacent to the nucleus being more basophilic [30]. In small cell carcinoma of the lung, the neoplastic cells are usually smaller than those of most carcinomas but are nevertheless still larger than haemopoietic blasts. They have scanty, weakly basophilic cytoplasm and nuclei with coarse chromatin and inconspicuous nucleoli. The nuclei may appear to be bare and 'moulded' by the nuclei of adjacent tumour cells (Fig. 10.9).

Non-haemopoietic neoplastic cells in a bone marrow aspirate must be distinguished from lymphoma cells, blast cells of acute leukaemia and the neoplastic cells of Langerhans cell histiocytosis or systemic mastocytosis. Other cells that are sometimes confused with malignant cells include osteoblasts, osteoclasts, stromal fibroblasts, endothelial cells, atypical megakaryocytes and crushed erythroblasts.

When the bone marrow is infiltrated by malignant cells there may be associated reactive changes including increased plasma cells or mast cells, gran-

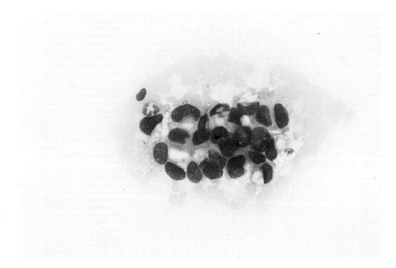

Fig. 10.8 BM aspirate, carcinoma of breast, showing adenocarcinoma cells with secretory globules. MGG ×40.

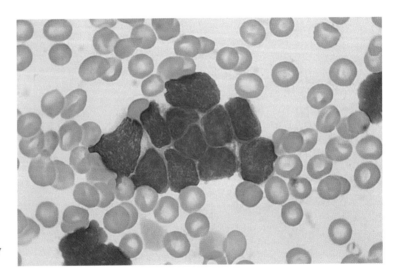

Fig. 10.9 BM aspirate, small cell carcinoma of lung, showing carcinoma cells with scanty cytoplasm and 'moulding' of cells by adjacent cells. MGG ×100.

ulocytic or megakaryocytic hyperplasia, increased macrophages and increased storage iron. Gelatinous transformation is rare but may be seen in severely cachectic patients.

Immunocytochemistry and flow cytometric immunophenotyping

Immunocytochemistry can be useful both to confirm the presence of carcinoma cells in a bone marrow aspirate and to detect infrequent cells (Fig. 10.10). A number of studies have been undertaken to assess the value and reliability of immunocytochemistry for epithelial antigens as a means of

assessing the extent of bone marrow involvement by metastatic carcinoma (see page 579).

On flow cytometric immunophenotyping, the failure of cells with cytological features resembling those of acute leukaemia to react with antibodies to CD45 should raise the suspicion of a non-haemopoietic tumour. A CD45-negative, CD56-positive phenotype can be used in bone marrow staging of a known neuroendocrine tumour [31].

Cytogenetic and molecular genetic analysis

Cytogenetic analysis may be useful in suggesting the non-haemopoietic nature of malignant cells

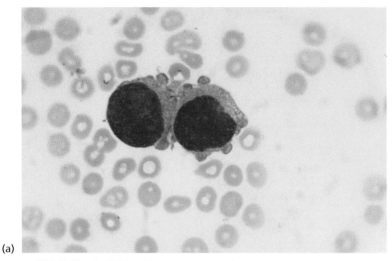

(a)

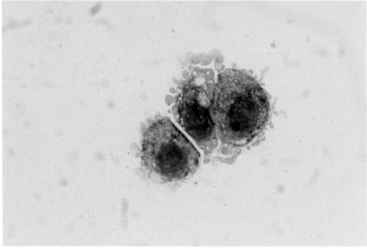

(b)

Fig. 10.10 BM aspirate, metastatic carcinoma of breast. (a) MGG ×100. (b) Immunoperoxidase with anti-cytokeratin antibody ×100.

infiltrating bone marrow and in confirming the specific diagnosis in paediatric small cell tumours (Table 10.3). For example, t(2;13)(q35;q14) can be demonstrated in many cases of rhabdomyosarcoma [32] and variant translocations in a minority [33]. In neuroblastoma, +7 and 17q+ are typical, the latter often resulting from an unbalanced translocation with chromosome 1 in which 1p is lost [34]. Ewing's sarcoma and other PNET may be associated with t(11;22)(q24;q12) or variants. Recurrent cytogenetic abnormalities have also been reported in several types of adult sarcoma but we have not

yet seen examples of these involving bone marrow. Bone marrow films can be used for fluorescence *in situ* hybridization (FISH) analysis to identify specific chromosomal abnormalities of diagnostic or prognostic significance.

Molecular genetic analysis in Ewing's sarcoma most often shows t(11;22)(q24;q12) with rearrangement of the *EWS* gene at 22q12 and formation of an *EWSR1-FLI1* fusion gene. In the minority of patients with a variant translocation other fusion genes are found. In alveolar rhabdomyosarcoma, the *PAX3* and *PAX7* genes at 2q35 and 1p36,

Table 10.3 Some characteristic acquired cytogenetic and molecular genetic abnormalities associated with specific tumours.

Tumour	Cytogenetic abnormalities	Molecular genetic abnormalities	Frequency
Alveolar rhabdomyosarcoma	t(2;13)(q35;q14)	*PAX3-FOXO1A* fusion	Common
	t(1;13)(p36;q14)	*PAX7-FOXO1A* fusion	Uncommon
PNET including Ewing's sarcoma	t(11;22)(q24;q12)	*EWSR1-FLI1* fusion	Common
	t(7;22)(p22;q12)	*EWSR1-ETV1* fusion	Uncommon
	t(17;22)(q21;q12)	*EWSR1-ETV4* fusion	Uncommon
	t(21;22)(q22;q12)	*EWSR1-ERG* fusion	Uncommon
	t(16;21)(p11;q22)		Uncommon
Neuroblastoma	Double minute or homogeneously staining regions on 2p	*MYCN* amplification	Common

PNET, primitive neuroectodermal tumours.

respectively, are rearranged resulting in the formation of *PAX3-FOXO1A* and *PAX7-FOXO1A* fusion genes [33]. Neuroblastoma may be associated with *MYCN* amplification; when present, such amplification is associated with an adverse prognosis. FISH is used for detection of *MYCN* amplification in bone marrow films.

Bone marrow histology

Marrow infiltration by metastatic tumour may be focal or diffuse. Stromal and bone reactions are frequent but not invariable. Frequent stromal reactions include: (i) fibroblast proliferation with deposition of reticulin with or without collagen; (ii) neoangiogenesis; (iii) an inflammatory response (presence of lymphocyte, monocytes, macrophages, mast cells); and (iv) necrosis. Bone changes include: (i) osteolysis, resulting from erosion by tumour cells or osteoclast activation; (ii) osteosclerosis with the presence of woven bone or increased lamellar bone formation; and (iii) mixed osteolysis and osteosclerosis. New bone formation can be either metaplastic (interstitial) or appositional. Any combination of stromal and bone changes can be seen. Marked fibrosis is most frequent in carcinomas of the breast and prostate gland but is also found relatively commonly in metastases from cancers of the stomach and lung [9,35,36]. In patients with fibrosis the number of tumour cells is variable (Figs 10.11 and 10.12) and they can be very infrequent. Failure to

recognize tumour cells within the fibrous stroma can result in a mistaken diagnosis of primary myelofibrosis. The degree of differentiation of metastatic tumour is very variable and it is often impossible to be certain of the site of the primary tumour on purely morphological grounds. Frequently, metastases are undifferentiated and the differential diagnosis includes poorly differentiated carcinoma, high grade non-Hodgkin lymphoma and malignant melanoma (Figs 10.13–10.15); immunohistochemistry is invaluable (see below) [37]. In undifferentiated or poorly differentiated carcinomas it is not usually possible to determine the site of origin of the tumour. In tumours showing differentiation it may be possible to determine the type of carcinoma and suggest the likely site of origin – for example, in metastatic squamous carcinoma, the lung is the most likely primary site. Squamous differentiation is recognized by the formation of keratin and the presence of intercellular bridges. A mixed pattern of differentiation, with squamous cell carcinoma, small cell carcinoma and adenocarcinoma in any combination, is highly suggestive of origin from the lung.

Metastatic adenocarcinoma can be diagnosed on the basis of the formation of glands (Fig. 10.16), the presence of signet ring cells and/or the presence of mucin (best detected using a combined diastase-treated Alcian blue/PAS stain). A mucin stain facilitates the detection of small numbers of carcinoma

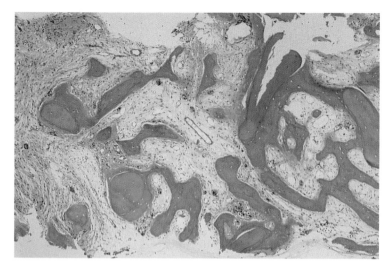

Fig. 10.11 BM trephine biopsy section, carcinoma of the breast, showing osteosclerosis and replacement of the marrow by dense fibrous tissue containing tumour cells. Paraffin-embedded, haematoxylin and eosin (H&E) ×4.

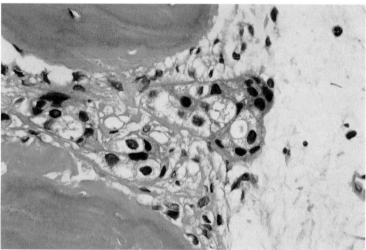

Fig. 10.12 BM trephine biopsy section, carcinoma of the breast (same patient as Fig. 10.11), showing a group of tumour cells with hyperchromatic nuclei and vacuolated cytoplasm. Paraffin-embedded, H&E ×40.

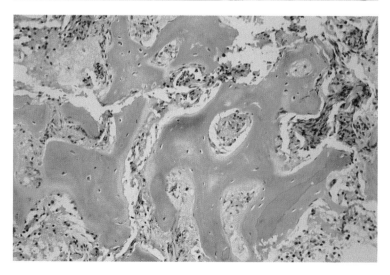

Fig. 10.13 BM trephine biopsy section, poorly differentiated prostatic carcinoma, showing osteosclerosis and replacement of the marrow by dense fibrous tissue containing tumour cells. Paraffin-embedded, H&E ×10.

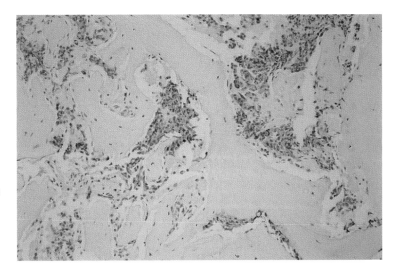

Fig. 10.14 BM trephine biopsy section, poorly differentiated prostatic carcinoma (same patient as Fig. 10.13), showing expression of cytokeratin by tumour cells. Paraffin-embedded, peroxidase/anti-peroxidase, anti-cytokeratin McAb ×10.

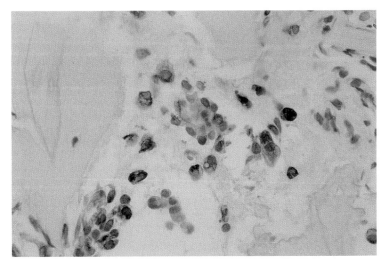

Fig. 10.15 BM trephine biopsy section, poorly differentiated prostatic carcinoma (same patient as Fig. 10.13), showing expression of cytokeratin by tumour cells. Paraffin-embedded, peroxidase/anti-peroxidase, anti-cytokeratin McAb ×40.

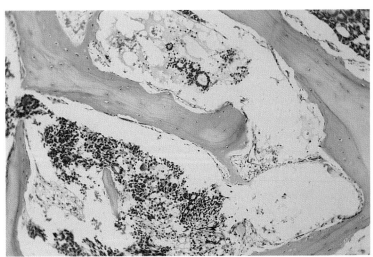

Fig. 10.16 BM trephine biopsy section, well-differentiated prostatic carcinoma, showing a tumour composed of small, well-defined glandular structures. Resin-embedded, H&E ×10.

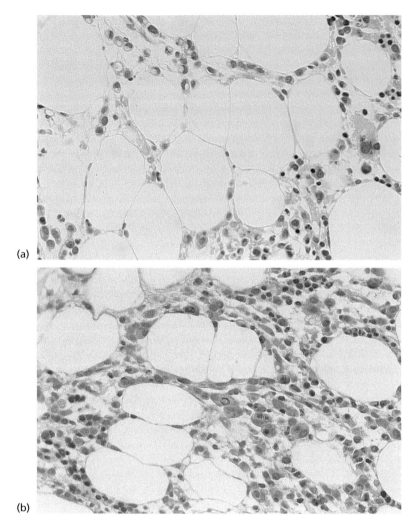

(a)

(b)

Fig. 10.17 BM trephine biopsy section, adenocarcinoma, showing interstitial infiltrate. (a) Paraffin-embedded, H&E ×40. (b) Paraffin-embedded, Alcian blue stain ×40. (By courtesy of Dr S. Wright, London).

cells which may be difficult to detect when they are present as an interstitial infiltrate (Fig. 10.17). Some adenocarcinomas produce large amounts of extracellular mucin, also detectable with a mucin stain (Fig. 10.18). It should be noted that, very rarely, signet ring cells occur in lymphomas [38]. Metastatic adenocarcinoma may arise from primary tumours in the gastro-intestinal tract, breast, prostate gland, ovary, endometrium, pancreas and many other sites. Primary sites whose identification is particularly important because of their sensitivity to hormonal therapy are the breast, endometrium, ovary and prostate gland. Prostatic origin is sug-

gested by a cribriform, microglandular pattern associated with fibrosis and new bone formation (Fig. 10.19). Occasionally a macroglandular pattern is present (Fig. 10.20), also usually accompanied by fibrosis and neo-osteogenesis. Identification of breast carcinoma is usually based on its morphological resemblance to primary breast cancers, including duct formation and, particularly in lobular carcinoma, the presence of cell columns forming 'Indian file' patterns (Fig. 10.21). Intracytoplasmic lumina are sometimes visible within individual breast carcinoma cells and these can be highlighted by combined Alcian blue/PAS

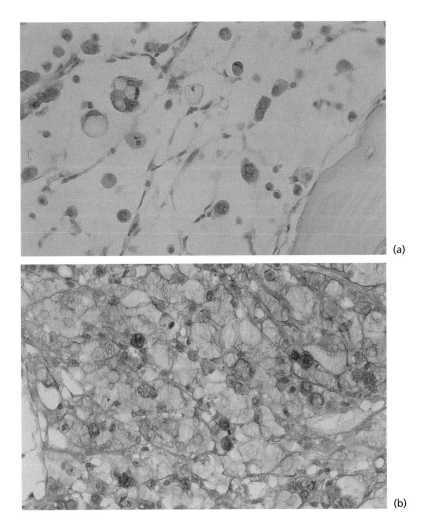

(a)

(b)

Fig. 10.18 BM trephine biopsy section, adenocarcinoma, showing intracellular mucin and abundant extracellular mucin. (a) Paraffin-embedded, H&E ×40. (b) Paraffin-embedded, PAS stain ×40.

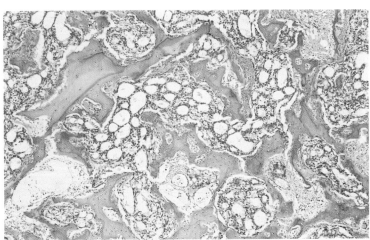

Fig. 10.19 BM trephine biopsy section, prostatic adenocarcinoma showing microglandular pattern with extensive new bone formation. Paraffin-embedded, H&E ×20.

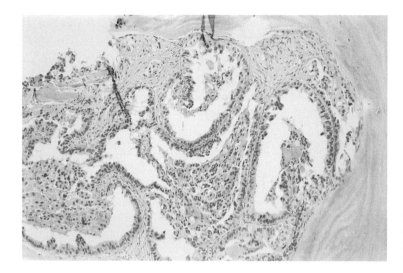

Fig. 10.20 BM trephine biopsy section, macroglandular pattern of prostatic adenocarcinoma. Paraffin-embedded, H&E ×20.

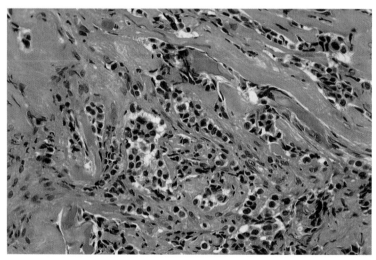

Fig. 10.21 BM trephine biopsy section, carcinoma of the breast, showing tumour cells with hyperchromatic nuclei arranged in cords and strands in a dense fibrous (desmoplastic) stroma. Paraffin-embedded, H&E ×40.

staining (Fig. 10.22). Most, but not all, bone marrow metastases from breast cancer are associated with fibrosis and new bone formation. Immunohistochemical staining can be helpful (see below). Because metastatic lobular carcinoma of the breast can produce an interstitial infiltrate with little cellular reaction, its detection can be difficult. Routine use of immunohistochemistry when a biopsy is carried out for staging purposes has therefore been advised [39]. Adenocarcinoma composed predominantly of ribbons or villous formations of columnar epithelium with intracellular mucin (goblet cells) is usually of large bowel origin (Fig. 10.23). Clear cell carcinomas have large amounts of pale cytoplasm due to the presence of abundant glycogen or lipid; mucin stains are negative. Likely primary sites of metastatic clear cell carcinoma include the kidney, ovary and lung. In rare cases when metastatic follicular carcinoma of the thyroid gland is present, it may be suspected on morphological grounds if follicles containing colloid are seen.

Metastatic small cell carcinoma of the lung commonly involves the bone marrow (see below). The cells are usually small with intensely hyperchromatic, round or oval nuclei and scant cytoplasm (Fig. 10.24). Nuclear moulding by adjacent cells is characteristic although not specific. Necrosis is

Fig. 10.22 BM trephine biopsy section, lobular carcinoma of breast, showing intracytoplasmic lumen formation. Alcian blue-positive material is present at the periphery of what appears to be a cytoplasmic vacuole and PAS-positive material is present in the centre. Electron microscopy has shown that these structures in lobular breast carcinoma represent true lumina, formed within individual cells, rather than simple secretory vacuoles. Paraffin-embedded, combined Alcian blue/PAS stain ×100.

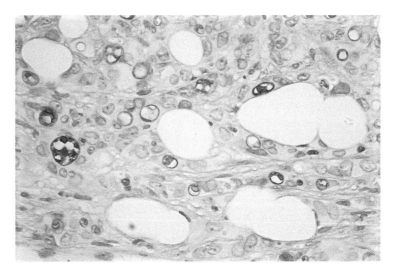

Fig. 10.23 BM trephine biopsy section, metastatic adenocarcinoma from a colonic primary tumour, showing a glandular and villous pattern. Paraffin-embedded, H&E ×40.

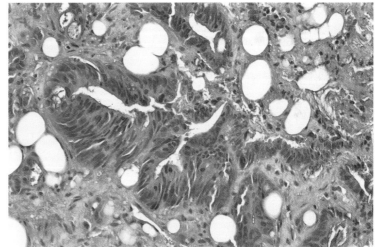

Fig. 10.24 BM trephine biopsy section, small cell carcinoma of the bronchus, showing a sheet of small cells with hyperchromatic ovoid nuclei and scanty cytoplasm; in places there is nuclear 'moulding'. Resin-embedded, H&E ×40.

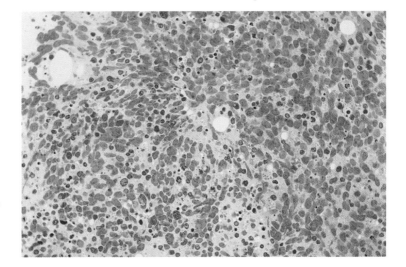

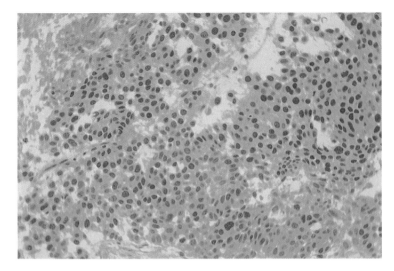

Fig. 10.25 BM trephine biopsy section, carcinoid tumour (unknown primary site), showing relatively uniform cells with ovoid hyperchromatic nuclei and eosinophilic cytoplasm; in some areas the cells are arranged in trabeculae. Resin-embedded, H&E ×40.

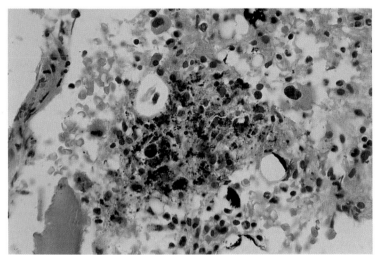

Fig. 10.26 BM trephine biopsy section, malignant melanoma, showing a focal tumour infiltrate composed of cells containing large amounts of melanin. The tumour cells have hyperchromatic nuclei, and some have prominent nucleoli. (It should be noted that it is unusual to see large amounts of melanin in metastatic malignant melanoma.) Paraffin-embedded, H&E ×40.

common and there is often smearing of nuclei which can render interpretation difficult. Morphological variants of small cell carcinoma also occur, in which the cells are slightly larger and have either a fusiform or polygonal shape. The principal differential diagnosis of metastatic small cell carcinoma is that of non-Hodgkin lymphoma. Metastases from other tumours with neuroendocrine differentiation, such as malignant carcinoid tumours, may also occasionally spread to bone marrow; these may have distinctive morphology, with nests and ribbons of monomorphic cells having nuclei with dense, evenly distributed chromatin (Fig. 10.25).

Malignant melanoma is found in the bone marrow in approximately 5% of patients with disseminated disease [40]. If melanin is present in the tumour cells (Fig. 10.26) or associated macrophages, the diagnosis is relatively easy although, if the patient is not already known to have melanoma, the nature of any pigment present should be confirmed by either a Masson–Fontana or a Schmorl stain for melanin. However, not infrequently, metastatic malignant melanoma is amelanotic (Fig. 10.27) and immunohistochemistry should then be considered for confirmation. Malignant melanoma should be suspected if the metastatic tumour is composed of polygonal or spindle cells with prominent nucleoli.

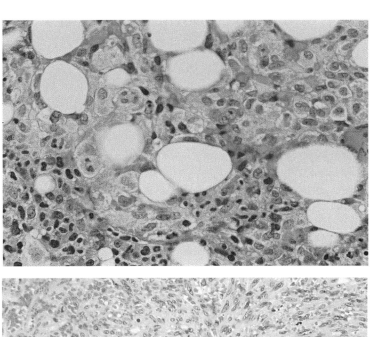

Fig. 10.27 BM trephine biopsy section, amelanotic melanoma composed of fairly bland epithelioid cells. Immunohistochemistry was required to confirm the true nature of this tumour; cells expressed S100 protein and the antigen recognized by HMB-45. Paraffin-embedded, H&E ×40.

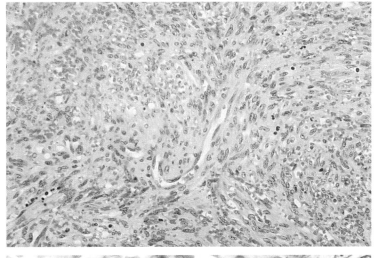

(a)

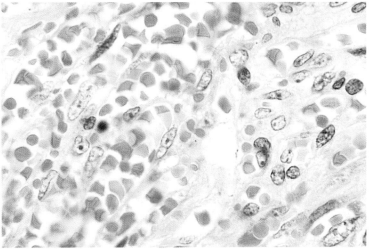

Fig. 10.28 BM trephine biopsy section showing Kaposi's sarcoma in a patient who did not have AIDS. (a) Paraffin-embedded, H&E ×25. (b) Paraffin-embedded, H&E ×100. (By courtesy of Dr R. M. Conran and Dr V. B. Reddy, Aurora, Colorado.)

(b)

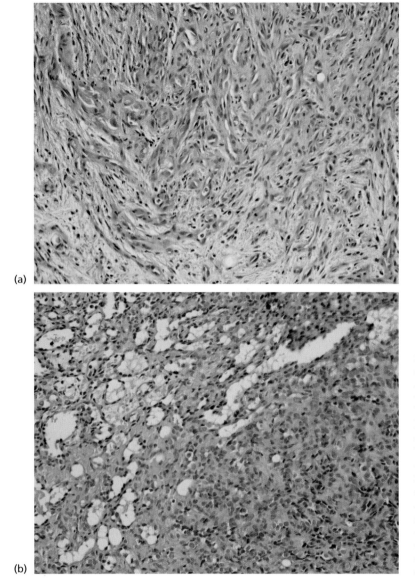

(a)

(b)

Fig. 10.29 BM trephine biopsy sections showing infiltration by angiosarcoma. A computerized tomography scan showed multiple bone lesions and hepatosplenomegaly. The primary site was not established definitively but the histology and distribution of disease suggested metastatic bone marrow spread from a primary splenic angiosarcoma. A mixture of angiomatous, solid and kaposiform growth is present with atypical endothelial cells in all components expressing CD31. (a) Paraffin-embedded, H&E ×20. (b) Paraffin-embedded, H&E ×20.

The differential diagnosis of metastatic spindle cell tumour within the marrow includes carcinoma showing spindle cell differentiation, malignant melanoma and various sarcomas. Sarcomas rarely metastasize to the marrow and, when they do, the primary tumour is usually readily apparent. Occasionally Kaposi's sarcoma and other angiosarcomas may present in the bone marrow or may be sampled when bone marrow is investigated for reasons other than staging in patients (e.g. individuals with AIDS) who have known primary tumours elsewhere. Bone marrow involvement by Kaposi's sarcoma is rare but has been observed both in AIDS [41] and in occasional HIV-negative patients [42]. The bone marrow may be extensively replaced by abnormal tissue composed of slit-like vascular channels lined by spindle-shaped endothelial cells (Fig. 10.28). Large, plump nuclei of neo-

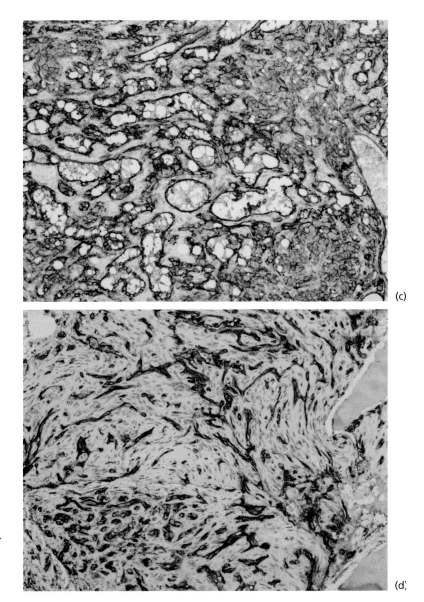

Fig. 10.29 (continued)
(c) Mixed area. Paraffin-embedded, immunoperoxidase for CD31 ×20.
(d) Kaposiform area. Paraffin-embedded, immunoperoxidase for CD31 ×20.

plastic endothelial cells protrude into the abnormal vascular channels, some of which are engorged with erythrocytes. Haemosiderin-laden macrophages are increased. Angiosarcomas, including Kaposi's sarcoma, show widely varying degrees of vascular differentiation and may form reticular or solid spindle cell areas (Figs 10.29 and 10.30). Immunohistochemistry to demonstrate expression of endothelial antigens may be helpful in cases lacking obvious vessel formation.

Many of the malignant tumours that occur in childhood are composed of small cells with relatively uniform, round nuclei. The differential diagnosis of bone marrow infiltration by such cells in a child includes non-Hodgkin lymphoma (usually lymphoblastic or Burkitt lymphoma), metastatic

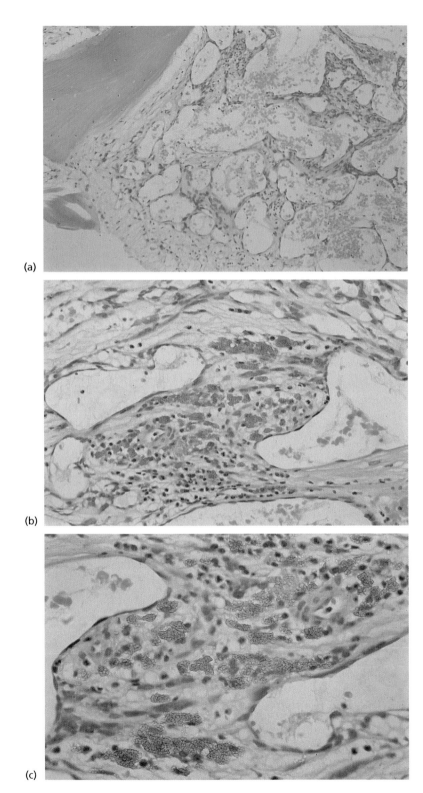

(a)

(b)

(c)

Fig. 10.30 BM trephine biopsy section, metastatic Thorotrast-induced angiosarcoma, showing refractile Thorotrast. Paraffin-embedded, H&E: (a) ×10; (b) ×20; (c) ×40.

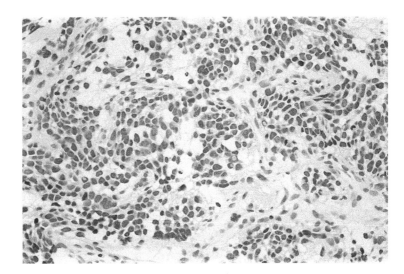

Fig. 10.31 BM trephine biopsy section, neuroblastoma, showing extensive, diffuse infiltration by small cells with scanty cytoplasm. Paraffin-embedded, H&E ×40.

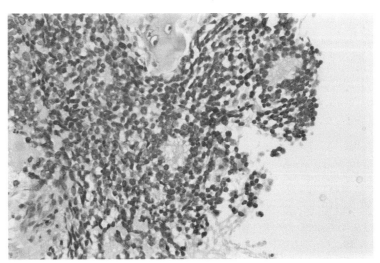

Fig. 10.32 BM trephine biopsy, neuroblastoma, showing rosette formation. Note the collections of pink material around which the neuroblastoma cells are clustered. Paraffin-embedded, H&E ×40.

neuroblastoma, rhabdomyosarcoma, Ewing's sarcoma, other PNET and retinoblastoma. In order to make a specific diagnosis the clinical features, morphological findings and histochemical and immunohistochemical staining characteristics all need to be considered. The marrow findings in lymphoblastic and Burkitt lymphoma are described on pages 305, 364 and 360; both express CD45 and B-cell immunophenotypic markers. Neuroblastoma is the most common malignant solid tumour in children and often metastasizes to the bone marrow. The majority of cases occur in children under 4 years of age. The neoplastic cells are slightly larger than small lymphocytes with regular, round, hyperchromatic nuclei and little cytoplasm [43] (Fig. 10.31). Rosettes are present in a minority of cases, consisting of tumour cells arranged around central fibrillary material which is pink in haematoxylin and eosin (H&E)-stained sections (Fig. 10.32). The cells of neuroblastoma may show focal PAS positivity but this is usually less marked than that seen in rhabdomyosarcoma and Ewing's sarcoma. In all of these neoplasms, PAS positivity is difficult to detect in fixed tissue sections; it should be sought by staining of aspirate films, as described above.

In one series, rhabdomyosarcoma was found to

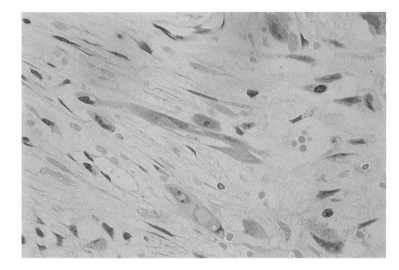

Fig. 10.33 BM trephine biopsy section, rhabdomyosarcoma, showing elongated cells with plentiful eosinophilic cytoplasm (rhabdomyoblasts). Resin-embedded, H&E ×40.

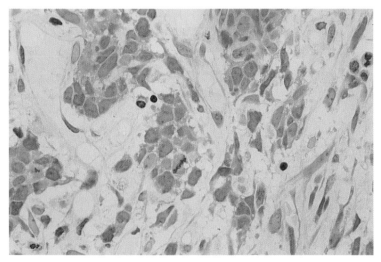

Fig. 10.34 BM trephine biopsy section, Ewing's sarcoma, showing irregular groups of cells in a fibrous stroma; the cells have ovoid nuclei with indistinct nucleoli and scanty cytoplasm. Resin-embedded, H&E ×40.

have metastasized to the bone marrow in 16% of cases [1]. Several histological variants are recognized: (i) embryonal, which may be further subdivided into myxoid, spindle cell or round cell patterns [44], with the round cell subtype being represented most commonly in bone marrow metastases; (ii) alveolar, characterized by a pattern of irregular spaces lined by tumour cells [45]; and (iii) pleomorphic, which is very rare and not usually seen in children. In any of these subtypes there may be a few multinucleated rhabdoid cells with peripheral nuclei. A pseudo-alveolar pattern may be produced by cells adhering to the margins of vascular channels [29]. Diagnosis depends on the

recognition of skeletal muscle differentiation. Rhabdomyoblasts may be oval, spindle, tadpole or strap shaped. They have abundant pink granular cytoplasm which may show cross-striations (Fig. 10.33). The number of rhabdomyoblasts present is highly variable; in many patients the majority of cells are undifferentiated round or spindle cells. Ewing's sarcoma and related PNET are malignant tumours that may arise in bone or soft tissue. Most patients are in the second decade of life and approximately 35% of cases develop bone marrow metastases [1]. The tumour cells are approximately twice the size of small lymphocytes and have round-to-oval vesicular nuclei (Fig. 10.34). They

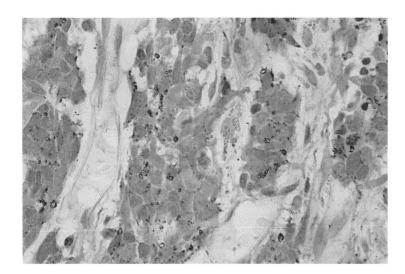

Fig. 10.35 BM trephine biopsy section, Ewing's sarcoma, showing large granules of glycogen in the cytoplasm. Resin-embedded, PAS ×40.

may show PAS-positive cytoplasmic staining for glycogen, either finely dispersed or forming large blocks of positively stained material (Fig. 10.35). Erythrophagocytosis [46] and haemophagocytosis by malignant cells can occur in rhabdomyosarcoma [47,48] but are not specific since they can also occur in other tumours (see above).

Immunohistochemistry

In bone marrow trephine biopsy sections containing metastatic poorly differentiated tumours, immunohistochemistry with a small panel of antibodies is useful to demonstrate lymphoid antigens (CD45, CD20 and CD3), epithelial markers (cytokeratins and epithelial membrane antigen) and melanoma-associated antigens (S100 protein, Melan A and the antigen recognized by antibody HMB-45) [20,37,49,50]. If an undifferentiated tumour is negative or yields equivocal results for all of these, the differential diagnosis includes anaplastic plasmacytoma/myeloma, large cell anaplastic lymphoma and undifferentiated carcinoma; further immunohistochemistry is needed to investigate these possibilities.

Differential expression of cytokeratins can help to establish the primary site of a carcinoma, particularly adenocarcinoma (see Table 10.2).

The prostatic origin of a metastatic adenocarcinoma may be confirmed by immunohistochemical staining with antibodies that react with prostate-specific antigen [51]. Since these antibodies may also react with some colonic tumours [52], the use of parallel immunostaining for prostate-specific acid phosphatase is recommended. Use of both antibodies considerably improves sensitivity and specificity in confirming the prostatic origin of metastatic cancer.

Unfortunately, there are no antigens with equivalent tissue specificity for breast carcinoma but differential cytokeratin expression is useful (see Table 10.2). Nuclear expression of oestrogen and progesterone receptors may be demonstrated immunohistochemically (Fig. 10.36) but these antigens are also expressed in a variety of other adenocarcinomas, particularly those arising in the endometrium or ovary. They may also be expressed in metastatic adenocarcinoma of the lung [53]. Expression of these antigens, irrespective of precise tumour origin, is important for selection of treatment. HER2 expression is also highly relevant to treatment choice and immunohistochemistry for this antigen is relevant in adenocarcinoma of unknown origin. However, if a biopsy specimen of the primary tumour is available HER2 analysis should be done on that tissue rather than on the bone marrow since fixation and decalcification make analysis of the bone marrow metastasis less reliable.

Immunohistochemical staining for thyroglobulin is useful in confirming the thyroid origin of metastatic tumour cells. Thyroid transcription factor 1 is also usually positive but it should be noted that positive reactions are usual in non-squamous cell

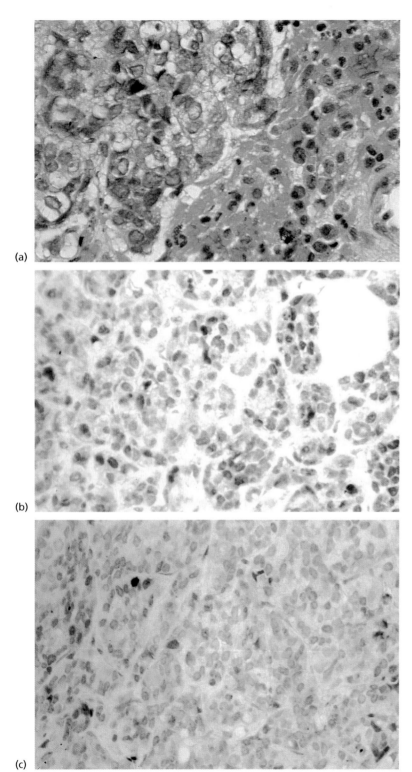

(a)

(b)

(c)

Fig. 10.36 BM trephine biopsy sections showing a poorly differentiated adenocarcinoma of the breast; there is nuclear expression of oestrogen receptor but not progesterone receptor.
(a) Paraffin-embedded, H&E ×50.
(b) Paraffin-embedded, immunoperoxidase for oestrogen receptor ×50. (c) Paraffin-embedded, immunoperoxidase for progesterone receptor ×50.

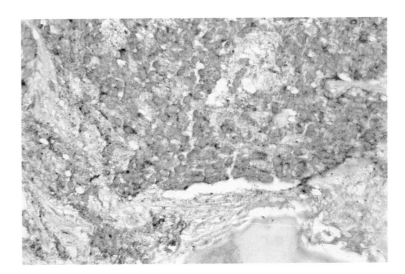

Fig. 10.37 BM trephine biopsy section showing neuroblastoma. Paraffin-embedded, immunoperoxidase for chromogranin ×40. (By courtesy of the late Professor D. Evans, London.)

carcinoma of the lung, which is more likely to present as a tumour of unknown origin.

Small cell carcinoma reacts positively with antibodies directed against CD56 and usually with some antibodies to cytokeratin (e.g. CAM5.2 and MNF116). Cytokeratin expression is distinctive with an intracytoplasmic dot-like or perinuclear ring pattern. Protein gene product 9.5 (PGP9.5), a further antigen expressed by neuroectodermal cells, may also be useful in diagnosis of small cell carcinoma but it should be noted that polyclonal anti-PGP9.5 antisera cross-react with some lymphomas [54] and with about 50% of myelomas [55]. Other tumours showing neuroendocrine differentiation, such as carcinoid tumours and medullary carcinoma of the thyroid gland, may metastasize to the bone marrow; immunohistochemical staining for CD56, chromogranin, synaptophysin, neurofilament protein and PGP9.5 can help to identify neuroendocrine differentiation in these tumours [56–58]. In addition, medullary carcinomas of the thyroid may express calcitonin.

In cases of metastatic melanoma, immunohistochemical staining for S100 protein is usually positive [37]. HMB-45 and Melan A also react well with metastatic malignant melanoma in bone marrow trephine biopsy sections. Spindle cell melanomas and spindle cells carcinomas can be confused; the former express S100 protein and the latter cytokeratins. However, a significant minority of breast carcinomas express S100 in addition to cytokeratins. Use of vimentin immunostaining to distinguish such spindle cell tumours from true sarcomas is unreliable, since many non-sarcomatous tumours with spindle cell morphology express vimentin; apart from variants of angiosarcoma, however, metastatic sarcomas are exceptionally rarely seen in bone marrow biopsies. In angiosarcoma and Kaposi's sarcoma, the endothelial origin of malignant cells can be demonstrated by immunohistochemical staining for von Willebrand factor, CD31 and CD34. The causative agent of Kaposi's sarcoma, human herpesvirus 8 (HHV8) [59], can de demonstrated by immunohistochemistry, confirming this specific diagnosis.

Neuroblastoma cells usually express neurone-specific enolase and PGP9.5; less consistently, chromogranin (Fig. 10.37) and the antigens detected by antibodies NB84 and NeuN are expressed. In rhabdomyosarcomas, immunohistochemical staining for desmin, myogenin and MyoD are usually positive [60] although staining for myoglobin, which is said to be more specific, is variable [44]. Ewing's sarcomas with t(11;22)(q24;q12) express CD99 (MIC2) [61,62], but expression is not specific for this tumour being seen also in a high proportion of cases of both T-lineage and B-lineage acute lymphoblastic leukaemia [63] and in some other neoplasms.

The role of bone marrow examination in the staging of solid tumours

Examination of the bone marrow by aspiration and trephine biopsy is an established part of the staging of neuroblastoma in children in most large centres. The bone marrow biopsy is positive at the time of initial diagnosis in approximately half of all patients, most of whom have evidence of metastatic spread at other sites [64]. Discordance between marrow aspirate and trephine biopsy findings is common. In one reported series, the trephine biopsy alone was positive in 20% of cases whereas neoplastic cells were seen in the aspirate films when trephine biopsy sections appeared normal in 7%. Taking bilateral bone marrow aspirates and trephine biopsies from the iliac crests increases the sensitivity of the staging procedure by approximately 10%. Particularly careful examination of aspirate films and trephine biopsy sections is necessary because infiltration is often extremely focal [65,66]. In cases in which the marrow appearances are suspicious but not diagnostic of infiltration, immunocytochemical staining of aspirate films using antibodies reactive with neuroectodermal antigens (UJ13A and UJ127.11, reactive with epitopes of the CD56 antigen) may be of value in confirming marrow involvement [67,68]. Immunohistochemical staining of paraffin-embedded sections of trephine biopsies for neurone-specific enolase has not been found to increase the sensitivity of marrow biopsy as a means of detecting tumour cells [57]. Detection of PGP9.5 expression is considerably more reliable and should be performed in all cases; its expression is predominantly nuclear with weaker cytoplasmic staining. Its use permits demonstration of tiny clusters and even single cells in patients with minimal bone marrow involvement (Fig. 10.38). Immunohistochemical staining with additional antibodies such as NB84 [69,70] and NeuN [71] can also be used but may be negative in cases with more primitive cells that are nevertheless detected by PGP9.5 expression. Assessment of marrow infiltration by neuroblastoma is more difficult in patients who have been treated with chemotherapy; it is essential that trephine biopsy specimens are of adequate size and quality [72–74]. It has been suggested that the appearances in post-treatment marrow trephine biopsy sections should be divided into four grades: grade 1, normal (or hypocellular) marrow; grade 2, marrow with reticulin fibrosis as the only abnormality; grade 3, distorted architecture with collagen fibrosis; and grade 4, marrow with obvious tumour cells, with or without other abnormalities [43]. Grades 2–4 were all considered by Reid and Hamilton [43] to be compatible with continued bone marrow involvement by tumour, even when individual neoplastic cells could not be identified with certainty. It remains unclear whether this is really true for grades 2 and 3 [75] and whether the different grades correlate with differences in clinical outcome. An important additional feature to recognize in follow-up bone marrow samples obtained during treatment of neuroblastoma is differentiation of the primitive small cells to produce large, ganglion-like cells and areas of pink, fibrillary tissue (neuropil) composed of neuronal and glial cell processes (Fig. 10.39). Ganglion-like cells may show superficial resemblance to megakaryocytes and neuropil requires differentiation from fibrous tissue. Immunostaining for PGP9.5 is positive in both types of differentiated neuroblastoma tissue and is very helpful in confirming their true nature.

In adults, examination of the bone marrow is not a routine staging procedure for most solid tumours and, although it has been advocated for small cell lung carcinoma and breast cancer, it is by no means practised universally, even for these tumours. In small cell carcinoma of the lung, bone marrow trephine biopsy is positive in 25–30% of cases [10,76,77]; the aspirate is only slightly less sensitive for detecting marrow involvement. It has been suggested that bone marrow examination is indicated in patients with small cell lung carcinoma in order to identify patients who may be suitable for attempted curative therapy [78]. However, some studies have shown no difference in survival between patients with and without marrow involvement [10,69], and the value of routine bone marrow examination has therefore been questioned [10]. Imaging techniques such as magnetic resonance imaging have been proposed as more sensitive alternative staging procedures [79].

Several studies have evaluated the use of marrow aspiration and trephine biopsy in the staging of breast cancer. Detection of subclinical metastatic disease may be useful in identifying patients with apparently localized disease who might benefit

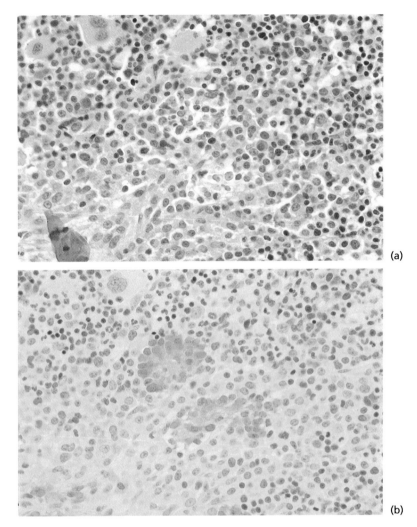

(a)

(b)

Fig. 10.38 BM trephine biopsy section showing minimal infiltration by neuroblastoma. (a) Paraffin-embedded, H&E ×40. (b) Paraffin-embedded, immunohistochemistry for PGP.9.5 ×40.

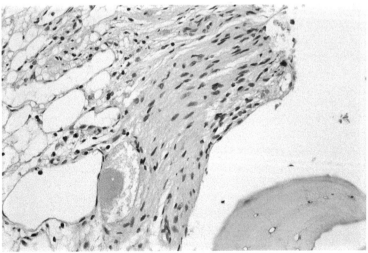

Fig. 10.39 BM trephine biopsy section, post-treatment follow-up for neuroblastoma. Cellular 'fibrous' tissue remains and the cytoplasm of at least one large ganglion-like cell can be seen. Paraffin-embedded, H&E ×40.

from adjuvant chemotherapy. Bone marrow biopsy is positive in 25–55% of patients with positive radio-isotope bone imaging, but only 4–10% of patients with negative radio-isotopic imaging have tumour detected by bone marrow biopsy [8,80]. In one reported series, 23% of all breast cancer patients had positive bone marrow biopsies at the time of first recurrence [80]. In an attempt to increase the sensitivity of bone marrow examination as a staging procedure, some studies have used immunocytochemical staining to identify micrometastases that would not be detected by conventional techniques. The method used has involved aspirating bone marrow from multiple (up to eight) sites under general anaesthesia at the time of initial surgery, pooling the material and preparing several films. Tumour cells are then detected by immunostaining with antibodies reactive with EMA [81,82] or cytokeratins [83] or with a cocktail of antibodies recognizing these antigens [84]. Using this approach, micrometastases have been found in 27–35% of cases at the time of diagnosis and correlation has been shown between their presence and the size of the primary tumour [81,82]. The presence of bone marrow micrometastases is a predictor of early relapse in bone. Despite these findings, application of immunocytochemistry to detect micrometastases in bone marrow aspirates performed for staging of breast cancer has not yet become standard practice. A similar approach has been suggested for detection of oral, oesophageal and gastric cancers [85–88], pancreatic cancer [89,90], non-small cell lung cancer [91], urological cancers [92] and malignant melanoma [93]. Use of reverse transcriptase polymerase chain reaction (RT-PCR) directed at carcino-embryonic antigen mRNA to detect occult involvement of aspirated bone marrow by carcinomas arising from breast or colon [94,95], and directed at cytokeratin mRNA in cases of breast cancer [96], has also proved successful in initial studies. The clinical value of detecting occult bone marrow micrometastases in such tumours by these techniques remains unproven [97]. In all cases, including breast carcinoma, technical problems with the immunocytochemical approach, including false-positive results due to skin contamination or non-specific haemopoietic cell reactivity, limit its applicability in routine practice [98,99].

The role of bone marrow examination in identifying the tissue of origin of metastases and markers of relevance to prognosis or treatment

Sometimes the detection of a bone marrow metastasis provides the first evidence that a patient has a neoplastic condition, with no primary tumour apparent. It is important to ascertain the tissue of origin when a specific treatment may be available, even in a patient with metastatic disease. It is therefore necessary to recognize carcinoma of the breast, endometrium, ovary, prostate, lung and thyroid and small cell tumours of childhood. Depending on the nature of the tumour, recognition of the tissue of origin may be contributed to by cytology, histology, immunophenotyping and cytogenetic or molecular genetic analysis, as discussed above. Information from all these types of investigation needs to be integrated and interpreted in the light of the age and gender of the patient.

Problems and pitfalls in identification of tumour infiltration of bone marrow

Normal components of bone marrow may be mistaken for non-haemopoietic malignant cells in aspirate films and biopsy sections. These include megakaryocytes, crushed erythroid cells, osteoblasts (Fig. 10.40), osteoclasts, stromal macrophages, endothelium and fibroblasts. Awareness of the appearances of stromal components in aspirate films is particularly important in avoiding confusion with malignant cells.

Artefactual inclusions of extraneous tissue in trephine biopsy specimens (e.g. skin, sweat glands, hair follicles or skeletal muscle) may mimic malignant non-haemopoietic cells (Fig. 10.41, and see also Figs 1.67–1.70, pages 47–48). Care should be taken to avoid such inclusions by making a small skin incision prior to insertion of the biopsy needle and using disposable needles to ensure a sharp cutting edge. Carry-over from other specimens into the paraffin block during tissue processing should be avoided by good laboratory practice with regard to preparation of small or friable biopsy specimens; such specimens should be wrapped in tissue paper or sponge, or placed in a wire mesh insert, before processing. If carry-over is suspected, it can be confirmed by molecular analysis to demonstrate the different patient origins of separate

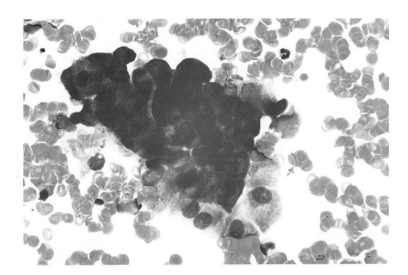

Fig. 10.40 BM aspirate showing a cluster of osteoblasts mimicking carcinoma cells. MGG ×40.

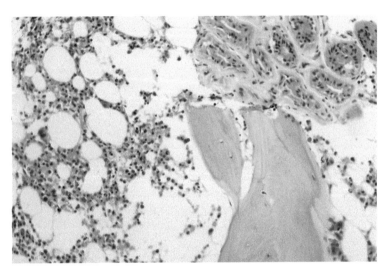

Fig. 10.41 BM trephine biopsy section, sweat gland interposition mimicking adenocarcinoma. Paraffin-embedded, H&E ×40.

tissue fragments in a single wax-embedded block [100,101]. However, formic acid decalcification limits the quality of DNA obtainable from trephine biopsy samples and this approach may therefore be unsuccessful in specimens decalcified in this way. Extraneous tissue may also appear to be present in histological sections due to contamination by a 'floater' from another tissue block as sections are cut, floated on a water-bath and picked up on individual glass slides (see Fig. 1.73). Good laboratory practice will ensure that fragments of previous sections are not allowed to contaminate the water-bath between cases. If such contamination is suspected, examination of the complete set of stained trephine biopsy sections should show that other sections are free of extraneous material. If doubt persists, new sections cut from the trephine biopsy specimen will be free of contamination.

Other pathological components in trephine biopsy specimens may occasionally be mistaken for non-haemopoietic malignant cells. These include macrophages (present singly or within granulomas), lymphoid cells in some types of non-Hodgkin lymphoma, Reed–Sternberg cells in Hodgkin lymphoma, neoplastic mast cells in systemic mastocy-

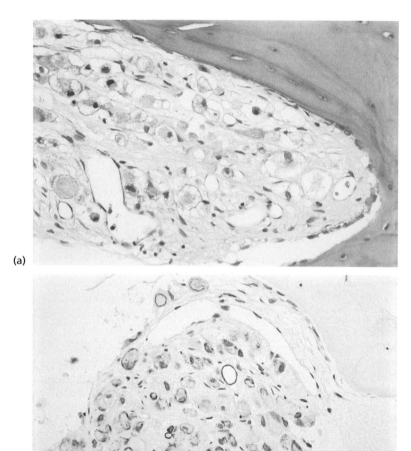

(a)

(b)

Fig. 10.42 BM trephine biopsy section, signet ring carcinoma of unknown primary origin. (a) In H&E-stained sections, malignant cells are indistinct and resemble macrophages. Paraffin-embedded, ×40. (b) Immunostaining for low molecular weight cytokeratins confirms their epithelial nature. Paraffin-embedded, ×40.

tosis and the cells of Langerhans cell histiocytosis. Immunohistochemistry will establish the nature of each of these types of cell. Macrophages are best demonstrated by the CD68R antibody PGM1 and lymphoid cells by their expression of CD3 (T cells) or CD20 (B cells). Reed–Sternberg cells express CD30, mast cell tryptase can be demonstrated with the monoclonal antibody AA1 and cells in Langerhans cell histiocytosis express CD1a.

Malignant cells of non-haemopoietic origin may be confused with normal bone marrow constituents or with neoplastic haemopoietic cells. Examples include undifferentiated carcinomas that may infil-

trate bone marrow without any stromal reaction, clear cell carcinoma, signet ring carcinoma (Fig. 10.42), malignant melanoma and the small cell solid tumours of childhood. Deposits of metastatic carcinoma eliciting a fibrotic response may also be confused with myelofibrosis, Hodgkin lymphoma or non-Hodgkin lymphoma. Among the non-Hodgkin lymphomas, those of T-cell lineage are most likely to produce significant stromal fibrosis. Immunohistochemistry will assist in making a correct diagnosis. Expression of low and high molecular weight cytokeratins is present in almost all carcinomas, S100 protein in melanomas, and

CD45 plus CD3 or CD20 in T- or B-cell lymphomas, respectively. Neoplastic plasma cells frequently lack CD45 and CD20 expression but their nature can be confirmed by expression of CD138 or p63 (detected using monoclonal antibody VS38c) in the absence of expression of cytokeratins; CD79a is expressed in many cases, but not all, and a negative result can therefore be misleading. Neoplastic plasma cells often express CD56 and in cases lacking mature plasma cell morphology this should not be taken for evidence of neuroendocrine differentiation. The diagnosis of some small cell tumours of childhood can be confirmed on the basis of expression of PGP9.5 (neuroblastoma) or desmin (rhabdomyosarcoma). However, the expression of CD99 is not specific for Ewing's sarcoma [63].

Detection of non-haemopoietic malignant cells in necrotic deposits can be very difficult. Reticulin staining may demonstrate a preserved pattern of nested cells or gland formation despite loss of cellular detail. Immunohistochemistry is often unhelpful in necrotic tissue and can be misleading due to `non-specific false-positive results as well as loss of antigen expression by dead or dying cells [102].

References

1 Anner RM and Drewinko B (1977) Frequency and significance of bone marrow involvement by metastatic solid tumours. *Cancer*, **39**, 1337–1344.

2 Singh G, Krause JR and Breitfeld V (1977) Bone marrow examination for metastatic tumour. *Cancer*, **40**, 2317–2321.

3 Finkelstein JZ, Ekert H, Isaacs H and Higgins G (1970) Bone marrow metastases in children with solid tumours. *Am J Dis Child*, **119**, 49–52.

4 Delta BG and Pinkel D (1964) Bone marrow aspiration in children with malignant tumours. *J Paediatr*, **64**, 542–546.

5 Kleinschmidt-Demasters BK (1997) Bone marrow metastases from glioblastoma multiforme: the role of dural invasion. *Hum Pathol*, **27**, 197–201.

6 Hoffmann M, Henrich D, Dingeldein G and Uppenkamp M (1999) Medulloblastoma with osteoblastic metastasis and bone marrow fibrosis. *Bone Marrow Transpl*, **23**, 631.

7 Dawson TP (1997) Pancytopaenia from a disseminated anaplastic oligodendroglioma. *Neuropathol Appl Neurobiol*, **23**, 516–520.

8 Ingle JN, Tormey DC and Tan HK (1978) The bone marrow examination in breast cancer. *Cancer*, **41**, 670–674.

9 Rubins JR (1983) The role of myelofibrosis in malignant myelosclerosis. *Cancer*, **51**, 308–311.

10 Tritz DB, Doll DC, Ringenberg S, Anderson S, Madsen R, Perry MC and Yarbro JW (1989) Bone marrow involvement in small cell lung cancer. *Cancer*, **63**, 763–766.

11 Becker FO and Schwartz TB (1973) Normal fluoride 18 bone scans in metastatic bone disease. *JAMA*, **225**, 628–629.

12 Suprun H and Rywlin AM (1976) Metastatic carcinoma in histologic sections of aspirated bone marrow: a comparative autopsy study. *South Med J*, **69**, 438–439.

13 Lang W, Stauch G, Soudah B and Georgii A (1984) The effectiveness of bone marrow punctures for staging carcinomas of the breast and lung. In: Lennert K (ed) *Pathology of the Bone Marrow*. Gustav Fischer Verlag, Stuttgart.

14 Savage RA, Hoffman GC and Shaker K (1978) Diagnostic problems involved in detection of metastatic neoplasms by bone-marrow aspirate compared with needle biopsy. *Am J Clin Pathol*, **70**, 623–627.

15 Wang NP, Zee S, Zarbo RJ, Bacchi CE and Gown AM (1995) Coordinate expression of cytokeratins 7 and 20 defines unique subsets of carcinomas. *Appl Immunohistochem*, **3**, 226–234.

16 Agoff SN, Lamps LW, Philip AT, Amin MB, Schmidt RA, True LD and Folpe AL (2000) Thyroid transcription factor-1 is expressed in extrapulmonary small cell carcinomas but not in other extrapulmonary neuroendocrine tumors. *Mod Pathol*, **13**, 238–242.

17 Arpino G, Bardou VJ, Clark GM and Elledge RM (2004) Infiltrating lobular carcinoma of the breast: tumor characteristics and clinical outcome *Breast Cancer Res*, **6**, R149–156.

18 Chu P, Wu E and Weiss LM (2000) Cytokeratin 7 and cytokeratin 20 expression in epithelial neoplasms: a survey of 435 cases. *Mod Pathol*, **13**, 962–967.

19 Lal P, Tan LK and Chen B (2005) Correlation of HER-2 status with estrogen and progesterone receptors and histologic features in 3,655 invasive breast carcinomas. *Am J Clin Pathol*, **123**, 541–546.

20 Gatter KC, Abdulaziz Z, Beverley P, Corvalan JRF, Ford C, Lane EB *et al.* (1982) Use of monoclonal antibodies for the histopathological diagnosis of human malignancy. *J Clin Pathol*, **35**, 1253–1267.

21 Athanasou NA, Quinn J, Heryet A, Woods CG and McGee JO'D (1987) The effect of decalcification on cellular antigens. *J Clin Pathol*, **40**, 874–878.

22 Mufti GJ, Flandrin G, Schaefer H-E, Sandberg AA and Kanfer EJ (1996) *An Atlas of Malignant*

Haematology: Cytology, histology and cytogenetics. Martin Dunitz, London, p. 368.

23 Spivak JL (1973) Phagocytic tumor cells. *Scand J Haematol*, **11**, 253–256.

24 Falini B, Bucciarelli E, Grignani F and Martelli MF (1980) Erythrophagocytosis by undifferentiated lung carcinoma cells. *Cancer*, **46**, 1140–1145.

25 DeSimone PA, East R, Powell RD (1980) Phagocytic tumor cell activity in oat cell carcinoma of the lung. *Hum Pathol*, **11** (Suppl. 5), 535–539.

26 Youness E, Barlogie B, Ahearn M and Trujillo JM (1980) Tumor cell phagocytosis – its occurrence in a patient with medulloblastoma. *Arch Pathol Lab Med*, **104**, 651–653.

27 Reid MM (1999) Erythrophagocytosis by rhabdomyosarcoma. *Br J Haematol*, **106**, 835–836.

28 Smith SR and Reid MM (1994) Neuroblastoma rosettes in aspirated bone marrow. *Br J Haematol*, **88**, 445–447.

29 Reid MM, Saunders PWG, Bown N, Bradford CR, Maung ZT, Craft AW and Malcolm AJ (1992) Alveolar rhabdomyosarcoma infiltrating bone marrow at presentation: the value to diagnosis of bone marrow trephine biopsy specimens. *J Clin Pathol*, **45**, 759–762.

30 Jonsson LL and Rundles RW (1951) Tumour metastases in bone marrow. *Blood*, **6** 16–25.

31 Farinola MA, Weir EG and Ali SZ (2008) CD56 expression of neuroendocrine neoplasms on immunophenotyping by flow cytometry: a novel diagnostic approach to fine-needle aspiration biopsy. *Cancer*, **99**, 240–246.

32 Stindl R, Fiegl M, Regele H, Gisslinger H, Breitenseher MJ and Fonatsch C (1998) Alveolar rhabdomyosarcoma in a 68-year-old patient identified by cytogenetic analysis of bone marrow. *Cancer Genet Cytogenet*, **107**, 43–47.

33 Anderson J, Gordon A, Pritchard-Jones K and Shipley J. (1999) Genes, chromosomes, and rhabdomyosarcoma. *Genes Chromo Cancer*, **26**, 275–285.

34 Bown N, Cotterill S, Lastowska M, O'Neill S, Pearson AD, Plantaz D *et al.* (1999) Gain of chromosome arm 17q and adverse outcome in patients with neuroblastoma. *New Engl J Med*, **340**, 1954–1961.

35 Kiely JM and Silverstein MN (1969) Metastatic carcinoma simulating agnogenic myeloid metaplasia. *Cancer*, **24**, 1041–1044.

36 Spector JI and Levine PH (1973) Carcinomatous bone marrow invasion simulating acute myelofibrosis. *Am J Med Sci*, **266**, 145–148.

37 Gatter KC, Ralfkiaer E, Skinner J, Brown D, Heryet A, Pulford KAF *et al.* (1985) An immunohistochemical study of malignant melanoma and its differential diagnosis from other malignant tumours. *J Clin Pathol*, **38**, 1353–1357.

38 Talbot DC, Davies JH, Maclennan KA and Smith IE (1994) Signet-ring lymphoma of bone marrow. *J Clin Pathol*, **47**, 184–186.

39 Bitter MA, Fiorito D, Corkill ME, Huffer WE, Stemmer SM, Shpall EJ *et al.* (1994) Bone marrow involvement by lobular carcinoma of the breast cannot be identified reliably by routine histological examination alone. *Hum Pathol*, **25**, 781–788.

40 Savage RA, Lucas PV and Hoffman GC (1978) Melanoma in marrow aspirates. *Am J Clin Pathol*, **79**, 268–269.

41 Karcher DS and Frost DR (1991) The bone marrow in human immunodeficiency virus (HIV)-related disease: morphology and clinical correlation. *Am J Clin Pathol*, **95**, 63–71.

42 Conran RM, Granger E and Reddy VB (1986) Kaposi's sarcoma of the bone marrow. *Arch Pathol Lab Med*, **110**, 1083–1085.

43 Reid MM and Hamilton PJ (1988) Histology of neuroblastoma involving bone marrow: the problem of detecting residual tumour after initiation of chemotherapy. *Br J Haematol*, **69**, 487–490.

44 Variend S (1985) Small cell tumours in childhood: a review. *J Pathol* **145**, 1–27.

45 Enzinger FM and Shiraki M. (1969) Alveolar rhabdomyosarcoma; an analysis of 110 cases. *Cancer*, **24**, 18–31.

46 Reid MM (1999) Erythrophagocytosis by rhabdomyosarcoma. *Br J Haematol*, **106**, 835–836.

47 Tsoi W-C and Feng C-S (1997) Hemophagocytosis by rhabdomyosarcome cells in bone marrow. *Am J Hematol*, **54**, 340–341.

48 Kounami S, Douno S, Takayama J and Ohira M (1998) Haemophagocytic ability of rhabdomyosarcoma cells. *Acta Hematologica*, **100**, 160–161.

49 Bacchi CE, Bonetti F, Pea M, Martignoni G and Gown A (1996) HMB-45 – a review. *Appl Immunohistochem*, **4**, 73–85.

50 Orchard GE (1998) Melan A (MART-1): a new monoclonal antibody for malignant melanoma diagnosis. *Br J Biomed Sci*, **55**, 8–9.

51 Nadji M, Tabei SZ, Castro A, Chu TM, Murphy GP, Wang MC and Morales AR (1984) Prostate specific antigen. An immunohistologic marker for prostatic neoplasms. *Cancer*, **48**, 1229–1239.

52 Wilbur DC, Krenzer K and Bonfiglio TA (1987) Prostatic specific antigen staining in carcinomas of non-prostatic origin. *Am J Clin Pathol*, **88**, 530.

53 Frisch B and Bartl R (1999) *Biopsy Interpretation of Bone and Bone Marrow: Histology and immunohistology in paraffin and plastic*, 2nd edn. Arnold, London.

54 Langlois NEI, King G, Herriot R and Thompson WD (1995) An evaluation of the staining of lymphomas and normal tissues by the rabbit polyclonal antibody to protein gene product 9.5 following non-enzymatic retrieval of antigen. *J Pathol*, **175**, 433–439.

55 Otsuki T, Yata K, Takata-Tomokuni A, Hyodoh F, Miura Y, Sakaguchi H et al. (2004) Expression of protein gene product 9.5 (PGP9.5)/ubiquitin-C-terminal hydrolase 1 (UCHL-1) in human myeloma cells. Br J Haematol, **127**, 292–298.

56 Lloyd RV, Cano M, Rosa P, Hille A and Huttner WB (1988) Distribution of chromogranin A and secretogranin I (chromogranin B) in neuroendocrine cells and tumour. Am J Pathol, **130**, 296–304.

57 Reid MM, Wallis JP, McGuckin AG, Pearson ADJ and Malcolm AJ (1991) Routine histological compared with immunohistological examination of bone marrow trephine biopsy specimens in disseminated neuroblastoma. J Clin Pathol, **44**, 485–486.

58 Erickson LA and Lloyd RV (2004) Practical markers used in the diagnosis of endocrine tumors. Adv Anat Pathol, **11**, 175–189.

59 Moore PS and Chang Y (1995) Detection of herpesvirus-like DNA sequences in Kaposi's sarcoma in patients with and without HIV infection. New Engl J Med, **332**, 1181–1185.

60 Wang NP, Marx J, McNutt MA, Rutledge JC and Gown AM (1995) Expression of myogenic regulatory proteins (myogenin and myoD1) in small blue round cell tumors of childhood. Am J Pathol, **147**, 1799–1810.

61 Fellinger EJ, Garin-Chesa P, Triche TJ, Huvos AG and Rettig WJ (1991) Immunohistochemical analysis of Ewing's sarcoma cell surface antigen p30/32[MIC2]. Am J Pathol, **139**, 317–325.

62 Lazda EJ and Berry PJ (1998) Bone marrow metastasis in Ewing's sarcoma and peripheral primitive neuroectodermal tumor: an immunohistochemical study. Pediatr Dev Pathol, **1**, 2–30.

63 Lucas DR, Bentley G, Dan ME, Tabaczka P, Poulik JM and Mott MP (2001) Ewing's sarcoma vs lymphoblastic lymphoma: a comparative immunohistochemical study. Am J Clin Pathol, **115**, 11–17.

64 Franklin IM and Pritchard J (1983) Detection of bone marrow invasion by neuroblastoma is improved by sampling at two sites with aspirates and biopsies. J Clin Pathol, **36**, 1215–1218.

65 Reid MM (1994) Detection of bone marrow infiltration by neuroblastoma in clinical practice: how far have we come? Eur J Cancer A General Topics, **30**, 134–135.

66 Cheung NKV, Heller G, Kushner BH, Liu CY and Cheung IY (1997) Detection of metastatic neuroblastoma in bone marrow: when is routine marrow histology insensitive? J Clin Oncol, **15**, 2807–2817.

67 Rogers DW, Treleavan JG, Kemshead JT and Pritchard J (1989) Monoclonal antibodies for detecting bone marrow invasion by neuroblastoma. J Clin Pathol, **42**, 422–426.

68 Carey PJ, Thomas L, Buckle G and Reid MM (1990) Immunocytochemical examination of bone marrow in disseminated neuroblastoma. J Clin Pathol, **43**, 9–12.

69 Thomas JO, Nijjar J, Turley H, Micklem K and Gatter KC (1991) NB84: a new monoclonal antibody for the recognition of neuroblastoma in routinely processed material. J Pathol, **163**, 69–75.

70 Miettinen M, Chatten J, Paetau A and Stevenson A (1998) Monoclonal antibody NB84 in the differential diagnosis of neuroblastoma and other small round cell tumors. Am J Surg Pathol, **22**, 327–332.

71 Wolf HK, Buslei R, Schmidt-Kastner R, Schmidt-Kastner PK, Pietsch T, Wiestler OD and Bluhmke I (1996) NeuN: a useful neuronal marker for diagnostic histopathology. J Histochem Cytochem, **44**, 1167–1171.

72 Reid MM and Roald B (1996) Adequacy of bone marrow trephine biopsy specimens in children. J Clin Pathol, **49**, 226–229.

73 Reid MM and Roald B (1996) Central review of bone marrow biopsy specimens from patients with neuroblastoma. J Clin Pathol, **49**, 691–692.

74 Reid MM and Roald B (1999) Deterioration in performance in obtaining bone marrow trephine biopsy cores from children. J Clin Pathol, **52**, 851–852.

75 Turner GE and Reid MM (1993) What is marrow fibrosis after treatment of neuroblastoma? J Clin Pathol, **46**, 61–63.

76 Lawrence JB, Eleff M, Behm FG and Johnston CL (1984) Bone marrow examination in small cell carcinoma of the lung. Cancer, **53**, 2188–2190.

77 Levitan N, Byrne RE, Bromer RH, Faling J, Caslowitz P, Pattern DH and Hong WK (1985) The value of the bone scan and bone marrow biopsy in staging small cell lung cancer. Cancer, **56**, 652–654.

78 Kelly BW, Morris JF, Harwood BP and Bruya TE (1984) Methods and prognostic value of bone marrow examination in small cell carcinoma of the lung. Cancer, **53**, 99–102.

79 Imamura F, Kuriyama K, Seto T, Hasegawa Y, Nakayama T, Nakamura S and Horai T (2000) Detection of bone marrow metastases of small cell lung cancer with magnetic resonance imaging: early diagnosis before destruction of osseous structure and implications for staging. Lung Cancer, **27**, 189–197.

80 Landys K (1982) Prognostic value of bone marrow biopsy in breast cancer. Cancer, **49**, 513–518.

81 Mansi JL, Berger U, Easton D, McDonnell T, Redding WH, Gazet J-C et al. (1987) Micrometastases in bone marrow in patients with breast cancer: evaluation as an early predictor of bone metastases. BMJ, **295**, 1093–1096.

82 Berger U, Bettelheim R, Mansi JL, Easton D, Coombes RC and Neville AM (1988) The relationship between micrometastases in the bone marrow, histopathologic features of the primary tumor in breast cancer and prognosis. Am J Clin Pathol, **90**, 1–6.

83 Braun S, Pantel K, Muller P, Janni W, Hepp F, Kentenich CRM et al. (2000) Cytokeratin-positive cells in the bone marrow and survival of patients with stage I, II or III breast cancer. *New Engl J Med*, **342**, 525–533.

84 Untch M, Harbeck N and Eiemann W (1988) Micrometastases in bone marrow in patients with breast cancer. *BMJ*, **296**, 290.

85 Mathew BS, Jayasree K, Madhavan J, Nair MK and Rajan B (1997) Skeletal metastases and bone marrow infiltration from squamous cell carcinoma of the buccal mucosa. *Oral Oncol*, **33**, 454–455.

86 Thorban S, Roder JD, Nekarda H, Funk A, Pantel K and Siewert JR (1996) Disseminated epithelial tumor cells in bone marrow of patients with esophageal cancer: Detection and prognostic significance. *World J Surg*, **20**, 567–573.

87 Heiss MM, Allgayer H, Gruetzner KU, Babic R, Jauch KW and Schildberg FW (1997) Clinical value of extended biologic staging by bone marrow micrometastases and tumor-associated proteases in gastric cancer. *Ann Surg*, **226**, 736–744.

88 Maehara Y, Hasuda S, Abe T, Oki E, Kakeji Y, Ohno S and Sugimachi K (1998) Tumor angiogenesis and micrometastasis in bone marrow of patients with early gastric cancer. *Clin Cancer Res*, **4**, 2129–2134.

89 Thorban S, Roder JD and Siewert JR (1999) Detection of micrometastasis in bone marrow of pancreatic cancer patients. *Ann Oncol*, **10**, 111–113.

90 Roder JD, Thorban S, Pantel K and Siewert JR (2000) Micrometastases in bone marrow: prognostic indicators for pancreatic cancer. *World J Surg*, **23**, 888–891.

91 Pantel K, Izbicki J, Passlick B, Angstwuan M, Häussinger K, Thetter O and Reithmüller G (1996) Frequency and prognostic significance of isolated tumour cells in bone marrow of patients with non-small cell lung cancer without overt metastasis. *Lancet*, **347**, 649–653.

92 Schwaibold H, Wenck S, Huland E and Huland H (1997) Immunocytologic staining of cytokeratin in bone marrow aspirates to detect micrometastatic cells fails in patients with metastatic urologic carcinoma. *Int J Oncol*, **11**, 1197–1201.

93 Thybusch-Bernhardt A, Klomp HJ, Maas T, Kremer B and Juhl H (1999) Immunocytological detection of isolated tumour cells in the bone marrow of malignant melanoma patients: a new method for the detection of minimal residual disease. *Eur J Surg Oncol*, **25**, 498–502.

94 Castells A, Boix L, Bessa X, Gargallo L and Pique JM (1998) Detection of colonic cells in peripheral blood of colorectal cancer patients by means of reverse transcriptase and polymerase chain reaction. *Br J Cancer*, **78**, 1368–1372.

95 Zhong XY, Kaul S, Thompson J, Eichler A and Bastert G (1998) Evaluation of the reverse transcriptase/polymerase chain reaction for carcinoembryonic antigen for the detection of breast cancer dissemination in bone marrow and peripheral blood. *J Cancer Res Clin Oncol* **125**, 669–674.

96 Vannucchi AM, Bosi A, Glinz S, Pacini P, Linari S, Saccardi R et al. (1998) Evaluation of breast tumour cell contamination in the bone marrow and leukapheresis collections by RT-PCR for cytokeratin-19 mRNA. *Br J Haematol*, **103**, 610–617.

97 Funke I and Schraut W (1998) Meta-analyses of studies on bone marrow micrometastases: an independent prognostic impact remains to be substantiated. *J Clin Oncol*, **16**, 557–566.

98 Lagrange M, Ferrero JM, Lagrange JL, Machiavello JC, Monticelli J, Bayle C et al. (1997) Non-specifically labelled cells that simulate bone marrow metastases in patients with non-metastatic breast cancer. *J Clin Pathol*, **50**, 206–211.

99 Borgen E, Beiske K, Traschel S, Nesland JM, Kvalheim G, Herstad TK et al. (1998) Immunocytochemical detection of isolated epithelial cells in bone marrow: non-specific staining and contribution by plasma cells directly reactive to alkaline phosphatase. *J Pathol*, **185**, 427–434.

100 Bateman AC, Leung ST, Howell WM, Roche WR, Jones DB and Theaker JM (1994) Detection of specimen contamination in routine histopathology by HLA class II typing using the polymerase chain reaction and sequence specific oligonucleotide probing. *J Pathol*, **173**, 243–248.

101 Giroti R and Kashvan VK (1998) Detection of the source of mislabeled biopsy tissue paraffin block and histopathological section on glass slide. *Diagn Mol Pathol*, **7**, 331–334.

102 Judkins AR, Montone KT, LiVolsi VA and van de Rijn M (1998) Sensitivity and specificity of antibodies on necrotic tumor tissue. *Am J Clin Pathol*, **110**, 641–646.

ELEVEN

DISEASES OF BONE

Trephine biopsy, particularly when the specimen includes cortex, is useful in assessing bone pathology. Diseases of bone are also not infrequently encountered when examining a specimen obtained for the investigation of haematological disease. The normal structure of bone is described in Chapter 1. Before discussing the more important diseases of bone that can be diagnosed by trephine biopsy it is necessary to consider briefly some aspects of normal bone physiology [1]. Advances in understanding of the molecular processes involved in normal bone turnover also provide new clues to the pathogenesis of bone disease [2,3].

Bone is in a constant state of turnover in adult life, by a process of remodelling during which resorption and formation are balanced in order to maintain the total skeletal mass [1]. Microscopic portions of the trabecular and cortical bone surface are resorbed by osteoclasts which form small resorption bays (Howship's lacunae). Bone formation starts soon after resorption ceases, with the deposition of unmineralized matrix (osteoid) in layers (lamellae) by osteoblasts. After a time lag of 10–15 days (the osteoid maturation time) the osteoid becomes mineralized along an advancing front (the mineralization front), starting at the base of the previous resorption bay (the cement line) [4].

For the study of metabolic bone disease, sections of undecalcified bone are essential. Osteoid seams, i.e. layers of non-calcified bone on the surface of trabeculae, are a feature of normal bone. In haematoxylin and eosin (H&E)-stained sections they appear paler and pinker than calcified bone but they can be recognized more easily in sections stained for calcium with alizarin red or von Kossa's silver stain. The mineralization front appears as a metachromatic granular line in toluidine blue-stained sections.

Morphometry of bone

Morphometric methods are commonly used in the diagnosis of diseases of bone. These may be divided into static and dynamic measurements. Static measurements include: (i) the proportion of trabecular surface that is resting, resorbing or covered by osteoid (by a perimeter intersect technique); (ii) the thickness of the osteoid seams; and (iii) the proportion of the section occupied by mineralized bone, osteoid, woven bone, lamellar bone or fibrous tissue (by a point-counting technique or by computerized image analysis). Dynamic studies may be performed using a tetracycline labelling method. When a single dose of tetracycline is administered it becomes incorporated at the mineralization front; this can be visualized as a single line in undecalcified sections examined under ultraviolet light. By giving two doses of tetracycline at a known interval and measuring the distance between the two lines of incorporation, it is possible to measure the mean rate of mineralization.

Osteoporosis

Osteoporosis is defined as a decreased amount of bone per unit volume. There is no decrease in the external dimensions of the bone, which is histologically normal, but there is a reduction in the amount of trabecular bone per unit volume of cancellous bone and there may also be thinning of the cortex (Fig. 11.1). Fragility of the bone may lead to spicules being fractured during the biopsy procedure [5]. Histomorphometry shows that approximately 60% of patients have reduced numbers of

Bone Marrow Pathology. By Barbara Bain, David Clark and Bridget Wilkins. © 2010, Blackwell Publishing.

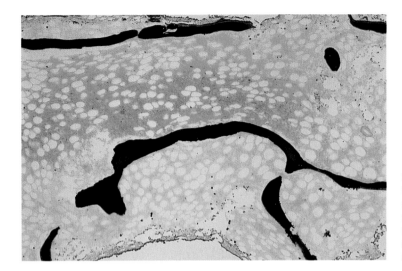

Fig. 11.1 Bone marrow (BM) trephine biopsy section, osteoporosis, showing a decrease in the total amount of bone with thinning of trabeculae. Paraffin-embedded (non-decalcified), Tripp and MacKay stain ×4.

osteoblasts [6]. The ratio of fat cells to haemopoi-etic and other cells is increased [7]. The disorder is common in the elderly, in whom it causes consid-erable morbidity as a result of increased susceptibil-ity to fractures. Osteoporosis is more common in women and its frequency increases progressively after the menopause. Severe osteoporosis has also been reported in men [8] and in children [9]. The cause of osteoporosis is not known but genetic factors have been implicated [10]. The mechanism is thought to be increased osteoclastic resorption in conjunction with a reduced rate of bone formation [11]. In a minority of cases, osteoporosis is second-ary to other disease such as Cushing's syndrome, thyrotoxicosis, hypopituitarism, malnutrition, mal-absorption and chronic heparin or corticosteroid administration. It is often present in thalassaemia major patients maintained on blood transfusion. Diffuse osteoporosis is also sometimes associated with myeloma, aplastic anaemia, chronic granulo-cytic leukaemia, systemic mastocytosis and poly-cythaemia vera. It may occur as an uncommon feature of dyskeratosis congenita, being seen in less than 5% of patients. Localized osteoporosis can occur following immobilization of a limb.

Plain radiographs of the vertebral column are usually only abnormal in advanced disease and are an unreliable means of diagnosing osteoporosis. An assessment of the severity of osteoporosis can be made by biopsy of the iliac crest [12]. The trabecu-

lae are usually thinned and are reduced to slender strands, often with complete transection, but they are otherwise normal and there is no increase in the width of osteoid seams. Rather, osteoid seams and the number of osteoblasts tend to be reduced. Four histological patterns have been described: (i) irregular thinning of trabeculae; (ii) generalized thinning of trabeculae; (iii) a reduction in the number of trabeculae but without thinning; and (iv) the presence of small islands of bone [13]. Accurate assessment of the severity of osteoporosis requires the use of static morphometric measure-ments. Iliac trabecular bone normally occupies approximately 23% (SD ± 3%) of the measured area in adults under 50 years of age, but this falls to 16% (SD ± 6%) in elderly individuals [14]. When the amount of trabecular bone falls below 11% (SD ± 3%), vertebral fractures tend to occur [4].

Recently, reliable non-invasive techniques for the measurement of bone mass at the sites most prone to fracture have become available; these include dual proton absorptiometry, quantitative computerized tomography and dual-energy X-ray absorptiometry [15]. Such techniques have made iliac crest biopsy unimportant in the diagnosis of osteoporosis.

The peripheral blood is normal in osteoporosis; the bone marrow is essentially normal, although increased numbers of mast cells have been reported

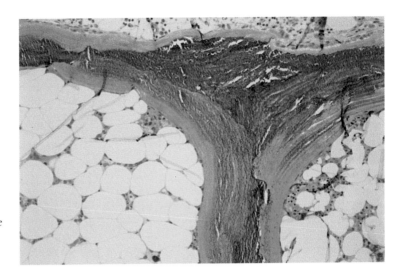

Fig. 11.2 BM trephine biopsy section, osteomalacia, showing wide osteoid seams on the surface of the bone trabecula. Resin-embedded, H&E ×10.

[16]. There may, however, be an appearance of hypocellularity since the loss of bone leads to an increased percentage of the marrow cavity being occupied by fat cells.

Osteomalacia

Osteomalacia literally means softening of the bones. It is a consequence of a failure of mineralization of bone matrix, resulting in abnormally wide osteoid seams around the bone trabeculae (Fig. 11.2). Numerous causes of osteomalacia have been described but the majority of cases result from a deficiency of vitamin D due, in turn, to reduced intake, to inadequate exposure to sunlight or to abnormalities of absorption or metabolism of the vitamin (as in renal disease). Rarely, osteomalacia is caused by a hereditary end-organ resistance to vitamin D and its metabolites. In adults, severe osteomalacia predisposes to fractures. In growing children, in whom the epiphyses have not yet closed, the clinical picture is that of rickets, with its characteristic skeletal deformities.

In normal adults, morphometry has shown that approximately 0.5% of the whole bone area (that is, bone plus marrow) is made up of osteoid, which covers 13% (SD ± 7%) of the trabecular bone surface. A mineralization front is seen in more than 60% of the surface osteoid. Under polarized light, normal osteoid seams are seen to be composed of between one and four lamellae [4]. In osteomalacia there is an increase in both total osteoid and the area of trabecular surface covered by osteoid; the osteoid seams are greater than five lamellae in thickness and the mineralization front is decreased. There may also be peri-osteocytic zones of osteoid [13]. Osteomalacia has been defined as osteoid comprising more than 10% of total bone with osteoid seams covering more than 25% of the trabecular surface [13]. Double tetracycline labelling shows a reduction in the mineralization rate (normal mean value 0.7 μm per day).

The peripheral blood and bone marrow are usually normal in osteomalacia. However, children with severe vitamin D deficiency rickets have been reported to develop a hypocellular bone marrow with fibrosis, thrombocytopenia and a leucoerythroblastic anaemia associated with extramedullary erythropoiesis [17].

Hyperparathyroidism

Skeletal changes occur in both primary and secondary hyperparathyroidism [18–21]. The extent of these changes depends on the severity and duration of the underlying disease. Primary hyperparathyroidism is usually the result of a parathyroid adenoma; primary hyperplasia is a less common cause. Very rarely, there is an underlying parathyroid carcinoma. Secondary hyperparathyroidism is usually a consequence of renal disease; less commonly the underlying cause is intestinal malabsorption and rare cases have been reported following gastric bypass surgery for treatment of severe obesity [22]. In one reported case, high levels of secretion of parathyroid hormone-related protein, by cells of adult T-cell leukaemia/lymphoma, produced bone disease indistinguishable from hyperparathyroid bone disease [23]. A rare cause of the histological features of hyperparathyroidism is pseudohypoparathyroidism [13].

Parathyroid hormone and related molecules increase osteoclast generation and function, resulting in increased bone resorption; more recently, parathyroid hormone has also been shown to increase bone formation [24]. Skeletal changes in hyperparathyroidism follow a predictable sequence. The earliest change is the presence of excess osteoid seams around bone trabeculae, an appearance that closely resembles osteomalacia. Later, osteoclasts are activated and there is increased bone resorption with both surface excavation (prominent Howship's lacunae containing osteoclasts) and tunnelling into trabeculae by fibrous tissue and osteoclasts. There is fibrosis of the paratrabecular marrow (Fig. 11.3). The Howship's lacunae may be filled by large bizarre osteoclasts and, as the lacunae enlarge, trabeculae may be transected. Fibrosis increases and fibrous tissue eventually fills some intertrabecular spaces completely. There is a moderate increase in the vascularity of the marrow. At this stage, macroscopic cysts may be visible. Haemosiderin-laden macrophages are frequently seen within the fibrous tissue, resulting from microhaemorrhages; foreign body-type giant cells may also be present. This final stage is sometimes referred to as osteitis fibrosa cystica. Blood vessel walls may become calcified as part of this process [13].

Only a minority of patients with hyperparathyroidism have significant bone disease and, with earlier diagnosis and treatment, severe manifestations (osteitis fibrosa cystica) are rarely seen nowadays. The features are important to remember, however, since bone marrow biopsy is occasionally performed to investigate either hypercalcaemia or radiographic lesions suspicious of metastatic carcinoma in patients with unsuspected severe hyperparathyroidism [25–27].

There are no specific peripheral blood or bone marrow aspirate abnormalities associated with primary hyperparathyroidism although mild anaemia may occur [28].

Renal osteodystrophy

The majority of patients with chronic renal failure have some abnormality of bone structure [20,21]. The manifestations are complex [29] and include combinations of bone disease due to secondary hyperparathyroidism (80–90% of cases), osteomalacia (20–40% of cases) and osteosclerosis (around 30% of cases) [4,30]. The most severe changes are seen in those patients with chronic renal failure

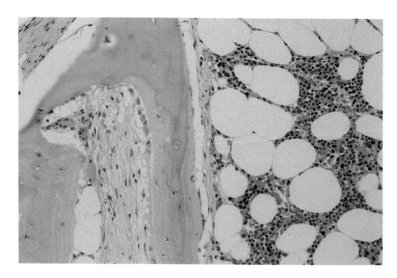

Fig. 11.3 BM trephine biopsy section, primary hyperparathyroidism, showing paratrabecular fibrosis. Paraffin-embedded, H&E ×20.

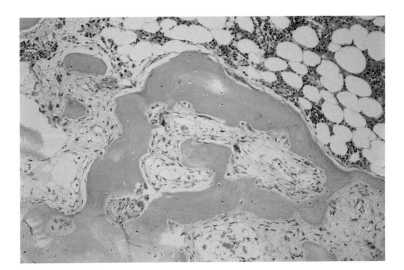

Fig. 11.4 BM trephine biopsy section, renal osteodystrophy, showing irregular bone trabeculae with prominent resorption bays (Howship's lacunae) and replacement of haemopoietic marrow by fibrous tissue. Paraffin-embedded, H&E ×10.

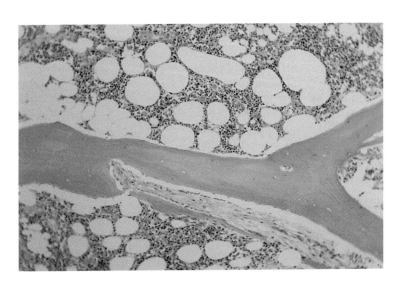

Fig. 11.5 BM trephine biopsy section, renal osteodystrophy, showing prominent tunnelling into a trabecula by fibrous tissue. Paraffin-embedded, H&E ×10.

who are maintained on dialysis. There is marked geographical variation in the nature of renal osteo-dystrophy, with hyperparathyroid bone disease predominating in the United States and osteomala-cia in the United Kingdom. In adults, the symptoms are rarely severe. Secondary hyperparathyroidism in renal failure is consequent on hypocalcaemia which is, in turn, caused by a combination of reduced hydroxylation of vitamin D and phosphate retention by the kidney [31]. The major cause of renal osteomalacia is the toxic action of aluminium derived from dialysate; geographical variations in

the incidence are related to the concentration of aluminium in water used for dialysis [31,32]. The use of de-ionized water has resulted in a fall in the incidence of renal osteomalacia in some centres [4].

The histological changes are identical to those previously described in hyperparathyroidism (ostei-tis fibrosa), often combined with those of osteomala-cia (Fig. 11.4). Bone trabeculae may have tunnels excavated within them by osteoclasts (Fig. 11.5) but the most severe changes of osteitis fibrosa cystica are seen only rarely. Osteosclerosis, due to increased formation of woven bone, may be widespread throughout the skeleton. With advanced renal osteodystrophy, the bone marrow may be hypocellular and extensively fibrosed with proliferation of blood vessels, particularly arterioles. Patients with renal osteodystrophy have been noted to have mononuclear cells within the haemopoietic marrow which are positive for tartrate-resistant acid phosphatase; these cells are probably osteoclast precursors [33,34]. Rarely the cause of renal failure is revealed by trephine biopsy, e.g. myeloma, amyloidosis or oxalosis (see Fig. 9.49).

There may also be abnormal deposition of aluminium or iron. Aluminium deposition occurs at the junction between osteoid and mineralized bone. It is detected as a red/purple line in an Irwin stain using an undecalcified biopsy [35] and provides evidence of exposure to an excessive aluminium concentration in the dialysate. Aluminium may also be detected inside bone marrow cells, possibly macrophages [36]. In dialysis patients who are iron-overloaded, iron may also be deposited at the mineralization front [37]; iron deposition may be aetiologically related to osteomalacia.

Renal osteodystrophy may contribute to the anaemia of chronic renal failure and may also cause leucopenia or thrombocytopenia [38]. There are no specific associated morphological abnormalities in the peripheral blood or bone marrow aspirate although a 'dry tap' may occur. Response to erythropoietin therapy is worse in those patients who have more severe secondary hyperparathyroidism [39] and iron overload [40].

Paget's disease of bone

Paget's disease of bone is a disease of unknown aetiology, characterized by increased osteoclastic resorption of bone followed by uncoordinated formation of disordered bone. Infection by a virus of the paramyxovirus group (including measles virus, respiratory syncytial virus and canine distemper virus) has been suspected as a cause of this disease but investigations have been inconclusive [41,42]. In one series of patients, molecular genetic analysis has failed to find evidence of paramyxovirus RNA sequences in tissue from pagetic bone [43]. Paget's disease of bone occurs with familial clustering in some instances [42,44] and genetic linkage to chromosome 18q21-22 has been established in some, but not all, families [44–46]. Occupational expo-

sure to lead has also been proposed as a possible contributory factor in development of the disease [47,48]. Paget's disease is uncommon before the age of 40 years and becomes progressively more common with increasing age. In approximately 15% of cases, the disease is confined to a single bone (monostotic). In the majority of cases, however, several bones are involved, most commonly the vertebral column, pelvis, femur, skull and sacrum. The clinical features are pain, due to microfractures, and neurological symptoms consequent on damage to nerves as they pass through the foramina of the skull and vertebrae. Rarely, there is high output cardiac failure as a result of the highly vascular bone lesions acting as arteriovenous shunts. The development of osteosarcoma is an uncommon, but well established, complication of Paget's disease.

In the initial stages of the disease, increased bone resorption is the dominant feature. Trabeculae have a scalloped appearance due to increased numbers of resorption bays containing very large osteoclasts with numerous nuclei (Fig. 11.6). The increased resorption of bone is followed by deposition of disordered woven bone. Osteoblasts are increased. At this stage, the marrow cavity is partly occupied by loose connective tissue; there is increased vascularity with arteries, arterioles, capillaries and sinusoids all being increased. There may be increased plasma cells, lymphocytes, mast cells and macrophages within the connective tissue adjacent to abnormal bone [13]. Eventually, new bone formation becomes the dominant feature and lamellar bone is laid down causing thickening of the bone trabeculae. However, the lamellar bone is laid down in an uncoordinated and haphazard fashion. The irregular cement lines, which appear more basophilic than the surrounding bone, form a characteristic mosaic or tesselated ('tile-like') pattern that is the hallmark of Paget's disease (Fig. 11.7). Each of the cement lines represents a surface where bone resorption has been followed by bone deposition. The trabeculae eventually become massively thickened and encroach upon the marrow cavity.

Severe Paget's disease may have an associated mild anaemia and occasionally pancytopenia. The bone marrow aspirate does not show any specific abnormality but increased osteoblasts and osteoclasts are sometimes seen.

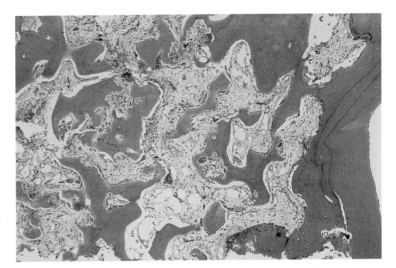

Fig. 11.6 BM trephine biopsy section, Paget's disease of bone, showing thickening of bone trabeculae, numerous resorption bays (Howship's lacunae) containing large osteoclasts and replacement of marrow by vascular connective tissue. Paraffin-embedded, H&E ×4.

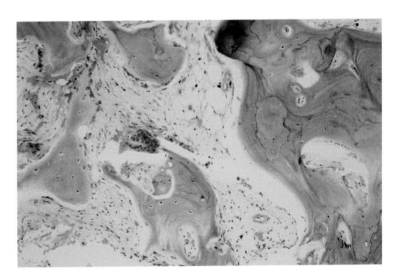

Fig. 11.7 BM trephine biopsy section, Paget's disease of bone (same patient as Fig. 11.6), showing thickening of bone trabeculae with a typical mosaic pattern and large osteoclasts. Paraffin-embedded, Giemsa ×10.

It should be noted that prolonged bleeding, consequent on the greatly increased vascularity, has been reported following trephine biopsy in a patient with Paget's disease [49].

Osteosclerosis

Osteosclerosis is the term used to describe a group of conditions in which there is an increase in the amount of bone per unit volume, usually resulting from increased bone formation. Osteosclerosis is most often seen in conjunction with severe bone marrow fibrosis, either in a myeloproliferative neo-

plasm or in metastatic carcinoma. It occurs in patients with systemic mastocytosis [50], who may also have mixed osteosclerotic and osteolytic lesions or osteoporosis. Osteosclerosis occasionally occurs in myeloma but osteolytic lesions are much more characteristic. It is also associated with plasma cell neoplasia in the POEMS syndrome (see page 452) and has been reported in patients with hairy cell leukaemia, in whom it has regressed or stabilized with treatment of the underlying lymphoproliferative disease [51,52]. Osteosclerosis may be a feature of fluorosis, heavy metal poison-

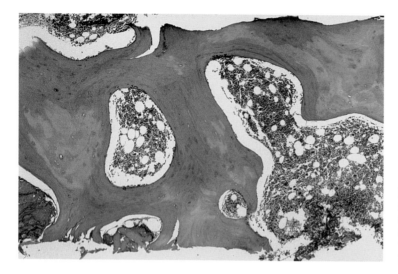

Fig. 11.8 BM trephine biopsy section, idiopathic osteosclerosis, showing marked thickening of bone trabeculae by mature lamellar bone. The intervening marrow is normal. Paraffin-embedded, H&E ×4.

ing (lead, mercury, phosphorus, bismuth) and hypervitaminosis A and D [13]. In fluorosis there may be features of both osteosclerosis and osteomalacia together with some disruption of normal lamellar structure [13]. Osteosclerosis may occur without primary bone marrow disease in the congenital condition designated osteopetrosis (see below) and also, rarely, in adults in the absence of any associated disease (Fig. 11.8). The cause of isolated osteosclerosis in adults is unknown; some reported cases have suggested an association with intravenous drug abuse [53].

In the myeloproliferative neoplasms (see Fig. 5.31), the term osteomyelosclerosis is sometimes used [54,55]. The new bone may be either bone formed on the endosteal surface of trabeculae, leading to marked trabecular thickening or, less commonly, irregular spicules of metaplastic woven bone within the fibrous tissue. Strands of woven bone may form an irregular network in the intertrabecular spaces and, in severe cases, the medullary cavity is almost completely obliterated. Some conversion of woven bone to mature bone occurs.

Metastases from various types of carcinoma may cause dense bone marrow fibrosis and osteosclerosis but these changes are most commonly associated with carcinomas of the breast and prostate (see Figs 10.11 and 10.13). When osteosclerosis is due to metastatic carcinoma, malignant cells can be detected within the fibrous tissue. The bone

changes do not differ from those associated with the myeloproliferative neoplasms.

In idiopathic osteosclerosis, the bone trabeculae are increased in thickness by mature lamellar bone.

Peripheral blood and bone marrow changes in osteomyelosclerosis are those of the underlying disease. In osteosclerosis associated with metastatic carcinoma, a leucoerythroblastic anaemia is usual and there is sometimes also thrombocytopenia or leucopenia; bone marrow aspiration may be impossible or the aspirate may contain tumour cells or increased osteoblasts and osteoclasts. In idiopathic osteosclerosis, the peripheral blood and the bone marrow aspirate are normal.

The bone may be so hard in osteosclerosis that penetration is impossible or needles bend or break. Open biopsy may then be necessary for diagnosis.

Thyroid disease [56,57]

Thyrotoxicosis has been found to be associated with osteoporosis, an increased percentage of osteoid and a marked increase in osteoclasts. Hypothyroidism is associated with osteosclerosis, normal or decreased osteoid percentage and reduced osteoclasts.

Bone necrosis and repair

Conditions causing bone marrow necrosis (see page 148) also cause necrosis of trabecular bone in many

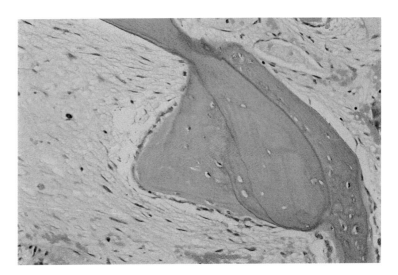

Fig. 11.9 BM trephine biopsy section showing newly deposited woven bone on the surface of a necrotic trabecula. Paraffin-embedded, H&E ×20.

instances. In the acute phase, necrotic bone is recognized by the absence of osteocytes from lacunae. It should be noted that occasional lacunae may appear empty in normal bone if the plane of section does not pass through an osteocyte nucleus.

Repair occurs by appositional new bone formation. Woven bone is deposited on the surface of the dead lamellar bone (Fig. 11.9). This is followed by the normal processes of bone remodelling in which the woven bone is replaced by lamellar bone.

Osteopetrosis (Albers–Schoenberg disease)

Osteopetrosis, also known as marble bone disease or Albers–Schoenberg disease, is a hereditary metabolic disease consequent on a defect in osteoclast function [58–60]. Osteoclasts may be increased (Fig. 11.10), decreased (Fig. 11.11) or present in normal numbers but they are always qualitatively abnormal [61,62]. The result is osteosclerosis with gradual obliteration of the marrow cavity by both bony encroachment and associated fibrosis. Although bone density is increased, the bone is more fragile than normal. Osteopetrosis occurs in an autosomal recessive form, which manifests itself either *in utero* or during infancy, and as an autosomal dominant form in adults. The autosomal recessive form is a severe disease with symptoms of marrow failure due to obliteration of the marrow cavity; the autosomal dominant form has much milder clinical manifestations with an increased

predisposition to fractures. Histologically, the trabeculae appear thickened due to increased amounts of mature lamellar bone with osteoclasts being prominent in some cases [61]. The narrow intertrabecular spaces are occupied by connective tissue. There is loss of the distinction between cortex and trabeculae. Masses of irregularly mineralized osteoid surrounding unresorbed cartilaginous cores have also been described [63].

In the severe infantile form of osteopetrosis there is increasingly severe leucoerythroblastic anaemia and thrombocytopenia associated with extramedullary haemopoiesis. Occasionally, the white cell count is increased and granulocyte precursors, including even blast cells, are present in the blood [64]. In the milder adult form of the disease there is only a minor degree of anaemia.

Features of osteopetrosis associated with renal tubular acidosis, cerebral calcification and developmental delay are seen in carbonic anhydrase II deficiency, a rare condition with autosomal recessive inheritance described in the Mediterranean region, the Middle East and Ireland [65].

Bisphosphonate therapy

Bone disease similar to the inherited form of osteopetrosis has been observed in a child treated with a bisphosphonate (pamidronate) [66]. Nitrogen-containing bisphosphonates (e.g. aledronate) reduce bone resorption and lead to cytological

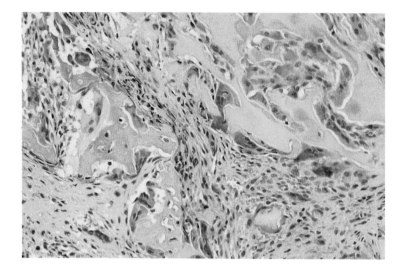

Fig. 11.10 BM trephine biopsy section from a child with osteopetrosis showing a marked increase in osteoclast numbers and bone marrow fibrosis. Paraffin-embedded, H&E ×20. (By courtesy of Adrienne Flanagan, London.)

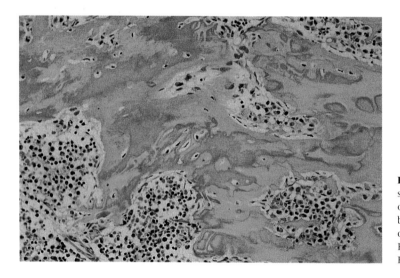

Fig. 11.11 BM trephine biopsy section from a child with osteopetrosis showing abnormal bone structure and no detectable osteoclasts. Paraffin-embedded, H&E ×20. (By courtesy of Adrienne Flanagan, London.)

abnormalities in osteoclasts; giant osteoclasts with pyknotic nuclei are often present, their number correlating with dose [67]. Osteoclasts appear detached from the bone and a proportion are apoptotic [67]. At higher doses osteoclasts, both cytologically normal and abnormal, are increased in number [67]. Some changes persist for at least a year after stopping treatment [67].

Osteogenesis imperfecta

Osteogenesis imperfecta comprises a group of related hereditary diseases due to abnormalities in the synthesis of type I collagen [68,69]. Several different biochemical defects have been identified, all of which are associated with increased fragility of the skeleton and a tendency to fractures. Other manifestations include blue sclerae, laxity of joints and abnormalities of dentition. The most severe variant (type II) has an autosomal recessive inheritance and is fatal in the perinatal period. Several other variants have been described that are compatible with survival into adult life; these usually have an autosomal dominant pattern of inheritance. Histologically, thinning of the cortex and trabeculae is seen [9]. In some cases there is loss of the normal lamellar structure of the bone [70]. Osteoblasts, osteoid-covered surfaces and osteocytes are increased [13]. Biopsies in young patients may show disorganization of the transitional zone between cartilage and bone, and islands of cartilage surrounded by woven bone [13].

The peripheral blood and bone marrow aspirate findings are normal.

Gorham's disease

Gorham's disease or 'vanishing bone disease', a condition of unknown aetiology, may affect the pelvis and thus be detected in a trephine biopsy specimen. This condition is characterized by a marked increase in osteoclastic activity with destruction of bone and its replacement by vascular connective tissue containing inflammatory cells [13].

Fibrous dysplasia

Fibrous dysplasia may affect the pelvis and thus be detected in a trephine biopsy section. The process starts in the marrow cavity and spreads to involve cortical and trabecular bone. The abnormal fibrous tissue contains whorls of spindle-shaped fibroblasts, osteoblasts, osteoclasts and foci of woven bone and cartilage [13].

Problems and pitfalls

Damage caused by torsion or crushing of the trephine biopsy core may generate fragments of bone that mimic Paget's disease or bone necrosis. The artefactual changes are usually limited to the inner end of the biopsy core and trabecular bone in areas with well-preserved architecture will be normal.

Incomplete decalcification may lead to basophilic staining of bone with H&E, particularly affecting central areas within trabeculae, which may suggest abnormal bone growth. If sections are examined from several levels through the biopsy specimen, it is usually clear that the incomplete decalcification is more extensive towards the centre of the core. When the sections are studied carefully, a normal pattern of lamellae and lacunae can be seen, even in partly calcified areas. If poor decalcification causes difficulty with cutting or staining of sections,

surface decalcification of the wax block can be used but the routine laboratory protocol for decalcification should also be reviewed.

Trabeculae of bone may become detached from trephine biopsy sections during staining (see Fig. 1.65) and, in particular, during proteolysis or wet-heat exposure for antigen retrieval in immunohistochemical techniques. The spaces remaining may mimic dilated sinusoids but careful attention to their contours and comparison of their position relative to any preserved trabeculae usually makes their true nature obvious.

Regenerating bone post-chemotherapy may mimic hyperparathyroid bone disease or renal osteodystrophy but does not show the tunnelling of trabeculae by fibrous tissue that is such a prominent feature of the latter conditions. A common finding after a period of intensive chemotherapy, which may also be found after an episode of severe systemic illness (particularly infection), is a single prominent cement line a short distance below a normal trabecular bone surface. This is likely to represent a pause in normal bone remodelling, followed by its resumption; it is most often visible between 2 weeks and 2 months after the causative clinical episode.

Newly made woven bone has large lacunae and the resident osteocytes may not all be apparent in a particular section. The bone may therefore appear to lack osteocytes and may be mistaken for an area of necrosis. However, only a few lacunae, at most, will appear acellular and the lack of lamellar structure (confirmed, if necessary, with a reticulin or trichrome stain) will show that woven bone is present.

The irregular bone of severe Paget's disease may mimic osteomyelosclerosis due to primary myelofibrosis or metastasis. The diagnosis of Paget's disease is confirmed by the presence of giant osteoclasts and the distinctive tesselated (mosaic) pattern of irregular bony plates with scalloped edges that make up individual trabeculae.

Reactivities of some monoclonal antibodies with normal bone cells should not be mistaken for reactions with other normal or abnormal cells (see Tables 2.6 and 2.7): VS38c and (less consistently) CD30 react with osteoblasts, while antibodies of the CD68 cluster react with osteoclasts, the latter being of macrophage origin.

References

1 Raisz LG (1999) Physiology and pathophysiology of bone remodeling. *Clin Chem*, **45**, 1353–1358.

2 Boyce BF, Hughes DE, Wright KR, Xing L and Dai A (1999) Recent advances in bone biology provide insight into the pathogenesis of bone diseases. *Lab Invest*, **79**, 83–94.

3 Clarke B (2008) Normal bone anatomy and physiology. *Clin J Am Soc Nephrol*, **3** (Suppl. 3), S131–S139.

4 Ellis HA (1981) Metabolic bone disease. In: Anthony PP and Macsween RNM (eds) *Recent Advances in Histopathology 11*. Churchill Livingstone, Edinburgh.

5 Gatter K and Brown D (1994) *An Illustrated Guide to Bone Marrow Diagnosis*. Blackwell Science, Oxford.

6 Byers RJ, Denton J, Hoyland JA and Freemont AJ (1997) Differential patterns of osteoblast dysfunction in trabecular bone in patients with established osteoporosis. *J Clin Pathol*, **50**, 760–764.

7 Verma S, Rajaratnam JH, Denton J, Hoyland JA and Byers RJ (2002) Adipocyte proportion of bone marrow is inversely related to bone formation in osteoporosis. *J Clin Pathol*, **55**, 693–698.

8 Kelepouris N, Harper KD, Gannon F, Kaplan FS and Haddad JG (1995) Severe osteoporosis in men. *Ann Intern Med*, **123**, 452–460.

9 Rauch F, Travers R, Norman ME, Taylor A, Parfitt AM and Glorieux FH (2000) Deficient bone formation in idiopathic juvenile osteoporosis: a histomorphometric study of cancellous iliac bone. *J Bone Miner Res*, **15**, 957–963.

10 Zmuda JM, Cauley JA and Ferrell RE (1999) Recent progress in understanding the genetic susceptibility to osteoporosis. *Genet Epidemiol*, **16**, 356–367.

11 Raisz LG (1988) Local and systemic factors in the pathogenesis of osteoporosis. *N Engl J Med*, **318**, 818–828.

12 Beck JS and Nordin BEC (1960) Histological assessment of osteoporosis by iliac crest biopsy. *J Pathol Bacteriol*, **80**, 391–397.

13 Frisch B and Bartl R (1999) *Biopsy Interpretation of Bone and Bone Marrow: Histology and immunohistology in paraffin and plastic*, 2nd edn. Arnold, London.

14 Ellis HA and Peart KM (1972) Quantitative observations on mineralised and non-mineralised bone in the iliac crest. *J Clin Pathol*, **25**, 277–286.

15 Fogelman I and Blake G (1990) How to measure osteoporosis. In: Smith R (ed) *Osteoporosis*. Royal College of Physicians, London.

16 Frame B and Nixon RK (1968) Bone marrow mast cells in osteoporosis of aging. *N Engl J Med*, **279**, 626–630.

17 Yetgin S and Ozsoylu S (1982) Myeloid metaplasia in vitamin D deficiency rickets. *Scand J Haematol*, **28**, 180–185.

18 Broadus AE (1989) Primary hyperparathyroidism. *J Urol*, **141**, 723–730.

19 Parisien M, Silverberg SJ, Shane E, Dempster DW and Bilezikian JP (1990) Bone disease in primary hyperparathyroidism. *Endocrinol Metab Clin North Am*, **19**, 19–34.

20 Dabbagh S (1998) Renal osteodystrophy. *Curr Opin Pediatr*, **10**, 190–196.

21 DeVita MV, Rasenas LL, Bansal M, Gleim GW, Zabetakis PM, Gardenswartz MH and Michelis MF (1992) Assessment of renal osteodystrophy in hemodialysis patients. *Medicine*, **71**, 284–290.

22 Shaker JL, Norton AJ, Woods MF, Fallon MD and Findling JW (1991) Secondary hyperparathyroidism and osteopenia in women following gastric exclusion surgery for obesity. *Osteoporos Int*, **1**, 177–181.

23 Yamaguchi T, Hirano T, Kumagai K, Tsurumoto T, Shindo H, Majima R and Arima N (1999) Osteitis fibrosa cystica generalizata with adult T-cell leukaemia: a case report. *Br J Haematol* **107**, 892–894.

24 Finkelstein JS, Klibanski A, Schaefer EH, Hornstein MD, Schiff I and Neer RM (1994) Parathyroid hormone for the prevention of bone loss induced by estrogen deficiency. *N Engl J Med*, **331**, 1618–1623.

25 Bassler T, Wong ET and Brynes RK (1993) Osteitis fibrosa cystica simulating metastatic tumor: an almost-forgotten relationship. *Am J Clin Pathol*, **100**, 697–700.

26 Joyce JM, Idea RJ, Grossman SJ, Liss RG and Lyons JB (1994) Multiple brown tumors in unsuspected primary hyperparathyroidism mimicking metastatic disease on radiograph and bone scan. *Clin Nucl Med*, **19**, 630–635.

27 Pai M, Park CH, Kim BS, Chung YS and Park HB (1997) Multiple brown tumors in parathyroid carcinoma mimicking metastatic bone disease. *Clin Nucl Med*, **22**, 691–694.

28 Zingraff J, Drueke T, Marie P, Man NK, Jungers P and Border P (1978) Anaemia and secondary hyperparathyroidism. *Arch Intern Med*, **138**, 1650–1652.

29 Llach F (1991) Renal bone disease. *Transplant Proc*, **23**, 1818–1822.

30 Teitelbaum SL (1984) Renal osteodystrophy. *Hum Pathol*, **15**, 306–323.

31 Lee DB, Goodman WG and Coburn JW (1988) Renal osteodystrophy: some new questions on an old disorder. *Am J Kidney Dis*, **11**, 365–376.

32 Iwamoto N, Ono T, Yamazaki S, Fukuda T, Kondo M, Yamamoto N *et al.* (1986) Clinical features of aluminum-associated bone disease in long-term hemodialysis patients. *Nephron*, **42**, 204–209.

33 Kaye M and Henderson J (1988) Nature of mononuclear cells positive for acid phosphatase activity in bone marrow of patients with renal osteodystrophy. *J Clin Pathol*, **41**, 277–279.

34 Hoyer JD, Li CY, Yam LT, Hanson CA and Kurtin PJ (1997) Immunohistochemical demonstration of acid phosphatase isoenzyme 5 (tartrate-resistant) in paraffin sections of hairy cell leukemia and other hematologic disorders. *Am J Clin Pathol*, **108**, 308–315.

35 McClure J, Fazzalari NL, Fassett RG and Pugsley DG (1983) Bone histoquantitative findings and histochemical staining reactions for aluminium in chronic renal failure patients treated with haemodialysis fluids containing high and low concentrations of aluminium. *J Clin Pathol*, **36**, 1281–1287.

36 Kaye M (1983) Bone marrow aluminium storage in renal failure. *J Clin Pathol*, **36**, 1288–1291.

37 Pierides AM and Myli MP (1984) Iron and aluminium osteomalacia in haemodialysis patients. *N Engl J Med*, **310**, 323.

38 Weinberg SG, Lubin A, Weiner SN, Deorus MP, Ghose MK and Kopelman SN (1977) Myelofibrosis in renal osteodystrophy. *Am J Med*, **63**, 755–776.

39 Rao DS, Shih M-S and Mohini R (1993) Effect of serum parathyroid hormone and bone marrow fibrosis on the response to erythropoietin in uremia. *N Engl J Med*, **328**, 171–175.

40 El Reshaid K, Johny KV, Hakim A, Kamel H, Sebeta A, Hourani H and Kanyike FB (1994) Erythropoietin treatment in haemodialysis patients with iron overload. *Acta Haematol*, **91**, 130–135.

41 Singer FR (1999) Update on the viral etiology of Paget's disease of bone. *J Bone Miner Res*, **14** (Suppl. 2), 29–33.

42 Gallacher SJ (1993) Paget's disease of bone. *Curr Opin Rheumatol*, **5**, 351–356.

43 Ralston SH, Digiovine FS, Gallacher SJ, Boyle IT and Duff GW (1991) Failure to detect paramyxovirus sequences in Paget's disease of bone using the polymerase chain reaction. *J Bone Miner Res*, **6**, 1243–1248.

44 Hocking L, Slee F, Haslam SI, Cundy T, Nicholson G, Van Hul W and Ralston SH (2000) Familial Paget's disease of bone: patterns of inheritance and frequency of linkage to chromosome 18q. *Bone*, **26**, 577–580.

45 Haslam SI and Ralston SH (1998) The genetics of Paget's disease of bone. *Curr Opin Orthop*, **9**, 17–20.

46 Haslam SI, Hul WV, Morales Piga A, Balemans W, San Millan JL, Nakatsuka K *et al.* (1998) Paget's disease of bone: evidence for a susceptibility locus on chromosome 18q and for genetic heterogeneity. *J Bone Miner Res*, **13**, 911–917.

47 Spencer H, O'Sullivan V and Sontag SJ (1994) Occupational exposure to lead: preliminary observations in Paget's disease of bone in women and in family members of affected patients. *J Trace Elem Exp Med*, **7**, 53–58.

48 Spencer H, O'Sullivan V and Sontag SJ (1995) Exposure to lead, a potentially hazardous toxin:

Paget's disease of bone. *J Trace Elem Exp Med*, **8**, 163–171.

49 Ben-Chetrit E, Flusser D and Assaf Y (1984) Severe bleeding complicating percutaneous bone marrow biopsy. *Arch Intern Med*, **144**, 2284.

50 De Gennes C, Kuntz D and De Vernejoul MC (1992). Bone mastocytosis: a report of nine cases with a bone histomorphometric study. *Clin Orthop Relat Res*, **279**, 281–291.

51 Van der Molen LA, Urba WJ, Longo DL, Lawrence J, Gralnick H and Steis RG (1989) Diffuse osteosclerosis in hairy cell leukemia. *Blood*, **74**, 2066–2069.

52 Verhoef GEG, De Wolf Peeters C, Zachee P and Boogaerts MA (1990) Regression of diffuse osteosclerosis in hairy cell leukemia after treatment with interferon. *Br J Haematol*, **76**, 150–151.

53 Whyte MP, Teitelbaum SL and Reinus WR (1996) Doubling skeletal mass during adult life: the syndrome of diffuse osteosclerosis after intravenous drug abuse. *J Bone Miner Res*, **11**, 554–558.

54 Burkhardt R, Frisch B and Bartl R (1982) Bone biopsy in haematological disorders. *J Clin Pathol*, **35**, 257–284.

55 Thiele J, Hoeppner B, Zankovich R and Fischer R (1989) Histomorphometry of bone marrow biopsies in primary osteomyelofibrosis/-sclerosis (agnogenic myeloid metaplasia) – correlations between clinical and morphological features. *Virchows Arch A Pathol Anat Histopathol*, **415**, 191–202.

56 Bordier Ph, Miravet L, Matrajt H, Hioco D and Ryckewaert A (1967) Bone changes in adult patients with abnormal thyroid function with special reference to ^{45}Ca kinetics and quantitative histology. *Proc Roy Soc Med*, **60**, 1132–1134.

57 Abu E and Compston J (1998) The impact of thyroid hormones on bone. *Curr Opin Endocrinol Diabetes*, **5**, 282–287.

58 Singer FR and Chang SS (1992) Osteopetrosis. *Semin Nephrol*, **12**, 191–199.

59 Shankar L, Gerritsen EJA and Key LL Jr. (1997) Osteopetrosis: pathogenesis and rationale for the use of interferon-gamma-1b. *BioDrugs*, **7**, 23–29.

60 Askmyr MK, Fasth A and Richter J (2007) Towards a better understanding and new therapeutics of osteopetrosis. *Br J Haematol*, **140**, 597–609.

61 Helfrich MH, Aronson DC, Everts V, Mieremet RHP, Gerritsen EJA, Eckhardt PG *et al.* (1991) Morphologic features of bone in human osteopetrosis. *Bone*, **12**, 411–419.

62 Flanagan AM, Sarma U, Steward CG, Vellodi A and Horton MA (2000) Study of the nonresorptive phenotype of osteoclast-like cells from patients with malignant osteopetrosis: a new approach to investigating pathogenesis. *J Bone Miner Res*, **15**, 352–360.

63 Strauchen JA (1996) *Diagnostic Histopathology of the Bone Marrow*. Oxford University Press, Oxford.

64 Toren A, Meyer JJ, Mandel M, Sohiby G, Kende G and Bassat I (1993) Malignant osteopetrosis manifesting as juvenile chronic myeloid leukemia. *Pediatr Hematol Oncol*, **10**, 187–189.

65 McMahon C, Will A, Hu P, Shah GN, Sly WS and Smith OP (2001) Carbonic anhydrase II deficiency: phenotype, genotype and marrow transplantation. *Br J Haematol*, **113** (Suppl. 1), 34.

66 Whyte MP, Wenkert D, Clements KL, McAlister WH and Mumm S (2003) Bisphosphonate-induced osteopetrosis. *N Engl J Med*, **349**, 457–463.

67 Weinstein RS, Roberson PK and Manolagas SC (2009) Giant osteoclast formation and long-term oral bisphosphonate therapy. *N Engl J Med*, **360**, 53–62.

68 Cole WG (1988) Osteogenesis imperfecta. *Baillieres Clin Endocrinol Metab*, **2**, 243–265.

69 Cole WG (1993) Etiology and pathogenesis of heritable connective tissue diseases. *J Pediatr Orthop*, **13**, 392–403.

70 Falvo KA and Bullough PG (1973) Osteogenesis imperfecta: a histometric analysis. *J Bone Joint Surg*, **55A**, 275–286.

APPENDIX

Many readers of the previous editions of this book have given helpful comments that have been incorporated into subsequent editions. One of the most common requests has been for methods used for processing and staining of bone marrow. The following section gives details of various methods, including the stains most commonly used for bone marrow trephine biopsy sections in the laboratories in which the authors work. We find these give good results. However, it cannot be stressed too strongly that the key to obtaining high quality sections and stains is close co-operation between pathologists and laboratory scientists. A more detailed discussion of the various techniques described may be found in the references at the end of this section.

Technical methods applicable to trephine biopsy specimens

Fixation

Adequate fixation of a trephine biopsy specimen is essential if one is to prepare sections that preserve the fine cytological detail needed for interpretation of haematological disorders. In most laboratories, 10% neutral buffered formol-saline is used as a general purpose fixative for all specimens and this gives satisfactory results with bone marrow trephine biopsy specimens. It is important to ensure that the formol-saline is not left for long periods at ambient or high temperature before being used because formic acid and formalin pigment may be produced. Use of stale fixative is one of the more common causes of poor quality sections. The pH should be checked before use. Trephine biopsy cores should be fixed in formol-saline for a minimum of 18 hours but fixation for longer periods, up to 48 hours, does not adversely affect subsequent processing or morphology and is desirable for large samples. Neutral buffered saline containing 0.5% glutaraldehyde but only 1% formaldehyde, rather than the 4% present in the standard 10% neutral buffered formol-saline, has also been used and is said to prevent shrinkage.

Other fixatives, such as Bouin's fixative and the mercury-based fixatives, Zenker's and B5, are also used with trephine biopsy specimens. These fixatives give excellent preservation of cytological detail but are less practical in laboratories processing a wide range of tissues, in which the majority of other specimens will be fixed in formol-saline. The use of fixatives containing mercury has now become impossible in some countries. The reactivity of antibodies used for immunohistochemical staining may also be affected by the choice of fixative (use of Bouin's solution is particularly limiting) and Zenker's fixative can destroy chloroacetate esterase activity. If Zenker's solution is used, the biopsy core should be fixed for a minimum of 4 hours but longer periods of fixation are perfectly acceptable. Fixation in Bouin's solution should be for 4–12 hours. If B5 fixative is used, the duration of fixation is more critical – 4 hours is optimal; if fixation lasts for more than 6 hours hardening of the tissue can make it difficult to cut sections. An alternative fixative has been adopted for trephine biopsy specimens in some laboratories, with excellent results and no impairment of tinctorial or immunohistochemical staining. This fixative is a combined aceto-zinc formalin solution; conditions for its use are essentially identical to those employed with standard formol-saline. It has been claimed that this is superior to formol-saline fixation for preservation of nuclear acids but, in our experience, polymerase chain reaction (PCR) analyses have been more satisfactory after conventional fixation and decalcification with the chelating agent, ethylene diamine tetra-acetic acid (EDTA).

Decalcification

The method of decalcification used depends on how the biopsy specimen is to be processed. If it is to be embedded in resin it may not be necessary to use any decalcification at all, although better results are often obtained by decalcifying the specimen using EDTA.

If the trephine specimen is to be embedded in paraffin wax, decalcification using EDTA, formic acid or acetic acid is required. Decalcification using inorganic acids, such as hydrochloric or nitric acid, should be avoided as this affects morphological preservation adversely and impairs metachromatic staining of sections, e.g. with Giemsa or toluidine blue. Some methods of decalcification can lead to artefactual staining with immunohistochemical techniques; for example, the use of nitric acid can cause megakaryocytes to give positive reactions with antibodies to CD34. Decalcification using EDTA may require longer incubation than methods using organic acids; speed may be increased by agitation and/or warming to 37°C or by use of ultrasound or microwaves. Decalcification of paraffin-embedded biopsy specimens using formic or acetic acid destroys chloroacetate esterase activity but use of EDTA preserves this. Both acid and chelation methods remove variable amounts of iron from the tissue, rendering assessment of iron stores unreliable in decalcified specimens.

Whichever method is preferred locally, it is essential to achieve good fixation before exposure of the tissue to any decalcifying agent. The use of proprietary combined decalcifying fixative solutions should be avoided unless absolutely necessary to obtain rapid haematoxylin and eosin (H&E)-stained sections in an exceptionally urgent situation. If they must be used, it must be recognized that many other staining techniques will be unsuccessful although reticulin is generally well preserved.

Processing

Paraffin embedding

One of the major advantages of this technique is that it can be used in virtually any diagnostic his-

topathology department using the automated processors employed routinely for other histopathology specimens. The cytological detail is not as good as that seen in high quality resin-embedded (often referred to as plastic-embedded) sections but, with care, excellent results can be obtained. The key to obtaining good results is co-operation between the pathologist interpreting the sections and the laboratory staff processing the sample, ensuring that careful attention is paid to the various steps involved in preparing histological sections. If sections are unsatisfactory, in most cases the problem lies in the fixation, decalcification, cutting or staining rather than in the processing itself.

Sections should be cut at no more than 3–4 μm thickness. If a focal lesion is suspected clinically, sections should be cut at multiple levels. H&E and a stain for reticulin (Gomori's or Gordon and Sweet's stains) are usually performed on all specimens. We also perform a Romanowsky stain (Giemsa or one of its variants) on all specimens. Although many pathologists do not use this routinely, it can be helpful in the identification of early erythroid precursors, plasma cells and mast cells and in distinguishing neutrophil and eosinophil granules. Almost all of the stains used routinely with other paraffin-embedded tissues may be employed with trephine biopsy specimens but, as mentioned previously, most enzyme histochemistry is unsuccessful because of irreversible denaturation of the enzymes during decalcification and processing. One exception is acid phosphatase activity which is sometimes retained. When hairy cell leukaemia is suspected, demonstration of tartrate-resistant acid phosphatase (TRAP) activity may be useful although the recent introduction of monoclonal antibodies for the immunohistochemical detection of this enzyme in fixed tissues offers a simpler technical alternative for many laboratories.

Resin embedding

Glycol methacrylate and methyl methacrylate are the most commonly used resins for embedding trephine biopsy specimens. Both allow sections to be cut without decalcification, with preservation of excellent cellular detail and without the shrinkage artefacts that are prominent in most decalcified specimens. Resin embedding allows staining by many enzyme histochemical techniques. All of the stains used routinely with paraffin-embedded sections can be employed with resin-embedded sections although many require modification of the method to optimize results. Because resins continue to polymerize over long periods of time, antigen retrieval techniques for immunohistochemistry need to be modified for older specimens. In general, progressively longer proteolysis or wet-heat exposure is needed as the resin becomes more highly polymerized.

Methods

Fixation, decalcification and paraffin embedding

1 The trephine biopsy core should be expelled from the needle and placed directly into fixative solution. If touch preparations are needed, the core should be transferred into fixative as quickly as possible after they have been prepared.
2 Leave the specimen to fix in 10% neutral-buffered (pH 7.6) formol-saline for 24 hours.
3 Decalcify overnight in 5% formic acid or 5% EDTA solution. Large cores may require up to 48 hours, particularly if EDTA is used.
4 Wash in 70% alcohol.
5 Place back into formol-saline until required for processing.
6 Process routinely in an automated tissue processor with other histological samples.
7 Embed specimen in paraffin wax. Use of a high melting point (hard) wax, if feasible within the laboratory routine, may assist section cutting.
8 Cut sections at no more than 3–4 μm.

Aceto-zinc fixative method

Fixative solution
• Zinc chloride: 12.5 g
• Formaldehyde (concentrated): 150 ml
• Distilled water: 1000 ml
• Glacial acetic acid: 7.5 ml
This can be prepared in advance and aliquotted into universal containers with appropriate hazard labelling. It is used in an identical manner to formol-saline, following the schedule described above.

Aceto-zinc fixative solution has a weak decalcifying action but the presence of zinc ions seems to stabilize nucleic acids and provides protection against the adverse effects on morphological preservation seen with some proprietary combined fixative/decalcifier solutions. Trephine biopsy cores still require further decalcification with organic acid or EDTA after fixation in aceto-zinc.

Resin embedding (glycol methacrylate)

Materials
1 Monomer:
  • 2-Hydroxyl ethyl methacrylate: 80 ml
  • 2-Butoxyethanol: 8 ml
  • Benzoxyl peroxidase: 1 g
2 Activator:
  • Polyethelene glycol 400: 15 parts
  • *N*-*N*-dimethylaniline: 1 part
3 Embedding mixture:
  • Monomer: 42 ml
  • Activator: 0.1 ml

Procedure
1 70% alcohol – two changes of 15 minutes each.
2 95% alcohol – two changes of 15 minutes each.
3 Absolute alcohol – two changes of 15 minutes each.
4 Glycol methacrylate monomer for 2 hours.
5 Glycol methacrylate monomer second change – leave overnight.
6 Embed in embedding mixture and leave for several hours to polymerize.

Histochemical staining for paraffin-embedded sections

Many laboratories use automated staining machines for bulk staining of histological sections with H&E. Bone marrow biopsy sections stained in this way can give perfectly acceptable results. Other laboratories prefer manual staining as this allows the timing of individual steps to be optimized for marrow sections. Many laboratories (including our own) also use automated staining machines that utilize kits to perform many of the other histochemical stains commonly used with bone marrow biopsy sections, giving very satisfactory results. The manual methods detailed below also work well; precise technical details such as incubation times may require refining in individual laboratories for best results.

Haematoxylin and eosin (H&E)

Solutions

1 Eosin 1% aqueous solution:
   • Eosin: 10 g
   • Distilled water: 1 litre
2 Harris's haematoxylin solution:
   • Haematoxylin: 5 g
   • Ethyl alcohol: 50 ml
   • Ammonium or potassium alum: 100 g
   • Distilled water: 1 litre
   • Mercuric oxide red: 2.5 g

Dissolve the alum in the distilled water, over heat, stirring frequently. Dissolve the haematoxylin in the alcohol and add to the alum solution. Bring to the boil while stirring. Remove from the heat and add the mercuric oxide. Mix and allow to cool. Filter into a glass stain bottle and the solution is ready for use. It is advisable to filter the solution at regular intervals of a few days, to avoid precipitates developing, and to prepare fresh solution on a weekly or fortnightly basis, depending on frequency of use.

3 Scott's tap water:
   • Sodium hydrogen carbonate: 3.5 g
   • Magnesium sulphate: 20 g
   • Distilled water: 1 litre
4 Acid alcohol:
   • 0.5% hydrochloric acid in 70% alcohol

Procedure

1 Dewax sections with two changes of xylene.
2 Rehydrate sections using two changes of absolute alcohol, followed by 95% alcohol and wash briefly in running tap water.
3 Stain with haematoxylin solution for up to 5 minutes.
4 Wash in running tap water.
5 Differentiate in acid alcohol for approximately 5 seconds.
6 Wash in running tap water.
7 'Blue' in Scott's tap water for a few seconds.
8 Wash in running tap water.
9 Stain with eosin for approximately 5 minutes.
10 Wash in running tap water.
11 Dehydrate, clear and mount sections.

Giemsa

Solutions

1 1% aqueous acetic acid.
2 10% solution of Giemsa stain (preferably Gurr's improved), freshly prepared in distilled water.

Procedure

1 Dewax sections with two changes of xylene.
2 Rehydrate sections with two changes of absolute alcohol, 95% alcohol and wash in running water.
3 Stain sections with Giemsa solution for 20 minutes. Staining may be improved if this step is conducted at 56 °C in a temperature-controlled water-bath.
4 Rinse in distilled water.
5 Dip sections quickly into 1% acetic acid.
6 Wash with distilled water.
7 Check the staining microscopically and, if required, re-stain.
8 Dehydrate, clear and mount sections.

Gordon and Sweet's technique for reticulin staining

Solutions

1 Acidified potassium permanganate solution:
   • 0.5% aqueous potassium permanganate: 95 ml
   • 3% sulphuric acid: 5 ml
2 2% aqueous oxalic acid.
3 5% aqueous ferric ammonium sulphate (iron alum).
4 5% aqueous sodium thiosulphate.
5 0.1% aqueous gold chloride.
6 Nuclear fast red.
   • 0.1 g nuclear fast red in 100 ml 5% aluminium sulphate
7 Ammoniacal silver solution.

To 5 ml of 10% silver nitrate add concentrated ammonia drop by drop, mixing continuously, until the formed precipitate just redissolves. Add 5 ml of 3% sodium hydroxide and mix and a black precipitate will form. Add concentrated ammonia, as described previously, until the precipitate just redissolves. Make the solution up to 50 ml with distilled water.

Procedure

1 Dewax sections with two changes of xylene.

2 Rehydrate sections with two changes of absolute alcohol followed by 95% alcohol and then wash in distilled water.

3 Treat with potassium permanganate solution for 5 minutes.

4 Rinse in distilled water.

5 Bleach sections in 2% oxalic acid solution for 1 minute.

6 Wash well in distilled water.

7 Treat sections with iron alum for 20 minutes.

8 Wash well in several changes of distilled water.

9 Treat with ammoniacal silver solution for approximately 10 seconds.

10 Wash well in distilled water.

11 Treat with 10% formalin for 1–2 minutes.

12 Wash well in distilled water.

13 Tone in gold chloride solution for up to 1 minute.

14 Wash well in distilled water.

15 Treat with sodium thiosulphate solution for 2 minutes.

16 Wash well in distilled water.

17 Stain nuclei with nuclear fast red for 2–3 minutes.

18 Wash in distilled water.

19 Dehydrate, clear and mount sections.

Results
• Reticulin fibres – black
• Collagen – yellow-brown (if sections are untoned; black, if toned)
• Nuclei – red

Note Microscopic examination of sections at stage 10 is important since the staining can vary from section to section. If the fibres are not adequately stained, steps 7–10 can be repeated if the sections have not been toned. If non-specific silver deposition is a persistent problem, which appears to be the case in some laboratories, toning will give a cleaner result at the expense of losing differentiation between reticulin and collagen. Since alternative stains for collagen can be employed in individual cases when needed, this approach can be greatly preferable to everyday poor quality reticulin staining.

Gomori's method for reticulin staining

Solutions

1 1% potassium permanganate solution.

2 1% aqueous oxalic acid.

3 Gomori's ammoniacal silver solution, prepared freshly, as follows. In a fume hood, add 4 ml of 10% aqueous potassium hydroxide to 20 ml of 10% aqueous silver nitrate solution; a precipitate will form. Add concentrated ammonia, dropwise, until the precipitate clears. Add further 10% aqueous silver nitrate until the solution develops a faint opalescence. Dilute with an equal volume of distilled water and then keep at 4 °C until used. Note: surplus solution must be discarded, following safe laboratory procedures, as it is unstable and potentially hazardous.

4 2.5% aqueous ferric ammonium sulphate (iron alum).

5 1% formaldehyde.

6 0.2% gold chloride.

7 3% potassium metabisulphite.

Procedure

1 Dewax sections with two changes of xylene. Rehydrate sections with two changes of absolute alcohol followed by 95% alcohol and then wash in distilled water.

2 Oxidize in 1% potassium permanganate for 1–2 minutes.

3 Wash well in distilled water.

4 Bleach in 5% oxalic acid for 30 seconds.

5 Rinse well in distilled water.

6 Sensitize in aqueous ferric aluminium sulphate (iron alum) for 20 minutes.

7 Wash well in tap then distilled water.

8 Impregnate in Gomori's ammoniacal silver solution (kept at 4 °C) for 1 minute.

9 Rinse well in distilled water to stop silver oxidization. Control the end-point microscopically using a control section first and then the individual test sections. Re-impregnate in ammoniacal silver if necessary.

10 Reduce in 1% formalin for 3 minutes.

11 Wash in tap water.

12 Tone in dilute 0.2% gold chloride for up to 10 minutes.

13 Wash in tap water.

14 Treat with 3% potassium metabisulphite for 1 minute.

15 Wash in tap water; dehydrate, clear and mount.

Results
• Reticulin fibres (and some pigments) – black

- Collagen – old rose (purplish-grey) when toned; gold when untoned
- Nuclei – grey (many laboratories use the nuclear counterstain nuclear fast red for added contrast)

Periodic acid–Schiff (PAS) stain

Solutions
1 1% solution of periodic acid in distilled water.
2 Schiff's reagent:
  - Pararosaniline C.I.: 1 g
  - Distilled water: 200 ml
  - Potassium metabisulphite: 2 g
  - Concentrated hydrochloric acid: 2 ml
  - Activated charcoal: 2 g

Boil the distilled water, remove from the heat and add the pararosaniline. Allow to cool to 50 °C and add the potassium metabisulphite. Mix and allow to cool to room temperature. Add the hydrochloric acid and activated charcoal, mix and leave overnight. Filter. The resulting liquid will be clear or straw-coloured. Store in a dark container at 4 °C.

Procedure
1 Dewax sections with two changes of xylene.
2 Rehydrate sections with two changes of absolute alcohol followed by 95% alcohol and then wash in distilled water.
3 Treat sections with periodic acid solution for 5 minutes.
4 Wash well in distilled water.
5 Treat with Schiff's reagent for 15 minutes.
6 Wash sections in running tap water for 10 minutes.
7 Counterstain the nuclei lightly with Mayer's haematoxylin (approximately 60 seconds).
8 Wash in tap water to 'blue' the haematoxylin (10 minutes).
9 Dehydrate, clear and mount sections.

Results
- PAS-positive material (neutral mucins and glycogen) – magenta
- Nuclei – pale blue

Note In histological sections of bone marrow, the following can be generally expected to be PAS positive: granulocytes (metamyelocytes and polymorphs of the neutrophil series), some megakaryocytes, inclusions such as Russell and Dutcher bodies in plasma cells, and connective tissue components of larger blood vessel walls.

Pre-treatment with diastase (see below) removes glycogen from the sections. Following diastase treatment, neutrophils and megakaryocytes are no longer PAS positive. The lack of neutrophil staining makes screening a section for small PAS-positive fungi such as histoplasma much easier, and we generally prefer pre-treatment with diastase when using PAS to demonstrate such organisms.

Perls' reaction for iron

Solutions
1 Nuclear fast red:
  - 0.1 g nuclear fast red in 100 ml 5% aluminium sulphate
2 Incubating solution:
  - Potassium ferrocyanide 2%: 25 ml
  - Hydrochloric acid 2%: 25 ml

Procedure
1 Dewax sections with two changes of xylene.
2 Rehydrate sections with two changes of absolute alcohol followed by 95% alcohol and then wash in distilled water.
3 Treat sections with incubating solution for 30 minutes.
4 Wash well with several changes of distilled water.
5 Counterstain nuclei with nuclear fast red for 2 minutes.
6 Dehydrate, clear and mount sections.

Results
- Ferric iron salts – blue
- Nuclei – red

Note Decalcification, whether by acid or EDTA, results in variable loss of stainable iron from tissue sections.

Histochemical staining for resin-embedded sections

Haematoxylin and eosin (H&E) for resin-embedded sections

Solutions
1 Mayer's haemalum:

- Haematoxylin: 1 g
- Distilled water: 1 litre
- Ammonium or potassium alum: 50 g
- Sodium iodate: 0.2 g
- Citric acid: 1 g
- Chloral hydrate: 50 g

Dissolve the alum, haematoxylin and sodium iodate in the distilled water by standing overnight at room temperature. Add the chloral hydrate and citric acid, mix and boil for 5 minutes. Mix and allow to cool. Filter into a glass stain bottle and the solution is ready for use.

2 All other solutions are prepared as described in the method for paraffin-embedded sections.

Procedure

1 Stain with Mayer's haemalum for up to 5 minutes.
2 Wash in running tap water.
3 Differentiate in acid alcohol for approximately 5 seconds.
4 Wash in running tap water.
5 'Blue' in Scott's tap water for a few seconds.
6 Wash in running tap water.
7 Stain with eosin for approximately 5 minutes.
8 Wash in running tap water.
9 Dehydrate, clear and mount sections.

Reticulin stain for resin-embedded sections

Solutions

1 Silver solution:
  - 10% silver nitrate: 20 ml
  - 10% potassium hydroxide: 4 ml
  - Concentrated ammonia

Mix the silver nitrate and potassium hydroxide solutions together and a brown flocculant precipitate will appear. Add concentrated ammonia drop by drop until the precipitate disappears. Add silver nitrate solution drop by drop until the solution just discolours to a pale yellow-brown colour. Add 6 drops of ammonia. Filter into a Coplin jar. Add approximately 25 ml of distilled water.

2 1% aqueous potassium permanganate.
3 1% aqueous oxalic acid.
4 4% aqueous ferric ammonium sulphate (iron alum).
5 5% aqueous sodium thiosulphate.
6 Nuclear fast red:

- 0.1 g nuclear red in 100 ml
- 5% aluminium sulphate

Procedure

1 Treat sections with potassium permanganate solution for 10 minutes.
2 Rinse in distilled water.
3 Bleach sections in 1% oxalic acid solution for 1 minute.
4 Wash well in distilled water.
5 Treat sections with iron alum for 10 minutes.
6 Wash well in several changes of distilled water.
7 Treat with silver solution for approximately 10 minutes.
8 Wash well in distilled water.
9 Treat with 10% formalin for 1–2 minutes.
10 Wash well in distilled water.
11 Treat with sodium thiosulphate solution for 2 minutes.
12 Wash well in distilled water.
13 Stain nuclei with nuclear fast red for 2–3 minutes.
14 Wash in distilled water.
15 Dehydrate, clear and mount sections.

Giemsa staining for resin-embedded sections

We have had great difficulty in obtaining satisfactory Giemsa staining of resin-embedded sections. However, incubation of sections in the Giemsa staining solution at 56°C rather than room temperature or brief microwave heating as detailed below produces excellent results.

Solutions

1 Staining solution:
  - Giemsa stain: 1 ml
  - Phosphate buffer: 2 ml
  - Distilled water: 47 ml
2 Phosphate buffer.

To 20 ml of 0.1 m sodium hydrogen orthophosphate add 0.1 m disodium orthophosphate drop by drop until the pH reaches 5.1. *The buffer should be freshly prepared.*

Procedure

1 Place slides in water then transfer to the Giemsa staining solution and microwave at 500 watts for 45 seconds. *Do not boil.*

2 Remove slide container from microwave and place in a preheated oven at 55 °C for 15 minutes.
3 Rinse slides briefly in a solution of 4 drops of acetic acid in 100 ml of distilled water.
4 Rinse slides in clean absolute alcohol.
5 Clear and mount sections.

Immunohistochemical staining of paraffin-embedded sections (which have been fixed in 10% neutral buffered formol saline)

Streptavidin–biotin–peroxidase method

Solutions
1 Antibody diluent:
- 0.01 m phosphate-buffered saline (PBS) or Tris-buffered saline (TBS) pH 7.6 prepared with ultra-pure or distilled water

If necessary, this may be modified by the addition of 0.1% bovine serum albumin and 0.1% sodium azide to reduce background staining. However, peroxidase-linked reagents should be diluted in PBS/TBS that does not contain azide, since azide inhibits peroxidase activity.
2 Peroxidase development solution (freshly made immediately before use):
- 0.05% diaminobenzidine tetrachloride (DAB) in PBS with 0.1% (w/v) hydrogen peroxide

Note: DAB is a possible carcinogen; for convenience and to minimize handling, it can be purchased ready-prepared with peroxidase in stabilized solution or tablet form.

Procedure
1 Mount paraffin-embedded sections on slides pre-coated with poly-l-lysine or other adhesive such as silane, or use proprietary electrically charged glass slides. If wet-heat pre-treatment is to be used, silanized slides are recommended. Negatively charged glass slides may also be used but do not always provide reliable adhesion with wet-heat antigen retrieval techniques.
2 Dewax paraffin-embedded sections in xylene and rehydrate through graded alcohols.
3 Block endogenous peroxidase activity by incubation at room temperature, in a humidified staining tray, with two changes of freshly prepared 0.3% (w/v) H_2O_2 in methanol, for 15 minutes each. It is important to make up fresh peroxidase-

blocking solution immediately before each incubation, as H_2O_2 activity is lost rapidly.
4 Pre-treat sections (antigen retrieval) with protease or wet-heat, as required for the antigen under investigation.* Proteolysis may be conducted at 37 °C with freshly prepared trypsin solution (in PBS/TBS, pH 7.6, with added $CaCl_2$) or, more conveniently, at room temperature using a commercially prepared solution of pronase (Dako, Ely, UK). Wet-heat methods generally employ a microwave oven at medium setting for approximately 25 minutes or a pressure cooker brought to full pressure for approximately 2 minutes; citrate solution at pH 6.0 or EDTA solution at pH 8.0 are used, depending on the particular antigen of interest. Precise conditions need to be established in each laboratory. It is important to note that decalcified bone marrow trephine biopsy sections, in general, require less intensive antigen retrieval than sections from non-decalcified tissues; it is usually most convenient to modify the various techniques by shortening the exposure time of sections.
5 Block possible non-specific background staining with 10% bovine serum albumin in PBS/TBS or non-immune serum from the species that is to provide the second antiserum (e.g. normal goat serum if the second antiserum is raised in a goat). Non-immune serum is usually diluted 1 in 20 (5%) in the standard antibody diluent. Sections should be incubated with blocking solution, in the humidified staining tray, at room temperature for 10–20 minutes.
6 Drain off the blocking serum solution but do not wash the sections. Apply the primary monoclonal antibody or polyclonal antiserum* at its optimal dilution (determined by prior titration) and incubate sections in the humidified staining tray for a predetermined standard time. The latter may vary from 30 minutes to overnight (e.g. 2 hours at room temperature or overnight at 4 °C).* Polyclonal antibodies are generally effective with relatively short incubations at room temperature; many monoclonal antibodies, when used with manual immunostaining techniques, require overnight incubation. Overnight incubation should always be carried out at refrigerator temperature (4 °C) to minimize non-specific background staining. Protocols for automated immunostaining equipment often permit considerably shorter incubations with primary antibodies.

7 Allow sections to re-warm to room temperature, if necessary, and then rinse in three changes of PBS/TBS (5 minutes each). Remove excess buffer but keep the sections moist.

8 Dilute the appropriate second layer (biotinylated) antiserum in the antibody diluent. The second layer antiserum is chosen according to the species from which the primary antibody is derived, e.g. biotinylated goat anti-mouse immunoglobulin (when the primary antibody is a murine monoclonal antibody) or swine anti-rabbit immunoglobulin (when the primary antibody is a polyclonal rabbit antiserum).

9 Apply the diluted second layer antiserum to the sections and incubate at room temperature in a humidified staining tray for a period which is normally between 30 minutes and 1 hour.* At this time, prepare streptavidin-biotin solution as described below in step 11, so that complexes have at least 30 minutes to form.

10 Rinse the sections in three changes of PBS/TBS (5 minutes each).

11 Add solutions of streptavidin and biotinylated peroxidase together in PBS/TBS at predetermined concentrations and leave the prepared solution to stand at room temperature for 30 minutes for

---

* Precise details of the use and duration of heat or protease pre-treatment, and of the appropriate antibody dilutions and duration for which they are applied, are not given in the above general method since these are variable. For example, there is considerable variation in the optimal dilution between antibodies supplied by different manufacturers and even between different batches of one antibody from a single source. We recommend that the manufacturers' directions be consulted but that, for any new batch of antibody, the optimal conditions are determined before diagnostic use. Empirically, it has been found that pre-treatment by either protease digestion or heating of sections may expose antigenic sites and permit immunohistochemical staining. The choice of pre-treatment method, the duration of exposure needed and the antigens requiring this treatment must be determined by experiment. Useful sources of additional reference are given in the list below. However, there is continuing rapid expansion in the range of antibodies and detection reagents available for immunohistochemistry and automated methods are extending immunohistochemistry even further; no published work in this field can be fully comprehensive. Current product catalogues from major commercial suppliers generally provide substantial technical guidance concerning techniques for use of their antibodies for immunohistochemistry in fixed tissue sections.

complexes to form. Apply this solution to the sections for a standard time (30 minutes to 1 hour) in the humidified staining tray. New third layer reagents are now available that potentially offer even greater sensitivity than streptavidin-biotin complexes. Tyramide catalysed biotinylation, mirror-image immune complex and continually emerging new proprietary techniques may be of considerable value for demonstration of antigens expressed at very low concentrations by cells of interest.

12 Rinse sections in three changes of PBS/TBS (5 minutes each).

13 Develop the final coloured product by incubation of sections with the peroxidase development solution for 10 minutes at room temperature. The end-product of the reaction is an insoluble, dark brown precipitate.

14 Rinse sections in running tap water. Counterstain lightly with haematoxylin (30 seconds to 1 minute) and allow to 'blue' in running tap water (5–10 minutes).

15 Dehydrate, clear and mount.

Acknowledgements

The aceto-zinc fixation method was kindly provided by Dr Robert Hasserjian, Department of Pathology, Massachusetts General Hospital, Boston.

Further reading

Bancroft JD, Cook HC and Turner DR (1994) *Manual of Histological Techniques and their Diagnostic Application.* Churchill Livingstone, Edinburgh.

Beckstead JH (1994) A simple technique for preservation of fixation-sensitive antigens in paraffin-embedded tissues. *J Histochem Cytochem*, **42**, 1127–1134.

Bonds LA, Barnes P, Foucar K and Sever CE (2005) Acetic-zinc-formalin: a safe alternative to B-5 fixative. *Am J Clin Pathol*, **124**, 205–211.

Brunning RD (1992) Bone marrow specimen processing. In: Knowles DW (ed) *Neoplastic Haematopathology*. Williams & Wilkins, Baltimore, pp. 1081–1095.

Erber WN, Willis JI and Hoffman GJ (1997) An enhanced immunocytochemical method for staining bone marrow trephine sections. *J Clin Pathol*, **50**, 389–393.

Gatter KC, Heryet A, Brown DC and Mason DY (1987) Is it necessary to embed bone marrow biopsies in plastic for haematological diagnosis? *Histopathology*, **11**, 1–7.

Islam A and Frisch B (1985) Plastic embedding in routine histology. I: Preparation of semi-thin sections of undecalcified marrow cores. *Histopathology*, **9**, 1263–1274.

Krenacs T, Bagdi E, Stelkovics E, Bereczki L and Krenacs L (2005) How we process trephine biopsy specimens: epoxy resin embedded bone marrow biopsies. *J Clin Pathol*, **58**, 897–903.

Leong AS-Y, Cooper K and Leong FJW-M (2003) *Manual of Diagnostic Antibodies for Immunohistology*, 2nd edn. Greenwich Medical Media Ltd, London.

Li C-Y and Yam LT (1992) Cytochemical, histochemical and immunohistochemical analysis of the bone marrow. In: Knowles DW (ed) *Neoplastic Haematopathology*. Williams & Wilkins, Baltimore, pp. 1097–1134.

Lykidis D, Van Noorden S, Armstrong A, Spencer-Dene B, Li J, Zhuang Z and Stamp G (2007) Novel zinc-based fixative for high quality DNA, RNA and protein analysis. *Nucleic Acids Res*, **35**, e85.

McCluggage WG, Roddy S, Whiteside C, Burton J, McBride H, Maxwell P and Bharucha H (1995) Immunohistochemical staining of plastic embedded bone marrow trephine biopsy specimens after microwave heating. *J Clin Pathol*, **48**, 840–844.

Mangham DC and Isaacson PG (1999) A novel immunohistochemical detection system using mirror image complementary antibodies (MICA). *Histopathology*, **35**, 129–133.

Mengel M, Werner M and von Wasielewski R (1999) Concentration dependent and adverse effects in immunohistochemistry using the tyramine amplification technique. *Histochem J*, **31**, 195–200.

Miller K (2002) Technical aspects of lymphoreticular pathology. *CPD Bull Cellular Pathol*, **4**, 47–51.

Naresh KN, Lampert I, Hasserjian R, Lykidis D, Elderfield K, Horncastle D et al. (2006) Optimal processing of bone marrow trephine biopsy: the Hammersmith protocol. *J Clin Pathol*, **59**, 903–911.

Polak JM and van Norden S (eds) (1986) *Immunocytochemistry: Modern methods and applications*, 2nd edn. John Wright Sons Ltd, Bristol.

Sabattini E, Bisgaard K, Ascani S, Poggi S, Piccioli M, Ceccarelli C et al. (1998) The EnVision++ system: a new immunohistochemical method for diagnostics and research. Critical comparison with the APAAP, ChemMate, CSA, LABC, and SABC techniques. *J Clin Pathol*, **51**, 506–511.

Toda Y, Kono K, Abiru H, Kokuryo K, Endo M, Yaegashi H and Fukumoto M (1999) Application of tyramide signal amplification system to immunohistochemistry: a potent method to localize antigens that are not detectable by ordinary method. *Pathol Int*, **49**, 479–483.

INDEX

Page numbers in **bold** represent tables, those in *italics* represent figures

611